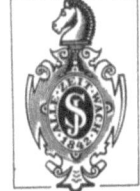

Leslie N. Pyrah

Renal Calculus

Foreword by D. Innes Williams

With 55 Figures

Springer-Verlag
Berlin Heidelberg New York 1979

Dr. Leslie N. Pyrah,
Emeritus Professor of Urological Surgery
at the University of Leeds,
Past President of the British Association of Urological Surgeons,
55 Weetwood Lane,
Leeds LS16 5NP, Great Britain

ISBN-13: 978-3-642-67126-5   e-ISBN-13: 978-3-642-67124-1
DOI: 10.1007/978-3-642-67124-1

Library of Congress Cataloging in Publication Data. Pyrah, Leslie Norman.
Renal calculus. Bibliography: pp. Includes index. 1. Kidneys—Calculi.
I. Title. [DNLM: 1. Kidney calculi. WJ356 P998r] RC916.P95 616.6'22
78-23788

2123/3321-543210

Contents

Contents   xiii

Foreword

Stone in the urinary tract has fascinated the medical profession from the earliest times and has played an important part in the development of surgery. The earliest major planned operations were for the removal of vesical calculus; renal and ureteric calculi provided the first stimulus for the radiological investigation of the viscera, and the biochemical investigation of the causes of calculus formation has been the training ground for surgeons interested in metabolic disorders. It is therefore no surprise that stone has been the subject of a number of monographs by eminent urologists, but the rapid development of knowledge has made it possible for each one of these authors to produce something new. There is still a technical challenge to the surgeon in the removal of renal calculi, and on this topic we are always glad to have the advice of a master craftsman; but inevitably much of the interest centres on the elucidation of the causes of stone formation and its prevention.

Professor Pyrah has had a long and wide experience of the surgery of calculous disease and gives us in this volume something of the wisdom that he has gained thereby, but he has also been a pioneer in the setting up of a research department largely concerned with the investigation of this complex group of disorders, so that he is able to present in terms readily intelligible to the general medical reader the results of extensive biochemical investigation in this area.

The urologist in practice, the urologist in training, the nephrologist and the physician with a metabolic interest should study calculous disease, not only for the practical benefits that such study will bring to their patients but also as an example of the methods of medical investigation and as a stimulus to undertake something further. Almost always the facts newly discovered pose as many questions as they answer and there is still in this field ample opportunity for further research, taking the investigator sometimes away from his original objective to other areas of medical science.

A feature of this work is the extensive lists of references, which should provide a stimulus to the post-graduate student to undertake wider reading. It is perhaps a criticism of modern medicine that too many papers are written and that the repetition of well known facts in many articles discourages the student from a prolonged study of the literature, but equally it is a criticism of surgical training in Britain as opposed to the United States that relatively little attention is given to background reading. The natural inclination of surgeons is to get on with the practical work, but the complexity of contemporary scientific medicine is such that a regular study of the journals is obligatory if the best service is to be offered to the patient. The habit of reading must be instilled into our post-graduate students; perhaps indeed if they were more familiar with what had already been written, they would not always find it necessary to publish yet another paper on what they believe to be rare conditions.

This book presents the results of a great many clinical, radiological and biochemical investigations: let us hope it will also prove to be the starting point of even more searching investigation.

Autumn 1978   D. INNES WILLIAMS

Acknowledgements

It is a pleasure to acknowledge the help I have received in discussions on the subject of stone with former colleagues in the Department, especially Dr. A. Hodgkinson and Dr. F.W. Heaton. Dr. W.E. Robertson helped in the preparation of the chapter dealing with idiopathic hypercalciuria. Mr. Irvine Smith was responsible for much of the information and script incorporated in the section dealing with recumbency calculi. I would like to thank Miss Mary D. Brown for some of the half-tone drawings, so carefully executed by her. I thank those friends and colleagues who have allowed me to reproduce illustrations and tables and also the publishers in whose journals such illustrations have appeared. Finally I thank my secretary, Miss M. Hart, for the enormous amount of work which she has done in collating and assessing the literature and in the preparation of the drafts and final typescript. To all these the author is very grateful. Finally, I thank my wife for her encouragement and forbearance during the period of preparation of the book.

Introduction

The book seeks to cover the entire field of renal calculous disease. The increase of knowledge available in recent years, however, has made it necessary to present the subject in abbreviated form and to omit reference to much of the known metabolic and crystallographic studies now available. Renal calculous disease is multifactorial in its etiology. The different chemical varieties of stone are often associated with a varied clinical picture and often call for different methods of surgical and non-surgical treatment.

Renal calculi are often found in association with many other intrarenal disorders and extrarenal diseases, covering a wide range of human pathology, from renal tumours and cystic conditions, to metabolic disorders which include hyperparathyroidism, Cushing's syndrome and hypercalciuria. These abnormalities are referred to in order to direct the attention of the clinician to possible abnormalities in the body as a whole and not merely to those in the kidney, on which the patient's symptoms are most commonly centred. Chemical substances which have been thought to contribute to stone formation or prevention (citrate, pyrophosphate, vitamin D) as well as such biochemical abnormalities as hypercalciuria and hyperoxaluria, which have been studied and characterized in detail only in recent years, are referred to. What I have called 'environmental calculi', resulting from the ingestion of substances taken as medicines or (to excess) in the diet, or have been received into the body during the patient's occupation, are referred to.

In the chapter dealing with the history and clinical features, stress has been laid, even in the non-infected cases, upon the almost life-long duration and the bilateral character of calculous disease in a high proportion of sufferers. It is therefore necessary for the urologist to deploy his efforts in the shorter and longer term, to remove the intrarenal and extrarenal contributory causes to stone formation, and not merely to regard a patient as being finally cured when a stone has been voided spontaneously or removed surgically. Since the book as a whole has been clinically orientated, the various surgical and non-surgical measures of treatment have been referred to in some detail. The possibility of the spontaneous voiding of many small calculi has been stressed in the hope that the number of instrumental and operative measures will be reduced. The available treatment of advanced calculous disease has been briefly described.

Chapter 1

Epidemiology of Urolithiasis

The study of the epidemiology of urolithiasis is concerned with the variable distribution or incidence of the disease throughout the countries and provinces of the world. This involves its incidence in the various ethnic divisions of the human race, its increased or decreased incidence during certain centuries, and its relationship to environmental factors such as climate, diet, economic conditions and occupation. Such enquiries have also thrown light upon the very different incidence of vesical calculi and calculi in the upper urinary tract during the last 150 years in different countries.

Vesical calculus had a high incidence in children (especially in boys) in some parts of England at the beginning of the last century, but this gradually disappeared as the diet of the population changed for the better; the stones were mostly uratic in composition. This former high incidence in England is today still paralleled by a similar high incidence in many countries which are less well-developed economically than our own, notably Thailand and parts of India. As a working hypothesis Andersen [4–6] suggested that a relative deficiency of animal protein and/or fats in the food, and too great a dependence upon vegetable protein as a principal article of diet could be the common factor in the diet of those populations which used to or still have a high incidence of vesical calculi.

The incidence of renal calculus in the economically highly developed western countries (referred to in more detail below) has undergone the opposite kind of change, in that there has been a considerable increase in adults, far greater than can be explained merely by the improved methods of diagnosis developed during the last seven decades. The stones are mainly calcium oxalate (with or without apatite) in composition. A possible clue to this generally increased incidence is the fact that it has undergone certain variations relevant to the great wars during the last 60 years (referred to later in this chapter).

The probability must be considered that dietary factors are the principal agents responsible for the generally increased incidence of renal stone; the richer diet, including a higher intake of calcium-containing foods, animal protein [5] and sugar [17] enjoyed by the people of the more wealthy communities, especially between and after the World Wars, is in a general sense probably conducive to renal stone formation.

I. Early Cases of Vesical Calculus

The incidence of vesical stone in 20 countries from 1830 was high in parts of France, England and some other European countries, low in Sweden, but reached 4.1 per 100,000 people in Denmark [16]. Not a single case had been reported from the General Hospital in Christiania during a 4-year period during which 3200 patients had been treated, nor in a 10-year period from the Oslo Hospital.

Stone in the bladder was much more common in England in the early and middle parts of the last century than it is now. The high incidence of stone in Norfolk, found mainly among farm labourers, probably resulted from their defective diet, which consisted mainly of wheat bread, water and tea with a little milk [23]. Stones were said to be five times more common in East

Norfolk, a wheat-growing area, than in West Norfolk, where there was mixed farming [6]. There had been a gradual reduction in the incidence of vesical calculi in the East Norfolk area from 1871 to 1947 following the change-over to mixed farming, which took place between 1916 and 1925, and vesical calculi in children had almost disappeared from the area by 1938 [58].

Of the period in England after 1834 it was stated that 'the premier surgical operation, especially amongst schoolboys, was for stone in the bladder'. There is available a descriptive catalogue of 642 calculi from English patients over 100 years ago, one-third of which were vesical calculi and 73% contained uric acid or urates [57]. A lithotrity hospital in Westminster was closed when the incidence of stone in the bladder fell.

In Russia it was reported that 77% of 630 cases of vesical stone operations done were in children under the age of 10 and only 13 were in females [9]. Little accurate information concerning the incidence of renal calculi exists for this early period, since the diagnosis by radiography only became possible in the early years of the century.

II. Ethnic Considerations

Renal stone is common among the white peoples of the western economically developed races, but the incidence is far from uniform; thus there are 'stone belts' in the United States and in the European countries in which the incidence is (or has been) considerably higher than the average. Similarly among brown-skinned peoples the incidence of calculus varies from country to country independently of the colour of the skin. Negroes appear to have a considerable degree of built-in immunity to renal calculus, an attribute which seems to apply whether they live in the country or the continent of their origin, or in a different

habitat (for example, the United States) and even after several generations. The apparent immunity, however, is more marked in the African than in the American Negro.

1. The African Negro

Among 1,091,000 coloured patients who had been treated in the native hospitals in Johannesburg between the years 1922 and 1935, urinary calculus was found in only 1 patient with unmixed Negro blood; by contrast, among 126,000 white patients, 1 in every 460 suffered from urinary stone. The incidence of stone among the Cape Coloured in South Africa, who are a half-caste race of mixed Negro and Caucasian blood, was almost as great as that among the members of the Caucasian race [60].

Although the diet of the South African Negroes is poor in calcium, they have good skeletons and good teeth with few caries [19]. Randall's plaques on the renal papillae (which are regarded as frequent precursors of renal stone) have been found in 17.2% of kidneys of Caucasian subjects examined in South Africa, and in only 4.3% of kidneys of Bantu Negroes [61].

Among 483,450 Bantu patients admitted to a hospital in Durban between 1951 and 1959, there was only one with renal calculus [63]. Similarly among 162,449 Bantu patients admitted to a hospital in Pietermaritzburg of Natal, South Africa, during 1954 to 1962, records of only 5 patients with renal calculi were found, in 3 of whom there had been a history of prolonged recumbency [18]. While renal calculi were very rare among the Bantu in South Africa, such cases numbered 9% among the white urological patients seen in Cape Town [44]. It seems to be irrelevant that the Bantu are not an entirely homogeneous group of people, and indeed they speak several languages (Swahili, Zulu, Sotho and Xhosa). Those who live in the

Reserves have a lower standard of living than the white population; yet in spite of such racial differences the low incidence of stone seems to hold. Ethnic differences have been observed in the incidence of diseases other than renal calculus; the diseases commonly encountered in the white population (coronary thrombosis, thyrotoxicosis, multiple sclerosis, gallstones, rheumatoid arthritis) are rarely encountered in the Bantu.

In searching for an explanation of the relative immunity of the Bantu, it has been thought that differences in the chemical composition of the urine in the Negro (with a higher sodium content) from that of the white races (often with a higher calcium content) might account for the differing incidence of calculous disease. The 24-h urinary magnesium in the normal Bantu did not differ significantly from that in white subjects, though the urinary citric acid level was significantly lower than that in the white group [44].

The incidence of urolithiasis in other parts of Africa has been shown to have variations, being extremely rare in Kenya, Tanzania and Uganda, though vesical calculi occurred sometimes in young boys. In the countries abutting on the White Nile (between Uganda and the confluence with the Blue Nile at Khartoum) urolithiasis was almost absent except for a few calculi found as complications of urethral stricture. Only three African patients with urinary calculi had been observed in 19 years of surgical practice in Uganda. In the region of the Blue Nile (which passes from east to west to its confluence at Khartoum with the White Nile) it was found that in Ethiopia urinary calculi appeared to be common, though with a lower incidence than that in the Sudan; such problems admit of no easy answer [15]. By contrast, over 100 patients with urinary calculi, many being young children, were seen by another observer during a period of 5 months in Khartoum [20].

2. The American Negro

There are differences in the incidence of calculous disease in the American Negro (some of whom have Caucasian blood) from that in the African Negro on the one hand, and that in the white American population on the other. In New Orleans urinary calculi have been encountered three times as often among white as among coloured patients; urinary calculous disease as a cause of death in the United States has been found to be one-quarter less common in the Negro than in the Caucasian. In the Jackson Memorial Hospital, Miami, Florida, a state in which the incidence of urinary calculus is high, only one Negro patient with urolithiasis was found; an occasional such patient was often a mulatto [31].

In a report of approximately 5900 necropsies between 1884 and 1935, during a study of the incidence of urolithiasis among white and coloured men, 79 cases of urinary calculi were found, of which only 4 were in the coloured people; when stone occurred in the coloured races it was in subjects of relatively advanced age [53]. Thus the African Negro seems to be almost immune from nephrolithiasis often in spite of inadequate or ill-balanced diet and defective sanitation, and despite transportation to other lands with varying climatic conditions. A higher incidence of urolithiasis in white than in Negro troops in the United States has been reported [48]. In a report of 15,919 autopsies and surgical specimens during a 22-year period in an exclusively Negro hospital only 13 cases of renal stone (0.08%) were found [51].

Medical records of World War I showed only 52 instances of nephrolithiasis among Negro troops, who had a mean annual strength of 286,548 (0.18 per thousand), whereas the ratio among white troops was 0.41 per thousand [43]. Boyce et al. [14] in their investigation of the incidence of urolithiasis in the United States found that it was lower among the Negro than among the white population; from the Tuskegee Institute, Alabama (the patients being principally Negro), only three diagnoses of urinary calculus among 15,954 discharges from the adult services had been made. The highest incidence among a mainly Negro population was that in the Freedman's Hospital, Washington, D.C., where 102 patients were reported with urinary calculi among 52,093 patients discharged from the adult services (1.9%).

III. Climate

It is not easy to attribute a high incidence of patients with urolithiasis in any given country or continent to climatic conditions alone, since in every country other factors such as diet, race and ethnic factors play their part. Dry heat or humid heat results in loss of water by way of the skin through sweating and by way of the breath through respiration, so that even with a high daily intake of liquid, subjects in hot countries pass highly concentrated urine (usually acid in reaction) perhaps only once in 24 h or even longer. Crystals may therefore be deposited in the urine which predispose to renal stone formation.

Paradoxically, however, even in very hot countries urolithiasis may be uncommon. During 1 year's hospital practice in Ecuador, a tropical country, among 60,000 people observed, Davalos [19] did not encounter a single patient with urinary calculus. The contradictions inherent in the problem are shown by his observation that in South America, stones were common in North-East Brazil but rare in the Amazon Valley and also in Panama, where the climate is hot and humid all the year round. In Northern Peru, with its warm dry climate, urinary calculi are rare.

An increased incidence of acute renal colic (with ureteric stones) was observed by one group during hot weather, 135 cases

annually during a 6-year period having been seen [50]. A 50% increase in the incidence of urinary calculi was observed in the Pensacola region of Florida, during the hot season [35].

The incidence of renal stone is sometimes increased to an abnormally high level in military and naval personnel who are moved for long periods (as during wars) from more temperate zones to tropical or subtropical regions. A high incidence of renal calculi has been found among American soldiers living in a desert area where the heat in summer was almost intolerable [48]. During World War II a high incidence of renal and ureteric stone among British troops in North Africa and Egypt, many of whom had not previously been exposed to tropical heat, was observed [54].

Studies of the incidence of urolithiasis among personnel of the British Royal Navy (534 men) showed the differing incidence of stone during periods of service in the Mediterranean (1.4 per 1000), in the tropics (1.39 per 1000) and in the United Kingdom (0.36 per 1000). The incidence in the Mediterranean and United Kingdom groups rose to 2.2 and 1.7 per thousand respectively, when the figures were corrected to include patients with urolithiasis who had developed stone within 1 year of returning home. Adaptation of the individual to climatic conditions has a bearing upon the incidence, since 43% of the patients were known to have served at a later date in warm areas without having had symptoms of recurrence, suggesting that during later periods of service the subject had become conditioned (by a higher fluid intake) against the possibility of further stone. On the other hand, 69% of those who developed urolithiasis in areas where the weather was unusually hot, had previously served in such areas with no evidence of stone formation [11, 12]. The high incidence of stone in Israel (a hot country) is referred to later.

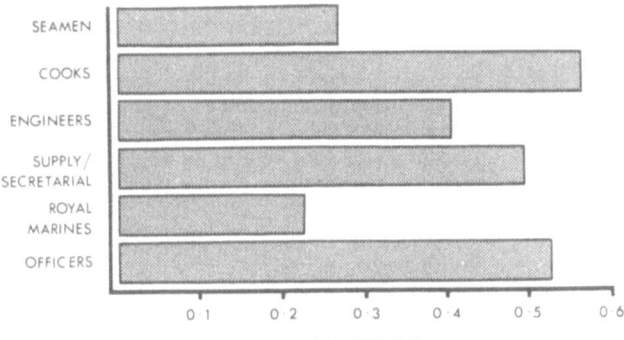

Fig. 1.1 Differential incidence of urolithiasis according to occupation in Royal Navy

IV. Occupation

Urolithiasis cannot strictly be described as an occupational disease though there is some evidence that people in some occupations are affected more than others. Foundry workers and miners have had a lower than average incidence of stone, possibly because of their physically strenuous work [13].

The incidence of stone in two groups of British naval personnel, namely cooks working in a ship's galley and engine room personnel (who were exposed to relatively high temperatures) was about twice that of the seamen who were not exposed to such temperatures (Fig. 1.1). There was a high incidence among officers, a significant proportion of whom were in the fourth and fifth decades of age, whereas many of the other ranks were much younger men. There was a low incidence in the Royal Marines (who have a high grade of physical activity) and a relatively high incidence among supply and secretarial staff, whose work was of a relatively sedentary character [11, 12].

In a study of the occupations of patients with urolithiasis in Czechoslovakia it was found that the majority were administrative employees and workers in other sedentary occupations, manual workers, transport workers, railwaymen, health workers and doctors; the condition was relatively rare among farmers. An increased standard of living was associated with a higher in-cidence of urolithiasis, while a large consumption of beer and of butter was associated with minimal calculous disease [41]. The avoidance of urination is a possible explanation of the reported frequency of urolithiasis in truck-drivers and air-pilots in the United States [38].

The incidence of renal calculi in members of the medical profession in Denmark has been found to be higher (at 8% of 100,000) than that in the general population [34]. The incidence of renal colic among doctors in the Glasgow area (6.7%) is lower than that in Denmark. The incidence was highest among those who work in proximity to a city or in a warm humid environment, as in an operating theatre [56]. The incidence of stone in city dwellers in Sweden has been shown to be higher than in the general population [1].

V. Incidence of Stone in Countries with Different Degrees of Economic Development

The United Kingdom, the Scandinavian countries, Finland, most other European countries, the United States and Israel have in common a high standard of economic development, so that an indifferent diet and under-nutrition are nowadays unlikely to be important factors giving rise to calculous disease in their peoples.

Table 1.1 Figures from Registrar-General's statistics showing deaths in England and Wales from calculus of the kidney and ureter

Sex	Urolithiasis of kidney and ureter													
	1959	1960	1961	1962	1963	1964	1965	1966	1967	1968	1969	1970	1971	1972
M	131	127	138	132	126	97	107	85	79	85	89	106	70	81
F	135	135	126	132	140	131	116	88	120	116	131	106	106	96

1. Great Britain

Urolithiasis is here a fairly common disease with a much greater predominance of renal over vesical calculi. The incidence of vesical calculi in East Anglia has been greatly reduced as a consequence of the dietetic changes and improved economic conditions of the last 60 years. Renal stone is common in the large area of Yorkshire served by the author's hospital and the incidence may be increasing. Thus a series of 1725 patients with renal calculi seen between 1951 and 1961 from the author's department probably did not include many patients who had voided calculi spontaneously or had had renal colic and were attended by their own general practitioner and were not seen in the hospital department [62].

The Registrar-General's statistics showing the annual death rate in England and Wales resulting from stone in the upper and lower urinary tract between 1959 and 1972 (Table 1.1) revealed a gradual decline in both groups. The figures have to be set against an increase in the total population during the period (which, if the incidence recurred constantly, would lead to the expectancy of a larger number of deaths) and also against a gradually improving standard of treatment for calculous disease, which has given a greater expectancy of life [54].

The incidence of stone in the upper urinary tract occurring among naval and marine personnel of the Royal Navy (numbering approximately 180,000; all males;

70% under the age of 25 years; a closed British community) during the 10-year period 1958–1967, was 534 (72% ureteric, 25% renal) [11, 12]. The proportion of the group who, by the age of 50 years, will have given evidence of urolithiasis on at least one occasion, was the relatively high figure of 35.5 per thousand (3.5%). The incidence among the patients of conditions known to predispose to urolithiasis (hydronephrosis, calyceal cysts, sponge kidney and congenital anomalies, but excluding urinary infection and hypercalciuria) was 7.5% and was comparable with the 9% recorded from the author's department [62]. Hypercalciuria was observed in 84 of 208 cases of renal stone investigated, bringing the incidence of known predisposing or etiological factors to nearly 50%. The majority of the stones were composed of calcium oxalate with or without an admixture of calcium phosphate.

In a survey of the incidence of urolithiasis in a limited island community of 25,000 in Stornoway (in the Outer Hebrides), it was found that during 1957–1961, of the 2693 adult patients admitted to the surgical wards, 86 were patients with calculi. The annual rate of admission to hospital of calculous patients was 68 per 100,000 of the population [8].

2. Sweden

During the last century the incidence of vesical stone in the Scandinavian countries was low [8]; the diet in those countries contained a good deal of fish and therefore of protein, which was the probable explanation. In Scandinavia the incidence of renal stone has increased considerably during the present century, when improved economic conditions have allowed a great improvement in the diet [45]. Others, however, have found little change in recent years [2]. The hospital incidence of urolithiasis (chiefly renal stones) during 1911–1931 in 42 Swedish hospitals was shown to have increased from 31 per 10,000 inpatients during the period 1911–1914, to 117 per 10,000 patients in the period 1927–1931 [30]. The incidence in the Uppsala province of Sweden (a selected area) had increased from 9.19 per 100,000 of the population during the period 1911–1914 to 82.9 in the period 1935–1938, falling slightly to 74.5 during the war period 1943–1946 [29]. In the district of Alvsborgs Län in South Sweden the incidence of urolithiasis was shown to be 80 per 100,000 [1]. Stone-formers have no greater risk of coronary heart disease than normal subjects [36].

3. Norway

The results of a survey covering a long period in Norway recorded by Andersen and his co-workers [3, 5, 7], showed that during the period 1910–1960 the incidence of stone in the lower urinary tract had diminished. In the records of the Oslo City Hospital they found between 1912 and 1917 only 3 cases of vesical calculus in which there was no obvious predisposing cause (urethral stricture, congenital abnormality of the bladder, spina bifida). They found records of 241 cases of vesical calculus, of which 64 had occurred between 1892 and 1940, only 3 being in children under the age of 15 (and none since 1940). Forty-seven were patients over the age of 40 years, 38 of whom had an enlargement of the prostate and were therefore not in the group of cases of endemic vesical calculi.

The number of patients with renal or ureteric stone in hospital between 1890 and 1960 had increased from one single patient in 1911, rising to 499 in 1955, and falling to 426 in 1960. The incidence of urolithiasis among patients diagnosed and treated either at home or in hospital among the insured population of Oslo rose from 118 in 1940 to nearly 300 in 1960 per 100,000. There had been a temporary fall in the incidence during the war years, when diet may have been less than perfect, but there was a rapid increase following the conclusion of hostilities when diet improved again.

The same rising trend in the incidence of calculi in the upper urinary tract, however, was observed in 10 other Norwegian hospitals. Between 1921 and 1960 the number of patients with urolithiasis in those hospitals in the south of Norway, where the inhabitants are better off economically, was higher than that in other parts of the country. Thus the incidence in Oslo in 1950 was about four times that in Bodô, the most northerly hospital to be studied, but by 1960, following considerable improvements in the economic condition of northern Norway (probably consequent upon greater industrial activity), the difference in the incidence of urolithiasis between the two places had been halved.

In assessing the significance of this apparent enormous increase, it was stated that the population of Oslo and Akar had doubled during the 60 years, that hospital admissions had quadrupled and now included many patients with renal colic who had formerly not been admitted to hospital, and that radiological diagnostic measures had been greatly improved.

4. Finland

The incidence of vesical calculi in Finland during the last century was lower than that in many other countries [55]; the national

Table 1.2. Urolithiasis in Finland

Series	Korhonen [33] 1918–1934		Sallinen [55] 1954–1956		National Board of Medicine (whole country) 1953–1954	
No. of patients	178		287		2399	
	No.	%	No.	%	No.	%
Urolithiasis in *upper* urinary tract	115	64.6	265	92.3	2250	93.8
Urolithiasis in *lower* urinary tract	63	35.3	22	7.5	149	6.2

Note: The number of patients with calculi in the upper urinary tract has increased considerably, while those with calculi in the lower tract has decreased during a 25-year period

diet was rich in milk, fish and cereals but contained little meat.

During the 50 years 1908–1958 the incidence of patients with calcium oxalate calculi in the upper urinary tract who were admitted to hospital had increased. The relative incidence of those with uric acid and infected phosphatic calculi had diminished. During the shorter period 1953–1954, when the mean population of Finland was 4,141,000, 0.3% of these were known to have been admitted to hospital for the treatment of urolithiasis, the number of such patients having increased one hundredfold in 47 years, probably because of economic and dietary improvement, though improved diagnostic facilities may have played a part together with the high magnesium content of the ingested food. The figure in the earlier series, compared with that of Sallinen [55] and that in the whole country (1953–1954) shows that there was a considerable proportionate increase in stones in the upper tract during a 23-year period (Table 1.2).

5. Czechoslovakia

Between 50 and 300 (average 100) per 100,000 patients with calculi in the upper urinary tract between 1930 and 1950 were admitted annually to hospital; a higher incidence of vesical stone was found in children in the poorer agricultural areas [42]. In an examination of 100 stones from Czechoslovakia considerably larger amounts of uric acid and urate and less of the calcium phosphates were found than in stones from comparable British series [38].

6. Israel

Urolithiasis is common in the Middle East; climatic conditions as well as diet influence the incidence. During 1955–1956 there was an incidence of 11.6 per 1000 in a group of 60,800 members of the state insurance scheme above the age of 14 [10]. The number of new patients with urolithiasis who were registered in 1955 was 8670 or 8.6 per 1000 of the total number of people insured [24]. It was found that the incidence of urolithiasis in drafted men aged 18–27 in Israel in 1956 was 3 per 1000. By comparison the incidence in drafted men between the ages of 18 and 30 in the United States in 1920 was 0.13, and in Florida, which is reputedly a stone belt, it was 0.4 [14].

A survey extending over 12 settlements in Israel comprising 30,292 people was carried out between July 1957 and March 1958, and showed an overall incidence of 11.8 per thousand with 357 cases of urolithiasis registered in all (232 male); only 8 had vesical calculi and 7 of these had had a history of renal colic. There were considerable differences in the incidence in various settlements, ranging from 1.6 to 34.1 per 1000, the highest being found in the warmer regions and the lowest in a temperate warm climate.

The Jews in Israel have emigrated from many different countries; those who were born in Israel and also immigrants from North Africa and the Middle East had a low incidence, while immigrants from European countries had the highest incidence. In a majority of patients with urolithiasis the disease became manifest within the first 5 years of living in the settlement; the highest incidence was in the age group 18–30.

The effects of a hot climate has a bearing on the incidence of stone. In the Jordan Valley, where the temperature may reach a high level, on a hot day an agricultural worker can only maintain a minimum output of urine of 1000 ml by a daily intake of fluid which may reach as much as 15 litres. Some subjects may void urine only once (a small amount) during a whole day, and unless a great deal of water is drunk the subject may lose weight. Many immigrants probably do not adequately alter their former habits in respect of the amount of fluid ingested, consequently they void urine of a high specific gravity, which is favourable for the deposit of crystalline matter.

7. Turkey

Urinary lithiasis is endemic in Turkish children; in 2.5 years Eckstein [22] encountered 119 cases in children from all parts of the country. The highest age incidence was between 2 and 4 years, though renal stones were evenly distributed to the age of 17. A deficiency of dietary protein and vitamin D were thought to be of etiological importance. The children were breast fed for a longer period than the average British

infant, cow's milk was not consumed by the village population, meat and eggs were eaten only rarely and the staple diet was *bulgur* (which is a boiled wheat product), vegetables and fruit; malnutrition was common.

8. Sicily

Whereas in 1910 vesical calculi (urates) were most common, stones in the upper urinary tract (calcium oxalate) are those most commonly seen and have increased considerably in number [25, 46, 47]. Sicily can be regarded as an area of intermediate economic development. The changed incidence and character of urolithiasis in Sicily probably followed an alteration in the diet and the introduction of a school feeding programme by the Italian Government, with a mixed diet incorporating an adequate proportion of protein and green vegetables instead of the old cereal diet (Fig. 1.2, see p. 12).

9. United States

It seems probable that there had been a high incidence of vesical calculi in the United States as in England during the early part of the nineteenth century. It was stated that 306 patients with vesical calculi had been operated on in the New York Hospital between 1820 and 1950, during which time the annual incidence of patients under the age of 30 had gradually decreased from 83% to 3.25% [49].

The stone-forming areas in the United States are said to be the south-eastern region, southern California and a longitudinal belt somewhat south of the Great Lakes. An investigation into the incidence of urolithiasis in a large group of general hospitals in the United States showed that in the country as a whole during the year 1952, 9.47 persons per 10,000 of the population had been admitted to hospital

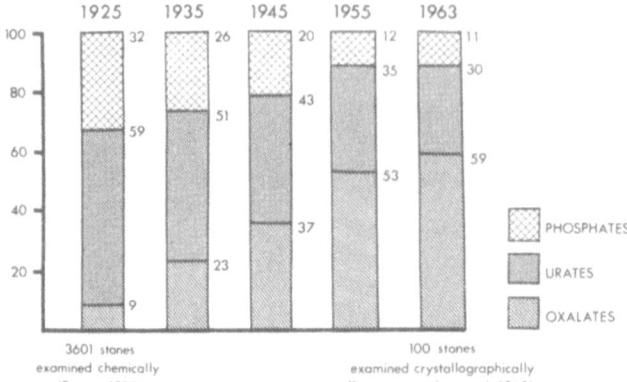

Fig. 1.2. Changes in composition of stones at Palermo, Sicily (adapted from M. Pavone, Macaluso)

with a diagnosis of urolithiasis [14]. There was considerable variation in the incidence of urolithiasis in different states and even in parts of the same state; thus at one extreme, the incidence was 19.25 and 18.42 per 10,000 of the population in South Carolina and Georgia respectively, whereas in Wyoming and Missouri it was 5.81 and 4.30 respectively. Similarly in the northern part of Alabama the incidence was less than half that in the southern part of the United States as a whole. There had been an increase in the incidence of stone between 1948 and 1952 in 5 of the 49 states; the proportion of vesical to renal and ureteric calculi was 5%, a figure which is in agreement with that from other parts of the world.

The record may not have represented the true incidence of urolithiasis, since many individuals must have voided small unreported calculi; moreover the proportion of white to Negro subjects (who have comparative immunity) in the population as a whole probably means that the true incidence of stone in the entire population is higher than that given in the figures.

10. India

In the Punjab and the northern portions of the United Provinces and in Sindh, stone is common but is less so in Madras and Southern India. As long ago as 1931 considerable variation was reported in the incidence of stone (mainly vesical) in different provinces of India [40]: Punjab, 438 per 100,000; Hyderabad, 266 per 100,000; Ahmednagar (Deccan), 13 per 100,000; Madras (Southern India), 0.3 per 100,000. The average incidence throughout India was estimated at 10 per 100,000 of population, which was 10 times that in Great Britain 100 years earlier.

An incidence was recorded during 1953–1955 which varied from 7 to 103 per 100,000 of the population in different parts of the Meheana District, Gujarat, India [52]. In the Ahmednagar District of India, from 1951 to 1957 the recorded incidence rose from 5.5 per 100,000 in 1953–1954 to 8.5 per 100,000 in 1955–1956 (which were famine years). The majority of the patients were children (peak incidence of 5 years) with vesical calculi (largely urate) and there was a smaller incidence of renal stone (mostly calcium oxalate) in adults between 50 and 60 [3–5, 7]. The patients were mainly from the poor rural agricultural class who had lived on a predominantly cereal and vegetarian diet. The poorer villagers were fed mainly on the local grains (hard millets known as *jowari* and *bhajeri*), salt and water being added, baked on an open fire and eaten with vegetables. The nuclei of the stones were usually composed of urates or oxalates.

It had been considered that vesical calculi in India were probably the result of a relative deficiency of vitamin A and an excess of calcium in the diet [39], though this view is no longer thought to be tenable; a general deficiency of animal protein is a more likely explanation.

11. Thailand

Government-sponsored epidemiological studies by Halstead and his co-workers [28] on the incidence, distribution and dietetic habits of children with vesical and renal calculi have given valuable information concerning a country which probably has the highest incidence of vesical stone in the world, and where it is considered to be a national disease.

Between 1953 and 1959 there was an average admission to hospital in Thailand of patients with urolithiasis of 23.1 per 100,000 of the population, regional differences varying from 0% to 102.9% [59]. In North-Eastern Thailand vesical calculi in children predominated by 20 to 1 while in other areas the incidence was only 8 to 1 (Fig. 1.3). In the city of Bangkok only did the incidence of renal calculi equal that of vesical calculi.

Investigations of the incidence of urolithiasis showed that there was an average annual hospitalization rate for patients with vesical and urethral calculi of 35.6 per 100,000 of the entire population in the Ubol Province (in Northern Thailand) between 1952 and 1962, a figure which excluded many who had voided stones spontaneously. During a 7-year period 3913 patients with vesical or urethral stones (nearly all children in the age group 3–4 years) but only 398 patients with renal or ureteric stones (nearly all over the age of 20) had been treated in hospital [28]. A striking finding was that the incidence of urolithiasis in three towns was only 210 per 100,000, while in 44 villages it was 1420

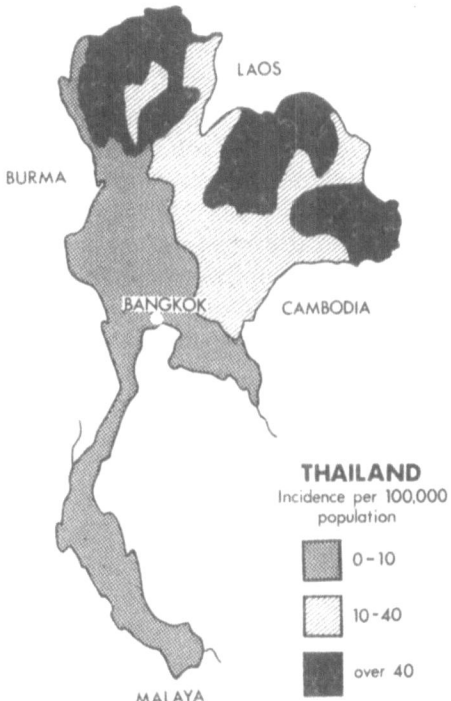

Fig. 1.3. Statistical survey of urinary stones for 1959 in North-eastern Thailand (by courtesy of the late Dr. D. A. Andersen, and J. & A. Churchill Ltd., London)

per 100,000 (most being vesical calculi in children).

The general unbalanced dietetic situation in Thailand is emphasized by the fact that among nutritional deficiency syndromes recognized in that country are iodine-deficiency goitre, kwashiorkor (in infants, resulting from protein deficiency) and occasionally beri-beri. Urolithiasis in Thailand occurs endemically in the north and north-east country regions (which are largely mountainous), mainly among the people of the Lao-Thai ethnic groups.

A survey of 16 farm families living in Nong Kohn (a Lao-Thai village in the north in which bladder stone was endemic) showed that the villagers had a monotonous diet consisting of glutinous rice, vegetables, uncooked fermented fish and a low intake of fat; 70% of the protein in the diet was of vegetable origin. In 15 families in the municipality of Ubol with a prevalence of disease which was 14 times less than in the country districts the diet was predominantly rice, cooked fermented fish and a variety of fruits and animal protein; the intake of calcium and of phosphorus was higher and that of vitamin A and vitamin C was lower in the diets of the villagers than in the inhabitants of the towns. Though the infants in the villages were breast-fed, most infants had feeds of glutinous rice, sometimes with mashed banana, from the first weeks of life, a type of feeding which may have reduced the daily amount of ingested breast milk. Of the urinary constituents in children from 2–10 years old in the villages, the daily urinary excretion of calcium and magnesium was found to be consistently higher than the corresponding values in children from Ubol city. Of village infants under 45 days old (but not city infants) 43% had oxalate crystalluria in freshly voided specimens, which was often eliminated by supplementation of the diet with orthophosphate and fat-free powdered milk.

By contrast in the towns only about 8% of mothers gave supplemental foods to the infants additional to the breast feeding during their first 4 weeks of life and only 52% were given glutinous rice in the first 3 months of life. In 30 city children no oxalate crystalluria was observed.

Vesical stones from a series of 200 from North-East Thailand were usually large (2.5–5 cm diameter) even in children; they had a central nucleus, were often laminated, light cream to brown in colour, and they consisted usually of ammonium acid urate and calcium oxalate monohydrate (either pure or mixed with each other). It was believed that poor nutrition was an important etiological factor in the stone formation, and that adequate animal protein in the diet offered a greater degree of protection against calculous disease than vegetable proteins [26]. At the Ubol Hospital in North Thailand, during the period 1960–1962, 1113 calculi had been removed from

boys under the age of 9 (the peak age incidence being 2.5 years), 161 from girls and 506 from adults [37].

Table 1.3 shows the incidence of stone in some countries which are well developed economically.

VI. The Stone Wave in Central Europe

The stone wave in Central Europe during the 1920s throws light upon epidemiological factors. Between 1924 and 1930 there had been a great increase in the incidence of (usually small unilateral nonrecurrent) calcium oxalate renal stones amounting in some districts to as much as 1000% in Central Europe, including all parts of Germany, Austria, Czechoslovakia, parts of Poland, Northern Switzerland and Sweden [27]. The stones appeared usually in males between the ages of 20 and 35; there was no corresponding increase in the incidence of vesical calculi. It was thought that the increased incidence began soon after the close of World War I and was greatly increased in the years after 1924 to 1937. The affected countries were those which had suffered most from the wartime blockade, which had led to hunger among many of the population. No similar increase in the incidence was reported in England, France, Belgium, Italy, the Baltic States and Denmark. A shortage of calcium (because of limited amounts of milk) in the wartime diet may have allowed the absorption of a greater amount of oxalate (from vegetables) from the intestine than usual.

The first post-war stone wave did not begin until several years after the war, by which time food had been plentiful. During the war years, prisoners of war in German prison camps, who had often had a reduced diet, had very few renal calculi. Switzerland and some Scandinavian countries not involved in the war had post-war stone waves though the inhabitants of those countries

Table 1.3. Incidence of stone in countries which are highly or moderately well-developed economically

Country	Incidence of renal calculi	Incidence of vesical calculi	Notes
Sicily	1965—renal calculi most common; number increased (Pavone et al., 1965)	In 1910 these were most common; in 1965, much less common	
Turkey	Renal stones common		
Israel	Renal stones common		
Czecho-slovakia	Renal stones: 1930–1950 average of 100 patients with calculi per 100,000 patients admitted to hospital		
Finland	1908–1958—considerable increase in renal calculi (calcium oxalate)	Incidence in last century lower than in most other countries (national diet rich in milk, fish and cereals)	
Norway	1890–1960: incidence of renal calculi increased	1910–1960—incidence of vesical calculi had diminished (Andersen, 1969)	
Sweden	1900–1960: incidence increased (Hellstrom, 1932; Hedenberg, 1951)	Incidence *low* (Andersen, 1969); diet contained much protein (fish)	
Great Britain	Fairly common. 1795 patients with renal calculus in author's department between 1951 and 1961	Common in East Anglia in last century; now much reduced deaths from renal and ureteric calculus	In England and Wales between 1959 and 1969 varied from 173 to 266 and from stone in other parts of the urinary tract from 20 to 48 (Registrar-General)

had not suffered except perhaps marginally from nutritional inadequacy. When nervous stresses resulting from the wars were at their highest, the incidence of renal stone was at its lowest [13].

It seems that the increased incidence of renal stone followed rather than accompanied a period of dietetic restriction resulting from rationing and shortage of foods in many countries during which the incidence of stone had been reduced.

The stone wave in Europe remained unchecked until the beginning of World War II when the incidence of urolithiasis again fell, only to rise once more several years after the war had ended. There is said to have been no stone wave after the wars in the United States [49]. A stone wave began in Japan in 1937 and was followed during the war years by a gradual decrease in the incidence of stone which lasted until 1944. Following the end of the war a second stone wave began after 1947 and the incidence of stone has been shown to be still increasing [32].

The suggestion therefore is that in times (as during wars) when there have been dietetic restrictions in many countries, the incidence of renal stone is diminished; but that when peaceful conditions restore dietary sufficiency the incidence of renal stone reaches a higher level.

References

1. Ahlgren,S.-A., Lorstad,M.: Renal and ureteral calculi in a Swedish district II and III. Acta Chir. Scand. Urol. *130*, 344–354 (1965)
2. Almby,B., Meirik,O., Schoneback,J.: Incidence, morbidity and complications of renal and ureteral calculi in a well-defined geographical area. Scand. J. Urol. Nephrol. *9*, 249 (1975)
3. Andersen,D.A.: The nutritional significance of primary bladder stones. Br. J. Urol. *34*, 160 (1962)
4. Andersen,D.A.: Patterns of incidence of stones of the urinary tract with special reference to endemic bladder stones. Urol. Treviso *34*, 385 (1967)
5. Andersen,D.A.: Historical and geographical differences in the pattern of incidence of urinary stones considered in relation to possible etiological factors. In: Renal Stone Research Symposium. Hodgkinson,A., Nordin,B.E.C. (eds.), p. 7. London: Churchill 1969
6. Andersen,D.A.: Environmental factors in the etiology of urolithiasis. In: International Symposium on Stone Research, p. 130. Madrid 1972
7. Andersen,D.A., Schiramachari,S., Khandagale,M.K.: Investigation into relationship between bladder stones and malnutrition. Indian J. Med. Sci. *17*, 617 (1963)
8. Anderson,G.S.: Urinary calculus in an island community. Br. Med. J. *35*, 556 (1964)
9. Assenfeldt,E.: Bericht über 630 stationar behandelte Stein-Kranke. Arch. Klin. Chir. *60*, 669 (1900)
10. Berman-Yeshurun,T.: Morbidity in the old population and in the newcomers since the establishment of the State of Israel. Dapim Refuim *15*, 3 (1956)
11. Blacklock,N.J.: The pattern of urolithiasis in the Royal Navy. J. R. Nav. Med. Serv. *51*, 99 (1965)
12. Blacklock,N.J.: The pattern of urolithiasis in the Royal Navy. In: Renal Stone Research Symposium. Hodgkinson,A., Nordin,B.E.C. (eds.), p. 33. London: Churchill 1969
13. Boshamer,K.: Morphologie und Genese der Harnsteine. In: Handbuch der Urologie. Vol. X/34. Berlin, Göttingen, Heidelberg: Springer 1961
14. Boyce,W.H., Garvey,F.K., Strawcutter, H.E.: Incidence of urinary calculi among patients in general hospitals. J. Am. Med. Assoc. *161*, 1437 (1956)
15. Burkitt,D.: Surgical pathology in the course of the Nile. Ann. R. Coll. Surg. Engl. *39*, 236 (1966)
16. Civiale,J.: Traité de l'Affection Calculeuse. Paris: Crochard 1838
17. Cleave,T.L., Campbell,G.D.: Diabetes, Coronary Thrombosis and the Saccharine Disease. Bristol: Wright 1966
18. Coetzee,T.: Urinary calculus in the Indian and African in Natal. S. Afr. Med. J. *37*, 1092 (1963)
19. Davalos,A.: The rarity of stone in the urinary tract in the wet tropics. J. Urol. *54*, 182 (1945)
20. Davidson,W.: Quoted Burkitt,D. (1966). Surgical pathology in the course of the Nile. Ann. R. Coll. Surg. Engl. *39*, 236 (1964)
21. Dix,V.W.: Stones in the lower third of the ureter: discussion. Proc. R. Soc. Med. *44*, 933 (1951)
22. Eckstein,H.B.: Endemic urinary lithiasis in Turkish children. Arch. Dis. Child. *36*, 137 (1961)
23. England,W.: Observations on the functional disorders of the kidneys which gave rise to the formation of urinary calculi; with remarks on the frequency in the County of Norfolk. London: Norwich, Bacon and Kinniebrook 1830
24. Frank,M., De Vries,A., Atsmon,A., Lazenbik,J., Kochwa,S.: Epidemiological investigation of urolithiasis in Israel. J. Urol. *81*, 597 (1959)
25. Gascio,G.: La calcolosi vesicale nell'infanzia. Riv. Pediatr. Silic. *10*, 1 (1955)
26. Gershoff,S.N., Prien,E.L., Chandrapanond,A.: Urinary stones in Thailand. J. Urol. *90*, 285 (1963)
27. Grossman,W.: The current urinary stone wave in Central Europe. Br. J. Urol. *10*, 46 (1938)
28. Halstead,S.B., Valyasevi,A. et al. (including Chubikorn,C., Pantuwatana,A., Tankayul, C., Dhanamitta,A., Van Reen,R.): Studies of bladder stone disease in Thailand. A symposium of nine papers. Am. J. Clin. Nutr. *20*, 1312 (1967)
29. Hedenberg,T.: Renal and ureteral calculi. Acta Chir. Scand. *101*, 17 (1951)

30. Hellstrom,J.: Forefinnes en stigande frekvens av urinvagskon krementen i Sverige? Hygiea (Stockholm) *94*, 337 (1932)

31. Holmes,R.J., Caplan,M.M.: A study of geographic incidence of urolithiasis with consideration of etiological factors. J. Urol. *23*, 477 (1930)

32. Inada,T., Miyasaki,S., Omori,T.: Statistical study on urolithiasis in Japan. Urol. Int. *7*, 150 (1958)

33. Korhonen,A.: Über die Harnsteine. Sonderabdruck aus den Acta Societatis medicorum Fenn. 'Duodecim' Ser. B. Tom. 22 Fasc. 3. (1936)

34. Larsen,J.F., Philip,J.: Studies on the incidence of urolithiasis. Urol. Int. *13*, 53 (1962)

35. Leonard,R.H.: Quantitative composition of kidney stones. Clin. Chem. *7*, 546 (1961)

36. Ljunghall,S., Hedstrand,H.: Renal stones and coronary heart disease. Acta Med. Scand. *199*, 481 (1976)

37. Lonsdale,K.: Human stones. Science *159*, 1199 (1968)

38. Lonsdale,K., Sutor,D.J.: X-ray diffraction studies of urinary calculi. In: Renal Stone Research Symposium. Hodgkinson,A., Nordin,B.E.C. (eds.), p. 105. London: Churchill 1969

39. McCarrison,R.: Urinary calculi in India. Br. Med. J. *1*, 72 (1927)

40. McCarrison,R.: The causation of stone in India. Br. Med. J. *1*, 1009 (1931)

41. Mates,J.: External factors in the genesis of urolithiasis. In: Renal Stone Research Symposium. Hodgkinson,A., Nordin,B.E.C. (eds.), p. 59. London: Churchill 1969

42. Mates,J., Krizek,V.: Urolithiasis. Statni Zdravotnicke Nakladatelstvi, Praha, 281 (1958)

43. Milbert,A.H., Gersh,I.: Urolithiasis in the soldier. J. Urol. *53*, 440 (1945)

44. Modlin,M.: Renal calculus in the Republic of South Africa. In: Renal Stone Research Symposium. Hodgkinson,A., Nordin,B.E.C. (eds.), p. 49. London: Churchill 1969

45. Norlin,A., Lindell,B., Granberg,P., Lindvall,N.: Urolithiasis: A study of its frequency. Scand. J. Urol. Nephrol. *10*, 159 (1976)

46. Pavone,M.: Cura medica e dietetic della calcolosi urinam. Rel. XVI Congr. Soc. Ital. Urol., *1*, 1 (1937)

47. Pavone,M., Macaluso,M., Piazza,B., Madonia,S.: Modificazioni di alcuni indici statistici nella urolitiasi in Sicilia (1965)

48. Pierce,L.W., Bloom,B.: Observations on urolithiasis among American troops in a desert area. J. Urol. *54*, 466 (1945)

49. Prien,E.L.: Personal communication (1970)

50. Prince,C.L., Scardino,P.L., Wolan,C.T.: The effect of temperature, humidity and dehydration on the formation of renal calculi. J. Urol. *75*, 209 (1956)

51. Quinland,W.S.: Urinary lithiasis; review of 33 cases in negroes. J. Urol. *53*, 791 (1945)

52. Rao: Deficiency syndrome in children of Hyderabad (Deccan). Preliminary report. Indian J. Med. Sci. (1953–1955)

53. Reaser,E.F.: Racial incidence of urolithiasis. J. Urol. *34*, 148 (1935)

54. Registrar-General's Statistical Review of England and Wales (1970). Medical Table. H.M. Stationery Office, 1972

55. Sallinen,A.: Aspects of urolithiasis in Finland. Acta Chir. Scand. *118*, 479 (1959)

56. Scott,R.: The incidence of renal colic in the medical profession in the West of Scotland. Health Bull. *29*, No. 1 (1971)

57. Taylor,R., Taylor,J.E.: A descriptive catalogue of the calculi and other animal concentrations in Museum of Royal College of Surgeons of England. Part I. London, 1842

58. Thomas,J.M.R.: Vesical calculus in Norfolk. Br. J. Urol. *21*, 20 (1949)

59. Unakul,S.: Urinary stones in Thailand. Siriraj Hospital Gazette *13*, 199 (1961)

60. Vermooten,V.: Occurrence of renal calculi and their possible relation to diet as illustrated in South African negroes. J. Amer. Med. Assoc. *109*, 857 (1937)

61. Vermooten,V.: Incidence and significance of the deposition of calcium plaques in the renal papilla as observed in the Caucasian and Negro (Bantu) population in South Africa. J. Urol. *46*, 193 (1941)

62. Williams,R.E.: Long-term survey of 538 patients with upper urinary tract stone. Br. J. Urol. *35*, 416 (1963)

63. Wise,R.D., Kark,A.E.: Urinary calculi and serum calcium levels in Africans and Indians. S. Afr. Med. J. *35*, 47 (1961)

64. Yelloly,J.: Sequel to remarks on the tendency to calculous disease. Philos. Trans. R. Soc. London. (Biol.) *120*, 415 (1830)

Chapter 2

Pathology of the Stone-Bearing Kidney

Renal calculi are solid concrements which form in the urine of the renal passages. Urine itself is a highly complex fluid containing crystalloid substances (usually in a state of supersaturation) and colloidal substances, hence the difficulty of pin-pointing not merely the multi-factorial causes but also the mode of stone formation.

The initiation of a calculus must be an event at molecular level and be followed by a period of growth to a tiny crystal or solid particle and later to a definitive stone. In addition to initiatory molecular changes there must also be an environmental setting; thus while most renal calculi have a metabolic origin, an unknown, but probably small, proportion result from infection. For example, the staphylococcus has occasionally been found inside renal calculi. The clinical importance of calculi concerns the changing behaviour of the calculus–kidney interrelationship.

I. Theories of Renal Stone Formation

How does a group of molecules (be they colloidal or crystalloid) within, say, the terminal renal tubules situated in the renal pyramid, become elaborated into the tiny solid particle which later becomes the mainly crystalloid calculus or the rarer matrix stone? Much experimental work and pathological enquiry has attempted to solve this problem.

There are three principal views: (1) That the first step is the formation of a tiny nucleus of organic colloidal material laid down in the urine (say in the ducts of Bellini or in the calyceal urine) according to recognized physicochemical principles, and that this is followed by the deposition of crystalloid substances on the nucleus. (2) That a stone results from the initial precipitation in the urine of crystals composed of inorganic crystalloid substances (as a consequence of supersaturation of the urine with the salt in question or of the urinary pH) followed by a gradual enmeshment of colloidal substances to bind the crystals together to give them permanent aggregation and stability. It is even possible that crystalloid and colloidal substances are thrown down in the urine at one and the same time, to participate simultaneously first in the initiation and then in the growth of calculi. (3) That there exist in the urine certain inhibitor substances or 'crystal-poisons' which, if present in sufficient quantities, inhibit stone formation, but if absent, allow stone formation to go ahead unimpeded.

1. Colloid Material

The view that the colloid in the matrix of renal calculi is of prime significance in their development (as held by many early pathologists) has been influenced by views concerning the development of cartilage and of bone in the animal body; but mineralogists would say that the rocks on the surface of the earth, which in many respects are analogous to calculi, do not contain a colloidal matrix.

The studies of Boyce and his co-workers [6, 8] on the urinary colloids and the laminar structure of matrix in urinary calculi and the relationship of the crystals to it, led them to the conclusion that the colloidal matrix is the determining factor in the siting and the composition of crystal deposits in calculi, and that concretions are never formed primarily as a mass of inorganic crystals. The architectural structure of calculi can only result from the deposition of crystals upon or within a preformed matrix; they concluded that the presence of crystallizable colloidal matrix is the essential factor and the initial phase of concrement formation. Crystallographic studies in the author's department have suggested that a relatively small group of calculi, namely the pisolitic calcium oxalate calculi, may have originated in colloid [27].

2. Crystals

The second and contrary view embodied in the crystalline theory of the origin of renal calculi is based upon the gradually increasing knowledge of the varied content, origin and metabolic behaviour of the principal crystalloid substances in the urine and of the physicochemical principles which are involved (for example, relative to their concentration and their reaction to the urinary pH). If this view is held, the presence of colloidal matrix within calculi could be a secondary phenomenon, or at least an example of co-precipitation, a process known to mineralogists.

A signpost pointing in the direction of the crystalline view of calculus formation is that the hyperexcretion of certain substances through the kidneys into the urine leading to its apparent supersaturation may be a determining cause of the formation of certain types of stone consequent upon the deposition of crystals in the urine. The presence in the urine of abnormally large amounts of uric acid (in hyperuricuria), of calcium (in primary hypercalciuria), of oxalates (in primary hyperoxaluria), of one of the sulphonamides (ingested for therapeutic purposes), of silicates (in some cattle and sheep), or of oxamide (fed to the experimental animal),

leading, so it would seem, to the formation of calculi composed wholly or mainly of those substances or their derivatives, suggests that an excess of such substances in the urine is of paramount importance.

The formation of cystine calculi can indeed "be used as a model in which one factor only, namely its increased output in the urine, is overwhelmingly important as against all the very many other factors (diet, infection, urinary tract abnormality) which are known to be concerned in the formation of many other kinds of stone" [16].

Vermeulen and his co-workers in a classic series of experimental studies on renal stone formation carried out over many years, gave support to the crystalline theory of the origin of renal stone. They considered that the stone-forming process falls into two stages: firstly the formation of a crystalline stone embryo, which has not only to be formed but also retained in a suitable site in the urinary tract; and secondly the subsequent maturation of the embryo into the mature stone [38].

These observers examined experimentally the conditions under which artificial concretions composed of the various stone-forming substances could be made, the composition of the experimental substrate or medium being varied so as to include or exclude non-dialysable urinary colloids as well as the various crystalline components of stone; they were able to form calculi comparable with those formed naturally [22]. By invoking the principle of the co-precipitation of crystalloids and colloids, they showed how it was possible for the urinary colloids to play a supporting rather than an initiating role in the formation of a urinary stone.

They showed how in the experimental animal the initiation of the stone-forming process could be touched off by a 'triggering' mechanism, which was of a degree of intensity different from the stimulus needed to secure the further growth of the stone. They emphasized the principle of 'habit' (as applied to rock minerals) in the formation of crystals of different shapes composed of the same chemical substances found in different media. They emphasized that the renal papilla is the part of the kidney of maximal importance in respect of the formation of concretions, the urine descending from the glomeruli, having by then achieved its maximum concentration and possibly being supersaturated in respect of the stone-forming components so that solid crystalline material may be thrown down. Such conditions are seen in the oxamide concretions made in the experimental animal [5, 38]. Vermeulen and his co-workers concluded that the physicochemical principles of the crystallization of crystalloid substances as applied to urine, afford an adequate explanation of stone formation [37].

3. Inhibitor Substances

The third view, embodying the possibility of inhibitor substances in the urine, has theoretical attractions and has been investigated experimentally in recent years by Howard and his co-workers and others. The possibilities that pyrophosphate might be such a crystal inhibitor has been explored by Fleisch and Bisaz [19], and the experimental results concerning the diphosphonate EHDP by Fraser et al. [20] raise interesting possibilities.

4. Calcific Foci

Moving from the molecular level to renal calcific particles which can be seen microscopically or macroscopically and which can be regarded as being not uncommonly the precursor of the definitive stone, are the calcific foci in the renal pyramids described by Randall [31], which were of two kinds: type I lesions were small calcified plaques located in the interstitial tissue beneath the surface epithelium of the renal papillae,

which gradually became exposed to the urine by the erosion of the epithelium overlying the plaque. Type II lesions consisted of calcific masses found in the terminal parts of the ducts of Bellini (Fig. 2.1). The presence of Randall's plaques has been confirmed by many workers including ourselves and they are believed to be the first or initiating lesion of many (but not all) calcium oxalate renal calculi. Crystallographic studies have shown them to be composed of calcium phosphate (apatite), calcium oxalate or both together [17].

Microscopic papillary calcific foci (such as oxamide concretions) have been shown by various observers to be possible precursors of definitive experimental calculi attached to a renal papilla [22].

Microscopic calcific foci are frequently found at various sites in the normal kidney (15% of 380 autopsy kidneys in the author's series [29]), commonly in the lumina or the membrana propria of the tubular epithelial cells of the renal papillae or in the adjacent connective tissue. In a series of stone-bearing kidneys such calcific foci were found in 38% (of 139 subjects) and were more numerous and in closer proximity to each other than those observed in normal kidneys. In mildly infected stone-bearing kidneys the calcific foci were often more widespread than in the non-infected kidney and situated mainly in the renal pyramids. Those calcific foci which are found in the terminal parts of the ducts of Bellini probably have a relationship to the origin of calyceal calculi. Some degree of correlation apparently exists between the presence of renal calcific foci (as described above) and hypercalciuria, which itself predisposes to stone formation [3].

In a study of calcific deposits in the human renal papilla Cooke [14] found deposits of calcium salts in 43 of 62 human kidneys examined, usually located in large amounts in the outer part of the renal medulla, where the vasa recta are grouped in bundles. Calcification was present in

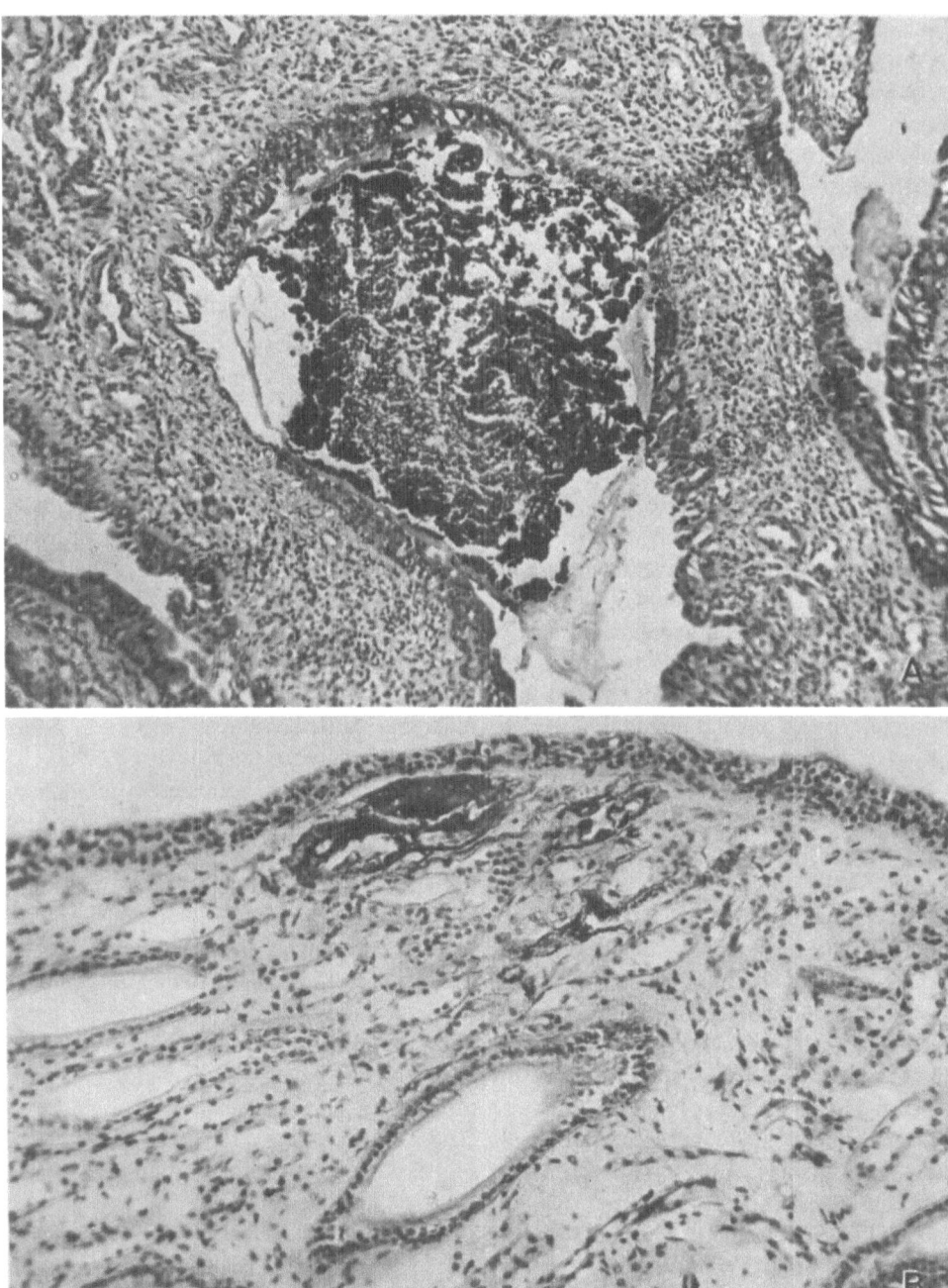

Fig. 2.1. The varieties of Randall's plaque from stone-bearing kidneys. **A.** A dense peritubular and intratubular plaque of calcium salts is seen in and around the terminal collecting tubules and ducts of Bellini at the tip of the renal pyramid; it is covered by a layer of hyperplastic transitional epithelium which separates it from the calyceal cavity and from the urine (H and E ×410). **B.** A plaque from a stone-bearing kidney seen as a small focus of calcification in the pyramidal connective tissues at the side of the pyramid and covered by a thin layer of single-cell attenuated epithelium (H and E ×600)

relation to the walls of the thinner limbs of the loops of Henle (confined to the immediate vicinity of the basement membrane) which, he concluded, were chiefly concerned with the calcification. It has been shown that in the renal papilla of the hamster, the dog and the rat, there is a high concentration of calcium, and in fact a concentration gradient between the calcium in the renal papilla (where there is the highest level) and that in the medulla and the cortex. In the rat and the dog there was also a gradient between the calcium concentration in the papilla (the higher) and that in the urine [21].

Carr [12, 13] suggested that renal calyceal stones are formed in a 'nest' leading off from a minor calyx and are at first separated from the stream of urine by a thin layer of urothelium which is ultimately eroded, the stone then being bathed in the urinary stream and enlarging by the addition of crystals of solid material passed to it by way of the renal lymphatics.

II. General Structure of Renal Calculi

The definitive stone is formed most commonly in the lowest calyx of one kidney, less commonly in more than one calyx more or less simultaneously, and not infrequently in one or more calyces of both kidneys at approximately the same time or separated by an interval of time.

Renal calculi are composed of one or more crystalline substances (probably reflecting their etiology) admixed with a colloidal matrix, usually 2.5% of the whole. The stone is at first small, usually solitary (but occasionally multiple), hard, flat, pyramidal or concavo-convex and often attached, at least at first, to a renal papilla and gradually enlarging to fill a calyx. A stone in the renal pelvis may at first be small (having migrated from a calyx) but gradually enlarges and often takes the shape of the pelvis. The 'staghorn' calculus

has prolongations (or separate calculi) in the calyces; the colour varies according to its chemical composition and may be modified by a superficial coating of blood pigment, pus or fibrin.

1. Crystalline Content

At least 11 different crystalloid substances may enter into the composition of the stone. Occasionally adventitious substances (including drugs such as sulphonamides, tetracycline, methylene blue or porphyrin) may also be incorporated into a calculus. The stone usually has an identifiable nucleus which may differ in composition from the remainder of the stone. When cut across, some stones show radial striation (calcium oxalate monohydrate, tri-calcium phosphate, uric acid) and also concentric lamination sometimes with crystalloid and colloidal laminae alternating, each being only a few microns thick.

The crystalline substances in human urinary calculi are recognized by standard physical methods, namely by the use of the polarizing microscope, X-ray crystallography [28] and microradiography, and by chemical analysis (which is a complementary method of detection though not necessarily the final test). The most common crystalline components are the calcium oxalates, the calcium phosphates, uric acid and urates, and cystine.

2. Colloid Content

The colloid content is a substance of greater complexity than the crystalloid content. The principal groups of substances of high molecular weight in the urine, namely the mucoproteins and the mucopolysaccharides, have not yet been fully characterized. The urinary biocolloids have been removed from urine by a combination of dialysis, ultrafiltration and perevaporation, their lyophilized daily dry weights averaging 0.09 g in the normal adult and 0.496 g in patients with calculous disease [9, 33].

Mucoprotein is composed of a protein molecule to which is attached a mucopolysaccharide, which contains hexosamine and usually hexuronic acid. In cartilage the protein (collagen) and a mucopolysaccharide (chondroitin sulphate, which is also found in urine) together form a complex which appears to be necessary for the calcification of cartilage, and to which are linked calcium ions which then react with phosphate to form apatite. A virus-inhibitory urinary protein insoluble in sodium chloride solutions of 0.58 M was discovered by Tamm and Horsfall [36].

It seems that both normal and calculous urine contain at least two mucoproteins which retain a negative charge throughout the entire pH range of urine, both of which are increased in the urine of patients with calcium-containing renal calculi and especially in some patients with primary hyperparathyroidism. A marked increase of the Tamm-Horsfall mucoprotein has been found in patients with renal calculous disease, a protein probably secreted by the transitional epithelium of the urinary tract [9].

The largest single component of the urinary colloids in normal and in calculous patients was 'uromucoid', which is a carbohydrate–protein conjugation, joined by polymer linkage to form a compound of high molecular weight, which is insoluble in molar sodium chloride. Some urinary mucoproteins known as glycoproteins contain appreciable amounts of hexosamine and usually sialic acid, and may have been derived from serum [2].

The colloidal matrix of a calculus is the non-dialysable remainder after the crystalline component has been dissolved. Stones can be decalcified by immersion for 40 days in a solution of EDTA when the matrix is available for study. Cross-sections show the matrix to have a concentrically laminated structure and to be composed of fibrils together with amorphous interfibrillary substances; the fibrils, which are arranged in broad bands or circular whorls of varying size, show parallel orientation of their long axes. The crystals are closely aligned with the margins of the fibrils and are embedded in the amorphous interfibrillary material [8].

There are variations in the spatial disposition of the crystals in relation to the fibrils in the different varieties of stone. The composition of stone matrix (a mucoprotein complex) seems to be fairly constant and consists of protein (amounting to about two-thirds), various sugars including glucose and mannose and also hexosamine and glucosamine (amounting to about 15%), and some inorganic substances including calcium and phosphate (amounting to about 10%). These substances combine together to form matrix, having been derived from the urine, the blood plasma and possibly the kidney [33].

Matrix substance A, which appears to originate in the renal parenchyma, has been demonstrated by immunological techniques to be present in the matrix of all types of stone. This mucoprotein is present in the urine of stone-forming patients, especially those forming infective stones, but not in patients with normal renal function [10]. The Tamm–Horsfall mucoprotein is a component of stone matrix in small amounts; uromucoid and also serum albumen and serum globulin are present in stone matrix. In urine, several workers have identified various small spheroidal colloidal particles, which are thought to have originated in the renal tubules, and which may relate to the formation of stone matrix. PAS-positive-staining granules have been identified in the kidneys of rats treated with parathormone [18].

In a study of renal biopsies from patients with renal calculi, in a high proportion of those with metabolic calculi, PAS-positive calcium-containing mucoproteinous particles having a laminar structure (regarded as evidence of intranephronic calculosis) have been found; while in biopsies from kidneys containing infected staghorn calculi, no such particles were found [7].

It is possible that calcium oxalate calculi (found usually in sterile urine) have a different mode of formation from the (usually) infective calculi generally composed of struvite or apatite. The former grow within the renal tubule as a result of crystals deposited in matrix deposited within the renal tubules; whereas the infective stone forms in the major renal collecting tubules from urinary mucoprotein, which unites with apatite to form, say, a staghorn type of infective stone [32, 39, 40].

III. Components of Renal Calculi

1. Calcium Oxalate

Calculi composed entirely or predominantly of calcium oxalates are the commonest renal stones; they are usually found in sterile acid urine and many contain varying amounts of apatite. The calcium oxalate occurs in two forms readily distinguished by their physical characteristics and by their powder pattern on X-ray diffraction [11, 23, 28]. The first form is calcium oxalate monohydrate (whewellite: $CaC_2O_4 \cdot H_2O$), which has monoclinic crystals; the second form is calcium oxalate dihydrate (weddellite; $CaC_2O_4 \cdot 2H_2O$), which has tetragonal crystals. Calcium oxalate trihydrate ($CaC_2O_4 \cdot 3H_2O$) has been recorded as a very rare component of calculi.

The varieties of calcium oxalate stones based on their external appearance include the hempseed calculi (small, round or ovoid, multiple, grey or brown with 'varnished' surfaces, and a concentrically laminated structure); the nodular or mulberry stones (rounded or ovoid, amber to dark brown, with numerous rounded bosses or mamillary processes corresponding to areas of different orientation resulting from

radial striation and lamination within the stone); and the jackstone (a variant of the nodular stone, having longish solid processes radiating from the centre). These calculi are usually composed of calcium oxalate monohydrate and may have nuclei of uric acid or apatite, and when thin sections are examined microscopically, they show well-marked lamination and radial striation, and are known as 'pisolitic calculi' (Fig. 2.2).

A fourth large group of oxalate stones is the 'crystalline stone', so called because the surface is covered with well-formed large 'envelope' crystals of calcium oxalate dihydrate easily visible to the naked eye. The interior may be composed of the monohydrate or apatite; this type of stone when sectioned shows only coarse lamination and no radial striation. There is also a mixed type consisting (in one single stone) partly of pisolitic and partly of crystalline elements [27, 35].

2. Phosphate

Four different phosphates occur commonly or not infrequently in urinary calculi, and their composition has been resolved by physical as well as by chemical methods; other rarer phosphates are found occasionally.

Apatite is the commonest constituent of urinary calculi and is found in two variants, namely hydroxyapatite ($Ca_{10}(PO_4)_6(OH)_2$) and carbonate apatite ($Ca_{10}(PO_4 \cdot CO_3OH)_6 \cdot OH_2$), which can only be identified by optical methods or by X-ray diffraction; the crystals are too small to be easily recognized microscopically. The apatites are often admixed with oxalates in the common oxalate stone.

Struvite or magnesium ammonium phosphate hexahydrate ($MgNH_4PO_4 \cdot 6H_2O$) is usually associated with varying proportions of apatite, the stone being creamy-white in colour, and is the main constituent of the stones found in alkaline infected urine, to

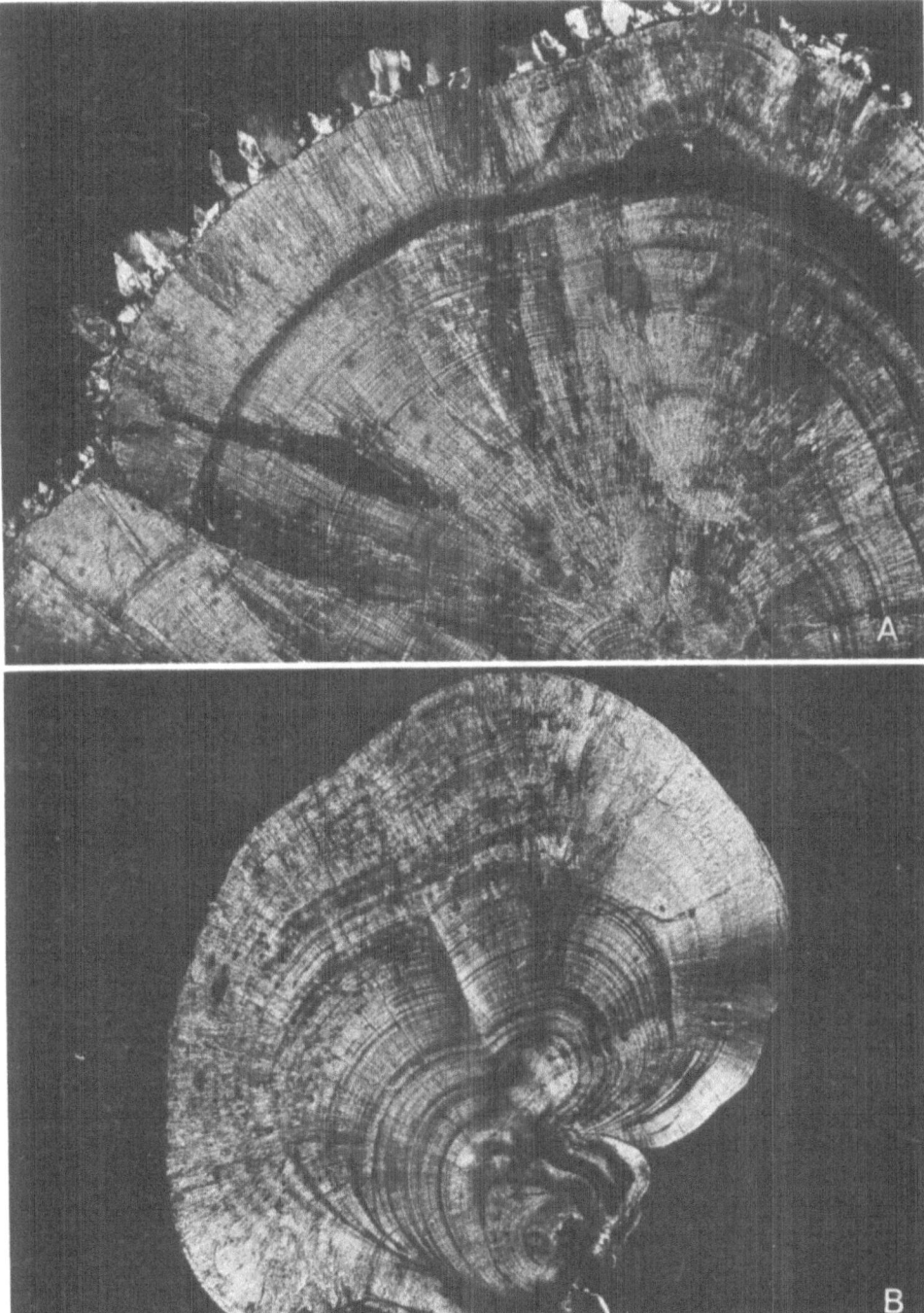

Fig. 2.2. **A.** Thin section of a pisolitic type of calcium oxalate calculus demonstrating the fine concentric laminations with numerous crystallites of whewellite perpendicular to the laminations giving the radial striation effect. There are a number of small weddellite crystals on the surface. **B.** Photomicrograph of a whewellite calculus which probably has originated from a Randall's plaque or from a crystalline mass in a duct of Bellini, the original nucleus being situated at the hilum of the stone. The nucleus of origin has affected the early growth of the stone and has resulted in its asymmetry

form one variety of the soft, friable, staghorn calculi. The crystals are short and prismatic and are formed in infected urine as 'knife-rest' or 'coffin-lid' crystals. Microscopically the stone shows the crystals to be arranged in a columnar or sometimes a laminar network. Brushite or calcium hydrogen phosphate dihydrate ($CaHPO_4 \cdot 2H_2O$), light yellow in colour, occurs as monoclinic crystals in an acid urine and is usually associated with oxalates and sometimes with apatite. Brushite tends to be precipitated from a saturated solution below a pH of 6.2; at higher pH levels phosphate is precipitated as apatite.

Whitlockite or β-tricalcium phosphate ($Ca_3(PO_4)_2$) occurs as long colourless rhombohedral crystals appearing as bristle-like structures radiating from a nucleus of apatite or calcium oxalate. Octocalcium phosphate or tetracalcium hydrogen tri-phosphate trihydrate ($Ca_4H(PO_4)_3 \cdot 2 \cdot 5H_2O$) was first detected by X-ray diffraction studies. It has been suggested that it may be the first of the phosphates to be precipitated during renal stone formation. There are several rare phosphate calculi including newberyite (magnesium hydrogen phosphate; $MgHPO_4 \cdot 3H_2O$), and several others which have been reported only a few times [23].

The calculi composed of uric acid and/or urates, and those composed of cystine are referred to in Chapters 15 and 16.

3. Rare Components

Sulphonamides ingested as drugs for therapeutic purposes may be incorporated in renal calculi or may be the sole constituent. Lead taken into the body during exposure to it has been recognized as a trace compound in stone. Porphyrin has been found in calculi in subjects who suffer from porphyrinuria. Silver, copper, zinc, and manganese have all been reported as trace elements. Fluorine has been shown by chemical tests to be present in many calculi. Gypsum (calcium sulphate dihydrate), calcium sulphide, indigo and tetracycline have been detected in renal calculi. Xanthine (Chap. 17) occasionally is the sole component of stones. Aragonite (or pure calcium carbonate) has been reported rarely as the sole constituent of stone. Silica has been found occasionally in human calculi and commonly in those found in animals. Haematin, fibrin and mucin have been identified in calculi. Bacterial calculi are rare and consist of densely packed masses of bacteria held together by some organic cement substance.

4. Matrix Calculi

A few renal calculi consisting almost entirely of colloidal matrix (65%–85% of matrix by weight) are occasionally found in kidneys in which there is an element of stasis, often with an associated infection (32, 39); these 'stones' are yellow-white to tan in colour and of a consistence which varies between jelly and putty and are gritty from a small content of crystalloid substance and are usually radiolucent. They can be cut with a knife and have concentric (and sometimes radial) lamination. Some matrix calculi may have initially been fully mineralized phosphatic calculi which have undergone partial dissolution of their crystalloid content, a change which may follow medicinal treatment to try to dissolve phosphatic calculi, as during the ingestion of acidifying drugs or aludrox (which reduces the urinary phosphate level). Possibly the converse may happen, as is suggested by the fact that at operation a soft matrix mass may be found adjacent to, or almost a part of a largely mineralized phosphatic stone, the urine being infected [40].

When a tiny concretion has been formed its late growth may (if the conditions within the medium are propitious) be determined by 'epitaxy', a term which is used to describe the phenomenon of the crystalline intergrowth of one crystal on a substrate of another. For this to happen the lattice spacings in the two crystal faces in contact must be almost identical with a near (though not necessarily exact) geometrical fit [25, 34].

IV. Morbid Anatomy

Changes take place in the stone-bearing kidney which differ in extent and with time, chiefly according to whether there is or there is not a resulting obstruction or an associated infection.

A calyceal calculus composed of calcium oxalate in a non-infected kidney may grow very slowly over many years with minimal structural change in the kidney, though sometimes a hydrocalycosis may develop when the stone partially obstructs the calyceal outlet. Similarly a larger stone in the renal pelvis may partially obstruct the pelviureteric outlet and give rise to a hydronephrosis, or if firmly impacted, ultimately to a varying degree of renal atrophy. The gradual conversion of the kidney under such circumstances into a functionless hydronephrotic sac is occasionally seen.

A stone passing down the ureter does not usually give rise to any lasting change. An uninfected calculus which comes to rest in the ureter may produce a considerable degree of obstruction to the downward drainage of urine for a short period after its arrest but it is rarely complete and there is some dilatation of the ureter above the stone. At the site of arrest the ureter is thick-walled and there is periureteric oedema but when the spasm has subsided urine flows fairly freely around the stone into the bladder and there may be relatively little back-pressure on the kidney. A stone lingering for a long time in the ureter may hollow out a bed in the wall of the ureter, which may become thinned and weakened

from the pressure of the stone with the formation of a false diverticulum or even a true saccule communicating with the lumen of the ureter by a constricted orifice [22]. Rarely a periureteric abscess may develop at that point.

Complete obstruction to the flow of urine if prolonged leads initially to dilatation of the renal pelvis; but if prolonged for several months the kidney may undergo a varying degree of atrophy until in the end all excretory tissue may be lost and there remains a mere fibrous shell covering a multiloculated hydronephrotic sac representing the greatly dilated calyces, the ureter also being considerably dilated above the stone.

1. Infection

The stone-bearing kidney, which is usually uninfected at first and may remain so for a long time if the stone increases in size only very slowly, usually sooner or later becomes infected but sometimes only after many years. Infection may reach the kidney by way of the blood stream (possibly from the colon), or from the bladder either by way of the lumen or the lymphatics of the ureter and may initiate the formation of renal stones.

E. coli may not be an originator of stone formation (except those varieties which can split urea), but it is commonly found in the kidney and the urine of patients with infected calculous disease, and often in association with other bacteria, probably as a secondary invader. *Bacillus proteus* and the other urea-splitting organisms including *Pseudomonas pyocyaneus*, by virtue of their capacity to form a strongly alkaline urine, often promote the gradual or rapid increase in the size of renal calculi which are then composed largely of ammonium magnesium phosphate deposited in layers upon a stone initially composed of calcium oxalate. Such a calculus may gradually fill several calyces as well as the renal pelvis (staghorn stone). Probably the majority of patients with a primary renal infection never have renal calculi. Some unusual renal infections, such as the rare gonococcal infection of the kidney, the not uncommon renal tuberculosis and the rare renal actinomycosis are sometimes associated with (but do not themselves initiate) renal calculi.

If the urine is able to drain freely down the ureter, changes in the renal parenchyma resulting from infection proceed more slowly than if a moderate grade of obstruction is present. A varying degree of calculous pyelonephritis, however, will probably develop slowly or quickly, the renal calyces become enlarged and the renal papillae flattened or partially destroyed; renal function will be increasingly impaired owing to a varying degree of renal atrophy.

When there is pelviureteric obstruction resulting from a partial or complete impaction of the stone associated with infection, the renal passages become gradually dilated, the changes waxing and waning with periods of improvement or relapse. Calculous pyonephrosis is usually a sequel to calculous pyelonephritis resulting from varying degrees of obstruction. The kidney is then usually moderately enlarged and may still retain a considerable amount of functioning parenchymatous tissue altered somewhat in appearance and structure because of back-pressure and infection. Individual stone-containing calyces may be enlarged, though the renal pelvis may be only moderately dilated and may contain calculi and pus; if the kidney is not removed surgically, the stones will probably continue to increase in size.

In another group, if pus is retained in the renal pelvis, an enormous pyonephrosis (the renal pelvis itself being massive) may develop, the obstruction here being usually intermittent and renal function being grossly impaired.

A renocutaneous sinus or fistula discharging pus and/or urine may be established between the kidney and the external surface of the body as a complication of an untreated ruptured pyonephrosis, a condition which may eventually be associated with multiple tracks and pockets of pus in the lumbar and iliac regions; such fistulae are rarely seen nowadays.

Very rarely a small pyonephrotic kidney (the 'atrophic' type), perhaps only 2 or 3 in. long is encountered, consisting of the renal pelvis with the dilated calyces joined together to form a cavity containing calculi and pus, and with still a small amount of renal tissue capable of limited function [24]. The presence of an impacted stone in the ureter, when the kidney is grossly infected and also contains calculi, leads to the changes of pyelonephritis and pyonephrosis already referred to; if the stone is not relieved the end-results must be destruction of the kidney.

2. Complications

The infected stone-bearing kidney in its advanced stages may present a varied range of pathological changes which are to some extent non-specific; such changes are rare nowadays because of earlier clinical recognition of calculous disease and the greater co-operation of patients [15].

Perinephric abscess, which may result from local atrophy of the renal cortex and subsequent rupture of a stone-bearing calyx of an infected kidney into the perinephric tissue, may complicate calculous pyelonephritis or a calculous pyonephrosis. If untreated, such an abscess may track widely in the retroperitoneal tissues, or rupture into the peritoneal cavity.

Occasionally a renobronchial fistula has resulted as a complication of a calculous pyonephrosis associated with a perinephric abscess which has gradually penetrated the diaphragm to enter the pleural cavity or a

Fig. 2.3. Renoduodenal, renocolic and other renal fistulae. **A.** Schematic drawing of the anatomical relations between the kidneys, the hepatic and splenic flexures and the colon and the duodenum; the perinephric fat is shown. When the fistulae form, the fat between the kidneys and the gut becomes quantitatively diminished (V.C., vena cava; Ao, Aorta). **B.** Diagrammatic representation of the various pathways through which renal fistulae penetrate the colon, the duodenum and the pleural cavity. **C.** Diagram to show the various fistulae (uretero-vesical, uretero-colic and uretero-vaginal) which can complicate a large untreated infected stone in the pelvic ureter

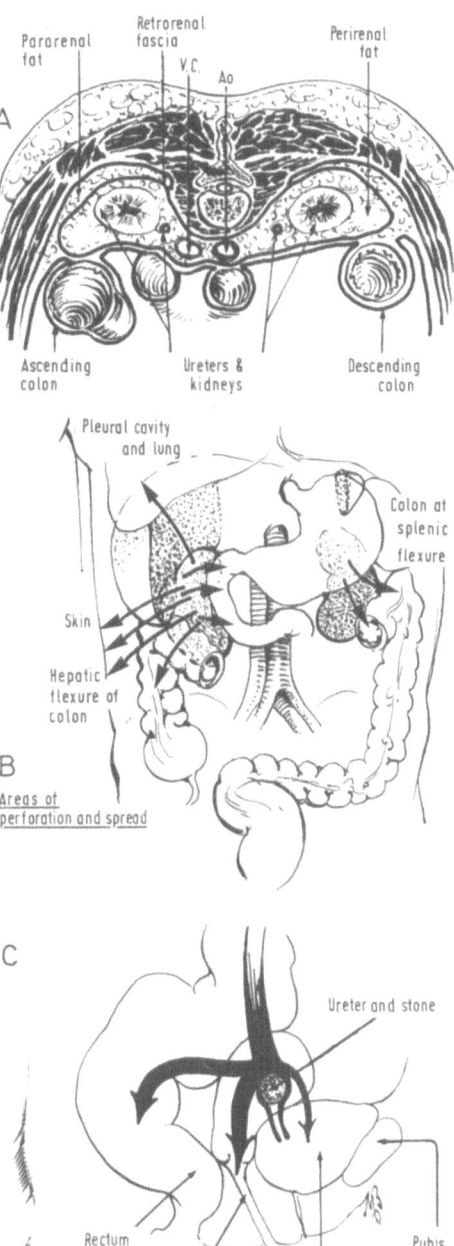

lung or a bronchus. Renoperitoneal fistula has usually been associated with a perinephric abscess complicating a stone in the renal pelvis or ureter. A fistulous communication between the kidney (renal pelvis or calyces) or the ureter and an adjacent organ or cavity may complicate renal and ureteric calculous disease (Fig. 2.3). Nephrocolic fistula, which is the most common type of spontaneous nephrovisceral fistula to complicate renal calculous disease occasionally, occurs usually between the lowest calyx of the right kidney (or occasionally the renal pelvis) and the hepatic flexure of the colon, which are in close anatomical relationship; the splenic flexure of the colon is involved only rarely.

Similarly, a pyeloduodenal fistula is occasionally found, a large stone in the renal pelvis ulcerating through into the lumen of the second part of the duodenum, the two viscera being in close anatomical relationship. The kidneys in such cases are badly infected and most of the renal parenchyma has been destroyed as a result of suppuration and pressure atrophy [1, 4].

Long-standing suppuration in an infected calculous kidney may give rise to renal amyloid changes which still further impair renal function. Xanthogranulomatous pyelonephritis, which is an occasional accompaniment of calculous pyelonephritis [26], results in tissue necrosis followed by phagocytosis of the liberated cholesterol; the condition may mimic renal cell carcinoma.

A kidney which has been largely or almost totally destroyed as a result of long-standing calculous disease may be the seat of a fatty or fibro-fatty replacement of the renal parenchyma, the resulting condition being known as renal fibrolipomatosis. The condition, which is non-specific in that it may complicate destruction of the kidney from other causes, is occasionally found at autopsy or at operation in cases of advanced renal calculous disease. A perirenal haematoma resulting from a gross haemorrhage from the infected renal parenchyma occasionally complicates advanced renal calculous disease [30]. The pathological process may proceed to subtotal or complete renal atrophy.

Various intrarenal conditions, including the renal obstructive lesions, various renal cysts and cystic conditions, and the neoplasia of the renal pelvis and parenchyma, may be associated with renal calculi (Chap. 3). Similarly several extrarenal diseases, which are occasionally or commonly associated with renal calculus, include primary hyperparathyroidism, Paget's disease, Cushing's disease, sarcoidosis, Wilson's disease and chronic peptic ulcer (Chap. 4).

References

1. Abeshouse,B.S.: Renal and ureteral fistula of visceral and cutaneous type; report of four cases. Urol. Cutan. Rev. *53*, 655 (1949)
2. Anderson,A.J., Lepper,M.H., Wincler,R.T.: The fractionation of urine colloids on anion-exchange cellulose. Biochem. J. *77*, 581 (1960)
3. Anderson,C.K., Hodgkinson,A., Pyrah, L.N.: Renal calcification, calculus formation and the urinary excretion of calcium. Lancet, *II*, 454 (1961)
4. Boardman,K.P.: Duodenal and common bile duct obstruction with a pyeloduodenal fistula caused by a renal calculous pyonephrosis. Br. J. Urol. *48*, 6 (1976)
5. Borden,T.A., Vermeulen,C.W.: The renal papilla in calculogenesis of oxamide stone. Invest. Urol. *4*, 125 (1966)
6. Boyce,W.H.: Organic matrix of human urinary concretions. In: Renal Stone Research Symposium. Hodgkinson,A., Nordin,B.E.C. (eds.), p. 93. London: Churchill 1969
7. Boyce,W.H.: Ultrastructure of human renal calculi. In: Urinary Calculi International Symposium. Renal Stone Research. Madrid, 1972, p. 247. Basel: Karger 1973
8. Boyce,W.H., King,J.S.Jr.: Crystal-matrix interrelations in calculi. J. Urol. *81*, 351 (1959)
9. Boyce,W.H., Garvey,F.K., Norfleet,C.M.: Proteins and other biocolloids of urine in health and in calculous disease. J. Clin. Invest. *33*, 1287 (1954)
10. Boyce,W.H., Stanton-King,J., Fielden, M.L.: Total non-dialysable solids in human urine XIII. Immunological detection of a component peculiar to renal calculous matrix and to urine of calculus patients. J. Clin. Invest. *41*, 1180 (1962)
11. Bunn,C.W.: Crystals, their role in nature and in science. New York, London: Academic Press 1964
12. Carr,R.J.: How do stones begin? World Med. *3*, 20 (1968)
13. Carr,R.J.: Etiology of renal calculi: microradiographic studies. In: Renal Stone Research Symposium. Hodgkinson,A., Nordin,B.E.C. (eds.), p. 123. London: Churchill 1969
14. Cooke,S.A.R.: The site of calcification in the human renal papilla. Br. J. Surg. *57*, 890 (1970)
15. Cox,C.E.: Symposium on renal lithiasis. Urinary tract infection and renal lithiasis. Urol. Clin. North Am. *1*, 279 (1974)
16. Dent,C.E., Senior,H.: Studies on the treatment of cystinuria. Br. J. Urol. *27*, 317 (1955)
17. Engfeldt,B., Lagergren,C.: Nephrocalcinosis: a roentgenologic, biophysical and histologic study. Acta Chir. Scand. *115*, 46 (1958)
18. Engfeldt,B., Gardell,S., Hellstrom,J., Ivemark,B., Rhodin,J., Strand,J.L.: Effect of experimentally induced hyperparathyroidism on renal function and structure. Acta Endocrinol. (Kbh.) *29*, 15 (1958)
19. Fleisch,H., Bisaz,S.: Mechanism of calcification: role of collagen, polyphosphates and phosphatase. Am. J. Physiol. *200*, 1296 (1962)
20. Fraser,D., Russell,R.G., Pohler,O., Robertson,W.G., Fleisch,H.: The influence of disodium, ethane-1-hydroxy 1,1-diphosphonate (EHDP) on development of experimentally-induced urinary stones in rats. Clin. Sci. *42*, 197 (1972)
21. Gains,N.A., Michaels,C.W., Thwaites,M., Trounce,J.R.: Calcium concentration in the kidney. Nephron *5*, 352 (1968)

22. Gill,W.B., Vermeulen, C.W.: Oxamide crystalluria and urolithiasis: rat and in vitro observations. Invest. Urol. *1*, 339 (1964)

23. Herring,L.C.: Observations on the analysis of 10,000 calculi. J. Urol. *88*, 545 (1962)

24. Joly,J.S.: Stone and calculous disease of the urinary tract. London: Heinemann 1929

25. Lonsdale,K.: Epitaxy as a growth factor in urinary calculi and gallstones. Nature (London) *217*, 56 (1968)

26. Malek,C.S., Greene,J.F., de Weerd,J.H., Farrow,G.M.: Xanthomatous pyelonephritis. Br. J. Urol. *44*, 296 (1972)

27. Murphy,B.T., Pyrah,L.N.: The composition, structure and mechanisms of the formation of urinary calculi. Br. J. Urol. *34*, 129 (1962)

28. Prien,E.L., Frondel,C.: Studies in urolithiasis. I. Composition of urinary calculi. J. Urol. *57*, 949 (1947)

29. Pyrah,L.N.: The calcium-containing renal stone. Proc. R. Soc. Med. *51*, 183 (1958)

30. Pyrah,L.N.: Various organic diseases. In: Encyclopaedia of urology. Alken,C.E., Dix,V.W., Weyrauch,H.M., Wildbolz,E. (eds.), Vol. XI/I, p. 155. Berlin, Heidelberg, New York: Springer 1967

31. Randall,A.: The initiating lesions of renal calculus. Surg. Gynecol. Obstet. *64*, 201 (1937)

32. Spector,A.R., Gray,A., Prien,Jr.E.L.: Kidney stone matrix. Differences in acidic protein composition. Invest. Urol. *13*, 387 (1976)

33. Stanton-King,J., Boyce,W.H.: In vitro production of simulated renal calculi. J.Urol. *89*, 546 (1963)

34. Sutor,D.J.: Crystallographic analysis of urinary calculi. In: Scientific foundations of urology. Williams,D.I., Chisholm,G.D. (eds.), Vol. I, p. 244. London: Heinemann 1976

35. Sutor,D.J., Brocken,J.: Crystallographic studies on the formation of renal calculi. Biochem. J. *122*, 6P (1971)

36. Tamm,I., Horsfall,F.: Characterisation and separation of an inhibitor of haemagglutination present in urine. Proc. Soc. Exp. Biol. Med. *74*, 108 (1950)

37. Vermeulen,C.W., Lyon,E.S.: Mechanisms of genesis and growth of calculi. Am. J. Med. *45*, 684 (1968)

38. Vermeulen,C.W., Lyon,E.S., Ellis,J.E., Borden,T.A.: Renal papilla and calculogenesis. J. Urol. *97*, 573 (1967)

39. Wickham,J.E.: Matrix and the infective renal calculi. Br. J. Urol. *47*, 727 (1975)

40. Wickham,J.E.: The matrix of renal calculi. In: Scientific foundations of urology. Williams,D.I., Chisholm,G.D. (eds.), Vol. I, p. 323. London: Heinemann 1976

Intrarenal, Pararenal and Ureteric Disorders Complicated by Renal Calculi and Calcification

Most calcium-containing calculi with which the urologist has to deal are initially the sole or the primary pathological abnormality in the affected kidney, which later undergoes the expected pathological changes. In some patients it emerges at once, or after investigation, that the renal stone is associated with one or other of a varied collection of intrarenal obstructive, cystic, neoplastic and vascular pathological conditions of the kidney and the ureter, and which pose problems of diagnosis. In such cases the clinical symptoms of the stone may be the first to present, or alternatively those related to the associated condition may be recognized first and the calculus discovered on investigation. A list of the conditions to be referred to is given below. Just as the pathological conditions within the kidney, in such cases, are biphasic, so also is the appropriate treatment if both conditions are to be relieved.

I. Renal and Ureteric Stone and Obstructive Conditions in the Urinary Tract

Partial or intermittent obstruction at the calyceal outlet, the pelviureteric junction, at any level of the ureter, at the ureterovesical junction and even at the neck of the bladder, leads to varying degrees of urinary stasis, difficulty in voiding crystalline particles into the bladder or to the exterior and hence to occasional stone formation above the obstruction. During the early stages the urine is usually sterile but stasis will encourage infection, which will still further promote stone formation.

1. Hydrocalycosis

A minor calyx, originally anatomically normal, may become gradually more and more dilated if its neck becomes narrow and partially obstructed from fibrosis resulting from infection or from trauma from a stone which has formed within it, and is then designated hydrocalycosis [158]. The calyx (usually the upper or middle ones) and the fornices become broader, the renal papilla which projects into it becomes flattened and the infundibulum wider and possibly shorter. If the narrow neck of the hydrocalycosis becomes sealed off as a result of infection or from the presence of a stone, one variety of renal cyst may result.

Hydrocalycosis may be symptomless; alternatively it may give rise to mild renal pain and haematuria if there is an associated calculus or infection. A moderately dilated calyx (which may contain one or more stones or sometimes none) may be seen on urography as a pouch which still retains a demonstrable communication with the major calyx. Symptomless hydrocalycosis does not require surgical treatment. Partial nephrectomy is the treatment of choice for a calyceal stone associated with hydrocalycosis which is thought to be causing symptoms. Several calyces in one kidney may be the seat of hydrocalycosis [158].

2. Pelviureteric Hydronephrosis

Hydronephrosis resulting from a primary partial pelviureteric obstruction (not uncommon in adolescents and young male adults) is not infrequently complicated by renal stone and occasionally by urinary infection, both being secondary to urinary stasis. The condition is essentially and clinically different from the hydronephrosis which is secondary to a primary renal pelvic stone impacted in the pelviureteric junction. In the second condition it is usually necessary only to remove the stone.

Primary pelviureteric obstruction is believed to result usually from a neuromuscular abnormality at the junction of the renal pelvis and the ureter. It is not uncommonly associated with an aberrant renal or lower polar artery, or with external fibrous bands, adhesions or kinks at the pelviureteric junction, all of which are usually believed to be secondary causes of the hydronephrosis. Less commonly there is a true stricture of the pelviureteric junction, congenital or acquired, or an abnormally high attachment of the ureter to the renal pelvis. The resulting enlarged renal pelvis may remain almost unchanged and clinically innocuous for years, though periodic attacks of renal colic, probably dependent upon kinking of the pelviureteric junction rather than on the presence of any associated stone, are usual. Less commonly there is discomfort in the lumbar region, haematuria and clinical symptoms of infection which may lead to pyonephrosis. The diagnosis is made by intravenous pyelography and occasionally retrograde pyelography is necessary.

Renal Calculi. The exact incidence of renal stone is unknown but it may be as high as 10%. The author has encountered a number of cases in a large series of cases of hydronephrosis. The stones were mostly biggish and spheroidal and located in the renal pelvis rather than in a calyx. They were found in non-infected hydronephrotic kidneys of only moderate size (Fig. 3.1, see p. 34). Hellstrom et al. [70] reported calculi (single or multiple) in 18 of 100 cases of hydronephrosis believed to be secondary to primary abnormalities at the pelviureteric junction of various kinds. The urine was uninfected in 12 and infected in 6 in several of which nephrectomy was done. If the stone is removed and the abnormality at the pelviureteric junction is not recognized and corrected, recurrent stone formation may be expected. Burns et al. [17] reported the presence of calculi in 23 cases of pelviureteric hydronephrosis.

Surgical treatment (a single operative procedure) is usually indicated to remove the stone and to revise or reconstruct the pelviureteric obstruction by one of the available plastic procedures, the hydronephrotic pelvis being reduced to normal size. Whereas in earlier years such plastic procedures usually failed because of the incidence of post-operative infection and secondary calculus formation, the improvement of surgical techniques (including the replacement of silk by catgut for suturing), the better control of infection and the general abandonment of the indwelling splint catheter and nephrostomy drainage have reduced the incidence of infection and improved the long-term results, including the prevention of stone formation. Four cases of calculi as long as 5–24 years after Y-plasty procedures for the relief of pelviureteric obstruction have been reported [26]. Of the various plastic procedures described, the author has favoured the Hynes–Anderson operation [11], the Culp procedure [29] and for small hydronephroses the Foley V–Y operation [52]. If renal function is seriously impaired and the kidney largely destroyed nephrectomy will be necessary.

3. Retrocaval Ureter

Retrocaval ureter, a comparatively rare condition, is sometimes complicated by renal or ureteric calculus. It arises as a consequence of a congenital anomaly of the abdominal venous vascular arrangements,

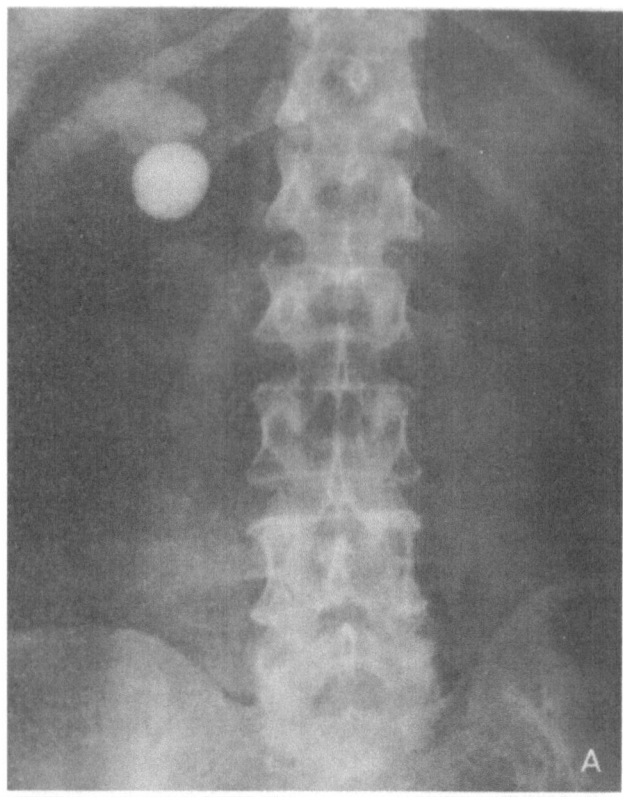

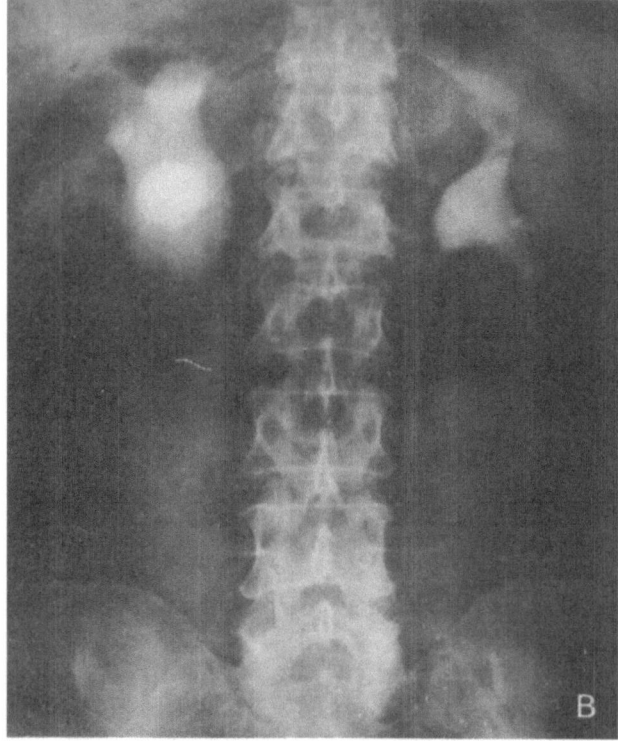

Fig. 3.1. Large calculus in a hydronephrotic right kidney in a male aged 35. **A**. The plain radiograph shows a large rounded stone in the right renal pelvis, the shape being characteristic of many in such a situation, though some are jackstones. **B**. The intravenous pyelogram shows typical dilatation of the renal pelvis and some of the calyces, the rounded lower end of the pelvic shadow being characteristic of pelviureteric obstruction. The medium is less dense than that in the other kidney (in keeping with early pelviureteric obstruction). The case was successfully treated by pyelolithotomy and a plastic operation (Hynes-Anderson) on the pelviureteric junction

resulting in an abnormal course of the ureter. In this anomaly instead of the right ureter descending to the brim of the pelvis, lateral to the inferior vena cava, it passes behind it, partially encircles it for a short distance and finally passes in front of it, continuing its descent to the bladder. Hydronephrosis, which is said to be present in three-quarters of the subjects, results from pressure of the inferior vena cava on the ureter, resulting in stasis and in consequence occasional urinary infection and stone. Heslin and Mamonas [71] stated that 40 cases, 32 male and 8 female, had been described by 1951, most from autopsies, only 18 having been observed antemortem.

Clinical symptoms relating to the abnormality may be completely absent. Symptoms which may occur as a consequence of the hydronephrosis, a renal stone or urinary infection when these are present, then include aching pain, renal colic and frequency of micturition, dysuria, haematuria and pyuria. The kidney may be palpably enlarged. The condition is readily recognized by the characteristic pyeloureterogram: Hydronephrosis of the pelvic type and dilatation of the upper part of the ureter above the compressed segment are seen, the shadow of the ureter turning inward at the junction of its upper and middle third to reach a position in front of the bodies of the vertebrae. A retrograde pyelogram may occasionally be necessary for diagnosis.

Renal Stone. The incidence of renal stone probably does not exceed 10%. Cases were reported by Rotter [130] (a male aged 49 with double post-renal vena cava associated with renal calculi, death following nephrolithotomy), and by Derbes and La Nasa [37] (a female patient aged 42 with hydronephrosis and renal calculi successfully treated by nephrectomy). Young's [169] patient had a calculus at the lower kink of the retrocaval ureter associated with some degree of hydronephrosis, the stone

being successfully removed and the anomaly corrected, with a good long-term result. Considine [23] reported two patients with retrocaval ureter, one of whom had a stone. The aim of surgical treatment in non-infected cases with good renal function must be to correct the congenital ureteric deformity and to remove the stone in the renal pelvis or the upper ureter if one is present. Nephrectomy is occasionally necessary when the kidney is disorganized from infection and/or calculi, or rendered functionally useless.

The following remedial measures have been used:

1. Following exposure of the kidney and the upper part of the ureter through an incision in the loin the ureter is freed from the inferior vena cava by blunt dissection and divided at the point where it crosses behind that vessel. The divided lower end is then transposed to the front of the inferior vena cava, cut obliquely, spatulated to avoid stricture and anastomosed directly to the upper segment [23, 80]. Stricture has occasionally followed.

2. In order to avoid stricture Harrill [68] and also Heslin and Mamonas [71] freed the ureter from the inferior vena cava and divided the lowest part of the renal pelvis transversely a little distance above the pelviureteric junction. The divided ureter with the stump of the renal pelvis was then passed round the inferior vena cava and brought to its natural position and was reanastomosed to the divided renal pelvis.

3. The same principle was used by Anderson and Hynes [11], who divided the ureter just below the pelviureteric junction and made a spatulated oval opening at the upper end of the lower segment of the ureter, which was then unwound from behind the inferior vena cava. The upper two-thirds of the enlarged renal pelvis was excised by vertical incisions and closed by continuous suture, while the lower third was cut away obliquely (including the pelviureteric junction) to leave a projecting

flap or spout of a suitable size to anasto-
mose to the spatulated upper end of the
ureter. This form of plastic procedure has
become the standard treatment for hydronephrosis due to pelviureteric obstruction in
the United Kingdom, and is most suitable
for the treatment of the retrocaval ureter.

4. Lowsley [90] divided the ureter close
to the bladder, freed it in an upward
direction, removed it from its abnormal
position behind the inferior vena cava and
reimplanted it into the bladder. In a
reported case the ureterovesical anastomosis was followed by a urinary fistula
possibly because of the failure of the blood
supply of the lower part of the ureter after
the prolonged dissection; a cutaneous ureterostomy was done.

5. A different principle was suggested by
Cathro [20] who, instead of dividing the
ureter at the point of obstruction, divided
the inferior vena cava, the ureter being first
dissected free from the cava. Two right
lumbar tributaries to the inferior vena cava
were divided between ligatures. After
separation of the various divided ends the
ureter and the vena cava respectively were
repaired by sutures.

4. Horseshoe Kidney

The incidence of renal calculi found in
association with horseshoe kidney has
varied from 10% to 30% of patients in
different series. Stone is related to the
presence of those anatomical abnormalities
in the kidney (especially hydronephrosis),
which predispose to stasis. Operative
removal of the stone and simultaneous
correction of the anatomical renal deformity and of any associated hydronephrosis
are frequently necessary.

The horseshoe kidney consists
anatomically of two kidneys fused by their
lower poles (95% of cases) or by their
upper poles (in less than 5%) and occasionally by their central parts. The fused

kidneys lie at a lower level in the abdomen
than do normal kidneys, each half lying
closer to the vertebral column than do
normal separate kidneys and seldom being
exactly similar to each other in size,
position or form. The isthmus, which is of
varying thickness, is grooved vertically
behind as it crosses in front of the great
abdominal vessels, usually consists of normal renal parenchymatous tissue but
occasionally merely of a band of fibrous
tissue. The renal pelves are situated on the
anterior surface of each kidney in front of
the blood vessels and face anteriorly,
medially or occasionally laterally, the
ureters being widely separated. The calyces
point inwards or downwards or both
towards the bodies of the vertebrae and
they extend into the parenchymal tissue of
the isthmus.

The curved ureters, which descend on the
anterior surface of the kidney and in front
of the isthmus, are attached to the renal
pelves at a higher level than in the normal
kidney. The renal arteries and veins vary in
their origins, position and number. The
abnormal origin and course of the ureters
over the isthmus, the pressure on them of
anomalous vessels and the impairment of
normal renal mobility because of the
attachment of the isthmus to adjacent
structures encourage urinary stasis, the
development of hydronephrosis and hence
of infection and calculus formation.

Horseshoe kidney may be symptomless
and be discovered during a routine radiological investigation or as the result of the
discovery by the patient of an abdominal
lump; in such cases no operative intervention is usually indicated. Alternatively,
as with any other kidney, it may be the seat
not merely of renal calculus but of renal
neoplasm or tuberculosis when there are the
appropriate clinical symptoms.

When important clinical symptoms exist
they most commonly relate to the presence
of a renal stone or to the hydronephrosis
which so often precedes it, and consist of

vague abdominal discomfort or renal pain [19]. In the 63 cases reported by Flocks and Stark [51] hydronephrosis of one or both kidneys was found in 24 (38%). Radiological examination usually demonstrates the outline of the horseshoe kidney and isthmus, with the associated pathological changes including the renal calculus (calyceal, isthmic or pelvic). The shadows of the calyces are seen on the inner rather than on the lateral side of the renal pelvis, lying near to or even in front of the bodies of the vertebrae. The axes of the renal pelves are directed obliquely downwards and inwards and their shadows lie further than normal from the middle line.

The existence of a hydronephrosis (unilateral or bilateral) giving rise to symptoms with or without a renal calculus is the commonest indication for operation (Fig. 3.2). If one-half of the horseshoe kidney is functionless because of severe hydronephrosis with or without stone or infection, it should be removed after dividing the isthmus. If both pelves are the seat of hydronephrosis giving rise to symptoms (with or without calculi) the isthmus should be divided, any renal calculi removed and the separated kidneys restored to as near a normal anatomical position in the loin as possible and fixed in that position (nephropexy). The pelviureteric junctions are examined for any associated stricture or other abnormality which, if present, may call for correction by some form of pyeloplasty.

The operation is usually done through an oblique incision in the loin similar to (but longer than) that used for the removal of a renal calculus from an otherwise normal kidney. The kidney is freed from the perirenal fat but mobilization of the lower pole is limited by the presence of the isthmus, which must be cleared of its surrounding fat and connective tissue in front and behind to a point beyond the middle line of the abdomen. A groove on the surface of the isthmus (renal tissue or fibrous tissue) may

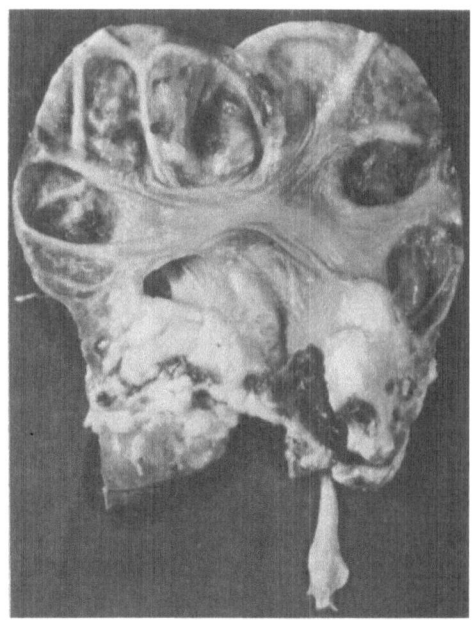

Fig. 3.2. Specimen of the right half of a horseshoe kidney from a male patient aged 50, containing a large pyramidal stone at the right pelviureteric junction; the urine was infected. The case was treated by removal of the right half of the kidney. There is an advanced degree of hydronephrosis and hydrocalycosis shown in the sagittal section of the kidney after removal

show the point of fusion of the two halves. After division of the isthmus sutures are inserted to arrest bleeding, the divided tissue being covered with a piece of fat. The kidney can then be mobilized into the loin. A radiograph of the exposed kidney to determine the precise localization of calculi is then taken before they are removed. A lower polar partial nephrectomy may be the appropriate treatment for a stone in a lower calyx. The anterior and posterior layers of the fascia of Gerota are stitched together below the kidney at the conclusion of the operation to form a shelf to help to retain it in position.

Renal Calculi. Table 3.1 shows the incidence of stone in a few series, with the method of treatment. Rusché and Bacon [137] successfully removed transperi-

Table 3.1. Calculi in horseshoe kidneys

Authors	Year	No. of cases	No. with calculi	Remarks
Rathbun	1928	108	29.4%	Cases of horseshoe and fused kidneys
Nation	1945	9	8	6 had unilateral calculi removed; 2 had hemi-nephrectomy for stone
Culp and Winterringer	1955	106 (all had renal operations)	63	Nephrectomy in 8; pyelo-lithotomy or nephrolitho-tomy in 38 (on 45 kidneys); 22 recurrences of stone in 19 patients
Flocks and Stark	1962	63	12	

toneally a stone from the right renal pelvis of a horseshoe kidney in which the two halves were fused by the upper pole. Peacock's [111] case had bilateral calculi for which a right pyelolithotomy and left partial nephrectomy were performed.

The author has operated on a small group of patients with calculous horseshoe kidneys, doing heminephrectomy in three of the worst cases, but removal of the stone with division of the isthmus in the others.

The varied results suggest that there is no single operative procedure which gives uniformly good results in the treatment of the calculous horseshoe kidney, and that the urologist must decide at the time of the operation which method in his judgment will give the best result.

5. Ureterocele

Calculi (single or multiple), often compli-cate a ureterocele and may give rise to the first clinical symptoms leading to the diagnosis. The calculi arise in the kidney and move into the pelvic ureter, where des-cent into the bladder is arrested by the pin-point ureterovesical orifice. One stone after another may move down from the kidney into the somewhat dilated ureter and remain there for a considerable time, enlarging gradually before giving rise to clinical symptoms.

A ureterocele is a cystic dilatation of the lower end of the ureter involving all the layers in its wall, and which projects into the bladder. It is the build-up of pressure behind this stenosed obstructed orifice which produces the ballooning seen cysto-scopically. Dilatation of the ureter above the opening may be limited to the lower third of the ureter or may extend to the pelvis and calyces. Total destruction of the kidney is a possibility because of back-pressure with or without infection. The cystic swelling seen in the bladder, which varies in size from 1 cm in diameter to one which completely fills the bladder (a type especially seen in the young) is oval, elongated or flat in shape. When bilateral as it often is, the cyst on one side may be larger than that on the other. Occasionally the entire cyst prolapses through the urethra in the female, or into the prostatic urethra or into the opening of a vesical diverticulum in the male.

A ureterocele may be symptomless, its presence being discovered accidentally dur-ing routine investigation. Symptoms when present are usually the result of inter-mittent ureteric obstruction by stone, of infection, or of irritation of the bladder from the presence of the cyst. Even when a stone is present there may be few symptoms, though pain along the course of the ureter or in the renal region may be complained of. Large ureteroceles may give rise to intermittent obstruction at the outlet of the bladder and hence to difficulty, hesitancy, dribbling or sudden cessation of the urinary stream. There may be incontinence or even retention of urine when the ureterocele prolapses into the urethra.

Urolithiasis. On radiography one or more calculi may be seen in the pelvic ureter just above the ureteric orifice and there may be a chain of stones in close juxtaposition, the entire group occupying a length of several inches. Stones may be present in the renal pelvis when none is found in the ureterocele (Fig. 3.3, see p. 40). In the excretion pyelogram a filling defect in the lateral part of the bladder may be observed due to the projecting intravesical head (cobra-head) of the ureterocele, the defect being surrounded by a halo which is best seen if the exposure is taken when the ureterocele is distended with opaque medium, sufficient of which has also entered the bladder. The halo results from the thickness of the wall of the ureterocele, which gives rise to a negative shadow in contrast with the normal filling in the cystogram.

The thin-walled translucent cyst at the ureteric orifice covered by fine superficial blood vessels on its wall and its pin-point orifice can be seen cystoscopically. As the cyst fills with urine it gradually enlarges to its maximum size when a jet of urine is expelled through the stenosed opening (easily demonstrated if indigo carmine has been given intravenously). The cyst then collapses considerably but does not disappear; slowly the process of filling and emptying recurs again and again. In large ureteroceles with thickened walls the cyst resembles a soft tumour and it never collapses completely. In infected cases with or without calculi the wall of the ureterocele appears to be soggy and rigid and is usually of a dull red colour.

Fifty cases (23 males, 27 females) of ureterocele mostly in adults, seen during a 10-year period in the author's department together with some patients treated by other surgeons, were reviewed [126]. The ages of the patients ranged from 2 to 79 years, 1 in 10 being children and 7 having bilateral ureteroceles; 10 patients had calculi in the ureterocele and 2 had stones in the corresponding kidney. The ureterocele had usually been observed during investigation for attacks of pain in the loin or of urinary infection; prolapse of the ureterocele into the urethra was observed in 2 patients. Dilatation of the upper urinary tract was observed radiographically in 20 patients, 4 of whom had calculi in ureteroceles. There was reduplication of the corresponding ureters in 3 patients.

Of Aas's [1] 52 adult patients (with 68 ureteroceles, several being bilateral), 28 had pyuria; 11 had haematuria; 18 had dysuria; and of 23 with renal colic, 20 had calculi (showing the frequency of urolithiasis), 13 being in the ureterocele, and 7 only in the corresponding kidney. The stones were usually composed of pure calcium oxalate or mixed calcium oxalate and apatite.

Treatment, when indicated because of symptoms, is directed to the relief of pain resulting from the calculi, and to the correction of the contracted ureteric orifice in order to prevent further stone formation.

Simple instrumental dilatation of the stenosed ureterovesical orifice is rarely successful. Incision of the top of the ureterocele down to the ureterovesical orifice, or a deliberate meatotomy using the diathermy electrode is usually satisfactory. The incision must be of sufficient size to allow the stone or stones when present to pass into the bladder whence they can be extracted by a lithotrite; multiple stones may need ureterolithotomy.

The principal drawback to treatment of this type is the possible destruction of the valve-like action of the ureterovesical orifice, when subsequent reflux and ascending infection may follow. The largest ureteroceles (mostly in children) should

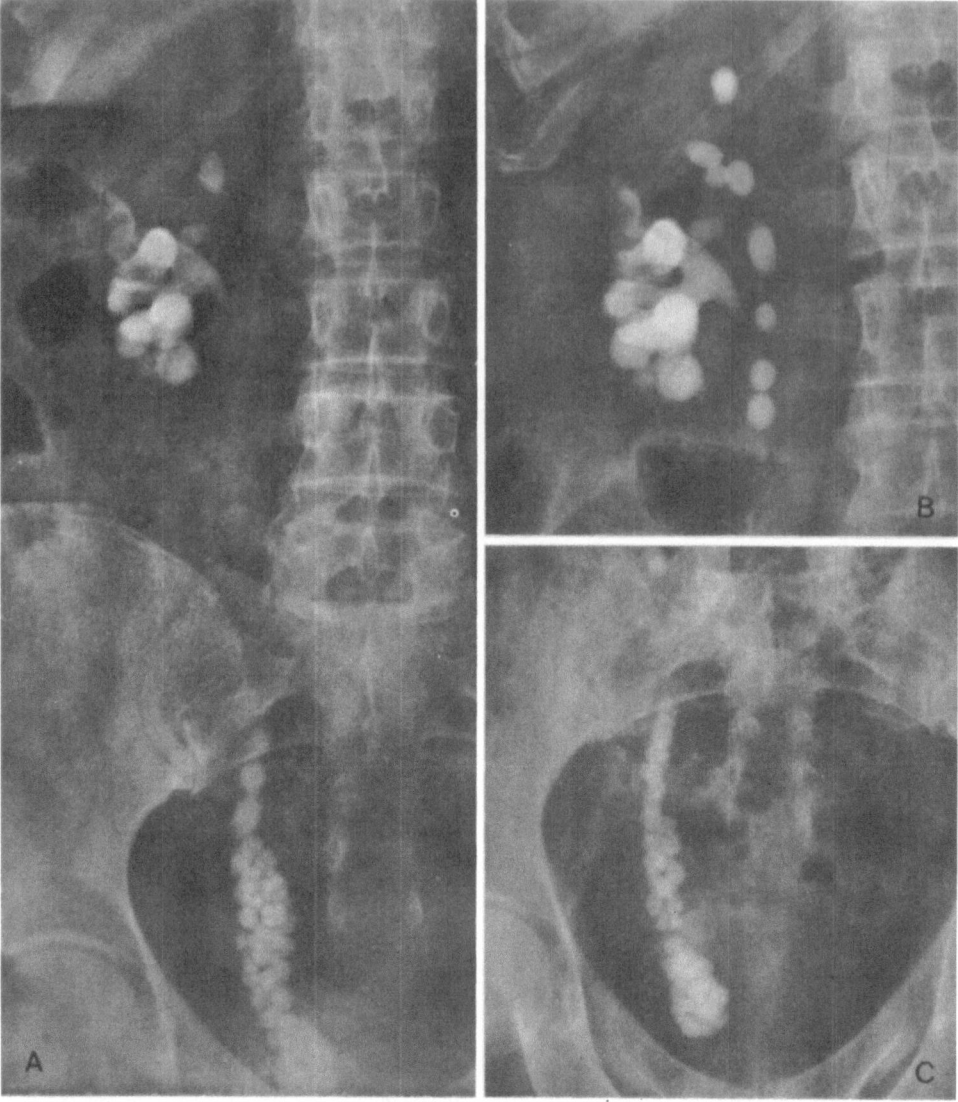

Fig. 3.3. Stones in the pelvis and calyces of the right kidney and in the ureter in association with a ureterocele in a female patient aged 58; the patient had had recurrent right-sided renal pain for several months. **A.** Multiple rounded stones in the renal pelvis, calyces and ureter. **B.** The plain radiograph shows a staghorn stone in the right renal pelvis and calyces and stones in the upper part of the ureter. **C.** A considerable number of rounded and faceted stones were present in the pelvic ureter, which was greatly dilated especially at its lower end where the stones lie in the ureterocele sac. The radiograph shows the appearance known as 'corn-cob' ureter. The case was treated by nephroureterectomy; because of the size of the ureterocele the bladder was opened and the part of it round the ureterocele was resected, the bladder then being repaired

usually be excised transvesically, the stones removed and the ureteric orifice reconstituted. Nephroureterectomy is rarely necessary except when the kidney has been damaged beyond repair and especially when gross infection is associated with multiple renal and ureteric calculi. The entire ureter with a small cuff of vesical mucosa must then be excised along with the kidney using, therefore, two incisions, one in the loin and one suprapubically.

In the author's departmental series referred to above [126], a few patients with minimal symptoms were not treated surgically and no sequelae were usually seen. Incision of the ureteric orifice by diathermy electrode or by a meatotome was done in 29 patients, 7 of whom had stones in the ureterocele. The late results of treatment were usually good, though subsequent attacks of pain in the loin were reported in 8, in 2 of whom nephrectomy was ultimately necessary because of renal damage. Open excision of the ureterocele with reconstruction of the orifice was done in 5 patients with good results.

6. Megaureter

Ureteric and occasionally renal calculi sometimes complicate the variety of megaureter in which there is partial obstruction at or near the lower end of the ureter. Megaureter which can be recognized radiologically may result from:

1. Back-pressure as a consequence of obstruction at the bladder neck or in the ureter.

2. Infection of the urinary tract, especially in neurogenic disorders affecting the bladder (resulting from spinal disease or injury when there may be ureteric reflux).

3. In association with duplication of the ureters.

4. As a result of organic ureteric obstruction.

5. In association with an apparently normal ureterovesical junction and lower urinary tract.

6. In the megaureter–megacystis syndrome, which occurs during childhood equally in boys and in girls (in which there is bilateral dilatation of the ureter, a bladder

of large capacity and widely gaping ureteric orifices [160, 161]).

Ureteric stone is not, generally speaking, a complication of these types of megaureter.

Urolithiasis. In patients with a simple megaureter, which may be unilateral or bilateral, and which usually occurs in adults in either sex, ureteric calculi are commonly found. The dilated hypertrophied ureter, which may be elongated and kinked, forms a bulb-like dilatation, which may lie at a level below that of the intramural ureter. The point of narrowing of the ureter which causes the partial obstruction lies a short distance above the bladder; the narrow zone below that point is of normal calibre.

The symptoms consist of recurrent attacks of urinary infection, colicky pain, haematuria (which may result from the complicating calculi) and occasionally a palpable renal swelling may draw attention to its presence. A moderate-sized stone impacted in the ureter may be palpable per rectum.

The diagnosis is made by urography, which demonstrates the point of obstruction and the extent of the ureteric dilatation. Cineurography may demonstrate active ureteric contractions or impaired ureteric motility. Ureteric calculi when present are round, or of the jackstone type and are freely mobile within the dilated ureter and there may be associated renal calculi. The ureteric orifice is usually normal on cystoscopy. The symptoms may call for surgical treatment, which may be nephroureterectomy in advanced unilateral cases in which the kidney has suffered from prolonged infection, or excision of the ureterovesical junction with removal of the stones and reimplantation of the divided ureter into the bladder; ureterolithotomy alone is illogical and inadequate. Replacement of the affected ureter by an ileal loop has been done [150].

7. Ureteric Stricture from Other Causes

A stricture of the ureter may result from external trauma from a penetrating or non-penetrating wound, from surgical intervention for the removal of a ureteric calculus, from long-standing impaction of a ureteric calculus, or from periureteric fibrosis (which produces stricture by external compression). In any of these conditions there is urinary stasis above the strictured segment of the ureter so that infection and stone formation may be seen as an occasional complication.

8. Renal Calyceal Diverticula

Diverticula of renal calyces which contain urine are sometimes complicated by calculus and urinary infection resulting from urinary stasis. A series of 345 cases mainly from the literature, collected by Abeshouse and Abeshouse [4], showed that the condition was found in patients of both sexes and usually between the third and sixth decades, the upper major calyx being affected most commonly.

The anatomical arrangements of the various sphincter muscles around the calyces may have a bearing on the formation of a calyceal diverticulum [99]. While the condition is sometimes congenital [103, 140], it may result from an acquired obstruction of the infundibulum of a minor calyx resulting from infection or calculus.

The diverticulum, which is spheroidal or ovoid in shape with a diameter between 0.5 and 7 cm, communicates with a minor calyx 2–4 mm in length and it is lined by transitional epithelium. Very often a calyceal diverticulum gives rise to no symptoms and is only of academic interest. Sometimes a calyceal diverticulum ruptures spontaneously [141].

Renal Calculi. There may be renal pain resulting from calculi or urinary infection,

haematuria and pyuria with frequency and scalding of micturition. Radiography may reveal a rounded, well-defined cystic cavity distal to a minor calyx and communicating with it by a narrow neck. A collection of many small renal calculi in close relation to each other overlying the peripheral part of the shadow of the kidney is suggestive of calculi in a calyceal diverticulum.

Calculi, which were present in 114 (36%) of the 345 cases collected by Abeshouse and Abeshouse [4], were sometimes multiple (when they were usually very small, 1–2 mm in diameter) and have been found to number from a few to very many; they are usually composed of calcium oxalate and apatite. An associated stone has occasionally been observed in the renal pelvis of the affected kidney; occasional stones migrate down the ureter resulting in ureteric colic. In the series of calyceal diverticula reported by Devine et al. [38], single or multiple calculi were present in 11 cases.

In the absence of symptoms no operative treatment is necessary but radiography at intervals is desirable. If calculi are present and are thought to be the cause of symptoms, a partial nephrectomy is appropriate, any infection being first brought under control. Small calyceal diverticula are not demonstrable or palpable on the surface of the kidney at operation, though larger ones may present on the convex border as in two cases described by Prather [117], which he treated by excision of the dome of the cyst, the walls of the cavity of the cyst being approximated by sutures to close the kidney. Simple excision of the diverticulum may be appropriate when it presents close to the surface of the kidney in the lower or upper pole, the neck of the diverticulum then being closed by non-chromic catgut sutures.

9. Ureteric Diverticula and Urolithiasis

Diverticula of the ureter are rare; some contain calculi; the diagnosis is not always easy. Richardson [128] collected from the literature 32 cases (and added 1 of his own) which be believed to be ureteric diverticula in living subjects, and which had been demonstrated at operation or by ureteropyelography; calculi were found in 8.

However, Culp [28] in a classic paper, reviewed critically 52 cases from the literature which had been reported unequivocally as being true ureteric diverticula, and he concluded that only 15 of these were authentic diverticula (10 congenital and 5 acquired). He considered that the remaining 37 were examples of other congenital anomalies which had simulated diverticula, and which included ureterocele, vesical diverticulum, blind-ending bifid ureter and segmental hydroureter. He defined a true diverticulum (congenital in origin) as a protrusion of the entire thickness of the wall of the ureter (including its muscular coat) which communicates with the lumen of the ureter by a small opening. He found in the literature records of 10 patients with this condition, the stomata being mostly located near the pelviureteric junction, or at the level of the sacro-iliac joint or in the juxtavesical segment of the ureter. Most were small, the larger ones being 8 cm, 18 cm and 5 in. in length respectively. Most of the patients had had pain (including renal colic), fever, infected urine, haematuria and pyuria; three of the diverticula contained calculi.

The diagnosis was made by radiography and retrograde pyelography in six cases (the opaque catheter usually coiling up in the diverticulum), and at operation in four. Treatment had usually consisted of excision of the diverticulum (with removal of the stone when present) and reconstruction of the ureter or uretero-neo-cystostomy, only two needing nephrectomy. In one patient the stone in the diverticulum was 8 cm long and was removed by transperitoneal ureterolithotomy [60].

Culp [28] defined an acquired or false diverticulum as a protrusion of the ureteric mucous membrane through its muscular wall above an obstruction in the ureter, the wall of the diverticulum being composed of fibrous tissue, and the site of the protrusion being determined by some previous trauma resulting from a previous operation (such as a ureterolithotomy) or from a calculus. He collected from the literature five cases in this group, in three of which previous operations for calculi had been performed. The symptoms were essentially the same as those found in patients with congenital diverticulum, those resulting from infection and calculi being most prominent.

Cases of ureteric diverticula probably unrelated to calculous disease have been reported by several observers [13, 38, 72, 98].

10. Obstruction of the Lower Urinary Tract, and Upper Tract Urolithiasis

Renal calculi may be found occasionally in patients who suffer from non-infected obstructive lesions in the lower urinary tract, which include simple and malignant enlargement of the prostate, fibrosis of the bladder neck and stricture of the urethra. Some calculous patients with these conditions have had infected urine (possibly by urea-splitting organisms) following intermittent catheterization, instrumentation or operative treatment. This may have been carried out, for example, for the relief of prostatic obstruction, the stone often then being of rapid growth and composed of ammonium magnesium phosphate. Such calculi nowadays, with adequate control of infection by the use of sulphonamides and antibiotics, are less common than a few decades ago. The diagnosis and treatment of such calculi is done in accordance with general principles.

II. Renal Calculi and Cystic Conditions of the Kidney

Renal calculi are not uncommonly found in association with the various localized renal cysts and the diffuse cystic diseases affecting a large part or the whole of the organ. Calculi may be found within the cysts, or in the parenchyma outside the cysts; calcific foci, small or diffuse, may be found in the fibrous wall of the cyst. Cysts may be classified in the present context as communicating cysts and non-communicating cysts, and they may be single or multiple.

The single communicating cysts, which communicate with a renal calyx or the renal pelvis and contain urine, are the pyelogenic cysts and the traumatic cysts; because of the imperfect drainage and the resulting urinary stones, they are liable to become infected.

The communicating multiple cystic diseases include polycystic disease of the kidney and medullary sponge kidney, both of which are commonly associated with renal stone. As with the obstructive lesions of the kidney and ureter these conditions call for treatment of the calculus as well as of the cystic condition if recurrent stone formation is to be avoided. In cases of multiple cystic disease with calculi radical treatment is not always possible.

The non-communicating cysts, which only exceptionally contain calculi, are the simple (or solitary) cysts, multilocular cysts, peripelvic cysts, hydatid cysts and pyelonephritic cysts. The walls of these cysts are sometimes partly calcified and calculi may be found elsewhere in the kidney in which they are present. Diffuse multiple non-communicating cysts include congenital unilateral multicystic disease (in which the walls of the cysts are sometimes calcified) and the rare cystic disease of the renal medulla and familial juvenile nephrophthisis. A full reference to the non-communicating cysts is beyond the scope of this book.

1. Pyelogenic Cysts

The term pyelogenic cyst was first used by Damm [33] to describe thin-walled, unilocular cysts lined by transitional epithelium, which usually lie in close relation to the posterior wall of the renal pelvis and extend into the renal sinus towards the central part of the kidney. They typically communicate with the renal pelvis or with the infundibulum of a major calyx by a narrow neck, which has sometimes been obliterated.

They are usually 3–5 cm in length and 1–2 cm in width, and their walls may contain collagenous material and plain muscle fibres. Since they communicate with the renal pelvis there is a considerable incidence of intracystic calculi consisting of either one biggish stone or a collection of small stones [48, 84] (Fig. 3.4). Pyelogenic cysts are usually recognized because of pain, notably when small stones are voided into the renal pelvis through the narrow neck; others have presented the picture of a renal infection. Hypertension is an occasional complication [49]. The cysts are not clinically palpable, some being dis-

Fig. 3.4. Calculi in a pyelogenic cyst. Patient, female aged 35, had had pain in the region of the right kidney. **A.** The plain radiograph shows a group of 30 or 40 rounded calculi lying close to each other and to the lower border of the second lumbar vertebrae. **B.** The intravenous pyelogram shows good secretion of the dye filling the calyces and also the cyst in which the calculi lay, causing the shadow of the cyst to be denser than that of the calculi alone. **C.** Intravenous pyelogram (semi-lateral view) showing good concentration of opaque medium; the cyst is now located in close relation to the upper border and posterior wall of the renal pelvis. **D.** The condition was treated by excision of the cyst, including the calculi and a thin wedge of renal tissue; the neck of the cyst communicated with the renal pelvis

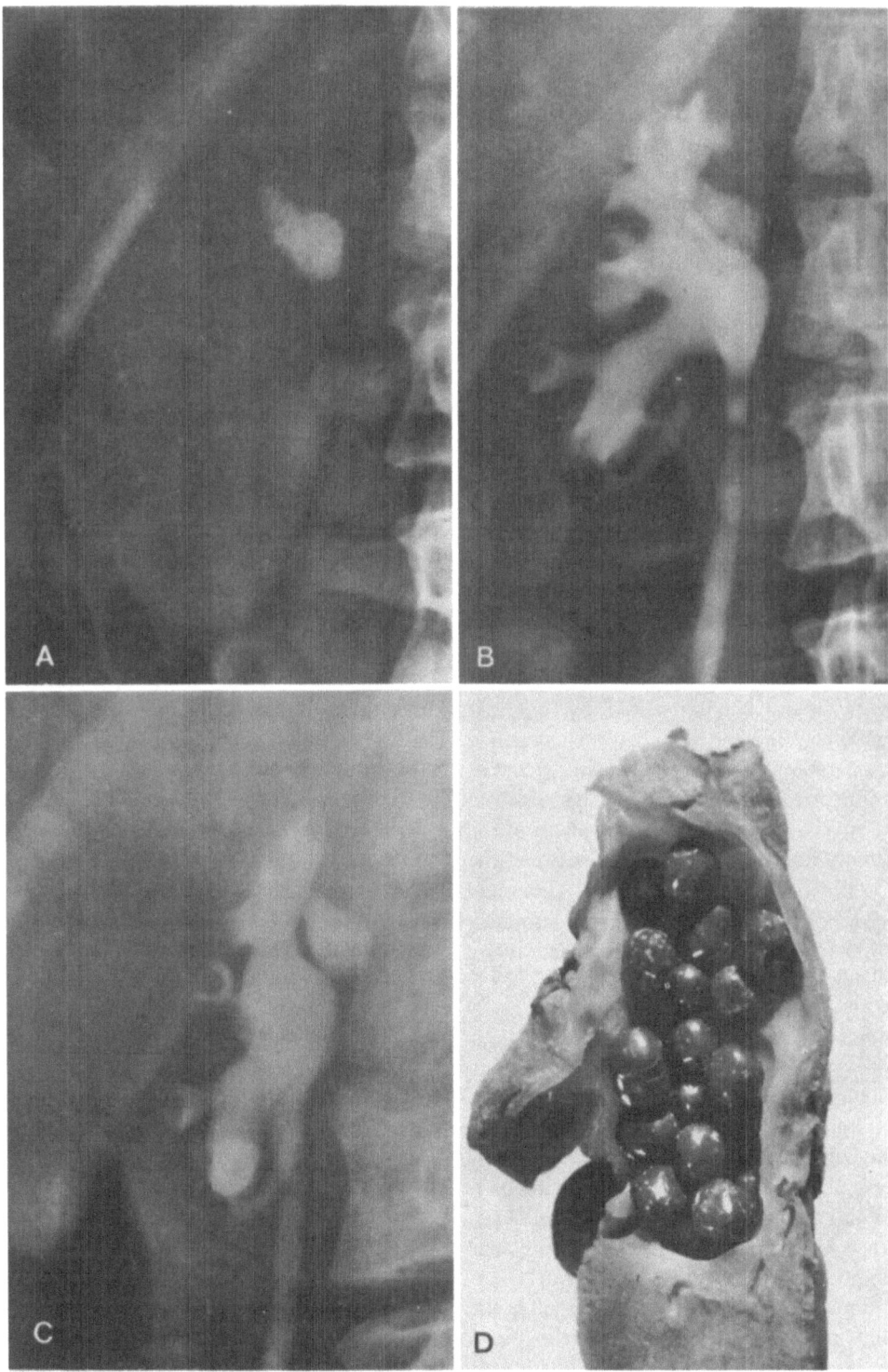

Fig. 3.4

covered accidentally during an operation for a supposed renal calculus.

The operative removal of the cyst, which is desirable if it is giving rise to symptoms (and especially if it contains calculi), may not be easy. After the kidney and its vascular pedicle have been mobilized, the cyst has to be dissected away from the renal pelvis and major calyces to which it is closely applied and from the renal artery and vein, which can easily be injured during the procedure; its patent neck is defined and closed by ligature or sutures. Nephrectomy is rarely necessary.

If the diagnosis has not been made before operation (as is frequently the case) difficulties may arise during the operation for their removal as in Yeates' case [168], in which the radiograph had shown an opacity in the left renal area which was seen on the intravenous pyelogram to be not completely contained within the shadow of the renal pelvis but which was nevertheless assumed to be a calculus obscured by contrast medium. When the renal pelvis was opened at operation no stone was found; a radiograph of the exposed kidney then showed an opacity in the region of the hilum of the kidney. Subsequent dissection between the posterior lip of the hilum and the renal pelvis disclosed a cyst of approximately 1 cm in diameter, which contained many calculi.

Milk of Calcium Cysts. These cysts constitute a sub-group of pyelogenic cysts which contain a number of tiny calculi or microliths (composed of calcium phosphate and calcium carbonate) with special characteristics giving rise to diagnostic difficulty. Some contain what appears on the radiograph to be a chalky suspension or precipitate.

Since these particles are suspended in the fluid medium of the cyst, they can move freely and settle into one layer in its lowest part. Therefore, when they are seen on the plain radiograph they appear collectively as a quarter-moon-shaped (crescentic) shadow, presenting the replica of a fluid level above and taking the crescentic shape of the wall of the cyst below. When the radiograph is taken in the lateral position, the calcific shadow is seen to have changed its position so that the sharp horizontal upper border between the calcific mass and the supernatant fluid in the cyst is now at right angles to that seen with the patient in the erect position. These accumulations of fine calcific microliths during the stage of formation have mostly been formed in cavities which contained urine and have had a communication with the renal pelvis or a calyx (which can sometimes be demonstrated by retrograde pyelography), which may or may not have been later obliterated [115]. The characteristic crescentic shadow seen on the radiograph has been confused with the fluid levels sometimes seen in a duodenal diverticulum, when it has been filled with opaque material or medium. It has also mimicked, because of its position, similar milk of calcium deposits in the gall bladder.

In one patient [135] more than 2000 microcalculi had migrated from the cyst into the renal pelvis whence they had been voided spontaneously. In another case the existence of a communication between the cyst and the renal pelvis was revealed by the excretory pyelogram. In yet another [118] a follow-up radiograph showed that the 'milk of calcium' content of the cyst seen at an earlier examination had become reduced in amount, many tiny concretions having been voided. A cyst may be filled with opaque medium several hours after an injection has been given for intravenous pyelography [100].

2. Traumatic Cysts

A ruptured kidney may in the longer term give rise to renal calculi (Fig. 3.5). Direct violence to the kidney which does not produce a partial or a complete tear of the renal parenchyma may result in the formation of an intrarenal haematoma, which usually gives rise to pain and also haematuria if the torn part of the renal parenchyma communicates with the renal pelvis or a calyx. In course of time such a haematoma may undergo gradual resolution by absorption and fibrosis. Alternatively, partial organization of the blood clots may lead to the formation of a thick-walled cyst, the wall of which may or may not become partly calcified, and which may communicate with the calyx when, since calcium salts are then available from the urine, calculi may form inside the cyst.

Under such circumstances a long period of freedom from clinical symptoms may follow the original injury, and the diagnosis of intracystic calculi or of a calcified cyst may only be made years after the accident, which it may sometimes be difficult to link with the calculous changes.

The group of calculi now referred to has to be distinguished etiologically from true recumbency renal calculi, which not uncommonly complicate spinal injury or fractured pelvis, the kidney itself not then suffering direct damage. If the initial trauma resulted in damage to the renal pelvis or to the pelviureteric junction, there may be some degree of hydronephrosis which could also contribute to stone formation and/or to infection.

Urologists have usually tended to treat renal injuries conservatively, operation being reserved for those cases adjudged to need nephrectomy because of the gradual increase in size of the swelling in the loin and because of continued haemorrhage. The occasional presence of late complications (including renal stones) raises the question as to whether some patients with renal injury should not be operated on at a relatively early stage in order to effect a primary repair of the damaged kidney and/or the renal pelvis to prevent such long-term sequelae.

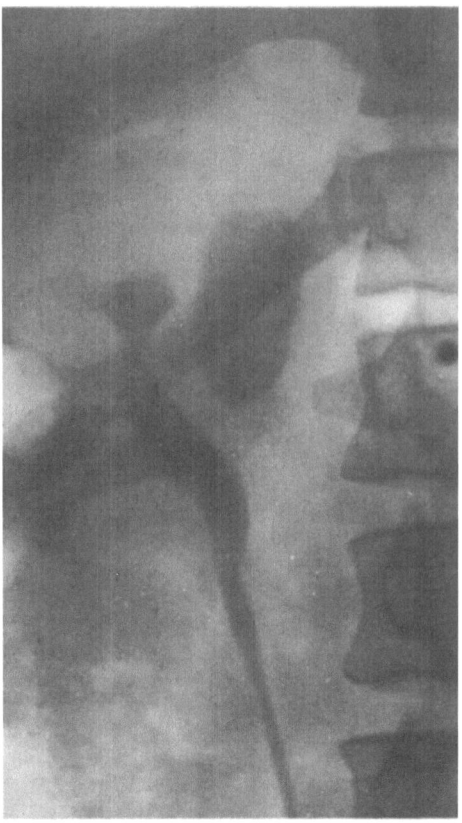

Fig. 3.5. Calcified traumatic cyst of the right kidney in a male patient aged 33, who had sustained an injury to the right loin followed at once by haematuria which had persisted for 2 months; a diagnosis of partial rupture of the right kidney was made. The intravenous pyelogram showed the calcified zone filled with opaque medium (thereby rendering the shadow more dense) though the actual connection with the upper renal calyx could not be demonstrated. The presence of gall stones was excluded by cholecystography. The clinical diagnosis was a renal cyst containing much calcified debris, which had resulted from the renal injury

Renal Calculi. Colston and Baker [22] reported a group of patients who had developed renal calculi or calcified cysts following injury to the kidney of the kind just described. In one case stones were found 15 years after the injury and in others stones were found 1 year and 5 years respectively after the injury.

A female patient aged 32 from the author's hospital, under the care of Mr. R. E. Williams, had had multiple fractures (pelvis and femur) which had necessitated several operations, and she was subsequently found to have developed recumbency calculi in the calyces of the left kidney. In the right kidney a diffuse opaque shadow in the radiograph of the lower part of the renal parenchyma, thought to be a haematoma undergoing some degree of calcification, was shown a year or more later to be a collection of calculi located in a cyst in the parenchyma, which had evidently followed the original injury.

3. Polycystic Disease

Renal calculi have been reported in 5%–10% of patients with the adult form of polycystic disease of the kidneys in different series; the infantile form does not appear to be so affected. In the adult form (in which the age varies between 30 and 70), the size of the kidneys varies from a moderate enlargement to two enormous and often unequal organs, each weighing several pounds and up to 15–19 in. in length.

The irregular external surface of the kidney is studded with closely packed, translucent cysts of various colours, bluish, yellowish or sometimes reddish from the presence within them of altered blood pigment so that the kidney as a whole resembles a bunch of grapes in appearance. In cross-section the remaining renal parenchyma seems to be almost obliterated. The walls of the cysts are lined by cuboidal or flattened epithelium. The renal pelvis and calyces undergo distortion and elongation though their general pattern is retained. Calculi occur most commonly within the calyces.

The clinical course of the disease includes a silent or latent period of indeterminate length, followed by a period usually of some years after diagnosis, when the patient may

enjoy reasonable health perhaps interrupted by incidents of renal infection, haematuria (in more than half of Dalgaard's [31] cases) or pain, and the clinical symptoms of calculus including renal colic may present. Finally there is a period of ill-health associated with deteriorating renal function with the characteristic symptoms of thirst, hypertension, indifferent appetite and some loss of well-being, followed by a terminal phase of increasing renal failure and uraemia lasting less than 2 years. The presence of infection and of calculi may accelerate the later stages, though calculi are not normally the chief cause of death, the function of the kidneys being already impaired.

The presence of palpably enlarged kidneys usually suggests the diagnosis. The plain radiograph usually shows the outline of the enlarged kidneys and sometimes their cystic structure. The urogram gives a characteristic picture of an elongated pelvicalyceal system, often with considerable distortion and a scalloped outline resulting from the bulging of cysts into some calyces, which may then be drawn out sometimes to great length, their normal cup-shaped ends being replaced by crescentic, flattened or bulbous tips.

Renal Calculi. The risk of stone formation has been considered to be as high as 24% by the time the patient has reached the age of 60 [32]. Renal calculi (usually calyceal) are found not infrequently because of stasis of urine in the renal pelvis and the lower calyces (and associated infection) resulting from pressure upon the outlets of these cavities by the enlarged cysts (Fig. 3.6). Table 3.2 shows the incidence of calculi in some published series.

Calcification of the whole or a part of the walls of one or more cysts giving rise to annular, crescentic or crenated calcific shadows on the plain radiograph is seen occasionally. In a reported case [164] in a unilateral polycystic kidney in a boy aged 7,

Table 3.2. Renal calculi with polycystic disease of the kidneys

Author	Year	Total cases	Renal calculi
Sieber [144]	1905	212	8
Oppenheimer [105]	1934	59	14
Walters and Braasch [157]	1934	85	5
Rall and Odel [124]	1949	207	29
Simon and Thompson [145]	1955		14.1%
Dalgaard [31]	1957	173	17 (autopsy)
Dalgaard [32]	1963	350	64

the plain radiograph showed many foci of calcification (suggestive of calculi) over much of the right renal area dispersed in linear or crescentic deposits or flakes (Fig. 3.7). The retrograde pyelogram showed much distortion of the pelvis and lower calyces, suggesting the presence of a renal neoplasm. The kidney after removal was found to be the seat of one variety of infantile polycystic kidney with partly calcified cysts of various sizes and of connective tissue which contained foci of calcified cartilage.

Rovsing [132, 133] in a classic contribution, in an attempt to check the onward course of the disease, exposed the affected kidney in the loin and punctured and emptied the cysts systematically, reducing the size of the kidney and relieving the pressure exerted by the cysts on the remaining unaffected renal tissue, the function of which was depressed; he reported encouraging results. Subsequent reports on this procedure were sometimes favourable [97, 145, 167], though sometimes less favourable or inconclusive.

The author has found the procedure useful for the relief of pain and for the arrest of severe recurrent unilateral haemorrhage, but remains unconvinced that there is any permanent material improvement in renal function or any prolongation of life expectancy. In a modification of the Rovsing procedure [57] the kidney is split along the convex border down to but not into the calyces, thereby enabling many more cysts to be punctured. The open halves of the kidney are sutured to the skin leaving it suspended and partly exposed in the wound, cysts being punctured at a later date through the scar tissue if thought desirable. In recent years, operative treatment has been supplemented by haemodialysis and occasionally by transplantation of a normal healthy kidney from a donor following bilateral nephrectomy.

The treatment of renal stones in these patients calls for a cautious and indeed a conservative approach, but it may be needed for the relief of symptoms. The urologist has to try to assess how much the calculi contribute to the patient's symptoms (infection, haemorrhage, obstruction and impairment of renal function) and whether removal of the stones would increase life expectancy at the given stage of the disease. It is believed that there is an average life expectancy after diagnosis of 10–15 years. The correction of associated urinary infection alone may produce clinical improvement even in a stone-bearing kidney. Moreover, the search for calyceal stones in a greatly enlarged kidney may be a matter of difficulty; the presence of pain, obstruction and infection, and haematuria attributable to the stone will incline the urologist towards its removal. Nephrectomy may occasionally be appropriate for a badly infected calculous kidney, if the function of the opposite kidney could justify it.

In one series [144] three renal calculi were removed by operation; and in another series of 60 cases [105] calculi were removed in 3. The author has removed

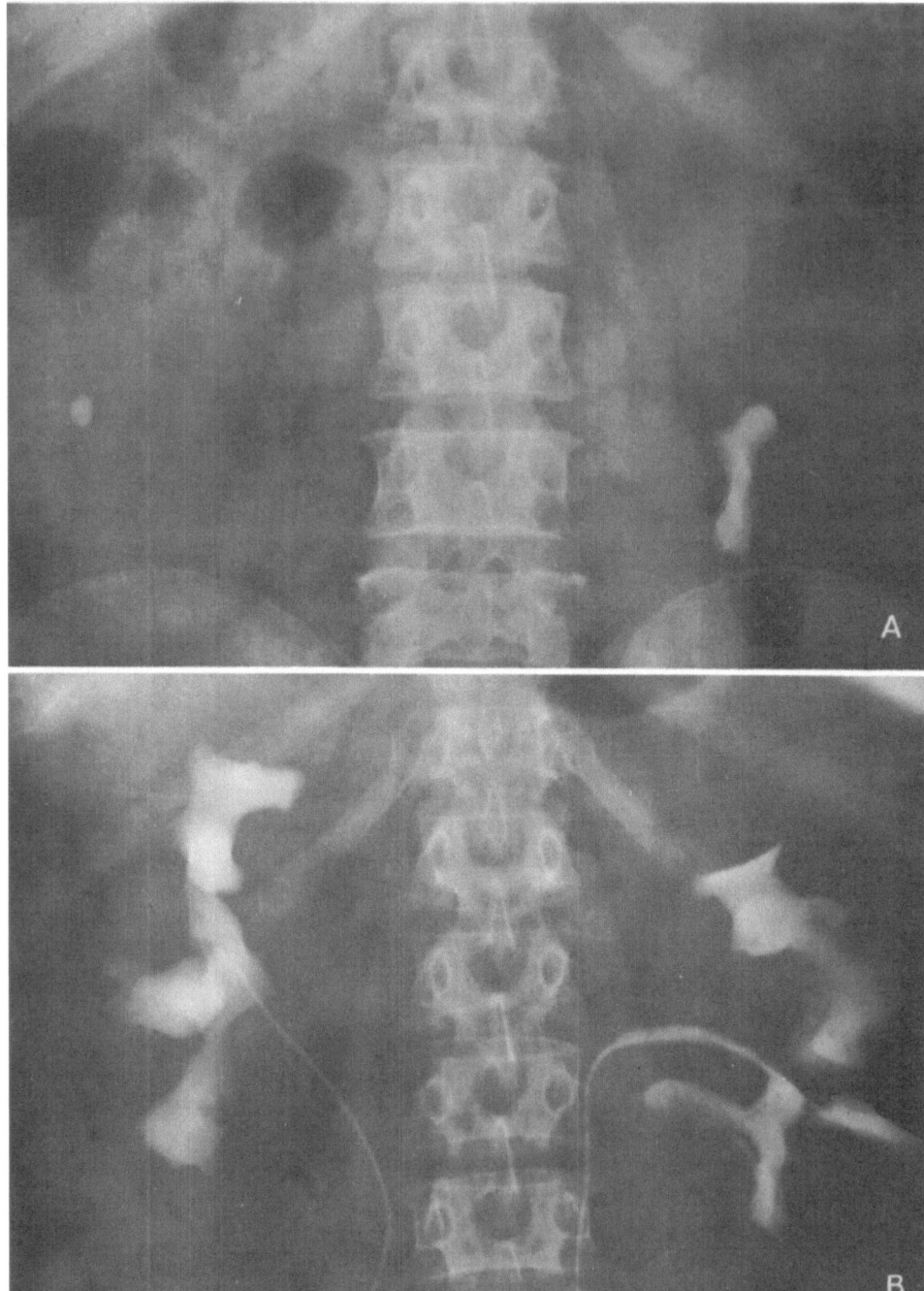

Fig. 3.6. Polycystic kidney with bilateral renal calculi in a female patient aged 40, who had had recurrent attacks of left-sided renal colic. **A.** The plain radiograph shows a rounded stone in the right kidney and a medium-sized irregularly shaped calculus in the left kidney. **B.** Retrograde pyelograms show the typical picture of bilateral polycystic kidneys with the gross distortion of the calyces. The stone in the right kidney is in a middle calyx; that in the left is in the lowest calyx and extends into the renal pelvis

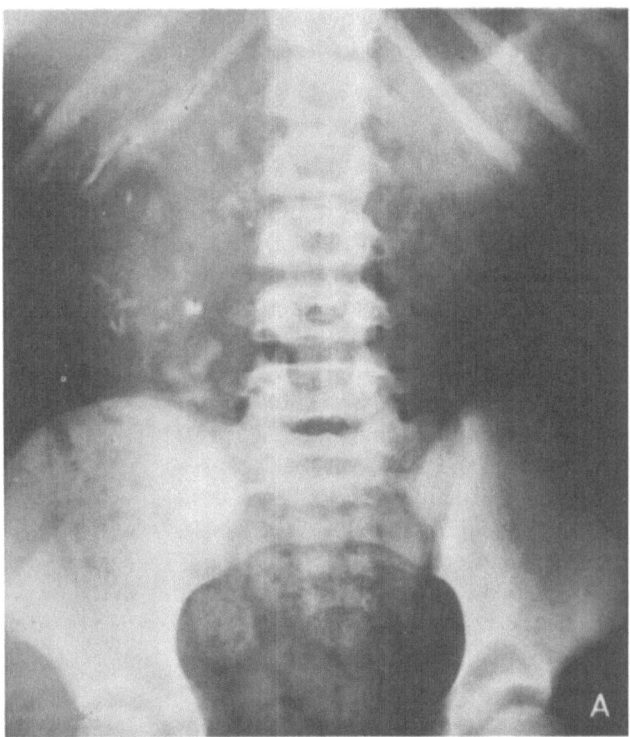

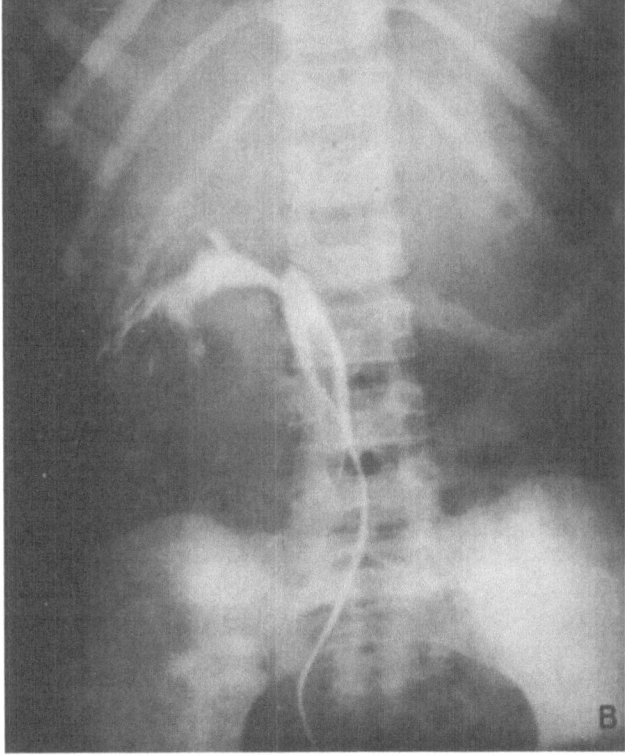

Fig. 3.7. Congenital cystic kidney of the infantile type removed from a boy aged 7, showing many cysts of variable size but with a considerable amount of fibrous-looking solid tissue, and showing widespread calcification of an unusual type. **A.** The plain radiograph shows diffusely scattered linear, crescentic and irregularly shaped foci of calcification in the right kidney. There was minimal excretion of medium in the intravenous pyelogram of the right kidney, the left being normal. **B.** The ascending pyelogram of the right kidney shows considerable deformity of the renal pelvis and considerable displacement of the ureter towards the middle line; the calcific foci lie mainly in relation to the calyces. (By courtesy of Mr. J.E. Willson-Pepper and Dr. D.A. Slade, and the Editor of the British Journal of Urology)

renal calculi from a number of patients whose symptoms seemed to demand it.

4. Medullary Sponge Kidney

This condition, which is a multi-cystic, usually bilateral, abnormality of the renal pyramids derived from dilated and obstructed ducts of Bellini, usually presents as a case of multiple renal calculosis (or nephrocalcinosis) discovered radiologically after the patient has voided stones in the urine [86, 87]. Though no age period is immune, most cases have been observed during the fourth, fifth and sixth decades of life, with males predominating over females.

The author reported a series of 21 acceptable cases of medullary sponge kidney [120–122]. Among the cases was a family in which six members who had the changes of medullary sponge kidney had presented clinically either with renal stones or infection.

Pathology. The pathological changes may affect both or only one kidney, or only one or more pyramids of one kidney; both were involved in 27 and one kidney only in 17 of 44 patients reported by Ekstrom et al. [44]. The affected kidney may in early cases be of normal size but more often either the entire kidney or only one pole is enlarged, depending on the size and degree of involvement of the renal papillae in the cystic changes.

The essential change is the presence of dilated ducts of Bellini, which sometimes remain patent or are altered into multiple small or medium-sized cysts located in the enlarged pyramid, imparting a spongy character to the otherwise solid medullary tissue. The cysts, which are 1–3 mm or more in size, are rounded, ovoid or irregular in shape and contain a dark brown collagenous substance as well as calcific particles or stones. They are located either at the tips of the renal papillae or they extend inwards towards the medulla, but never into the cortex.

The calculi vary in size from tiny gritty deposits to pea-sized stones usually composed of apatite sometimes admixed with calcium oxalate (Fig. 3.8). Some cysts do not contain stones and some stones ulcerate into the corresponding calyx. The affected papilla is larger than normal with a flattened tip and is surrounded by a splayed-out calyx. In long-standing cases the renal cortex may be reduced in thickness, the kidney as a whole then being smaller than normal; at this stage renal function may be impaired.

Microscopically the dilated tubules and cysts are lined with tall columnar, or transitional or low cuboidal epithelium. The cysts are surrounded by cellular connective tissue, usually sharply divided from the normal medulla.

Changes resulting from associated infection have included bullous oedema, epithelial hyperplasia and pyelitis cystica affecting the urothelium around the cysts and that lining the calyces, renal pelvis and ureter. Medullary sponge kidney has been reported in association with other disorders of congenital origin including polycystic disease of the liver [125], congenital pyloric stenosis [101], and renal tubular acidosis [35].

Symptoms. When symptoms are present they are related to the presence and/or migration of small or large calculi and less commonly to the presence of infection. The cases may be recognized in three clinical groups: (1) Following intravenous pyelography in a patient with cystic changes in the renal papillae probably of congenital origin and no renal calcification [116]; these are clinically early cases. (2) As one example of nephrocalcinosis, often showing unusually small as well as large multiple calculi; the case then presents a diagnostic problem. (3) As an unexpected histopathological finding in pyramidal renal tissue following the operative removal of the

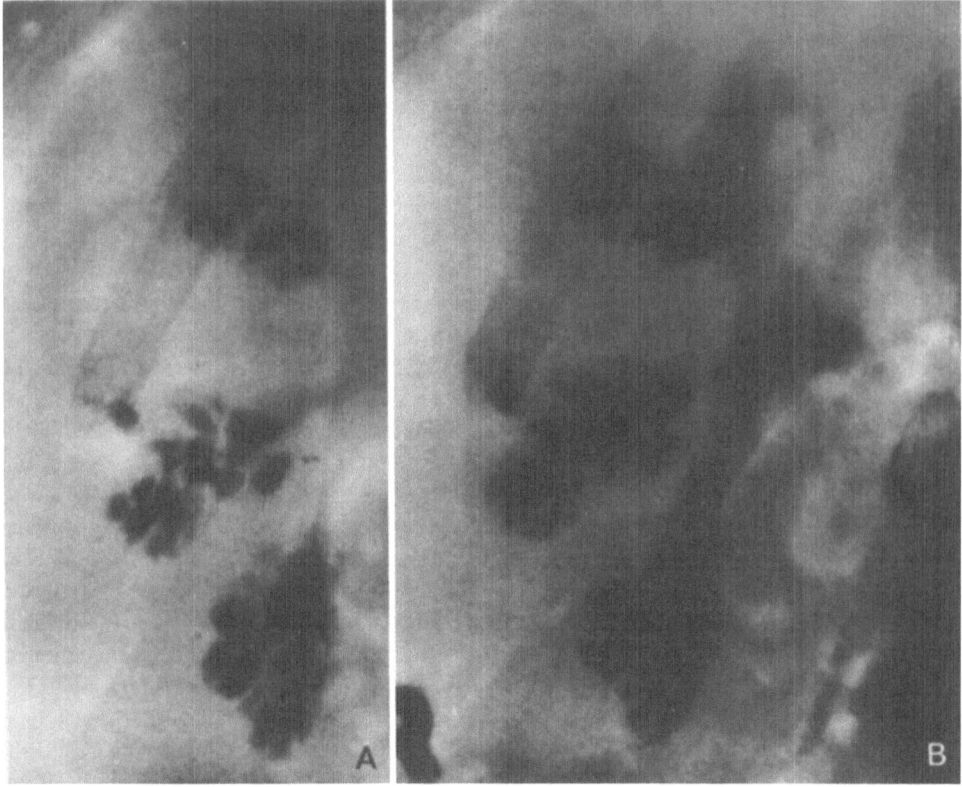

Fig. 3.8. Medullary sponge kidney in a 47-year-old man who had had recurrent attacks of renal colic. **A.** The control radiograph of the right kidney shows groups of medium-sized and large calcareous masses disposed in the region of the renal pyramids. **B.** The excretory urogram locates the position of the calcific masses in relation to the pyramids, the calyces being enlarged

whole or part of the kidney for the treatment of a renal stone which has given rise to clinical symptoms [120].

The condition exhibits the usual symptoms of renal calculus (renal colic, persistent renal pain). Some patients experience troublesome persistent pain in relation to one or other affected kidneys. Occasionally large numbers, and even hundreds, of calculi are voided spontaneously [125]. Intermittent haematuria is common and has sometimes been severe enough to merit nephrectomy [39, 40]. Associated infection may be an early manifestation; hypertension is an occasional complication.

The radiological changes seen in the kidney really determine the diagnosis and it is only occasionally appropriate to carry out renal biopsies. The combination of multiple pyramidal (or calyceal) calculi with cystic pyramidal changes is diagnostic; occasionally the radiograph demonstrates the dilated ducts of Bellini filled with opaque medium but without calculi. The enlargement of the renal papillae and the splayed-out renal calyces are characteristic, though reduction in the thickness of the renal cortex is unusual. The pyramidal cavities or cysts leading from the calyces (seen on pyelography) vary in size and shape and present as a bunch of rod-like or rounded projections leading from the calyces into the pyramids as far as their bases, and remain filled with contrast medium even when the renal pelvis has been emptied or when pressure has been removed from the ureters. There is usually good concentration of contrast medium, suggesting little interference with renal function. Rounded or oval stones or microconcrements of varying size, which are present in most cases, vary from very few to several hundreds and have probably formed secondarily in pre-existing cavities. They tend to be massed in small groups along with the closely packed cystic cavities. Hypercalciuria has been reported.

Diagnosis. Medullary sponge kidney has to be differentiated from the various cystic conditions found occasionally in the renal pyramids. These include solitary calyceal cysts and diverticula, pyelitis and ureteritis cystica. In this latter condition, the punched-out defects in the outline of the calyces, renal pelvis and ureter should not be mistaken for the extracalyceal cystic cavities seen in medullary sponge kidney, or with the (usually only one or more) cysts resulting from acute and chronic pyelonephritis, which originate from small abscesses in the renal pyramids or cortical parts of the kidney, and which may communicate with a calyx [3, 12].

When the characteristic pyramidal microliths (or bigger pyramidal calculi) are seen on the plain radiograph, medullary sponge kidney must be differentiated from primary hyperparathyroidism, in which the calcification is sometimes seen as a feather-like stippling of the renal pyramids or as coarser calcific deposits, but without the existence of enlarged and cavitied renal pyramids and splayed-out calyces. More-over, the biochemical findings of raised serum calcium and sometimes the typical skeletal changes are conclusive. Nor must it be confused with renal tubular acidosis, in which the pyramidal calcific foci are small, ovoid or rod-shaped and biochemically are found in association with a raised serum chloride, a reduced CO_2-combining power and often a low serum potassium level. This

occurs in the late stages of primary hyper-oxaluria, in which there is a high level of urinary oxalate, in addition to recurrent calculi, and radiologically demonstrable nephrocalcinosis.

The stippled calcification seen in the few patients with chronic glomerulonephritis who have an addiction to milk and alkalis has a total renal distribution in both kidneys, the cortex being affected to a greater extent than the medulla.

In renal tuberculosis calcific foci may be seen in relation to cavities in the renal papilla which are related to actual calyceal ulceration. The splayed-out calyces with the intrapapillary cavities and the more regularly sited calcific deposits of medullary sponge kidney should enable the differen-tiation to be made.

In renal papillary necrosis (associated with calculi) cavities or excavations may be observed on intravenous pyelography in the tips of the renal papillae. The calyceal fornices in the early stages of the condition remain normal. The clinical course of the two conditions (phenacetin addiction some-times being present) is different and mis-takes in diagnosis are unlikely.

Treatment. Active treatment of medullary sponge kidney (not usually necessary) is sometimes needed for the removal of stones which have ulcerated through from the pyramidal cystic cavities into the renal pelvis and have descended the ureter, causing pain and obstruction. Occasionally nephrectomy (total or partial) has been done for the treatment of recurrent severe unilateral bleeding or persistent severe pain [120, 121].

III. Renal and Ureteric Calculi Associated with Other Congenital Anomalies of the Urinary Tract

Complete duplication of the renal pelvis and the kidney with complete or incomplete relation to one or other affected kidney. duplication of the ureter is a common anatomical anomaly, the diagnosis being made following urography and cystoscopy, when two ureteric orifices may be seen. Calculi may be found in one or both segments of a duplicated kidney, in either ureter, or in the common ureter formed by the union of two ureters from the duplicated pelves, when obstructive changes may result in the two renal segments.

The clinical symptoms may call for a simple ureterolithotomy or for a partial nephroureterectomy if the affected segment of the kidney has suffered damage from infection or obstruction. A series was reported from the Mayo Clinic during a 10-year period of 131 patients with complete or incomplete duplication of the ureter [63]. The various pathological changes in the affected segments included renal or ureteric stones or both in 36 (4 being bilateral). In another series of 141 patients with re-duplication of the renal pelvis and ureter, calculi were present in 10 [110].

Calculi have been reported in fused kidneys, usually in one of the components [103, 140] and an incidence of calculus in 12% of 25 patients with fused kidneys has been found [128]. Fergusson [47] had experience of a patient with a cystine stone who presented with left renal colic and who was shown to have crossed renal ectopia, both kidneys being fused into one mass, lying in the right loin. The stone was located in the renal pelvis of the left component [43]. Calculi are occasionally found in ectopic kidneys [34, 147].

IV. Metaplastic Conditions and Tumours of the Kidney, the Ureter, and Calculi

1. Metaplasia (Squamous and Glandular) and Leukoplakia

With squamous metaplasia part of the normal transitional epithelium of the renal pelvis is replaced by squamous epithelium; the condition is sometimes found in association with calculi. The epithelial changes may arise de novo from an unknown cause or may be found in association with and possibly secondary to infection and/or nephrocalcinosis [46]. Some observers believe that squamous metaplasia is a precursor of squamous carcinoma of the renal pelvis.

In pyelitis and ureteritis glandularis, the transitional epithelium is replaced by columnar epithelium containing goblet cells and later by gland formation resembling that seen in the intestinal mucosa. The abnormality is probably derived from the epithelial cell nests first described by Von Brunn (1893) [155], the cells extending downwards and appearing to sink into the lamina propria, becoming detached and losing their continuity with the epithelium [46]. Pyelitis glandularis in association with renal calculi has also been described [15, 50, 109, 153].

Leukoplakia of the renal pelvis probably starts in the epithelium as a focal squamous metaplasia followed by keratinization of the superficial cells and by the formation of the characteristic pearly opaque plaques. The condition has been found as an independent abnormality but sometimes in association with long-standing calculi in the renal pelvis. In a series of 67 cases 28 had calculi [83]. The condition may give rise to clinical symptoms in its own right, including haematuria and the voiding of gritty flakes of calcified epithelium in the urine, the diagnosis sometimes being made possible by the observation of small localized pelvic filling defects on the pyelogram.

2. Carcinoma of the Renal Parenchyma

Renal calculi are occasionally found probably as a coincidence in a kidney which is the seat of a parenchymal carcinoma [156]. The clinical symptoms, which usually include pain as well as haematuria, may not suggest the complete diagnosis, though the intravenous pyelogram may reveal a filling defect in addition to the stone [30]; there is often a palpable swelling in the loin. In some cases the association has only been discovered at operation [1, 16, 56, 59, 119, 165].

Calcification in the kidney in association with renal carcinomata is a common finding and is of importance in the radiological differential diagnosis of the various calcific changes which are found in the kidney. It has been reported in 15%–38% of cases of renal carcinoma in different series [112]. It is seen on the plain radiograph as fairly dense streaks, flecks, whorls or stippling, and may be disposed in linear fashion throughout the tissue, or most characteristically as a clearly delineated ring-like shadow, presumably surrounding a necrotic mass or a hyaline zone of tumour tissue. Such a finding should always suggest a renal neoplasm [81].

3. Sarcoma of the Kidney

Sarcoma of the kidney (which is rare) is occasionally associated with renal calculus, probably coincidentally [82, 112].

Osteogenic sarcoma of the kidney usually gives rise to dense calcific shadows seen on the plain radiograph; the condition does not appear to have been reported in association with renal calculus, but its presence gives rise to diagnostic difficulties (from stone and renal calcification) because of the radiological appearances [50, 66, 75].

4. Epithelial Tumours of the Renal Pelvis

The papillary tumours of the renal pelvis, simple and malignant [162], are occasionally associated with renal stone, while the solid malignant tumours (transitional cell and squamous cell carcinoma of the renal pelvis) are commonly associated with stone.

The clinical picture of patients in this group often combines that of neoplasia of the renal pelvis with that of calculous disease, the final diagnosis often being possible from the straight radiograph and the pyelogram and possibly by the discovery of malignant cells in the urine. Joly's [77] collected series of 337 cases of tumours of the renal pelvis provides valuable information of the pathology and clinical behaviour.

Renal Calculi. Renal calculi were reported in 14 of 22 patients with epithelial tumours of the renal pelvis [95]. The average duration of the symptoms resulting from the calculi was about 19 years, while that from the tumour was estimated at 5 months.

In Joly's [77] analysis of 337 collected cases with tumours of the renal pelvis, of the papillary tumours, renal calculi were present in 11 of 120 cases of benign papilloma (9%) and in 8 of 138 cases of papillary carcinoma (5.8%), averaging 6%. But the incidence of calculi with the solid malignant tumours of the renal pelvis was much higher: in 5 of 29 patients (17.2%) with transitional cell carcinoma in 4 of whom there was an associated pyonephrosis; and in 26 of 50 patients (52%) with squamous carcinoma, in 22 of whom there was a calculous pyonephrosis. He concluded that as calculous disease is usually a more chronic condition than is an infiltrating tumour of the renal pelvis, the former is the primary lesion and the growth secondary. A urinary infection was frequently present even in some patients in whom there was no stone. Gahaghan and Read [54] reported 48 with stone in 100 collected cases. Utz and McDonald [154] found stones in 13 of their 23 cases (57%) of squamous carcinoma of the renal pelvis; they thought that the circumstances seemed to point to infection and stone together as the initiatory factors in the formation of carcinoma.

Willis [162], however, stated that calculi in patients with squamous carcinoma of the renal pelvis 'are secondary to the tumour and of no causative significance'. It is certainly the case, however, that the solid transitional cell carcinoma and the squamous cell carcinoma of the renal pelvis are found not infrequently in renal pelves known to have harboured large calculi for many years, especially when the urine has been infected for a long time.

Adenocarcinoma of the renal pelvis, which presumably originates from areas of pelvic mucosa affected by pyelitis glandularis, has been reported in association with renal calculi [5, 114, 123].

5. Epithelial Tumours of the Ureter

It would be expected by analogy with squamous carcinoma of the renal pelvis, that calculi would occasionally be found in association with the relatively uncommon tumours of the ureter; prolonged urinary obstruction with stagnation and infection possibly predisposing to stone formation above the level of the growth.

The clinical picture may be a summation of that of the separate symptoms of both conditions; or a ureteric tumour may be found at operation for the removal of a ureteric stone. Series of cases of carcinoma of the ureter in the literature include that reported by Joly [77], who collected 133 cases classified as benign papillomata and papillary carcinoma (101 cases) and transitional cell and squamous cell carcinoma (32 cases); and that by McIntyre et al. [96], which was a series of 40 cases from the author's department.

Ureteric calculi have been reported in association with ureteric tumours in 16% of cases of squamous carcinoma of the ureter and in other series in 6 of 49 cases [13]. Lazarus [85] reported ureteric calculi in

association with malignant tumour of the ureter in 10 cases; and in a second series he found calculi in 32 cases among 183 patients with carcinoma of the ureter. Squamous cell carcinoma has been found not infrequently in a ureteric stump following nephrectomy for calculous pyonephrosis, often many years after the operation; in such patients there has been persistent pyuria and/or haematuria [9, 149].

V. Renal Tubular Acidosis

Renal tubular acidosis is a disorder of the renal tubules in which there is a derangement of the local renal acid-base mechanism, resulting in a failure of the tubules to secrete hydrogen ion and sometimes a failure to form ammonium. The defects lead to the production of urine which is relatively alkaline, and also to a systemic hyperchloraemic acidosis, which, in the adult type of the disease, is often secondarily associated with hypercalciuria, nephrolithiasis or nephrocalcinosis, rickets or osteomalacia, and potassium deficiency. There are two principal groups.

1. In Infants (Lightwood's Syndrome)

This condition, first described by Lightwood [88], occurs in infants (usually during the first 18 months of life) who show a failure to thrive, loss of appetite and weight, polyuria, usually constipation and vomiting, wasting and usually muscular hypotonia. Biochemically there is an elevated serum chloride level and a reduced serum CO_2-combining power [18] and usually an alkaline urine, the kidneys being unable to form urine which is sufficiently acid to maintain the pH of the blood at its normal level.

The administration of sodium bicarbonate or citrate is generally followed by complete recovery after several months of treatment. In fatal cases the kidneys at autopsy show macroscopically a heavy deposit of insoluble calcium salts disposed in radial whitish lines in the renal pyramids, the remainder of the kidney being normal. Microscopically the collecting tubules contain masses of calcium salts and occasionally hyaline or calcium casts. No renal calculi are found.

Symptomless nephrocalcinosis (shown radiologically) is seen occasionally in older children who have had a history in keeping with earlier infantile primary renal acidosis, possibly an example of late dystrophic calcification.

2. In Adolescents and Adults

The adult (or persistent) primary type of renal tubular acidosis, first described by Albright et al. [7], usually starts in adolescence and may present either with renal colic resulting from the nephrocalcinosis or calculi, or bone pain or deformity from rickets or osteomalacia, or with attacks of hypokalaemic paralysis from an excessive urinary loss of potassium.

Early symptoms have included loss of appetite, listlessness, fatigue, general weakness and in adolescents a failure to achieve normal growth. Not all patients have renal calculi or nephrocalcinosis in the early stages of the disease, though the voiding of renal calculi with or without attacks of renal colic or infection may be the principal symptom (Fig. 3.9). The presence of nephrocalcinosis is believed to be favoured by urinary alkalinity, by hypercalciuria, which is often present, and possibly by the reduced urinary excretion of citrate. The nephrocalcinosis is demonstrated by the presence in all the renal pyramids of bilateral, spotty, radiologically demonstrable calcific particles or tiny calculi, which may escape from the ducts of Bellini, and which if they are not voided spontaneously may gradually enlarge

into biggish calculi and either remain in the calyces or move into the ureters giving rise to a hydronephrosis calling for surgical relief because of recurrent attacks of pain.

In some adolescents there is occasionally gross calcification in the medullary part of the kidney [7, 8, 18, 136].

In another group, early symptoms of flaccid paralysis, seen especially in the forearm muscles, may occur as the result of excessive urinary potassium excretion with hypokalaemia. A hypokalaemic crisis may be precipitated by starvation and vomiting, and a period of profound weakness and drowsiness or near-coma may then be associated with respiratory difficulty [142]. This syndrome may be followed at a later date by radiologically demonstrable nephrocalcinosis. In some patients there is a family history [36, 139].

As the disease advances, and presumably as a consequence of the hypercalciuria and calcium loss resulting from the acidosis, rickets with fractures, epiphyseal deformities and diminished stature may develop in adolescents, while osteomalacia with spontaneous fractures of long bones may be a dominant symptom in adults. Any patient presenting with symptoms limited to one group may over the years develop the complete clinical picture.

Smith [146] reported a series of 28 patients with renal tubular acidosis whose average age at the time of diagnosis was 29 (though symptoms often preceded the diagnosis by some years). The incidence of the principal clinical features was as follows: skeletal symptoms in 48%, renal calculi in 65%, nephrocalcinosis in 70%, hypokalaemia giving rise to clinical symptoms in 32%; one or more of these symptom groups may dominate the clinical picture. Whereas these patients formerly died in early adult life, nowadays with appropriate treatment they remain in reasonable health with adequate renal function, provided that obstructive symptoms are relieved.

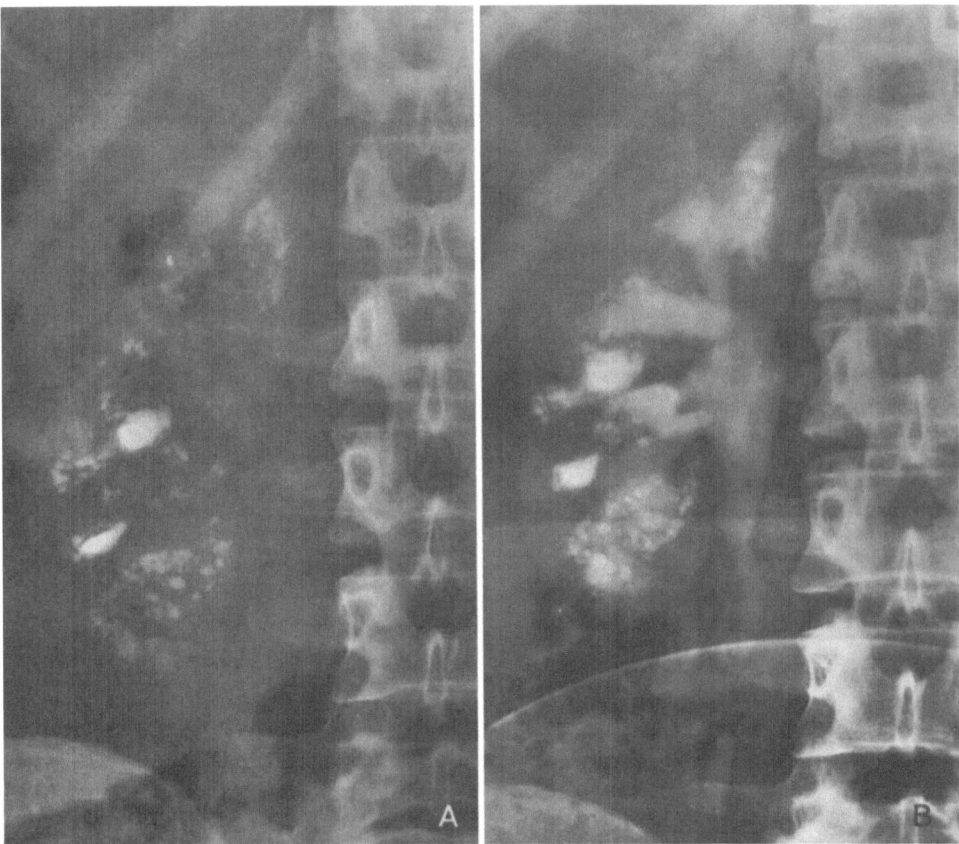

Fig. 3.9. Case of renal tubular acidosis; bilateral nephrocalcinosis; subsequent nephrolithiasis and ureterolithiasis; hypokalaemia, osteomalacia (female, aged 41). She had had several attacks of bilateral renal colic during some of which she had voided small calculi. She subsequently complained of muscular weakness of the forearm muscles and to a lesser extent, of those of the legs. She was found to have renal tubular acidosis with hypokalaemia. When treated with modified Shohl's solution (with potassium partly replacing the sodium), her condition greatly improved. Several years later radiography revealed calculi in the left ureter and the left renal pelvis, necessitating left ureterolithotomy and pyelolithotomy. The ureteric stones were composed of apatite. Several years later (1972) further calculi were again removed from the left kidney to relieve pain and recurrent ureteric colic. Clinically she has remained well, having enjoyed good health for 21 years, during which time she co-operated carefully with the medical alkaline treatment advised. A. Plain radiograph of right kidney showing the characteristic nephrocalcinosis; the left kidney was similarly affected. B. Intravenous pyelogram showing the site of the calcification in the renal pyramids, the calyces not being dilated; renal function is well maintained

The principal biochemical changes in the adult type of the disease are a fall in the plasma CO_2-combining power and an elevation of the plasma chloride level. The serum potassium level is often subnormal. The minimal urinary pH is usually about 6.0–6.8 (the normal being around pH 4.5). The urinary titratable acidity and the ammonium content are low. Since glomerular function is normal in the early and intermediate stages of the disease there is no azotaemia, the syndrome having been appropriately designated 'tubular-insufficiency - without - glomerular - insufficiency' by Albright and Reifenstein [6]; in the late stages glomerular function may become impaired. The biochemical pathogenesis of renal tubular acidosis and the normal and abnormal renal mechanism concerning the regulation of the acid-base balance have been described by several observers [113, 142, 166].

Several adult cases have been described in detail [6, 14]. Several cases have come under the author's observation, all except one presenting with nephrocalcinosis and/or voiding of calculi. One case, presenting with severe hypokalaemia which led to dangerous coma from which the patient was rescued by the administration of alkali and potassium, was found some years later to have bilateral nephrocalcinosis and the spontaneous voiding of calculi in the urine. All the patients had the characteristic biochemical findings and the daily urinary calcium was subnormal in all cases except one. The effect of treatment by alkalis (Shohl's solution) in all the patients gave satisfactory results.

Renal tubular acidosis has been found in association with a wide variety of diseases, including autoimmune hepatic disease, thyrotoxicosis and medullary sponge kidney. The renal histological changes in adult patients with renal tubular acidosis were reported by Govan [61], but later reports are very few. The renal pelves and calyces were found to be dilated and filled with small brown stones. A characteristic finding was seen in the epithelial cells of the first convoluted tubules, which were swollen and contained large vacuoles characteristic of the changes associated with hypokalaemia, the nuclei being pushed to the base of the cells, some of which were desquamated or even necrotic.

Incomplete Form. In a description of this condition Wrong and Davies [166] referred to a group of patients with nephrocalcinosis who had no systemic acidosis but

who were unable to excrete a highly acid urine when 'challenged' with an oral load of ammonium chloride (0.1 g/kg b. wt.). These patients could excrete ammonium normally and their glomerular function was satisfactory. In the author's department a small group of renal calculous patients with this variant of the syndrome came under observation and were regarded as examples of 'masked' renal acidosis [122]. If a series of patients with idiopathic renal calculi are examined using the short ammonium chloride loading test it is found that some do not possess the power to acidify the urine to a normal degree, an abnormality which may contribute to the stone formation. The long-term treatment of such patients by alkalis may help to prevent recurrent stone formation by correcting the abnormality, which may be a masked renal tubular acidosis. Cochran et al. [21] found such an abnormality in 24 of 600 patients with renal calculous disease. Possibly the abnormality may be the result of mild pyelonephritis, which is sometimes associated with calculous disease [94, 148, 151].

Treatment. The administration of Shohl's solution (140 g citric acid, 98 g sodium citrate, in 1 litre of water, given in 50–100 ml daily in 8-hourly divided doses) has enabled these patients to live on in reasonable health, whereas formerly most died before the age of 30. The treatment must be strictly adhered to through life in the adult patient. In the early stages (after diagnosis) the blood electrolytes should be examined at frequent intervals to establish the appropriate dose of alkali.

In the presence of hypokalaemia a similar dose of a mixture containing 50 g potassium citrate with 50 g sodium citrate and 140 g citric acid is effective treatment; but in such patients the serum levels of potassium and bicarbonate should be frequently examined and adjusted as indicated to prevent alkalosis or hyperkalaemia.

Some observers doubt the necessity for the long-term administration of potassium. Patients admitted to hospital with drowsiness or coma from hypokalaemia should be given infusions of sodium bicarbonate and potassium chloride as an emergency treatment. An induced alkalosis may cause respiratory trouble and tetany especially in the presence of hypocalcaemia [142]. A diet low in chloride is indicated if oedema develops.

It is not usually necessary to give vitamin D and calcium salts, since the hypercalciuria ceases when the acidosis (upon which it is dependent) has been corrected, though such measures may be used if there is severe demineralization.

No surgical treatment is indicated for the correction of the nephrocalcinosis as such, and indeed it would be impracticable. Some patients void small calculi for a long time during their period of treatment; in a few cases (as in one patient of the author's) calculi of considerable size come to rest in the ureter and cause pain and hydronephrosis and require pyelolithotomy or ureterolithotomy.

3. Acetazolamide (Diamox) and Renal Calculi

Acetazolamide (which is a heterocyclic sulphonamide: 2-acetylamino-1,3,4-thiadrazole-5-sulphonamide) acts as a diuretic and has been used in the treatment of glaucoma. The substance is an inhibitor of the enzyme carbonic anhydrase and consequently gives rise to a condition which closely mimics renal tubular acidosis. Normal acidification of the urine is prevented. Young rats experimentally fed with acetazolamide and a high calcium, high phosphorus diet, have been shown to develop nephrocalcinosis [69]. There are several reports in the literature of renal calculi in human patients who had received acetazolamide [58, 91, 93, 107].

VI. Infective Conditions of the Kidney and Calculous Disease

1. Renal Tuberculosis

Parenchymal renal calcification is often present in moderately advanced tuberculous kidneys, and true renal calculi are also not infrequently present in such kidneys; the coincidence of such conditions may give rise to difficulty in radiological diagnosis [42, 79].

Calcification in the tuberculous kidney results from the deposition of insoluble calcium salts in degenerative diseased tissue; it may develop even after treatment has rendered the diseased process inactive, when it may then be regarded as a continuation of the healing process [129]. The calcific foci may be single or multiple small calcified masses or a diffuse calcification affecting a large part or almost the whole of the kidney. Hanley [67] found radiological evidence of calcification in 37 of 87 tuberculous kidneys removed by operation and caseation was also present in the kidneys he examined. In a series of 740 patients with renal tuberculosis reported by Gow [62] calcification was found in 183 (24%).

Renal Calculi. When renal calculi and renal tuberculosis are found in the same kidney, one disease has originated before the other. Olsen [104] observed stone formation in 3 of 113 kidneys removed for tuberculosis; Crenshaw [27] found calculi in 1.8% of cases in a series of nearly 2000 patients with tuberculous kidneys at the Mayo Clinic; and Wershunt [159] gave the incidence of renal calculus in tuberculous kidneys as being between 0.9% and 2.7%.

Shucksmith [143] reported a male patient who had multiple calculi and also tuberculosis in the left kidney, the condition being complicated by an external renoinguinal fistula; he stated that 6 such cases had been reported since 1930. Couvelaire and Brizon [25] reported 29 cases (4%) of urinary calculi in 765 patients with genito-urinary tuberculosis. Of 740 patients with renal tuberculosis reviewed by Ross [129] between 1952 and 1969, 5 had staghorn calculi, in 14 calculi were found to be moving into the ureter and 7 had vesical calculi. The author has seen at least 4 patients with renal calculi among about 150 patients with renal tuberculosis.

2. Renal Actinomycosis

Renal actinomycosis, which is rare (Cope [24], finding only 20 cases in the literature to 1952) occurs as a localized suppurative lesion resembling a renal carbuncle, as diffuse pyelonephritis or as a pyo-nephrosis; in a few cases there have been associated calculi. Willson–Pepper's [163] patient had a staghorn calculus in a pyonephrotic kidney which was removed, *Actinomycosis bovis* being cultured from the pus.

3. Typhoid Infections of the Kidney

The kidney may be involved during the course of typhoid fever, during convalescence, or many years after as a true typhoid infection, presenting as multiple foci of suppuration or as a pyonephrosis. It is thought that the disease is sometimes primary in the kidney, the organism arriving there by way of the colonic lymphatics. Renal calculus occasionally complicates a typhoid kidney. Young and Lehr [170] found typhoid bacilli in the nucleus of a stone. Among several cases reported in the literature was one of typhoid calculous pyonephrosis [76, 78].

4. Bilharziasis of the Urinary Tract

Bilharziasis, the result of infestation by the worm *Schistosoma haematobium*, affects especially the urinary tract of Egyptians, Africans and also Europeans resident in Africa. The pathology has been described by Honey and Gelfand [73]. The common symptoms are haematuria, hypogastric discomfort and occasionally bilateral colicky pain and frequency of micturition as the fibrosis and contraction of the bladder increases. The diagnosis is made following examination of the urine (to recover the bilharzial ova), radiography and cystoscopy.

The characteristic radiological picture of the bladder wall in the fully developed state is that of a continuous or segmental thin calcific linear shadow 0.5–3 mm thick. Similar deposits may extend up the walls of the lower third of both ureters, occasionally as far as the renal pelvis and there may be ureteric calculi; urography may show dilatation and tortuosity of part or the whole of the calcified ureter in the advanced stages.

Renal calculi seem to have a proportionately higher incidence in the European than in the African population [73], and soft phosphatic calculi have been observed in the dilated renal pelvis in patients with an associated urinary infection [55]. In an infected subject pinkish bilharzial tubercles, sometimes in large numbers, may be seen distributed either in patches or over the entire wall of the bladder. In time the affected patches become firmer and look like grains of sand in the fibrosed mucous membrane; the ureteric orifices may be partly concealed by granulation tissue, and papilloma-like masses may be seen.

On radiography, punctate calcification in lengthy segments of the walls of one or both ureters may occasionally be seen, which Ghorab [55] designated ureteritis calcinosa. The calcified foci vary in size from that of a pinhead to a few millimetres and may mimic ureteric calculi. Not uncommonly small calculi are voided in the urine following attacks of colic, and with the passage of time the calcific masses may even diminish numerically and may eventually disappear.

With increasingly severe symptoms various surgical procedures are sometimes indicated for the relief of symptoms. Ileocystoplasty for the treatment of a severely contracted and partly calcified bladder has been used by Honey and Gelfand [73] in 25 patients. In some of Ghorab's [55] cases of ureteric calcinosa, ureteric catheters were passed at intervals to dilate the ureter and to dislodge concretions. When this treatment did not entirely relieve symptoms he exposed one or both ureters surgically and opened them by a longitudinal incision, dislodging calcific particles or masses from long segments of the ureter with a scoop. Renal and ureteric calculi may call for removal and occasionally ureteric strictures or a contracted bladder neck call for surgical treatment.

5. Gonococcal Infection of the Kidney

Infective changes in the kidney similar to those caused by the pyogenic organisms have been observed following the rare gonococcal infection of the kidney, and calculi have occasionally been reported. Five cases have been recorded by Parmenter et al. [108]. Mack and Buchanan [92], who collected 14 proven cases, recorded a case of their own of gonococcal pyonephrosis, in which several calculi were found in a dilated lower calyx.

6. Renal Brucellosis

A number of cases have been reported in which chronic pyelonephritis caused by the micro-organism *Brucella abortus* has resulted in nephrocalcinosis. Greene et al. [64, 65] described a patient who had suffered from the disease for 4 years prior to the onset of urinary symptoms. The brucella

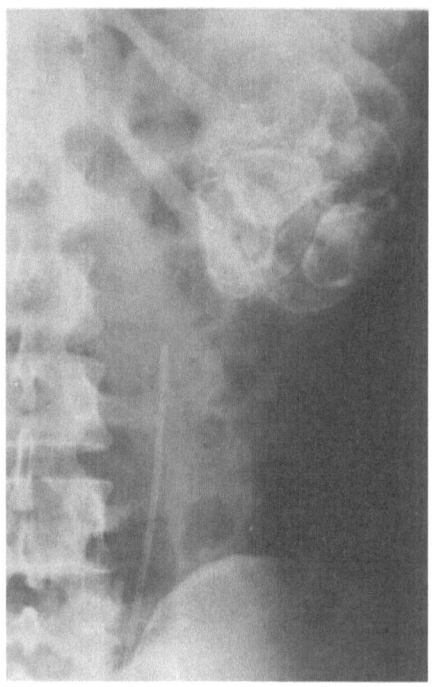

Fig. 3.10. Multiple calcified hydatid cysts of the kidney in a male patient aged 28, who was under treatment in hospital for haematemesis, when radiography revealed the cysts in the region of the left kidney; there were no renal symptoms. The clinical diagnosis was multiple primary hydatid cysts of the left kidney. (By courtesy of Mr. Alban Gee, F.R.C.S., Sydney, Australia)

organism was cultured from the blood and from the urine (which contained pus), and a plain radiograph showed calcific shadows throughout the renal parenchyma. They reported a second patient who had had the disease 10 years previously and who now showed extensive zones of calcification in each kidney. Abernathy et al. [2] reported a similar case. The patient reported by Honey et al. [74], a male aged 50, had had intermittent symptoms for some years including an infected hip joint and suppurative lesions in the leg. With the subsequent onset of urinary symptoms and pyuria, patchy bilateral nephrocalcinosis (most marked around some of the renal calyces) was observed radiographically, the brucella organism being recovered from the pus from a sinus in the tibia.

7. Hydatid Disease of the Kidney

Hydatid disease is only rarely seen in the kidney and may be recognized radiologically by the presence of calcified cysts seen on the plain radiograph (Fig. 3.10).

References

1. Aas,T.N.: Ureterocele: a clinical study of 68 cases in 52 adults. Br. J. Urol. *32*, 133 (1960)
2. Abernathy,R.C., Price,W.E., Spink,W.W.: Chronic brucellar pyelonephritis simulating tuberculosis. J. Am. Med. Assoc. *159*, 1534 (1935)
3. Abeshouse,B.S., Abeshouse,G.A.: Sponge kidney: a review of the literature and a report of five cases. J. Urol. *84*, 252 (1960)
4. Abeshouse,B.S., Abeshouse, G.A.: Calyceal diverticulum: a report of 16 cases and review of the literature. Urol. Int. *15*, 329 (1963)
5. Ackerman,L.V.: Mucinous adenocarcinoma of the pelvis of the kidney. J. Urol. *55*, 36 (1946)
6. Albright,F., Reifenstein,E.C.: Parathyroid glands and metabolic bone diseases. Baltimore: Williams and Wilkins 1948
7. Albright,F., Consolazio,W.V., Coombs, F.S., Sulkowitch,H.W., Talbot,J.H.: Metabolic studies and therapy in a case of nephrocalcinosis with rickets and dwarfism. Bull. Johns Hopkins Hosp. *56*, 7 (1940)
8. Albright,F., Burnett,C.H., Parsons,W., Reifenstein,E.C., Roos,A.: Osteomalacia and late rickets. Medicine *25*, 399 (1946)
9. Amar,A.D.: Squamous cell carcinoma of ureteral stump 30 years after nephrectomy. J. Urol. *91*, 337 (1964)
10. Anderson,C.K.: Personal communication (1971)
11. Anderson,J.C., Hynes,W.: Retrocaval ureter: a case diagnosed pre-operatively and treated successfully by a plastic operation. Br. J. Urol. *21*, 209 (1949)
12. Arena,G.C.: On sponge kidney. Presentation of several personal cases. Notes on the nosographic classification and differential diagnosis of the morbid form. Minerva Urol. *23*, 111 (1971)
13. Baines,G.H.: Diverticulum of the ureter. Br. J. Urol. *34*, 193 (1962)
14. Baines,G.H., Barclay,J.A., Cooke,W.T.: Nephrocalcinosis associated with hyperchloraemia and low plasma bicarbonate. Q. J. Med. (new series) *14*, 113 (1945)
15. Brutt,H.: Über Pyelitis Glandularis. Z. Urol. Chir. *14*, 157 (1923)
16. Bugbee,H.G.: Primary carcinoma of the kidney with impacted ureteral calculus. J. Urol. *5*, 267 (1921)
17. Burns,C.N.,Drew,J.E.,Dean,A.L.:Ureteropelvic obstruction with hydronephrosis: treatment by pyeloplasty in 23 cases. J. Urol. *70*, 846 (1953)
18. Butler,A.M., Wilson,L.L., Farber,S.: Dehydration and acidosis with calcification of renal tubules. J. Pediatr. *8*, 489 (1936)
19. Castro,J.E., et al.: Complications of horseshoe kidney. Urology *6*, 344 (1975)
20. Cathro, A.J.McG.: Section of the inferior vena cava for retrocaval ureter: a new method of treatment. J. Urol. *67*, 464 (1952)
21. Cochran,M., Peacock,M., Smith,D.A., Nordin,B.E.C.: Renal tubular acidosis of pyelonephritis with renal stone disease. Br. Med. J. *2*, 721 (1968)
22. Colston,J.A.C., Baker,W.W.: Late effects of various types of trauma of the kidney. Arch. Surg. *34*, 99 (1937)
23. Considine,J.: Retrocaval ureter. Br. J. Urol. *38*, 42 (1966)
24. Cope,V.Z.: Human Actinomycosis. London: Heinemann 1952
25. Couvelaire,R., Brizon,J.: Tuberculose genitourinarie et lithiase. J. Urol. *52*, 429 (1956)
26. Creevy,C.D., Bolt,H.K.S.: The results of Y-plasty after 5 to 24 years: a review of 73 operations. J. Urol. *77*, 388 (1957)
27. Crenshaw,J.L.: Renal tuberculosis with calcification. J. Urol. *23*, 515 (1930)
28. Culp,O.S.: Ureteral diverticulum. J. Urol. *58*, 309 (1947)
29. Culp,O.S., Winterringer,J.R.: Surgical treatment of horseshoe kidney. J. Urol. *73*, 747 (1955)
30. Czerniawski,J. et al.: A case of clear-cell renal carcinoma coexisting with renolithiasis diagnosed prior to surgery. Pol. Przegl. Chir. *48*, 277 (1974)

31. Dalgaard,O.Z.: Bilateral polycystic disease of the kidneys: a follow-up of 284 patients and their families. Acta Med. Scand. (Suppl. 328) *158*, 13 (1957)

32. Dalgaard,O.Z.: Polycystic disease of the kidneys. In: Diseases of the kidney. Strauss,M.B., Welt,L.G. (eds.), Ch. 31, p. 925. Boston: Little, Brown & Co. 1963

33. Damm,E.: Solitärcysten der Niere. Z. Urol. Chir. *35*, 103 (1932)

34. Davies,J.L.: Calculus in an ectopic kidney. Br. Med. J. *II*, 1031 (1931)

35. Deck,M.D.F.: Medullary sponge kidney with renal tubular acidosis: a report. J. Urol. *94*, 330 (1965)

36. Dedmon,R.A., Wrong,O.: The excretion of organic anion in renal tubular acidosis with particular reference to citrate. Clin. Sci. *22*, 19 (1962)

37. Derbes,V.J., La Nasa,M.J.: Postcaval ureter and hydronephrosis: case report. Urol. Cut. Rev. *41*, 172 (1937)

38. Devine,C.J., Guzman,J.A., Devine,P.G.: Calyceal diverticulum. J. Urol. *101*, 8 (1969)

39. Di Sieno,A., Guareschi,B.: Ill rene a spugna midollare concalcolosi multipla endocavitaria ed i suoi possibili rapporti con la nefrocalcinosis. Radiol. Med. *42*, 167 (1956a)

40. Di Sieno,A., Guareschi,B.: Il quadro radiologico del rene a spugna midollare (Revisione della letterature e presentazione di due casi). Radiol. Clin. *25*, 80 (1956b)

41. Dolan,P.A., Kirkpatrick,W.E.: Multiple ureteral diverticula. J. Urol. *83*, 570 (1960)

42. Ducasson,J. et al.: Renal tuberculosis and lithiasis. A case followed for 13 years. J. Urol. Nephrol (Paris) *77*, 644 (1971)

43. Eichwald,M., Wolfe,L.A.: Nephrolithiasis connected with hydronephrosis of a crossed renal ectopia. J. Am. Med. Assoc. *211*, 117 (1970)

44. Ekstrom,T., Engfeldt,B., Lagergren, C., Lindvall,N.: Medullary sponge kidney. Stockholm: Almquist and Wikswell 1959

45. Engel,W.J.: Nephrocalcinosis. J. Am. Med. Assoc. *145*, 288 (1951)

46. Evans,W.: Histological Appearances of Tumours. 1st ed. Edinburgh: Livingstone 1956

47. Fergusson,J.D.: Pers. comm. (1972)

48. Ferguson,G., Ward-McQuaid,J.N.: Stones in pyelogenic cysts. Br. J. Surg. *42*, 595 (1954–55)

49. Fetter,T.H., Yunen,J.R., Bogaev,J.H.: Parapelvic renal cyst. J. Urol. *88*, 599 (1962)

50. Fine,G., Stout,A.P.: Osteogenic sarcoma of extraskeletal soft tissues. Cancer *9*, 1027 (1956)

51. Flocks,R.H., Stark,T.E.: A review of 63 cases of horseshoe kidney from State University of Iowa Urology (Sectional) Conference of Surgeons of India: Christian Medical College Hospital, Vellore, S. India 1962

52. Foley,F.E.B.: Surgical correction of horseshoe kidney. J. Am. Med. Assoc. *115*, 1945 (1940)

53. Foot,N.C.: Glandular metaplasia of the epithelium of the urinary tract. South Med. J. *37*, 137 (1944)

54. Gahagan,E.Q., Read, W.K.: Squamous cell carcinoma of the renal pelvis; 3 case reports and review of literature. J. Urol. *62*, 139 (1949)

55. Ghorab,M.M.El: Ureteritis calcinosis: a complication of bilharzial ureteritis and its relation to primary ureteric stone formation. Br. J. Urol. *34*, 33 (1962)

56. Gigli,V.: Renal carcinoma associated with stone. Arch. Ital. Urol. *33*, 138 (1960)

57. Goldstein,A.E.: Polycystic renal disease with particular reference to the author's surgical practice. J. Urol. *66*, 163 (1951)

58. Gordon,E.E., Shepps,S.G.: Effect of acetazolamide on citrate excretion and formation of renal calculi. N. Engl. J. Med. *256*, 1215 (1957)

59. Gordon-Taylor,G.: Association of renal calculi and hypernephroma. Br. J. Urol. *7*, 41 (1935)

60. Gottlieb,J.: Zur Arbeit über Frage über Pathogenese und Therapie der Ureterocele. Z. Urol. Chir. *19*, 345 and *20*, 1 (1926)

61. Govan,A.D.T.: Renal tubular acidosis: autopsy findings. Q. J. Med. *19*, 277 (1950)

62. Gow,J.G.: Renal calcification in genito-urinary tuberculosis. Br. J. Urol. *52*, 283 (1965)

63. Goyanna,R., Greene,L.F.: Pathological and anomalous conditions associated with duplication of the renal pelvis and ureter. J. Urol. *54*, 1 (1945)

64. Greene,L.F., Albers,D.D.: Brucellosis of urinary tract. Proc. Mayo Clin. *25*, 638 (1950)

65. Greene,L.F., Weed,L.A., Albers,D.D.: Brucellosis of urinary tract. J. Urol. *67*, 765 (1952)
66. Hamer,H.G., Wishard,W.N.: Osteogenic sarcoma involving right kidney. J. Urol. *60*, 10 (1948)
67. Hanley,H.G.: Some observations on the treatment of calcifying renal tuberculosis. Br. J. Urol. *24*, 188 (1952)
68. Harrill,H.C.: Retrocaval ureter. J. Urol. *44*, 450 (1940)
69. Harrison,H.E., Harrison,H.C.: Inhibition of urine citrate excretion and production of renal calcinosis in the rat by acetazolamide (diamox) administration. J. Clin. Invest. *34*, 1662 (1955)
70. Hellstrom,J., Giertz,G., Lindblom,K.: Pathogenesis and treatment of hydronephrosis. VIII. Congr. Soc. Int. Urol. *1*, 163 (1949)
71. Heslin,J.E., Mamonas,C.: Retrocaval ureter: report of 4 cases and review of literature. J. Urol. *29*, 87 (1951)
72. Holly,L.E., Suncad,B.: Diverticular ureteral changes: a report of 4 cases. Am. J. Roentgenol. *78*, 1053 (1957)
73. Honey,R.M., Gelfand,M.: The urological aspects of bilharziasis in Rhodesia. Edinburgh: Livingstone 1960
74. Honey,R.M., Gelfand,M., Myers,N.H.: Chronic brucella pyelonephritis with calcification. Cent. Afr. J. Med. *3*, 465 (1957)
75. Hudson,H.C.: Osteogenic sarcoma involving the left kidney. J. Urol. *75*, 21 (1956)
76. Huggins,C.B., Roome,N.W.: Typhoid pyonephrosis. J. Urol. *31*, 587 (1934)
77. Joly,J.W.: Tumours of renal pelvis and ureter. Br. J. Urol. *5*, 327 (1933)
78. Kahle,P.J., Beacham,H.T.: Typhoid pyonephrosis with report of case. J. Urol. *30*, 299 (1933)
79. Kato,T.: Bilateral staghorn calculi associated with renal tuberculosis. Acta Urol. Jpn. *18*, 233 (1972)
80. Kimbrough,J.C.: Surgical treatment of hydronephrosis. J. Urol. *33*, 97 (1935)
81. King,R.L., Storasli,J.F., Dolandi,R.P.: Neuroblastomas: review of 28 cases and presentation of two cases with metastases and long survival. Am. J. Roentgenol. *85*, 733 (1961)
82. Kretschmer,H.L.: Sarcoma of the kidney and stone: report of a case and review of the literature. J. Urol. *36*, 99 (1936)
83. Kutzmann,A.A.: Leukoplakia of the renal pelvis. Arch. Surg. *19*, 871 (1929)
84. Kutzmann,T.J., Sauer,H.R.: A consideration of the problems presented by unilateral cystic kidney disease. J. Urol. *63*, 34 (1950)
85. Lazarus,J.A.: Primary tumour of the ureter with special reference to the malignant tumour; report of three cases. Ann. Surg. *99*, 769 (1934)
86. Lenarduzzi,G.: Reporto pielografico poco commune dilatazione delle view urinarie intrarenali. Radiol. Med. *26*, 346 and *26*, 884 (1939)
87. Lenarduzzi, G.: Sugli aspetti radiologici del rene a spugna. Commun. alla II Riunione Ass. Rad. Pad. Padova, 2 marzo (1958)
88. Lightwood,R.: Calcium infarction of kidneys in infants. Arch. Dis. Child. *18*, 205 (1935)
89. Lower,W.E., Belcher,G.W.: Renal infundibular stricture producing hydrocalyx. J. Urol. *12*, 121 (1924)
90. Lowsley,O.S.: Postcaval ureter, with description of a new operation for its correction. Surg. Gynecol. Obstet. *82*, 549 (1946)
91. MacDiarmid,J., Wallace,M.R., Reeder,J.: Exacerbation of nephrolithiasis by a carbonic amylase inhibitor. New Zealand Med. J. *79*, 687 (1974)
92. Mack,W.S., Buchanan,G.B.: Gonococcal infection of the upper urinary tract. Br. J. Urol. *10*, 150 (1938)
93. Mackenzie,A.R.: Acetazolamide-induced renal stone. J. Urol. *84*, 453 (1960)
94. Marquardt,H.: Incomplete renal tubular acidosis with recurrent nephrolithiasis and nephrocalcinosis. Urologe (A) *12*, 162 (1973)
95. Martin,H.H., Mertz,H.O: Tumours of the kidney and stone: report of a case of primary alveolar carcinoma of the pelvis associated with multiple stone. Mississipi Valley Med. J. *24*, 101 (1917)
96. McIntyre,D., Pyrah,L.N., Raper,F.P.: Primary ureteric neoplasms with a report on forty cases. Br. J. Urol. *37*, 160 (1965)
97. Meltzer,M.I.: Surgical polycystic kidney. Am. J. Surg. 7, 42 (1929)
98. Mims,M.M.: Multiple acquired diverticulosis of the ureter. J. Urol. *84*, 297 (1950)
99. Moore,T.: Hydrocalicosis. Br. J. Urol. *22*, 304 (1950)
100. Morin,L.J., Albert,D.J.: Milk-of-calcium stone in a renal cyst. J. Urol. *96*, 869 (1966)

101. Morris,R.C., Yamauchi,H., Palubinskas, A.J., Howenstine,J.: Medullary sponge kidney. Am. J. Med. *38*, 883 (1965)

102. Nation,E.F.: Horseshoe kidney: a study of 32 autopsy and 9 surgical cases. J. Urol. *53*, 762 (1945)

103. Newman,H.R.: Pelvic fused kidney with surgical removal of calculi. J. Urol. *56*, 169 (1946)

104. Olsen,S.: Associated renal pathology in renal tuberculosis. J. Urol. *23*, 81 (1930)

105. Oppenheimer,G.D.: Polycystic disease of the kidney. Ann. Surg. *100*, 1136 (1934)

106. Osathanondh,V., Potter,E.L.: Development of human kidney as shown by micro-dissection. V. Development of vascular pattern of glomerulus. Arch. Path. *82*, 403 (1966)

107. Parfitt,A.M.: Acetazolamide and renal stone formation. Lancet *II*, 153 (1970)

108. Parmenter,F.J., Foord,A.G., Leutenegger, C.J.: Gonococcal pyelonephritis. J. Urol. *24*, 359 (1930)

109. Paschkis,R.: Beiträge zur Pathologie des Nierenbeckens. Folia Urol. Leipz. *7*, 55 (1912)

110. Payne,R.A.: Clinical significance of re-duplicated kidneys. Br. J. Urol. *31*, 141 (1959)

111. Peacock,A.H.: Nephrolithiasis with infection. J. Urol. *49*, 370 (1943)

112. Phillips,T.L., Chin,F.G., Palubinskas,A.J.: Calcification in renal masses, an 11-year survey. Radiology *80*, 785 (1963)

113. Pitts,R.F., Alexander,R.S.: The nature of the renal tubular mechanism for acidifying the urine. Am. J. Physiol. *144*, 239 (1945)

114. Plaut,F.: Diffuses deckharne bulisches Adenom des Nierenbeckens mit gesch-wulstartiger Wucherung von Gesfäss-muskulatur. Z. Urol. Chir. *26*, 562 (1929)

115. Pomerantz,R.M., Kirschner, L.P., Twigg, H.L.: Renal milk-of-calcium collection: review of literature and report of a case. J. Urol. *103*, 18 (1970)

116. Potter,E.L., Osathanondh,V.: Medullary sponge kidney: two cases in young infants. J. Pediatr. *62*, 901 (1963)

117. Prather,G.C.: Calyceal diverticulum. J. Urol. *45*, 55 (1941)

118. Pullman,R.A.W., King,R.J.: Milk of calcium renal stone. Am. J. Roentgenol. *87*, 760 (1952)

119. Pyrah,L.N.: The calcium-containing renal stone. Proc. R. Soc. Med. *51*, 183 (1958)

120. Pyrah,L.N.: Medullary sponge kidney. Trans. Am. Assoc. Genito-urin. Surg. *57*, 67 (1965)

121. Pyrah,L.N.: Medullary sponge kidney. J. Urol. *95*, 274 (1966)

122. Pyrah,L.N., Hodgkinson,A.: Nephrocalcinosis. Br. J. Urol. *32*, 361 (1960)

123. Ragins,A.B., Rolnick,H.C.: Mucus-producing adenocarcinoma of the renal pelvis. J. Urol. *63*, 66 (1950)

124. Rall,J.E., Odel,H.M.: Congenital polycystic disease of the kidney. Review of literature and data on 207 cases. Am. J. Med. Sci. *218*, 399 (1949)

125. Ram,M.D., Chisholm,G.D.: Cystic disease of renal pyramids (medullary sponge kidney). Br. J. Urol. *41*, 280 (1969)

126. Raper,F.P.: Ureterocele in adults. Proc. R. Soc. Med. *51*, 781 (1958)

127. Rathbun,N.P.: Horseshoe kidney: infected hydronephrosis. Ann. Surg. *87*, 471 (1928)

128. Richardson,E.H.: Diverticulum of the ureter: a collective review with report of a unique example. J. Urol. *47*, 535 (1942)

129. Ross,J.C.: Calcification in genitourinary tuberculosis. Br. J. Urol. *42*, 656 (1970)

130. Rotter,H.: Dorsale Ureterverlagerung bei Abnormalien der unteren Hohlvene. Z. Anat. Entwicklungsgesch. *104*, 456 (1935)

131. Rousselot,L.M., Lamon,J.D.: Primary carcinoma of ureter: report of case and review of literature. Surg. Gynecol. Obstet. *50*, 17 (1930)

132. Rovsing,T.: Behendlung af det multiloculaere myrekysbon med multiple punktiner. Hospitalstid *4*, 105 (1911)

133. Rovsing,T.: Die Behandlung der multilokularen Nierencysten nebst Bemerkungen über die Art dieses Leidens. Dtsch. Med. Wochenschr. *52*, 614 (1926)

134. Rubin,E.L., Ross,J.C., Turner,D.P.B.: Cystic disease of the renal pyramids ('sponge kidney'). J. Fac. Radiol. *10*, 134 (1959)

135. Rudstrom,P.: Ein Fall von Nierenzyste mit eingenartiger Konkrementhildung. Acta Chir. Scand. *85*, 501 (1941)

136. Rule,C., Grollman,A.: Osteonephropathy: a clinical consideration of 'renal rickets'. Ann. Int. Med. *20*, 63 (1944)

137. Rusché,C.F., Bacon,S.K.: Congenital renal anomalies. Calif. Med. *50*, 344 (1939)

138. Sangree,H.K.: The management and prevention of renal and ureteric calculi. J. Urol. *59*, 842 (1948)

139. Schreiner,G.E., Smith,L.H., Kyle,L.H.: Renal hyperchloraemic acidosis. Familial occurrence of nephrocalcinosis with hyperchloraemia and low serum bicarbonate. Am. J. Med. *15*, 122 (1953)

140. Schwartz,A., Pfau,A., Weinberg,H.: Association of calyceal diverticulum and butterfly vertebra. J. Urol. *84*, 32 (1960)

141. Seery,W.H. et al.: Spontaneous rupture of pyelocaliceal diverticula. Urology *5*, 100 (1975)

142. Seldin,D.W., Wilson,J.D.: Renal tubular acidosis. In: The metabolic basis of inherited diseases. 2nd ed. Stanbury,J.B., Wyngaarden,J.B., Fredrickson,D.S. (eds.), p. 1230. New York: McGraw-Hill 1966

143. Shucksmith,H.S.: Spontaneous renoinguinal fistula in calculous tuberculous pyonephrosis. Br. J. Surg. *29*, 256 (1941–42)

144. Sieber,F.: Uber cystennieren bei Erwachaenen. Z. Chir. *79*, 406 (1905)

145. Simon,H.B., Thompson,G.J.: Congenital renal polycystic disease. A clinical and therapeutic study of 366 cases. J. Am. Med. Assoc. *159*, 657 (1955)

146. Smith,L.H.: Renal tubular acidosis. In: The metabolic basis of inherited diseases. Stanbury,J.S., Wyngaarden,J.B., Fredrickson,D.S. (eds.). New York: McGraw-Hill 1960

147. Smith,R.: Personal communication 1972)

148. Sommerkamp,H. et al.: Incomplete renal tubular acidosis in recurrent urinary phosphate calculi. Urologe (A) *12*, 167 (1973)

149. Sozer,J.T.: Squamous cell carcinoma and calculi. J. Urol. *99*, 264 (1968)

150. Swenson,I., MacMahon,H.E., Jaques, W.E., Campbell,J.S.: New concept of the etiology of megaloureter. N. Eng. J. Med. *245*, 41 (1952)

151. Tannen,R.L., Falls, W.F., Brackett,N.C.: Incomplete renal tubular acidosis: some clinical and physiological features. Nephron *15*, 111 (1975)

152. Thompson,G.J., Priestley,J.T.: Unilateral fused kidney complicated by stone in the 'left' ureter. J. Urol. *30*, 491 (1933)

153. Torassa,G.L.Jr.: Pyelitis glandularis. J. Urol. *60*, 393 (1948)

154. Utz,D.C., McDonald,J.R.: Squamous cell carcinoma of the kidney. J. Urol. *78*, 540 (1957)

155. Von Brunn,A.: Über drusenähnliche Bildingen in der Soleinhaut des Nierenbeckens des Ureters und der Harnblase beim Menschen. Arch. Mikrosc. Anat. *41*, 294 (1893)

156. Wagenknecht,L.V.: Association of hypernephroma and kidney calculus. Z. Urol. Nephrol. *67*, 121 (1974)

157. Walters,W., Braasch,W.F.: Surgical aspects of polycystic disease. A clinical and therapeutic study of 366 cases. J. Am. Med. Assoc. *159*, 657 (1934)

158. Watkins,K.H.: Cysts of the kidney due to hydrocalycosis. Br. J. Urol. *11*, 207 (1939)

159. Wershunt,L.P.: Calculi in tuberculous kidney. Q. J. Sea View Hosp. *1*, 441 (1935–36)

160. Williams,D.I.: The chronically dilated ureter. Ann. R. Coll. Surg. Engl. *14*, 107 (1954)

161. Williams,D.I.: In: Encyclopedia of urology. Alken,C.E., Dix,V.W., Weyrauch, H.M., Wildbolz,E. (eds.), Vol. 15. Berlin, Göttingen, Heidelberg: Springer 1958

162. Willis,R.: Pathology of tumours. 3rd ed. (1960)

163. Willson-Pepper,J.K.: Report on renal actinomycosis. Br. J. Urol. *23*, 160 (1951)

164. Willson-Pepper,J.K., Slade,D.A.: Calcification in a polycystic kidney. Br. J. Urol. *27*, 172 (1955)

165. Winsbury-White,H.P.: Renal calculus and hypernephroma. Br. J. Surg. *12*, 797 (1924–25)

166. Wrong,D., Davies,H.E.F.: The excretion of acid in renal disease. Q. J. Med. *28*, 359 (1959)

167. Yates-Bell,J.G.: Rovsing's operation for polycystic kidney. Lancet *I*, 126 (1957)

168. Yeates,W.K.: Personal communication (1961)

169. Young,J.N.: Retrocaval ureter with description of case complicated by ureteric calculus. Br. J. Urol. *19*, 22 (1947)

170. Young,H.H., Lehr,L.C.: Pyonephrosis due to B. typhosus. Johns Hopkins Hosp. Bull. *13*, 455 (1906)

Chapter 4

Some Extrarenal Diseases Associated with Renal Stone or Nephrocalcinosis

The commonest extrarenal diseases which are frequently or occasionally associated with renal calculi and/or nephrocalcinosis are a group of disorders of varied etiology in which there is some disturbance of calcium metabolism. The bony skeleton is frequently involved, either in the form of single or multiple localized pathological changes or as a generalized skeletal rarefaction. The renal stone or nephrocalcinosis is a kind of by-product of diseases with metabolic overtones, though either the symptoms associated with the renal calculus and/or the nephrocalcinosis, or the manifestations of the skeletal abnormality may present first.

The common etiological factors which are chiefly responsible for the incidence of calculi and/or nephrocalcinosis in this group of patients are hypercalcaemia and/or hypercalciuria, neither of which, however, are always present.

Hypercalcaemia is usually found in patients with primary hyperparathyroidism, frequently in patients with multiple myelomatosis and sarcoidosis and very occasionally (and temporarily) in those with immobilization osteoporosis (recumbency), but is usually absent in those with Cushing's syndrome and Paget's disease.

Hypercalciuria is present in a proportion of patients with primary hyperparathyroidism, during the early weeks of enforced recumbency, during the osteoclastic phase of Paget's disease and often in patients with Cushing's syndrome, myelomatosis, sarcoidosis and Wilson's disease. The two clinical conditions in this group of diseases of greatest practical importance to the urologist are primary hyperparathyroidism and recumbency calculi. The possibility of primary hyperparathyroidism presents itself with every patient with a calcium-containing renal stone, and in varied and sometimes disguised clinical form.

I. Primary Hyperparathyroidism

1. Pathology

The pathological types of hyperfunctioning parathyroid glands, knowledge of which emerged gradually between 1925 and 1958, give rise to an identical picture of clinical hyperparathyroidism including renal calculi and are as follows:

Single adenoma of one of the (usually) four parathyroid glands

Multiple adenomata affecting more than one gland

Primary wasserhelle or water-clear hyperplasia of all four glands

Primary chief-cell hyperplasia of all four glands

Carcinoma of the parathyroid gland

The single adenoma is the most common.

Renal Changes. The kidney is exposed to the action of an abnormally high level of circulating parathormone, which exercises a deleterious action on the renal cells. Parathormone injected into the experimental animal gives rise to calcification of the cells of the renal tubules, to PAS-staining casts within their lumina, to calcification of the basement membrane of the cells of Bowman's capsule, and probably to certain

Table 4.1. Incidence of principal symptoms in some series of cases of primary hyperparathyroidism

Authors	Skeletal changes only	Skeletal changes with renal calculi or nephrocalcinosis	Renal calculi or nephrocalcinosis only	No skeletal and no renal changes	No record	Total
Norris [68]	191	101	17	5	8	322
Albright and Reifenstein [1]	11	24	28	1		64
Black [6]	16	16	73	7		112
Hellstrom and Ivemark [42]	17	43	76	2		138
Dent [21]	27	11	73	14		125
Pyrah et al. [80]	17	20	26	3	2	68

changes in the renal ground substance including the accumulation of increased amounts of polysaccharides.

In the human kidney, microscopic changes observed in partial nephrectomy specimens obtained during the removal of calyceal calculi in patients with hyperparathyroidism are often slight. But in renal autopsy specimens from patients with advanced hyperparathyroidism, irreversible renal changes including fibrosis, cellular destruction and calcification have been found in keeping with the clinical deterioration of renal function gradually seen during life. According to some observers there is a release of protein from the bone matrix, which is excreted through the kidney and which may contribute to the observed changes.

Stone formation and nephrocalcinosis are encouraged by the existence of the calcific foci, themselves resulting from the hypercalcaemia and the frequently associated hypercalciuria. Similar changes can be found in other diseases in which there is hypercalcaemia (sarcoidosis, hypervitaminosis D). In advanced cases the surface of the kidney is furrowed and scarred and the organ somewhat reduced in size, the changes resembling those seen in chronic pyelonephritis. In patients who have died from acute hyperparathyroidism,

the renal changes are intensified, especially the calcification.

2. Clinical Picture

Primary hyperparathyroidism affects patients between the ages of 10 and 70 and the incidence in females in relation to that in males is approximately in the ratio of two to one. The patients when investigated may exhibit symptoms confined to one system only (skeletal, renal, abdominal or mental) or they may be deployed simultaneously or in sequence in breadth as a range of symptoms affecting several different organs and systems (Table 4.1). The presenting symptoms are often those of a general malaise, which may be difficult to relate to any syndrome but can be explained by the presence of hypercalcaemia.

The length of history before a diagnosis has been made has varied in reported series but it must usually depend upon how soon the clinician has become alerted to the possibility. In many patients nowadays the diagnosis is made following a single attack of renal colic. However, it is a measure of the chronicity of the disease that some patients apparently escape the worst effects of renal deterioration for a long time; some patients with renal calculus in the author's series had histories extending to 17, 20 (three cases) and 26 years respectively before they were referred for diagnosis.

Renal Manifestations. In the historical development of our knowledge of clinical primary hyperparathyroidism, it was the skeletal changes (including deformities and spontaneous fractures) to which the attention of surgeons was first drawn. An early report of Albright et al. [1], who had observed urinary calculi as a leading symptom in 10 of 17 patients, in 7 of whom they were the only manifestation of the disease, appears to have been largely overlooked.

Thus in the collected cases of primary hyperparathyroidism from the world literature published by Norris in 1947 [68], 332 in all, there were only 17 in which renal stone or nephrocalcinosis was the sole manifestation (skeletal disease being absent) though in 101 patients renal calculi or nephrocalcinosis were found in association with skeletal disease. However, during the last 30 years renal calculus (and sometimes nephrocalcinosis) has been recognized as the most common clinical manifestation of primary hyperparathyroidism.

Conversely, the true incidence of primary hyperparathyroidism in patients with calcium-containing renal calculi is still not known with certainty. Moreover, the figure probably varies in accordance with the special interest in any given clinic. In several published series the incidence has varied between 2% and 12%, though in McGeown's [63] series the incidence was 16.8%. Possibly the greater technical accuracy and availability of the appropriate biochemical tests sometimes determines the high incidence, as probably does the devotion of the urologist. Many patients with renal stone who also have a suspicion of skeletal changes or who are known to have had chronic duodenal ulcer or pancreatitis must especially be suspected of having hyperparathyroidism. The incidence

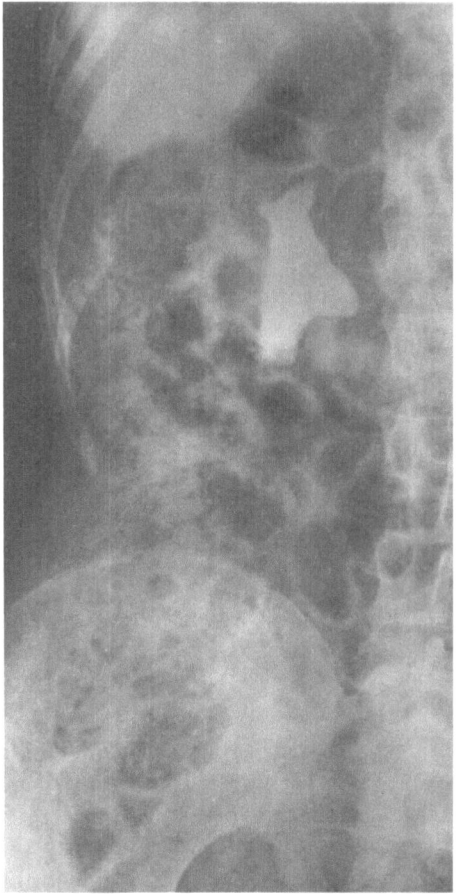

Fig. 4.1. Primary hyperparathyroidism in a woman of 45; the plain radiograph showed a massive staghorn stone in the left kidney, the urine being infected. There is generalized rarefaction of the bones and extensive cystic changes in the pelvic bones, especially the right side. The patient had had an amputation of the right leg some years before for a massive osteoclastoma at the lower end of the femur either for rupture of the tumour or spontaneous fracture, but the diagnosis of hyperparathyroidism had not been made at the time of the amputation

of that condition among patients with renal calculi is certainly higher than was thought to be the case two decades ago.

Patients with renal calculi present in a similar way to those with non-parathyroid renal calculi, namely with renal colic or pain, spontaneous voiding of calculi and occasionally haematuria (Fig. 4.1). Bilateral

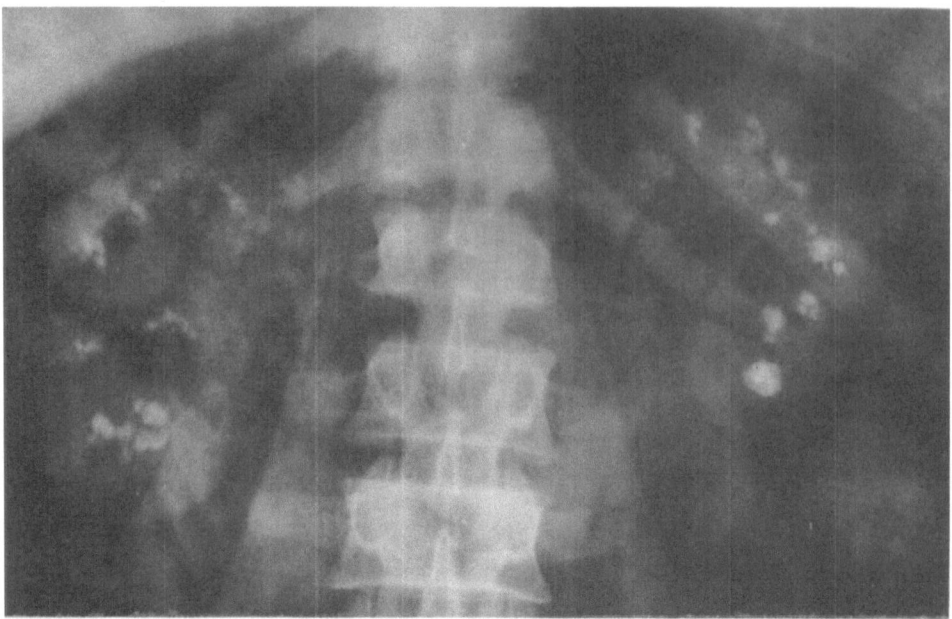

Fig. 4.2. A case of proven primary hyperparathyroidism with bilateral nephrocalcinosis; the calcific deposits are biggish and affect every renal pyramid

and recurrent renal calculi are common in any series of patients, and probably many such patients have hyperparathyroidism if it is looked for carefully. While usually the radiological appearance of the stone in the parathyroid patient does not differ from that in the non-parathyroid patient, occasionally the demonstration of a small group or cluster of small stones (which may be a variant of localized nephrocalcinosis) around one or more calyces may suggest hyperparathyroidism.

In earlier years, the author saw some advanced cases in which the disease had been active for a very long time, and bilateral calculi forming a cast of the renal pelvis and/or of some of the calyces were found. Such calculi, which are not usually of infective origin but are probably composed of apatite with much added organic matter are, in fact, soft, pasty masses existing in a sterile urinary tract. Following parathyroidectomy and a return of the serum calcium level to normal, such stones may disintegrate spontaneously and be voided completely within a few weeks, especially if the patient is given abundant oral fluids and ammonium chloride to acidify the urine.

Nephrocalcinosis, by which is meant the presence of multiple calcific radiologically demonstrable particles in or around the renal pyramids and the adjacent part of the medulla of one or both kidneys is a not infrequent variant of the more characteristic renal stone formation in hyperparathyroid patients. The condition may be found in association with calyceal or pelvic calculi (Fig. 4.2). The term nephrocalcinosis was first used by Albright et al. [1] to indicate in hyperparathyroid patients this occasional renal abnormality, which is now recognized in several other syndromes (of which medullary sponge kidney and renal tubular acidosis are the commonest).

Any patient with nephrocalcinosis from whatever cause, including hyperparathyroidism, may present clinically with backache, renal colic, the spontaneous voiding of calculi and haematuria, or a combination of these symptoms; in some patients it is symptomless at least for a long period. A patient who has nephrocalcinosis together with a spontaneous fracture of a long bone, may have either primary hyperparathyroidism or renal tubular acidosis (with which hypokalaemia is also associated). If it is found in association with a chronic gastric or duodenal ulcer, hyperparathyroidism or the milk-alkali syndrome may be the correct diagnosis.

In patients with primary hyperparathyroidism, more than the usual amount of urine is passed each day. A few patients void very large daily amounts (sometimes several litres) of urine of low specific gravity, so that the presence of diabetes insipidus is sometimes suspected. A continuous high daily intake of fluid (because of thirst) helps these patients to compensate in part for the loss of fluid; yet they feel ill and tired, lose weight and in the end may become dehydrated and acutely ill, when the level of the blood urea may rise. In some patients the polyuria persists for years with only mild symptoms. Following parathyroid adenomectomy, the output of urine falls dramatically and its specific gravity rises (sometimes gradually) and the feeling of well-being returns.

In patients with primary hyperparathyroidism the evidence suggests that the impaired renal function commonly found may be of two kinds, namely partly functional and reversible, and partly the consequence of an organic progressive and irreversible tubular lesion dependent upon renal fibrosis and calcification [26]. In the functional group there is interference with the power of the kidneys to concentrate the urine normally, probably because of renal tubular damage which has interfered with the normal tubular reabsorption of water. Such an abnormality may gradually disappear after parathyroid adenomectomy, though the return to normal is not always as striking nor as rapid as that seen in the extreme cases of polyuria. It is believed that the impairment of renal function is not entirely or chiefly the result of the renal stones and/or nephrocalcinosis; it is most marked in those patients with osteitis fibrosa in whom the renal parenchymal organic changes are most marked [29, 41, 42].

Because of the frequency of impairment of renal function and the known changes in the renal parenchyma, it is inevitable that hypertension should often complicate the middle and later term of the disease. Hypertension, which may have been observed long before the patient is operated on, may prevent a complete clinical recovery even after an apparently successful operation and may provide the background for an ultimate fatal ending many years after parathyroidectomy, from cerebro-vasculo-renal incidents.

Studies of hypertension in patients with hyperparathyroidism have shown that the percentage incidence of hypertension was lower in patients with renal stone or nephrocalcinosis alone, than in those who exhibited osteitis fibrosa [43]. Several late fatalities in patients who had hypertension both before and after parathyroidectomy were recorded, while patients who were normotensive both before and after operation survived. In the author's series of 68 patients with primary hyperparathyroidism, hypertension was present before operation or during follow-up in 19, no age-group being completely immune. Patients with renal calculi as well as those with combined renal and skeletal symptoms were affected; at least 3 patients died in later years from conditions believed to have been associated with the hypertension [80].

Non-renal Manifestations. Since many non-renal symptoms are often found in patients with primary hyperparathyroidism who also have renal calculi, the urologist has to be aware of the not infrequent skeletal, abdominal (peptic ulcer and pancreatitis) and mental symptoms. The condition occurs occasionally in children, some of whom have had calculi or nephrocalcinosis; the youngest case in the author's series was a girl aged 15.

A number of patients (several with renal calculi) had had a familial incidence [16]. The condition has been recognized in pregnant women, with important consequences on the newly born infant (maternal hyperparathyroidism).

Gout has been not infrequently associated with hyperparathyroidism. In another group the disease has been discovered by chance (serendipity). It is beyond the scope of this chapter to refer to these groups in detail but they have been described elsewhere by the author [80].

Acute Hyperparathyroidism. Primary hyperparathyroidism in most patients pursues the slow clinical course of a chronic illness with skeletal, renal, abdominal, hypertensive or mental symptoms or a combination of them. Relevant to this sequence is the fact that in such patients the levels of the serum calcium are usually between 10.6 and 13.0 mg/100 ml, only rarely exceeding 14 or 15 mg. Following successful operative removal of the parathyroid abnormality the patient escapes what would otherwise have been the severe terminal stage of the disease, namely, either cardio-vasculo-renal disease with one of the usual terminal events of that syndrome, or the acute form of the disorder with severe and urgent symptoms which may precipitate a rapidly fatal ending in the absence of urgent treatment, and known as 'acute hyperparathyroidism'.

Patients with renal calculi and nephrocalcinosis as well as those with the other manifestations of the disease have been found to develop this condition. The biochemical evidence suggests that in such cases the onset of the acute phase is determined by a critical high level of the serum calcium of 16–20 mg/100 ml and that such symptoms are most likely to arise if the renal function is moderately or seriously impaired as a consequence of the prolonged hypercalcaemia.

A similar acute syndrome is occasionally found in association with other diseases in which hypercalcaemia is present (sarcoidosis, hypernephroma with or without skeletal metastases, hypervitaminosis D and myelomatosis). Females are affected more than males. Occasionally acute hyperparathyroidism appears to have been precipitated in patients known to have been moderately but not desperately ill, following parathyroid adenomectomy or some other surgical operation (such patients having had a high level of serum calcium before operation).

It follows that no such operation, not even, for example, the removal of a stone in the kidney, should be done until the severe hypercalcaemia has been corrected as far as possible by the appropriate medical treatment, when the operation can be carried out with comparative safety. Usually the patient has for a long time had renal and other symptoms in keeping with a diagnosis of hyperparathyroidism which, however, may have remained unrecognized. Urgent symptoms gradually appear, including fatigue, transient loss of consciousness, increasing drowsiness, muscular weakness, mental confusion, passing into fatal coma accompanied by circulatory collapse. In another group acute symptoms are ushered in by nausea, anorexia and vomiting, so that subacute intestinal obstruction may be suspected.

Cases of acute hyperparathyroidism have been described by several observers [69, 91]. A fatal case with bilateral renal calculi was reported by Thomas et al. [94], who collected 19 cases from the literature. Of the 3 fatal cases of acute hyperparathyroidism in the author's series one, a female aged 61, who died following an emergency partial gastrectomy for recurrent haematemesis from a peptic ulcer, had at autopsy a calyceal calculus, nephrocalcinosis and an unsuspected chief-cell parathyroid adenoma. In the most striking case the patient was subsequently shown to have had not only a massive infected stone but also a carcinoma of the left kidney, both conditions being shown to have contributed to the high serum calcium level and to the ultimate fatal issue [80]. In the series of 42 cases collected from the literature by Lehmann and Donatelli [57] nephrolithiasis or nephrocalcinosis was present in 14.

3. Biochemical Diagnosis

Since most patients with renal stones and primary hyperparathyroidism seen by the urologist have no radiological evidence of skeletal disease, the diagnosis must depend entirely on the biochemical investigations [5]. Of the routine tests the finding of a raised serum calcium level is still the most important; the normal range in the author's department is 9.3–10.7 mg/100 ml. Any level above the upper limit has been thought to be consistent with a possible diagnosis of hyperparathyroidism, if other causes of hypercalcaemia have been excluded. Other laboratories work within slightly different ranges.

In an analysis of 71 proven cases Yendt and Gagne [106] regarded the normal level as being between 8.9 and 10.3 mg/100 ml (that for females being slightly lower than that for males). The remarkable constancy of the serum calcium level in their patients has been stressed by some workers. On the other hand in some of our patients with proven hyperparathyroidism, the serum calcium levels estimated, say, during a 12-month period have shown some variation within narrow limits and in one patient the mean value never exceeded 10.7 mg/100 ml [80].

In a few reported patients there have been spontaneous variations in the level of the serum calcium shown subsequently to have been the result of infarction of the

parathyroid adenoma, resulting from interference with the blood supply, leading to variations in its functional activity. The average levels of the serum calcium and the mean weight of the parathyroid adenoma are significantly lower in patients with renal stones than in those with skeletal disease [59] and it would be expected that the level in patients with stone in association with very small tumours would only slightly exceed the normal level. The daily oral administration of 150 mg cortisone for 10 days has been found to reduce a high level of serum calcium to normal in patients with hypervitaminosis D and sarcoidosis whereas the hypercalcaemia of hyperparathyroidism remains unaffected]20].

It has been shown in recent years that a few patients with renal calculi and normocalcaemia have proven adenomata or hyperplasia of the parathyroids; such patients have usually been within certain clinical groups (idiopathic hypercalciuria; recurrent renal calculi). Since comparatively few patients with normocalcaemia have so far been submitted to an exploratory operation on the neck to search for a possible hyperfunctioning parathyroid, it is not yet possible to assess the number of such patients. It is not yet known with certainty how long a time must pass before a functioning adenoma gives rise to sustained hypercalcaemia.

Patients with hyperparathyroidism and normocalcaemia have been reported by several observers [48, 64, 104, 106]; such reports have mostly referred to patients with renal calculi and have been reviewed by Wills [103], though a few have had skeletal changes (see Chap. 8 on Idiopathic Hypercalciuria). In some patients with hyperparathyroidism the proportion of serum-ionized calcium and of protein-bound calcium may be changed, and a normal total serum calcium reading may hide an abnormal ultrafilterable or ionized calcium [60]; however, the level of the serum-ionized calcium is perhaps of limited value in routine clinical investigations though valuable in research.

While the clinical history and physical examination, together with a careful use of diagnostic tests, will usually enable the cause of the hypercalcaemia in a given patient to be established, the problem of diagnosis is occasionally complicated by the presence in the same patient of more than one cause of hypercalcaemia, as in one patient of the author's who had massive renal calculi and renal carcinoma and another who had renal calculi with hyperparathyroidism and sarcoidosis [80].

The normal range of the serum inorganic phosphate level in the author's laboratory is 2.5–4.3 mg/100 ml (mean $\pm$ S.D.). The mean preoperative values in 48 proven cases of primary hyperparathyroidism (most having renal calculi) were below 2.5 mg/100 ml in 26 (54%) and within the lower normal range in 22. Low levels of the inorganic phosphate have also been found in some patients with idiopathic hypercalcaemia [27] and in many patients with calculi with normocalciuria.

The serum alkaline phosphatase level is usually raised when there is radiological evidence of skeletal disease, in patients with or without renal calculi.

The level of the urinary calcium was found to be elevated in many early reported (skeletal) cases of hyperparathyroidism with or without renal calculi. But in patients with predominantly renal symptoms hypercalciuria is not a constant finding. Thus in the author's series of cases (most having renal calculi) 12 of 37 patients with primary hyperparathyroidism (32%) had values within the normal range; similar findings were recorded by Yendt and Gagne [106]. The calcium balance is usually negative in patients with severe hyperparathyroidism (especially in those with skeletal changes) while those with milder grades (including many patients with renal calculi) are frequently in calcium balance on a normal diet.

The electrophoretic pattern of the serum proteins is usually normal unless there is extensive renal glomerular damage. Some of the more specialized biochemical tests including the phosphate clearance test, the phosphate deprivation test and the calcium infusion test were reviewed by the author [80].

Parathyroid hormone is an amino acid single-chain polypeptide with a molecular weight of approximately 9500 and its synthesis and secretion are controlled chiefly by the level of the ionized calcium in the circulating blood. Attempts to assay the level of parathormone in the blood, reviewed by Parfitt [71], have made progress in recent years using immunological techniques but have not yet reached the stage of easy application in the clinically difficult case of hyperparathyroidism [82].

4. Treatment

When primary hyperparathyroidism has been considered proven by clinical examination and biochemical tests, early operation to remove the hyperfunctioning parathyroid tissue (adenoma or hyperplasia) if the patient is fit, is indicated, since it is the only method of treatment known to be satisfactory.

In the patients with renal calculi, we have had, as have others, a number of cases in which the diagnosis of hyperparathyroidism has been in doubt, the serum calcium levels being in the upper normal range, with an occasional reading above the upper normal level for our laboratory. In such cases the surgeon has to decide whether to continue to keep the patient under observation for months or even years doing serum calcium estimations at intervals, or whether to do a deliberate exploratory operation on the neck. Otherwise he may regard the patient as having very mild hyperparathyroidism, hoping that little harm may result from leaving a small adenoma in the neck, at least until such time as a firm biochemical diagnosis has been made; such problems admit of no easy answer.

In the author's department the neck has been explored in a few patients with renal stone, in whom the diagnosis was doubtful, and sometimes a parathyroid tumour has been found. Many have been kept under long-term observation and some eventually have had a worthwhile operation. The author has usually felt it inadvisable to carry out exploratory operations on the neck in many patients with bilateral or recurrent renal calculi who have been thought by others to have hyperparathyroidism on the grounds of supposed high serum calcium levels, but which we ourselves have been unable to confirm.

The recent reports concerning some patients with renal stone who have normocalcaemic hyperparathyroidism may show that such a course has not always been completely justified, or at least that there is still room for closer study and for exploration of the neck in some doubtful cases.

Operation should not, generally speaking, be refused to any patient because of advanced skeletal deformities (with or without renal stone); in fact such patients usually withstand operation on the neck reasonably well. Detailed studies of the anatomy of the parathyroids were made by Gilmour and Martin [30]. Description of the operation to remove parathyroid tumour (which is beyond the scope of this book) has been given by several authors [11, 19, 80, 97].

Operative treatment for the renal calculi in patients with proved hyperparathyroidism is usually necessary. The wisest course is to remove the parathyroid adenoma or the hyperplastic glands before dealing surgically with the stones, the normal physiology then having been restored. It is necessary in every case to take a radiograph of the exposed kidney in the operating theatre, since it is more likely than in patients with non-parathyroid calculi that small pericalyceal calcific particles or small calculi (scarcely visible on the plain radiograph), will be present in addition to the stone for the removal of which the operation is being done.

Most renal calculi removed from patients with hyperparathyroidism are composed of calcium oxalate with or without an admixture of calcium phosphate; a few stones have had a nucleus of uric acid surrounded by mixed calcium oxalate and phosphate. If the parathyroid adenoma is removed and the calculi are not subsequently removed (apart from the soft pasty calculi in patients with skeletal symptoms previously referred to) they may continue to increase in size as do non-parathyroid calculi.

Parathyroid adenomectomy reduces the chance of recurrence following the operative removal of renal stone. In patients with nephrocalcinosis it is not possible by surgical means to remove the calcific masses so that operative treatment is not indicated unless there are associated obstructing renal or ureteric calculi. Moreover, even when a successful parathyroid adenomectomy has been carried out, the nephrocalcinosis does not disappear, though it does not appear to become worse, as shown by inspection of periodic successive radiographs. Renal function, however, may show gradual deterioration in such patients.

In patients with hypercalcaemia above the level of 15 mg/100 ml, operation for removal of the hyperfunctioning parathyroid should be postponed until measures have been applied to reduce the level of the high serum calcium. The patient should be given a low-calcium high-phosphorus diet (100 mg calcium/day or less). Dehydration should be corrected by the intravenous infusion of saline, and abnormal serum electrolyte levels (which may vary from a hypokalaemic alkalosis to a hyperchloraemic acidosis) should be corrected.

The administration of thyrocalcitonin may be tried.

Sodium phosphate in daily oral doses of 10–15 mg has been shown to result in a prompt and sustained fall in the level of the serum calcium [22], and this treatment is probably the best available. In one case the intravenous administration of sodium phosphate was followed by tetany, thereby demonstrating its effectiveness in reducing the level of the ionized calcium; the daily dose of phosphate should therefore be carefully controlled. In fact ectopic calcification may be aggravated by the long-term use of phosphate treatment in such patients. Good results following the treatment of 20 patients with hypercalcaemia from various causes using phosphate either orally or intravenously have been reported by Goldsmith and Ingbar [31]; the serum calcium level usually fell promptly to normal.

The intravenous infusion of sodium sulphate has been shown to increase the urinary excretion of calcium in the experimental animal and may be useful in the treatment of human hypercalcaemia. Ethylene-diamine tetra-acetic acid (EDTA) is a chelating agent which will incorporate a metal to form a stable ring structure and has an effect in reducing the ionized calcium, and may be used when hypercalcaemia is threatening life.

Haemodialysis may be useful in some patients. Once stable readings of serum calcium at a near normal level have been achieved, the immediate danger of acute hyperparathyroidism has passed and operative removal of the tumour may be carried out with safety.

II. Immobilization Osteoporosis and Recumbency Urolithiasis

1. Incidence

The formation of renal stones is amongst the more serious complications of recumbency. Though theoretically preventable and though less common than formerly, stones still occur among patients with traumatic paraplegia, poliomyelitis and orthopaedic disease necessitating prolonged rest or treatment in a respirator. The declining incidence of these stones owes much to the development and facilities of the spinal injuries centres.

Early reports of a high incidence of renal stone in paraplegics coming to autopsy appeared nearly 100 years ago, and also in patients undergoing treatment in recumbency for Pott's disease. During the 1914–1918 war, many paraplegic soldiers who survived for a long time, formed renal calculi. The possible relationship of such calculi to osteoporosis during recumbency was pointed out by Watson-Jones and Roberts [99], who stated that during immobilization 'generalized disuse depletes the calcium store of the whole skeleton' and that 'nephrolithiasis is the result of skeletal decalcification and is comparable with the nephrolithiasis of hyperparathyroidism'. An early attempt to prevent the formation of recumbency calculi was introduced by Pugh [76], who designed a tilting frame which enabled children with tuberculous spinal disease to be turned regularly from the supine to the prone position in order to interrupt the daily period of total recumbency. Reports of cases of recumbency calculi were published by the author [79], who described the most important etiological factors, and by Pulvertaft [77].

In spite of increasing awareness of the condition, many paraplegic patients during World War II developed calculi, there being at first no special facilities for the reception and treatment of such patients. Spinal injuries centres were made available in Great Britain from 1944 onwards and many were established in the United States [36, 37], the patients being placed under the care of one clinician. This led to the gradual improvment in facilities for mobilization, physiotherapy, occupational therapy, sport

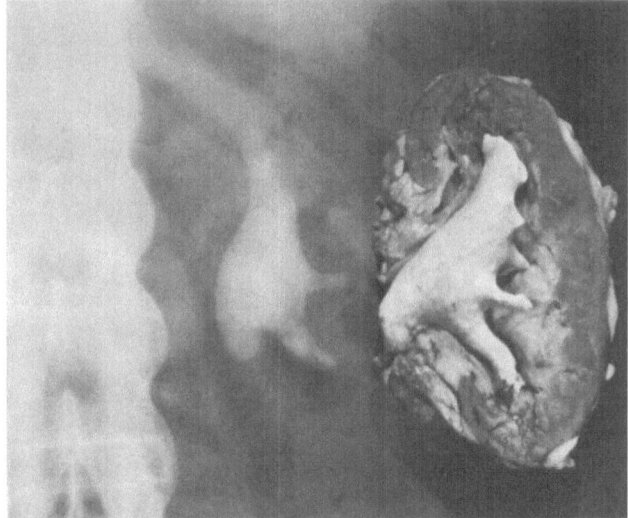

Fig. 4.3. A male patient aged 37, with ankylosing spondylitis, who had been treated in recumbency for a prolonged period. He developed a staghorn infected calculus in the left kidney, which had to be removed because of his clinical symptoms. The kidney showed infective changes around the large stone, which occupied the renal pelvis and most of the calyces

and laboratory and bacteriological services, all of which gradually relieved the lot of the patient [9].

Among early records Wilson [105] reported renal colic in 10% of 105 patients immobilized in 1919 with fractured femora, and Key [50] found renal calculi in 20% of 162 children immobilized for over 3 months for the treatment of surgical tuberculosis. Pulvertaft [77] reported a series of 184 cases of recumbency calculi including 60 of his own patients.

Examples began to be reported of calculi in patients with spinal injuries (with infected urine) especially in those with quadriplegia [37]. With the establishment of units for the early treatment of patients with spinal injuries the incidence of recumbency calculi began to fall; thus in one series a decrease from 12% in 1945–1950 to 1% in 1950–1955 was noted [12], and similar improvements were noted by other observers. The incidence of recumbency calculi fell in patients with poliomyelitis (for example, during epidemics in North America in 1951–1955) and especially in those receiving artificial respiration [28], up to 80% of such patients being so affected during some epidemics [74]. Trauma alone (other than war injury) still accounts for a considerable

annual number of patients with recumbency calculi (Fig. 4.3).

2. Causes

The state of recumbency is the all-important cause, and the various and detailed contributory factors all stem from that single cause, and may be considered under the headings of urinary stasis, urinary infection and alteration in the metabolism of bone and calcium.

Urinary Stasis. Recumbent patients in bed (unless carefully supervised) have a lower fluid intake than usual and have a consequently low urinary output, a factor which contributes to urinary stasis and which should be countered by diuresis (which also assists in the mechanical removal of particles and cellular debris) (Fig. 4.4, see p. 80).

The posture of the recumbent patient is not favourable to urinary drainage, the renal calyces then being situated well below the renal pelvis, which can only empty through its highest point into the ureter, and even here the urine has to flow uphill as far as the brim of the bony pelvis. The combined effects of posture and gravity

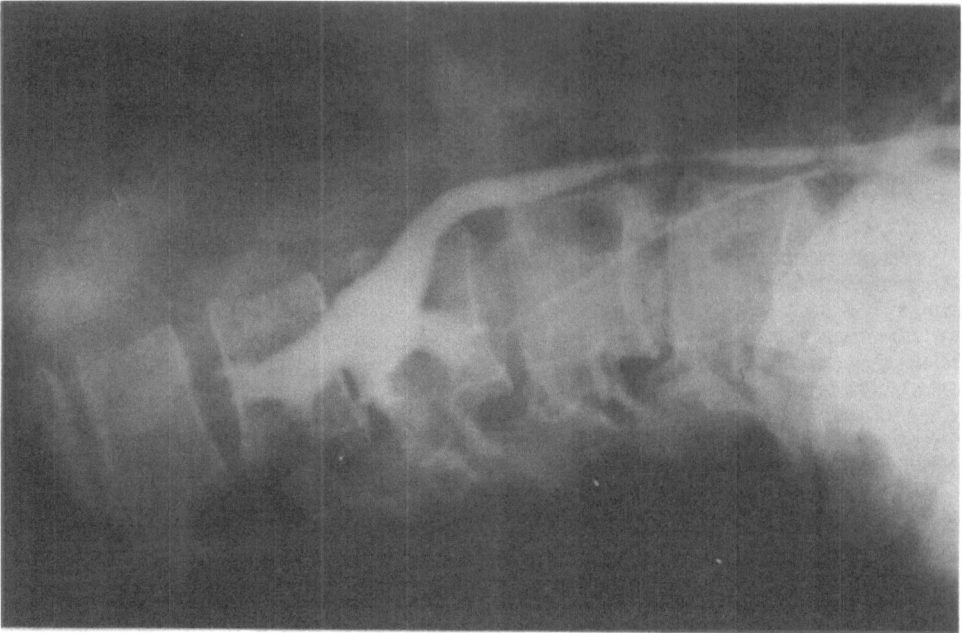

Fig. 4.4. The X-ray shows the lateral pyelogram of a normal kidney taken with the patient lying flat on his back. The film illustrates that the calyces in a recumbent patient occupy the lowest part of the pelvis-calyx system. The ureter in its descent lies on a plane which is inclined upwards. The radiograph illustrates that crystalline particles would be voided with difficulty into the bladder against the force of gravity

account for the accumulation of calcific debris in the renal calyces (especially in the upper calyx), as well as for ineffective suprapubic drainage when this has been instituted; the first clinical symptom of a stone may be renal colic experienced only when the patient first gets up.

Impaired function of the bladder (with a variable amount of residual urine) is by far the most important cause of urinary stasis; the after-care of the bladder is designed to minimize the deleterious effects. Ureteric reflux and hydroureter. (shown by cystography), which has been reported in frequencies ranging from 12% to 66% in several series [7, 8] is ultimately responsible for much ascending infection and dilatation of the upper urinary tract, and increases the chance of stone formation.

Urinary Infection. The most common and the most frequently fatal complication in

the paraplegic patient, urinary infection is usually the result of catheterization and is almost invariable if suprapubic cystostomy is done. Various forms of *B. proteus* and *Ps. pyocyaneus*, which are the most common infecting organisms, are dangerous, since they render the urine strongly alkaline by splitting urea into ammonia and therefore providing a urinary pH favourable to the precipitation of calcium phosphate. Infection has the effect of converting a less harmful phosphatic cast of the renal calyces into a definitive calculus. Infection is also deleterious in respect of returning vesical function (Fig. 4.5).

Metabolic Factors. With the change from full activity to complete bed rest, the most significant change concerned with the possibilities of renal stone formation is the great increase of the urinary calcium, resulting from its removal from the bones,

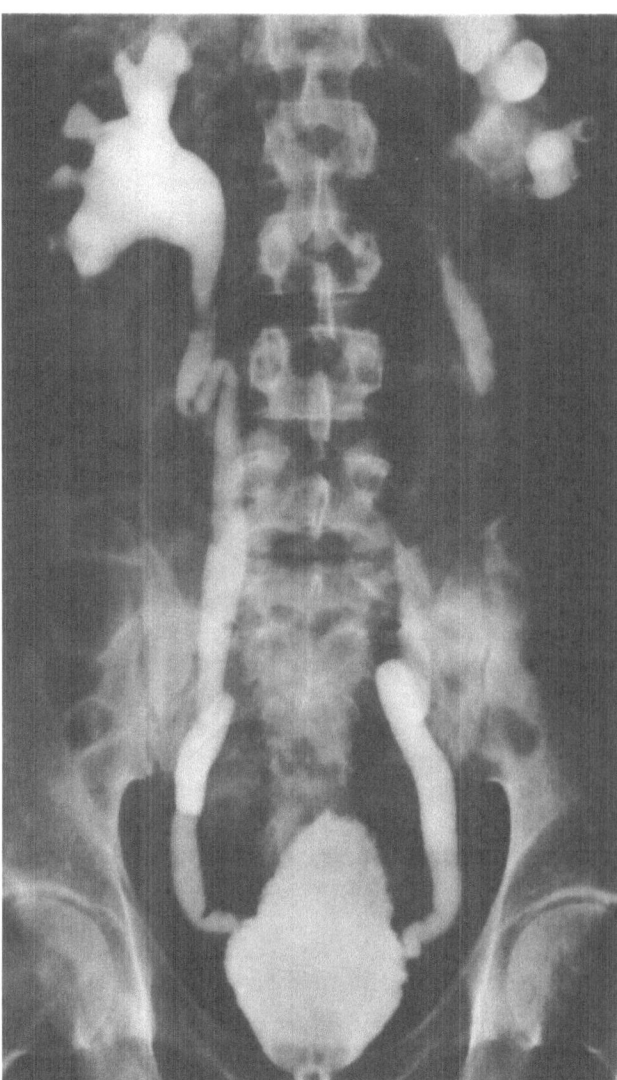

Fig. 4.5. R.H., male. This patient sustained a complete paraplegia from a stab wound in July 1969. Rehabilitation was satisfactory but he developed a bilateral hydronephrosis. A micturating cystogram 10 months after the injury showed bilateral vesicoureteric reflux. Following treatment with an indwelling catheter his kidneys returned virtually to normal radiologically. (By courtesy of Mr. P. Smith, F.R.C.S.)

which gradually become porotic. The 1 kg calcium contained in the bony skeleton, stored as tiny crystals of apatite, bathed in extracellular fluid to which they expose a surface area of about 100 m^2/g bone, or a total surface even exceeding 100 acres, is in a state of ceaseless activity during life so that small changes of bone metabolism materially affect the urinary excretion of calcium extensively, and if acute enough, may affect the serum calcium level.

Allison and Brooks [3] divided the brachial plexus of experimental animals and found that 30% of calcium was lost from the bones of the affected limb in 24 days. Dietrich et al. [25] examined the metabolic changes of calcium and other elements in four healthy conscientious objectors during 7 weeks of immobilization in plaster casts and compared the results with equivalent data obtained during similar periods of activity before and afterwards. It was found that while the active healthy adult just maintains a positive calcium balance, strict rest precipitates a loss of calcium by way of the urine within 48 h, a loss which reaches a peak in 4–5 weeks, lasts for at least 10 weeks during immobilization and even continues for 2–3 weeks after the resumption of full activity [45]. When healthy men on a fixed intake were immobilized for 7 weeks, the average calcium balance changed from +128 to −100 mg daily; the urinary calcium was more than doubled (up to 275 mg/day).

During immobilization associated with fractures the peak loss occurs earlier and the total loss may be twice as great (presumably due to adrenocorticoid activity). When immobilization follows serious paralysis the loss of calcium is even greater, the urinary calcium reaching as much as 1 g daily and may exceed 0.5 g/day for many months, with a negative balance lasting sometimes for a year or more [102]. The introduction of exercise during recumbency (such as the use of a bed bicycle for 5 min or more per day) will reduce the hypercalciuria in recumbent children. Recumbency may produce some rise of serum calcium (varying from 0.5 to 1.4 mg/100 ml) though not necessarily above the normal range. Hypercalcaemia, which was found in recumbent children by Howard et al. [45] and in 10 of 11 children with severe poliomyelitis [70], is a contributory cause to renal stone formation. While the amount of urinary phosphate is closely related to the dietetic intake of phosphate it has been found that when healthy men on a fixed intake of phosphorus were immobilized, their average urinary phosphate rose by 120 mg/day and their overall phosphate balance remained negative until physical activity was resumed. Although recumbency during health raised the urinary pH of volunteers by only 0.15, recumbency because of poliomyelitis caused a greater rise in pH, which was more difficult to influence by drugs and diet [28], and resultant alkalinity in such cases can greatly influence stone formation.

In a study by Poole-Wilson [75] of 61 patients with poliomyelitis who had survived with the aid of long-term respiratory support, it was found that renal calculi were much commoner in patients supported by the tank respirator or cuirass than in those treated by intermittent positive-pressure ventilation. Most of the calculi had developed in the first 5 years after the onset of the poliomyelitis and there was no obvious difference in the extent or severity of the paralysis. The plasma bicarbonate level in patients treated with intermittent positive-pressure ventilation (14–18 mEq/litre) was lower than that in those treated using the tank (19–292 mEq/litre): this difference was thought to be the result of hyperventilation, possibly resulting in a rise of the urinary pH, which itself would probably increase the chance of calculous disease.

3. Special Characteristics

A faint opacity outlining one or more renal calyces, later becoming denser and goblet-shaped from the deposition of a fine phosphatic cast on the calyceal wall, are the earliest findings of recumbency calculi to be seen on the radiograph. Such a cast may grow to fill the lumina of the calyces and/or pelvis with a pultaceous 'mud-stone', often so big as to suggest large staghorn calculi, parts of which may break away and descend down the ureter. In the absence of infection, such masses may undergo spontaneous disintegration when the patient achieves mobility and is given fluids generously. If the urine becomes infected, for example with *B. proteus*, with consequent urinary alkalinity, the soft material hardens to form a true struvite or apatite staghorn stone.

In any given series, single small or medium-sized rounded or ovoid calculi are most common and are mostly phosphatic, though pure calcium oxalate calculi have been found in sterile urine [77]. The calculi, in addition to causing pain and possibly haematuria, may lead to impairment of renal function, especially if there is associated urinary infection; and indeed may contribute to a fatal ending. The presence of urinary calculi in paraplegic patients may be camouflaged by sensory paralysis consequent upon the spinal injury.

4. Treatment

The prevention of the formation of recumbency calculi in the paraplegic patient depends essentially upon the successful management of the bladder. Paralysis of the urinary bladder resulting from spinal cord injury carries a high risk of urinary infection (and of ultimate stone formation and renal failure) because of the necessity to relieve urinary retention. The objectives of prevention of infection, low residual urine and high urinary flow are not easy to obtain; the patient with a spinal cord injury should be admitted within a short time to a special unit, and because of the tendency for urinary output to be reduced following injury, catheterization may generally be deferred until such admission has been achieved.

Intermittent catheterization every 6–8 h is most commonly employed (using every precaution against the introduction of infection including urinary antiseptics), the aim being to produce a reflex bladder with satisfactory emptying in the presence of a spinal cord lesion, or satisfactory emptying of the bladder by straining, in the presence of a lower motor neurone lesion. The precise timing of catheterization and the daily fluid intake should be arranged in such a way that the bladder is drained when it contains sufficient urine to promote reflex contraction but not so much as to cause distension.

The patient must be trained to appreciate abnormal sensations which indicate fullness of the bladder, and be instructed to attempt to empty his bladder by suprapubic pressure. Antibiotics instilled into the bladder at the end of every catheterization may lead to a urine virtually free from infection [73]. Intermittent catheterization may be reduced (or eventually stopped) when residual urine after voiding has reached a satisfactory level. Further details of the management of the urinary tract including the operative methods sometimes needed in intractable cases of retention should be obtained from special papers [13].

The treatment of established recumbency calculi varies from patient to patient. The urine should be kept acid by appropriate medicines and the level of urinary calcium be kept low by available measures. The administration of phosphates may be helpful. It has been shown that some soft non-infected calculi will disintegrate and be voided when the patient has achieved mobility. Small asymptomatic calculi in mobile patients may safely be left in the hope that they will be voided. Larger renal calculi associated with persistent renal infection should be removed surgically earlier rather than later in paraplegics, who usually withstand such operations quite well.

III. Diseases of Other Ductless Glands

1. Cushing's Syndrome

Cushing's syndrome results from the excessive production of cortisol by the adrenal cortex, which is stimulated to secrete the hormone by corticotrophin (ACTH) secreted by the anterior lobe of the pituitary gland, which in turn is stimulated by a corticotrophin-releasing factor (CRF) produced by the hypothalamus. Basophil or chromophobe adenomata of the anterior lobe of the pituitary, which have been found to be present in about half the patients with Cushing's syndrome examined at autopsy, are not usually recognizable during life. Locally malignant invasive pituitary adenomata are found occasionally; in

Table 4.2. Renal calculi in patients with Cushing's disease

Author	Year	No. of cases with Cushing's disease	Cases of urinary calculi	Remarks
Cope and Raker [14]	1955	46	11	The calculi were symptomless in 3 patients
Soffer et al. [91]	1955	40	3	Six additional patients had radiologically demonstrable cholelithiasis
Wang and Robbins [97]	1956	38	13 (24%)	Calculi were small and were unilateral or bilateral. Nephrocalcinosis was not observed
Scholz et al. [88]	1957	17	11 (65%)	
Horwith and Stokes [44]	1960	44	4 (11%)	
Ross et al. [87]	1966	50	8	Five of the 8 patients also had gallstones
Welbourn [100]	1969	52	8	Two patients needed operation for renal calculi; 21 had radiological evidence of osteoporosis. Nine had pathological fractures

patients without demonstrable pituitary adenomata, there is believed to be an overaction of the pituitary resulting in hyperplasia of the adrenal glands, which may be enlarged to twice their normal size or more. Alternatively the adrenal may be the site of a benign adenoma or of a carcinoma, tumours which are believed to be largely autonomous and no longer under the control of the pituitary.

The presenting symptoms include obesity, moon-face, menstrual irregularity, weakness, acne, hirsutism and bruising. The symptoms of the developed disease are general muscular weakness, backache, obesity, a florid complexion associated with purpura and bruising, oedema of the ankles, pigmentation of the skin and hypertension; supraclavicular pads of fat and the 'buffalo hump' are prominent features. In advanced cases there are bone changes and sometimes mental symptoms.

Renal Calculi. The serum calcium level is usually normal though occasionally above normal. Horwith and Stokes [44] recorded a negative calcium balance in 3 of 12 patients examined, with excessive urinary calcium loss on a low-calcium diet; presumably this factor is the chief contribution to the common renal stone formation. The administration of ACTH, cortisone and desoxycorticosterone cause a negative calcium balance with an increase in the urinary and faecal excretion of calcium in man [92].The pituitary may not act directly on the kidney in this respect but in humans after hypophysectomy, there is a fall in the urinary excretion of calcium.

Symptoms and signs similar to those in Cushing's syndrome are produced in nonendocrine patients by the prolonged administration of cortisone or hydrocortisone; the hypercalciuria following prolonged high dosage with cortisone may be counteracted by the administration of large doses of oestrogens to females and of androgens to males.

The incidence of renal stone in various reported series of cases of Cushing's disease has varied from 4% to 65% (Table 4.2); the stones may be symptomless and only discovered on routine radiography. A stone was present in Cushing's first patient [15].

Stones causing symptoms must usually be removed surgically but the calculous disease is unlikely to be cured permanently unless the presence of Cushing's disease is recognized and given radical treatment. Shortland and Crane [90] in a study of renal biopsies from 19 patients with Cushing's syndrome observed microscopic renal calcification, which may partly explain the origin of the calculi.

While subtotal adrenalectomy has been used in the treatment of Cushing's disease, adrenalectomy with cortisone replacement is the most satisfactory form of treatment in patients with adrenal hyperplasia. The removal of unilateral hyperfunctioning adrenal tumours can prove curative. Patients with pituitary adenoma may be treated with Yttrium 90 introduced directly into the gland, in order to reduce its size and functional activity; it is probably not so reliable as total adrenalectomy [100].

2. Acromegaly

Acromegaly, resulting from an adenoma of the anterior lobe of the pituitary gland, may exist as a clinical entity on its own, or be one of the several manifestations of the syndrome of multiple endocrine adenomatosis; it is occasionally complicated by renal calculi. It is a disease affecting both sexes equally, usually in the third and fourth decades, and is occasionally familial.

The onset of the disease is insidious and the diagnosis is often made from the patient's general appearance; characteristic symptoms are excessive sweating, paraesthesiae of the hands and feet, pain in the digits and joints, loss of libido, amenorrhoea or impotence, polyuria, visual disturbances. Objectively there is enlargement of the hands and feet, bowing of the legs (with a rolling gait), enlargement and protrusion of the lower jaw with thickening of the skin especially on the face, lips and brows, and enlargement of some of the

bones (ribs, clavicles, vertebral bodies) and of the viscera. In spite of these changes the patient may live to old age, life usually being terminated by degenerative vascular disease.

Renal Calculi. Patients with renal calculi and acromegaly were reported by Zubrod et al. [107], Vancil and Locke [95] and by Hartog [40]. In the author's own experience, a male patient, aged 69, who had acromegaly but no clinical or biochemical evidence of hyperparathyroidism, had bilateral renal calculi, which were successfully removed by operation.

In patients in whom there is an association with hyperparathyroidism, hypercalcaemia and hypercalciuria contribute to renal stone formation. A patient with acromegaly and a parathyroid adenoma reported by Hadfield and Rogers [38] had renal calculi, and a similar patient (with hypercalcaemia and hypercalciuria) was reported by Moldawer et al. [66]. Hypercalcaemia was observed in 2 of 6 patients with renal calculi among 100 with acromegaly observed by Gordon et al. [33]; three hyperplastic parathyroid glands were removed from 1 patient.

3. Multiple Endocrine Adenomatosis

This condition is a familial disorder affecting men and women equally, most patients being in the third and fourth decades. It is characterized by the simultaneous occurrence of hormonally active single or multiple tumours or hyperplasias involving two or more of the following endocrine organs in any combination: the parathyroids, the pancreatic islets of Langerhans and the anterior pituitary are most commonly involved; the adrenal glands and the thyroids are less commonly affected. The combinations confirm Wermer's [101] concept of dominant inheritance in multiple endocrine adenomata. A type of intractable chronic peptic ulcer is found in many patients, and renal calculus and/or nephrocalcinosis are commonly found, especially in those patients in whom the parathyroids, adrenals and pituitary are affected.

The early symptoms usually relate to hyperfunction of one single endocrine gland and may remain thus limited for some years. In the end a complex picture results from different metabolic disturbances; sometimes it may not be clear which of these abnormalities is responsible, for example, for the renal calculus formation. These patients are sometimes discovered during the investigations leading to a diagnosis of primary hyperparathyroidism; the subject has been discussed by the author [80].

IV. Sarcoidosis

Sarcoidosis, a disease of unknown etiology, has widely disseminated lesions affecting almost any tissue or organ in the body but most frequently the lymph nodes, lungs, skin, eyes, bones and kidneys, and characterized pathologically by the development of granulomatous tubercle-like lesions consisting of epitheloid cells and showing minimal or no necrosis. The kidney is affected in various ways in some 10% of recorded cases, and sometimes by nephrocalcinosis and renal calculi. In cases of generalized sarcoidosis, there may be renal insufficiency (possibly resulting from the hypercalcaemia), often associated with thirst, polyuria, frequency of micturition, loss of mental concentration and loss of weight. Sarcoid granulomatous nodules may be found in a kidney in which function is virtually normal.

Renal Calculi. The incidence of renal calculi must be largely determined by the existence of hypercalcaemia and hypercalciuria in many patients. Hypercalcaemia was first recorded by Harrell and Fisher [39] in 6 of

11 cases, and has been reported in many series in a varying proportion from 10% to 40%; levels of serum calcium have been recorded as high as 17.4 mg/100 ml [52]. The serum calcium level usually falls to normal following the administration of cortisone. The hypercalcaemia does not always run in parallel with the local (and occasionally generalized) skeletal rarefaction. The plasma phosphate level is usually normal but occasionally low, though elevated in cases with severe renal impairment. Sometimes the amount of calcium absorbed from the gut exceeds that found in normal individuals [46]. Several observers have considered that patients with sarcoidosis appear to have an abnormal sensitivity to vitamin D.

The stones found in patients with sarcoidosis are usually composed of calcium oxalate with or without an admixture of calcium phosphate. In many autopsy cases, microscopic renal calcification in association with renal calculi and nephrocalcinosis has been observed. Examples of renal calculi in 7 of 8 patients with sarcoidosis (some of whom had hypercalcaemia) were reported by Scholtz and Keating [88] and by several other observers [2, 4, 51, 61, 93]. Nephrocalcinosis (demonstrable radiographically) in association with hypercalcaemia was reported in seven cases of sarcoidosis (three being autopsy studies) by Davidson et al. [18]. In a review of 152 patients with sarcoidosis Lebacq et al. [56] reported that 11% had hypercalcaemia, 62% had hypercalciuria, and 13.8% had at least one renal stone.

V. Paget's Disease

Paget's disease (osteitis deformans) is a chronic disorder of unknown causation affecting sometimes nearly all the bones of the skeleton (though occasionally only one bone). Probably the not inconsiderable incidence of urolithiasis can be explained on

Table 4.3. Incidence of urolithiasis in Paget's disease

Author	Year	No. of cases of Paget's disease	No. of cases with urinary calculi	Remarks
Goldstein and Abeshouse [32]	1935	50	6	Bilateral renal and left ureteric, 1; bladder and ureteric, 2; left ureter, kidney and urethra, 1; right ureter, 1; left kidney, 1
Moehlig and Adler [65]	1937	26	4 (15.6%)	14 male; 12 female; 30% were diabetic
Dickson et al. [24]	1945	367	22 (6%)	Renal calculi, 11; ureteric calculi, 4; vesical calculi, 7
Newman [67]	1946	82	4	
Rosencrantz et al. [85]	1952	111	6	
Ridlon [83]	1962	438	22 (5%)	

the basis of the metabolic and skeletal changes. The early osteoclasis is succeeded by a type of osseous hyperplasia. In some areas there are large focal zones of rarefaction; the calcium content of the bone is relatively low during the active stage of the disease, though during remissions calcification with sclerosis outstrips bone resorption. The mosaic pattern of the bone is characteristic.

The disease is usually observed between the ages of 40 and 60, the condition often being symptomless at first; headache, fatigue, pains in the back and limbs, deafness and vertigo, and deformities in the chest and pelvis and bowing of the tibiae, sometimes with spontaneous fractures and in some patients with osteosarcoma.

Renal Calculi. Occasionally the serum calcium level has been reported as being high normal or above normal, though it is usually within the normal range. Rarely hyperparathyroidism (in which there would be a raised serum calcium level) has been found in association with Paget's disease; and occasionally there may be a negative calcium balance and hypercalciuria during those stages of the disease when the rate of bone resorption exceeds that of bone formation [23]. The 'mean incidence' of

urolithiasis among 1382 patients with Paget's disease was found by de Deuxchaisnes and Krane [23] to be 5% (Table 4.3).

The 22 patients with urolithiasis in the series of 438 with Paget's disease collected by Ridlon [83] were between the ages of 36 and 76, only 2 being female (Table 4.3). The author has seen a number of patients with Paget's disease and urolithiasis (kidney, ureter, bladder) but has not evaluated the incidence statistically (Fig. 4.6, see p. 88). Some patients with urolithiasis and Paget's disease are found to have prostatic enlargement so that it may not be easy to decide whether a vesical stone (which is not uncommon) is due to the Paget's disease or to the prostatic enlargement.

VI. Myelomatosis

Myelomatosis, a disorder of the reticuloendothelial system which gives rise to abnormal proliferation of plasma cells in the bone, spleen, lymph glands and liver, and occasionally in the general circulation, is often associated with hypercalcaemia, hypercalciuria, decalcification of the bony skeleton and occasionally with renal calculi and microscopic renal calcification (seen at

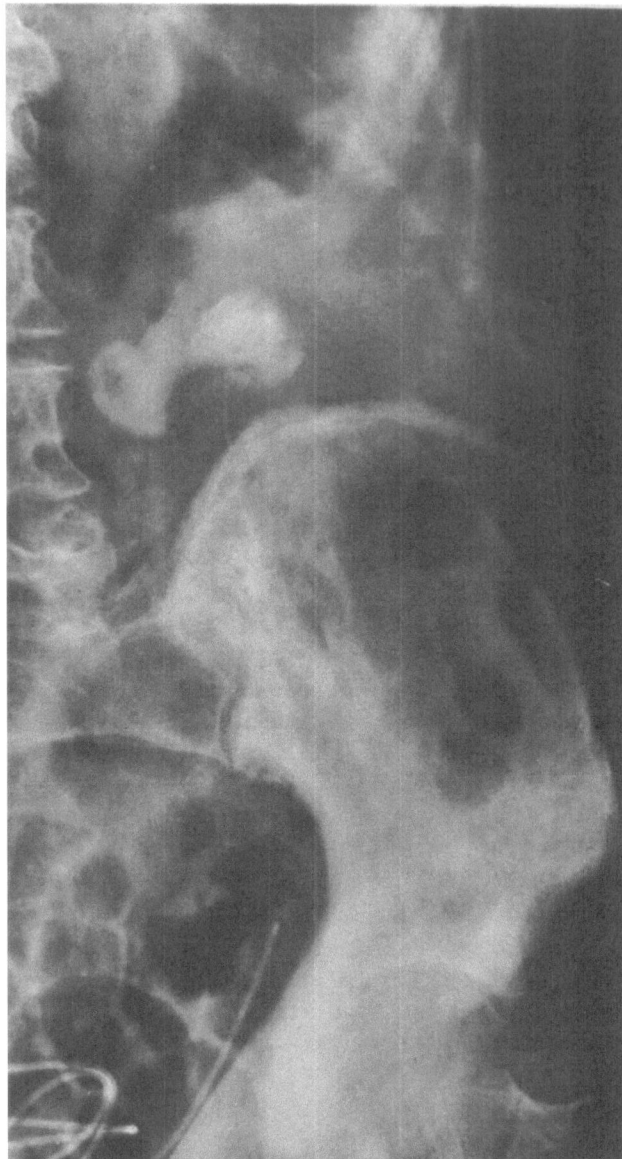

Fig. 4.6. A.M., female aged 50. The patient had had pain in the left kidney with pyuria. Radiography showed a large lobulated stone in the left renal pelvis extending into the lowest calyces in a non-functioning kidney; there was a small stone in the left pelvic ureter; there was fairly extensive osteosclerotic Paget's disease of the left pelvic bones. Left nephroureterectomy was done for a calculous pyonephrosis

autopsy). Degenerative changes in the kidneys in the later stages ultimately lead to fatal renal failure.

Early symptoms are pains in the bones, headache and sometimes a pathological fracture of a long bone or rib; with the advance of the disease there follow thirst, polyuria, fatigue, general weakness and pulmonary symptoms. Radiological changes **are** commonly demonstrable in the verte-brae, long bones, ribs and skull (where there may be punched-out foci or rare-faction). Red cell anaemia with the presence of myelocytes and myeloblasts, and an increase in plasma cells in the peripheral blood are commonly found.

Renal Calculi. Hypercalcaemia, which was found in 34 of 78 patients with myelo-matosis reported by Gutman and Gutman

[35], and in 31 of 78 cases recorded by Vix [96], must be a contributory cause of stone formation, and probably (as in primary hyperparathyroidism) to the renal impairment seen in the later stages of the disease. The hypercalcaemia usually falls to normal after 2 or 3 days, following the daily administration of 200 mg cortisone, thereby enabling the condition to be differentiated from primary hyperparathyroidism. Hypercalciuria may accompany the hypercalcaemia; the level of the plasma protein is increased and Bence-Jones proteinuria is present in about half the cases.

Renal calculi were found in patients reported by Kutzman and Sauer [53], by Jones et al. [49], and in 2 of 27 autopsied cases of myelomatosis recorded by Carson et al. [10].

The patient recorded by Macalister and Addison [62] illustrates the process of renal stone formation synchronizing with the earliest renal changes resulting from myelomatosis and therefore probably dependent upon them. The patient had had renal colic in 1946 (when calculi were removed from the lower pole of the left kidney by partial nephrectomy) and from the pelviureteric junction of the right kidney, nephrectomy subsequently being necessary. Myelomatosis at that time was not suspected. Following a fatal anuria some years later resulting from what was shown at autopsy to be myelomatosis affecting the remaining left kidney (which contained a stone), examination of the microscopic slides from the segment of the kidney removed by partial nephrectomy several years before revealed what were regarded as the early changes of myelomatosis. The association may be more common than has been suspected.

VII. Wilson's Disease

Wilson's disease (hepatico-lenticular degeneration) is the result of a rare autosomal recessive genetic defect in consequence of which there is degeneration of the basal ganglia and an associated portal cirrhosis. There is a failure of the formation of caeruloplasmin and an increased deposition of copper in the tissues. The neurological symptoms include torsion spasm, tremor, dysarthria and mental deterioration, though the cirrhosis may give rise to little disability.

Renal Calculi. Some patients with Wilson's disease have hypercalciuria and varying degrees of osteoporosis with pseudofractures. A few patients have renal calculi or nephrocalcinosis. Other biochemical changes which have been reported have included hyperphosphaturia, hypophosphataemia, aminoaciduria, glycosuria and uricosuria. The picture suggests a renal tubular leakage of several substances, and bears a resemblance to Fanconi's disease. The renal tubular defect has been regarded as being secondary to the renal tubular deposition of copper, the metabolism of which is abnormal in Wilson's disease [54].

Litin et al. [58] observed hypercalciuria in 4 of 5 patients with Wilson's disease, 1 of whom had a stone in the left kidney and another had bilateral nephrocalcinosis with a history of having voided two renal stones. In a report of 10 patients with Wilson's disease 4 had radiodemonstrable osteoporosis and 1 had nephrocalcinosis [86]. The daily urinary calcium in 7 patients with a normal daily calcium intake of 600–800 mg/day varied between 244 and 575 mg. Hypercalciuria (with no radiological evidence of osteoporosis) was observed in 4 of 9 patients with Wilson's disease by Randall et al. [81]; 1 patient in the series (without hypercalciuria) had a renal stone.

VIII. Ureterocolic Anastomosis, Ileal Ureterostomy and Cutaneous Ureterostomy

The operation of ureterocolic anastomosis, frequently performed in association with total cystectomy for the treatment of vesical neoplasms, and also as a diversion in patients with ectopia vesicae, is frequently complicated by electrolyte imbalance and its associated symptoms, which have been reduced in severity in recent years by appropriate treatment.

In the untreated patient, general weakness, fatigue, distaste for food, and thirst, may be followed after an interval by nausea, vomiting, drowsiness and fatal coma. The symptoms were shown to be the result of hyperchloraemic acidosis, which was present in a high percentage (80%) of untreated patients. It was subsequently shown that the electrolyte imbalance is the result partly of a differential absorption of electrolytes (chloride more than sodium ions) from the urine in the colon, across the colonic mucosa into the blood stream; and partly from impairment of renal function arising from ascending infection from the colon and resulting directly from the ureterocolic anastomosis [72, 78].

If the acidosis is uncorrected for a long time, there is a continued loss of calcium salts from the bones, which may lead to generalized bone rarefaction and osteomalacia in the adult (sometimes with pain and spontaneous fractures), and to rickets-like changes in the bones in infants and adolescents. The excess of calcium excreted in the urine, together with the renal infection, may lead to the presence of organic debris in the upper urinary tract and to the formation of renal (and ureteric) calculi. Grey Turner [34] recorded three cases of renal calculi in 13 patients who had ureterocolic anastomosis for ectopia vesicae.

Jacobs and Stirling [47] reviewed 1673 cases of ureterocolic anastomosis, among which were 15 instances of stone in the upper urinary tract. The author has observed a child with ureteric calculus following ureterocolic anastomosis and cystectomy for ectopia vesicae. The use of alkalis to correct the hyperchloraemic acidosis in these patients has improved their health and reduced the incidence of calculi.

Following the operation of ileal ureterostomy (a urinary diversion practised with cystectomy), calculi are occasionally found in the upper urinary tract; large calculi have occasionally been observed in the isolated loop of ileum into which the ureters have been transplanted. Renal calculi occasionally complicate the operation of cutaneous ureterostomy.

IX. Renal Calculi Complicating Renal Transplants

Renal calculi are occasionally observed in subjects with transplanted kidneys who have developed hypercalcaemia, believed to be secondary to hyperparathyroidism; a few such patients have developed renal tubular acidosis [17, 55, 84]. Patients seem to benefit by parathyroidectomy. One-third of 64 patients followed up by David and co-workers [17] for some years after kidney transplantation developed hypercalcaemia.

References

1. Albright,F., Bloomberg,E., Castleman,B., Churchill,E.D.: Hyperparathyroidism due to diffuse hyperplasia of all parathyroid glands rather than adenoma of one; clinical studies on three such cases. Arch. Intern. Med. 54, 315 (1934)
2. Albright,F. Reifenstein,E.C.: The Parathyroid glands and metastatic bone disease. Baltimore: Williams and Wilkins 1948
3. Allison,N., Brooks,S.: Bone atrophy, an experimental and clinical study of changes in bone which result from non-use. Surg. Gynecol. Obstet. 33, 250 (1921)
4. Anderson,G.S., Graham,A.G.: Renal sarcoidosis and nephrolithiasis. Scott. Med. J. 5, 392 (1960)
5. Bernheim,J. et al.: Evaluation of hyperparathyroidism and recurrent renal lithiasis. J. Urol. Nephrol. (Paris) 81, 824 (1975)

6. Black,B.K.: Carcinoma of parathyroid. Ann. Surg. *139*, 355 (1954)

7. Bors,E.: Neurogenic bladder. Urol. Surv. 7, 177 (1957)

8. Bors,E., Comarr,A.E.: Vesicoureteral reflux in paraplegic patients. J. Urol. *68*, 691 (1952)

9. Burr,R.G. et al.: Urinary calcium and kidney stone in paraplegia. Report of an attempted prospective study. Paraplegia *12*, 38 (1974)

10. Carson,C.P., Ackerman,L.Y., Maltby, J.A.: Plasma cell myeloma; clinical, pathologic and roentgenologic review of 90 cases. Am. J. Clin. Pathol. *28*, 849 (1955)

11. Churchill,E.D.: Operative treatment of hyperparathyroidism. Ann. Surg. *100*, 606 (1934)

12. Comarr,A.E.: A long-term survey of the incidence of renal calculosis in paraplegia. J. Urol. *74*, 447 (1955)

13. Cook,J.B., Smith,P.H.: Long-term urethral catheterisation after spinal cord injury. Paraplegia *6*, 11 (1968)

14. Cope,O., Raker,J.W.: Cushing's disease, surgical experience in the care of 46 cases. N. Engl. J. Med. *253*, 119 (1955)

15. Cushing,H.: The basophiladenomas of the pituitary body and their clinical manifestations (pituitary basophilism). Bull. Johns Hopkins Hosp. *50*, 137 (1932)

16. Cutler,R.E., Reiss,E., Ackerman,L.V.: Familial hyperparathyroidism in a kindred involving eleven cases with a discussion of primary chief-cell hyperplasia. N. Engl. J. Med. *270*, 859 (1964)

17. David,D.S., Sakai,S., Brennan,L., Riggio, R.A., Cheigh,J., Stenzel,K.H., Rubin, A.L., Sherwood,L.M.: Hypercalcaemia after renal transplantation: long-term follow-up data. N. Engl. J. Med. *289*, 398 (1973)

18. Davidson,C.N., Dennis,J.M., McNich, E.R., Willson,J.K.N., Brown,L.H.: Nephrocalcinosis associated with sarcoidosis. Radiology *62*, 203 (1954)

19. Davies,D.R.: Operative surgery. Rob,C., Smith,R. (eds.). London: Butterworth 1962

20. Dent,C.E.: Cortisone test for hyperparathyroidism. Br. Med. J. *I*, 230 (1956)

21. Dent,C.E.: Personal communication (1964)

22. Dent,C.E. Harper,C.M.: Plasma alkaline phosphatase in normal adults and in patients with primary hyperparathyroidism. Lancet *I*, 559 (1962)

23. Deuxchaisnes,C.N.de, Krane,S.M.: Paget's disease of bone; clinical and metabolic observations. Medicine *43*, 233 (1964)

24. Dickson,D.D., Camp,J.D., Ghormley, R.K.: Osteitis deformans: Paget's disease of bone. Radiology, *44*, 449 (1945)

25. Dietrich,J.E., Whedon,D.G., Shorr,E.: Effects of immobilization upon various metabolic and physiologic functions of normal men. Am. J. Med. *4*, 3 (1948)

26. Edvall,C.A.: Renal function in hyperparathyroidism. Acta Chir. Scand. (Suppl. 229) (1958)

27. Edwards,N.A., Hodgkinson,A.: Studies of renal function in patients with idiopathic hypercalciuria. Clin. Sci. *29*, 97 (1965)

28. Elliott,J.S., Todd,H.E.: Calculous disease in patients with poliomyelitis. J. Urol. *86*, 484 (1961)

29. Fourman,P., McConkey,B., Smith,J.W.G.: Defects of water reabsorption and of hydrogen ion excretion by the renal tubules in hyperparathyroidism. Lancet *I*, 619 (1960)

30. Gilmour,J.R., Martin, W.B.: The weight of the parathyroid glands. J. Pathol. Bacteriol. *44*, 431 (1937)

31. Goldsmith,R.S., Ingbar,S.H.: Inorganic phosphate treatment of hypercalcaemia of diverse etiologies. N. Engl. J. Med. *27*, 1 (1966)

32. Goldstein,A.E., Abeshouse,B.A.: Urinary calculi in Paget's disease. Am. J. Surg. *30*, 359 (1935)

33. Gordon,D.A., Hill,F.M., Ezrin,C.: Acromegaly; a review of 100 cases. Can. Med. Assoc. J. *87*, 1106 (1962)

34. Grey Turner,G.: Treatment of congenital defects of bladder and urethra by implantation of ureter in bowel with record of 17 personal cases. Br. J. Surg. *23*, 580 (1939)

35. Gutman,A.B., Gutman,E.D.: Calcium-protein relation in hyperproteinuria; total and diffusible serum calcium in lymphogranuloma inguinale and myeloma. Proc. Soc. Exp. Biol. Med. *35*, 511 (1936)

36. Guttman,L.: The treatment and rehabilitation of patients with injuries of the spinal cord. In: Medical history of the Second World War. Macnalty,A.S. (ed.). Surgery Volume, p. 422. Z. Cope 1953

37. Guttman,L.: Statistical survey on 1000 paraplegics. Proc. R. Soc. Med. *47*, 1099 (1954)

38. Hadfield,G., Rogers,H.: Two parathyroid tumours, one associated with acromegaly. J. Pathol. Bacteriol. *35*, 259 (1932)

39. Harrell,C.T., Fisher,S.: Blood chemical changes in Boeck's sarcoid with particular reference to protein, calcium and phosphatase values. J. Clin. Invest. *18*, 687 (1939)

40. Hartog,M.: Acromegaly and hyperparathyroidism. Proc. R. Soc. Med. *60*, 477 (1967)

41. Hellstrom,J.: Primary hyperparathyroidism. Observations on a series of 50 cases. Acta Endocrinol. (KbH) *16*, 30 (1954)

42. Hellstrom,J., Ivemark,B.I.: Primary hyperparathyroidism. Clinical and structural findings in 138 cases. Acta Chir. Scand. (Suppl.) *294*, 1 (1962)

43. Hellstrom,J., Birke,G. Edvall,C.A.: Hypertension in hyperparathyroidism. Br. J. Urol. *30*, 13 (1958)

44. Horwith,M., Stokes,P.E.: Cushing's syndrome. Experience with total adrenalectomy. Ann. Int. Med. *10*, 259 (1960)

45. Howard,J.E., Parson,W., Bigham,R.S.: Studies on patients convalescence from fracture. III. The urinary excretion of calcium and phosphorus. Bull. Johns Hopkins Hosp. *77*, 291 (1945)

46. Jackson,L.P.U., Dancaster,C.: A consideration of the hypercalciuria in sarcoidosis, idiopathic hypercalciuria and that produced by vitamin D: a new suggestion regarding calcium metabolism. J. Endocrinol. Metab. *19*, 658 (1959)

47. Jacobs,A., Stirling,W.B.: Late results of ureterocolic anastomosis. Br. J. Urol. *24*, 259 (1952)

48. Johansson,H. et al.: Normocalcaemic hyperparathyroidism, kidney stones and idiopathic hypercalciuria. Surgery *71*, 691 (1975)

49. Jones,T.N., Monto,R.W., Buck,R.E.: Thrombocytopenia and abnormal bleeding in multiple myeloma. Ann. Int. Med. *39*, 1281 (1953)

50. Key,L.A.: Urinary tract complications in the prolonged immobilization of children. Br. Med. J. *I*, 1150 (1936)

51. Klatskin,G., Gordon,M.: Renal complications of sarcoidosis and their relationship to hypercalciuria; with a report of two cases simulating hyperparathyroidism. Am. J. Med. *15*, 484 (1953)

52. Klinfelter,H.F., Salley,S.M.: Sarcoidosis simulating glomerulonephritis. Bull. Johns Hopkins Hosp. *79*, 333 (1946)

53. Kutzman,N., Sauer,H.R.: Consideration of problems presented by unilateral cystic kidney. J. Urol. *63*, 34 (1950)

54. Leading Article: Copper, kidneys and calcium. Lancet *II*, 867 (1952)

55. Leapman,S.B., Vidne,B.A., Butt,K.M.H., Waterhouse,K., Kountz,S.L.: Nephrolithiasis and nephrocalcinosis after renal transplantation: a case report and review of the literature. J. Urol. *115*, 129 (1976)

56. Lebacq,E., Verhaegen,H., Desmet,V.: Renal involvement in sarcoidosis. In: Sarcoidosis, proceedings of a conference. Postgrad. Med. J. *46*, 463 (1970)

57. Lehmann,J.Jr., Donatelli,A.A.: Calcium intoxication due to primary hyperparathyroidism. Lancet *II*, 406 (1964)

58. Litin,R.B., Goldstein,N.P., Randall,R.V., Diessner,G.R.: Hypercalciuria in Wilson's disease with data on the effect of DL-penicillamine on the urinary excretion of calcium and copper. J. Clin. Lab. Med. *52*, 923 (1958)

59. Lloyd,H.M.: Primary hyperparathyroidism. An analysis of the role of the parathyroid tumour. Medicine *47*, 53 (1968)

60. Lloyd,H.M., Rose,G.: Ionized protein-bound and complexed calcium in the plasma in primary hyperparathyroidism. Lancet *II*, 1258 (1958)

61. Longcope,W.T., Freiman,D.G.: A study of sarcoidosis based on a combined investigation of 160 cases including 30 autopsies from the Johns Hopkins Hospital and Massachusetts General Hospital. Medicine *31*, 1 (1952)

62. Macalister,C.L.O., Addison,N.V.: Renal aspects of myelomatosis. Br. J. Urol. *33*, 141 (1961)

63. McGeown,M.G.: Hyperparathyroidism. Br. J. Urol. *32*, 389 (1960)

64. McGeown,M.G., Morrison,E.: Hyperparathyroidism. Postgrad. Med. J. *35*, 330 (1959)

65. Moehlig,R.C., Adler,S.: Carbohydrate metabolism disturbance in osteoporosis and Paget's disease; associated soft tissue disturbances and results of various therapeutic procedures. Surg. Gynec. Obstet. *64*, 749 (1937)

66. Moldawer,M.P., Nardi,G.L., Raker,J.W.: Concomitance of multiple adenomas of parathyroids and pancreatic islets with tumour of pituitary: syndrome with familial incidence. Am. J. Med. Sci. *228*, 190 (1954)

67. Newman,F.W.: Paget's disease: statis-

tical study of 82 cases. J. Bone Joint. Surg. (Am.) *28*, 79 (1946)

68. Norris,E.H.: Collective review. Parathyroid adenoma; study of 322 cases. Int. Abstr. Surg. *84*, 1 (1947)

69. Oliver,W.A.: Acute hyperparathyroidism. Lancet *I*, 240 (1939)

70. Orr: Quoted by J.E. Howard (1942). Editorial on hypercalcaemia and renal injury. Ann. Int. Med. *16*, 176 (1942)

71. Parfitt,A.M.: Investigation of disorders of the parathyroid glands. Clin. Endocrinol. Metab. *3*, 451 (1974)

72. Parsons,F.M., Pyrah,L.N., Powell,F.J.N., Reed,G.W., Spiers,F.W.: Chemical imbalance following ureterocolic anastomosis. Br. J. Urol. *24*, 317 (1952)

73. Pearman,J.W., England,E.J.: The urological management of the patients following spinal cord injury. Springfield, Ill.: Thomas 1973

74. Plum,F., Dunning,M.F.: The effect of therapeutic mobilization on hypercalciuria following acute poliomyelitis. Arch Int. Med. *101*, 528 (1958)

75. Poole-Wilson,P.A.: A new factor in urolithiasis: long-term effects of severe respiratory poliomyelitis. Br. J. Urol. *45*, 335 (1973)

76. Pugh,W.T.G.: The prevention of calculus formation in the treatment of tuberculosis of spine and hip. Ann. Rep. London C.C. 4, pt. III, p. 38 (1933)

77. Pulvertaft,R.G.: Nephrolithiasis occurring in recumbency. J. Bone Joint. Surg. (Am.) *21*, 559 (1939)

78. Pyrah,L.N.: Ureterocolic anastomosis. Ann. R. Coll. Surg. Engl. *14*, 169 (1954)

79. Pyrah,L.N., Fowweather,F.S.: Urinary calculi developing in recumbent patients. Br. J. Surg. *26*, 98 (1938)

80. Pyrah,L.N., Hodgkinson,A., Anderson, C.K.: Primary hyperparathyroidism: a critical review. Br. J. Surg. *53*, 245 (1966)

81. Randall,R.N., Goldstein,N.P., Gross,J.B., Rosevear,J.W.: Hypercalciuria in Wilson's disease. Am. J. Med. Sci. *252*, 718 (1966)

82. Reiss,E., Canterbury,J.M.: Blood levels of parathyroid hormone in disorders of calcium metabolism. Ann. Rev. Med. *23*, 217 (1973)

83. Ridlon,H.C.: Urinary calculi associated with Paget's disease of bone. J. Urol. *87*, 499 (1962)

84. Rosenberg,J.C., Arnstein,A.R., Ing,T.S., Pierce,J.M., Rosenberg,B., Silva,Y.,

Walt,A.J.: Calculi complicating a renal transplant. Am. J. Surg. *129*, 326 (1975)

85. Rosencrantz,J.A., Wolf,J., Knicher,J.J.: Paget's disease: review of 111 cases. Arch. Int. Med. *20*, 610 (1952)

86. Rosenoer,V., Mitchell,R.C.: Skeletal changes in Wilson's disease (hepatolenticular degeneration). Br. J. Radiol. *32*, 805 (1959)

87. Ross,E.J., Marshall-Jones,P., Friedman, M.: Cushing's syndrome; diagnostic criteria. Q. J. Med. *35*, 149 (1966)

88. Scholz,D.A., Keating,F.R.: Renal insufficiency, renal calculi and nephrocalcinosis, in sarcoidosis. Am. J. Med. *21*, 75 (1956)

89. Scholz,D.A., Sprague,R.G., Kernohan, J.W.: Cardiovascular and renal complications of Cushing's Syndrome. N. Engl. J. Med. *256*, 833 (1957)

90. Shortland,J.R., Crane,W.A.L.: Histology and ultrastructure of renal biopsies in Cushing's syndrome. J. Pathol. *98*, 209 (1969)

91. Smith,F.G., Cooke,R.T.: Acute fatal hyperparathyroidism. Lancet *II*, 650 (1940)

92. Soffer,L.J., Eisenburg,J., Iannaccone,L., Gabrililone,J.L.: Cushing's syndrome. Ciba Found. Coll. Endocrinol. *8*, 487 (1955)

93. Spencer,J., Warren,S.: Boeck's sarcoid; report of a case with clinical diagnosis confirmed at autopsy. Arch. Intern. Med. *62*, 285 (1938)

94. Thomas,W.G., Connor,T.B., Morgan, H.G.: Some observations on patients with hypercalcaemia exemplifying problems in differential diagnosis, especially in hyperparathyroidism. J. Lab. Clin. Med. *52*, 11 (1958)

95. Vancil,M., Locke,W.: Acromegaly, hyperparathyroidism and probably mammary fibroadenoma in a man. Am. J. Surg. *110*, 495 (1965)

96. Vix,V.A.: Intravenous pyelography in multiple myeloma. A review of 52 studies in 40 patients. Radiology *87*, 896 (1966)

97. Walton,A.J.: Surgical treatment of parathyroid tumours. Br. J. Surg. *19*, 285 (1931)

98. Wang,C.C., Robbins,L.L.: Cushing's disease: its roentgenological findings. Radiology *67*, 17 (1956)

99. Watson-Jones,R., Roberts,R.E.: Calcification, decalcification and ossification. Br. J. Surg. *21*, 461 (1934)

100. Welbourn,R.B.: Cushing's syndrome. A review of 50 patients in 15 years. Ann. R. Coll. Surg. Engl. *44*, 182 (1969)

101. Wermer, P.: Genetic aspects of adenomatosis of endocrine glands. Am. J. Med. *16*, 363 (1954)

102. Whedon,G.D., Shorr,E.: Metabolic studies in paralytic acute anterior poliomyelitis. J. Clin. Invest. *36*, 966 (1957)

103. Wills,M.R.: Role of parathyroid hormone in acid base homeostasis. Lancet *I*, 142 (1971)

104. Wills,M.R., Pak,C.Y., Hambro,W.G.: Normocalcaemic primary hyperparathyroidism. Am. J. Med. *47*, 384 (1969)

105. Wilson,W.E.: Renal colic and haematuria during recumbency. Br. Med. J. *2*, 101 (1931)

106. Yendt,E.R., Gagne,R.J.: Detection of primary hyperparathyroidism with special reference to its occurrence in hypercalciuric females with 'normal' or borderline serum calcium. Can. Med. Assoc. J. *98*, 331 (1968)

107. Zubrod,C.G., Pieter,W., Hibbish,T.E., Smith,R., Dutcher,T., Wermer,P.: Acromegaly, jejunal ulcer and hypersecretion of gastric juice; clinical pathological conference at the National Institute of Health. Ann. Int. Med. *49*, 1389 (1958)

Chapter 5

Renal Calculi and Nephrocalcinosis Contributed to by Ingestion of Certain Substances: Environmental Calculosis

A group of patients develop renal calculi as a result of the ingestion of abnormally large amounts of the principal chemical substances contained in the stone, for example, silica or sulphonamides. Another group of patients form renal stones as a result of the toxic action on the renal epithelium of a substance (for example, phenacetin) which has been orally ingested, or taken into the body during the patient's occupation; the stones are then probably dystrophic in origin.

The term 'environmental calculi' is suggested as a collective title for this group of stones. The term 'iatrogenic stones' could be applied to stones which result from the ingestion of drugs taken during the treatment of an illness, but would not cover all the examples in the group. The over-enthusiastic ingestion of sodium bicarbonate (with or without calcium taken in milk or in tablets) for the relief of peptic ulcer and indigestion, has sometimes given rise to clinical symptoms, and microscopic renal calcification and calculi have been observed in some cases. It is appropriate to discuss the relationship between renal calculi and peptic ulcer.

There may be other substances taken in the food which are still undetected, and which may occasionally give rise to renal stone formation. It is known that hamsters fed with certain food emulsifiers sometimes develop stones in the bladder; no harmful sequelae from the use of such substances in man seem so far to have been reported.

I. Silicate Calculi

Silicate has been observed occasionally as a major component of renal calculi in man, and very frequently in calculi in some domestic animals. In man very small amounts of silica are ingested in vegetables and absorbed from the gut and it is said to occur in the blood and the urine to the extent of 10 mg per day. Certain silicates have been prescribed medicinally in recent years; the human renal calculus composed of silica which occasionally follows is probably an example of a hyperexcretory type of calculus, the kidneys excreting any silica which is presented to them above the normal level in the blood.

Certain forms of silica have physico-chemical properties which are relevant to the problem of renal calculus. Thus, a soluble polymerized silicate known as 'activated silica' can block the chelating effect of polyphosphate water conditioners and has been used for the purification of public water supplies [85]. Silica added in suitable amounts to normal urine has enabled it to mineralize collagen in vitro, and to block the effect of inhibitor peptides but not that of pyrophosphate [115].

1. In Man

Silicate in tiny amounts is an occasional component of renal calculi; thus in 14 renal calculi from different patients, Thomas [115] found that small amounts of silicate (0.02%–0.3% of the dry weight) were regularly present, and that urine from many patients receiving 'a restricted dairy-product-free diet' contained silicate usually in the monomeric form, but sometimes in a polymerized state (20%–30%). The public water supply in his area contained soluble (monomeric) silicate in amounts of 20 mg/litre. It is just possible, therefore, that polymerized silicate (as in the in vitro conditions just referred to), may contribute to calculus formation.

Renal Calculi. Renal calculi composed mainly of silica have been reported in a few patients who have had treatment for peptic ulcer with magnesium trisilicate (in one of its several preparations such as Zeolite), which was introduced as an antacid for the treatment of peptic ulcer by Mutch [86]. He stated that neither the salt itself nor the hydrated silica, formed when the trisilicate comes into contact with hydrochloric acid, are soluble; it would not be expected, therefore, that it would be absorbed.

When acid reacts with a silicate, part of the silica so formed is precipitated as a gel and part remains in solution as a colloid. The breakdown products in the digestive tract include various silicic acids, which are soluble and can therefore be absorbed and excreted in the urine. The excretion of silica in the urine of 5 healthy subjects before and after the administration of 5 g magnesium trisilicate daily was found to be 80 mg, which was higher than that in the controls [94].

Hammarsten et al. [49] first reported the presence of bilateral silica-containing stones in a man aged 49 who had had attacks of renal colic and who had taken five or six Zeolite tablets at intervals for nearly 2 years for the treatment of duodenal ulcer; each tablet contained 0.4 g synthetic magnesium–sodium–aluminium silicate, which was equivalent to a daily intake of 0.5 g silicon and 1.08 g silicic acid [57]. Some small stones were voided, one of which was shown to contain large quantities

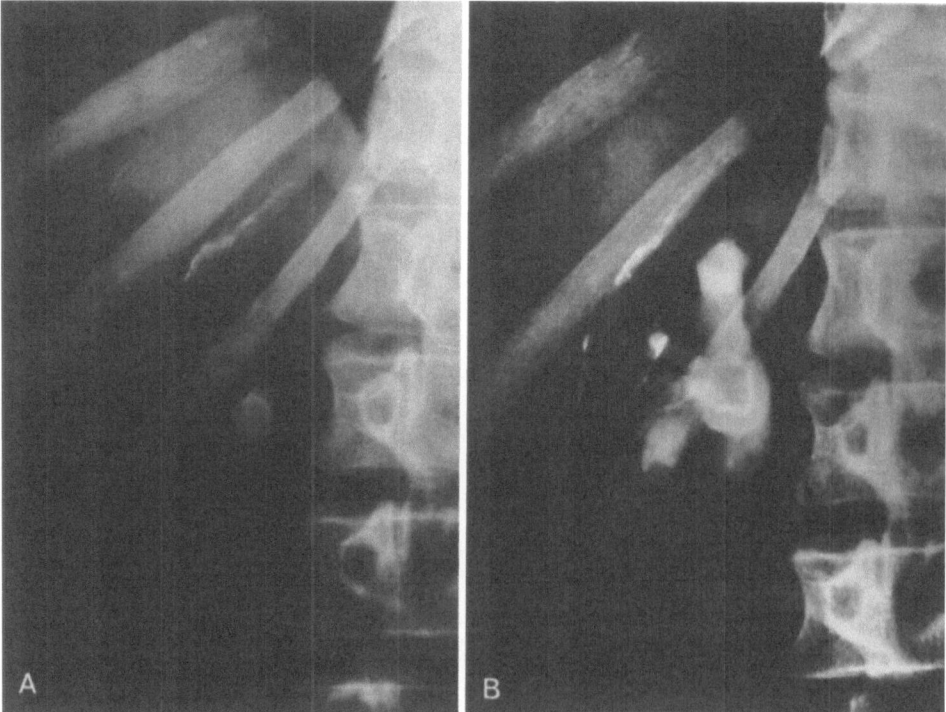

Fig. 5.1. **A.** Plain radiograph showing a laminated stone composed mainly of silica in the pelvis of the right kidney. **B.** Intravenous pyelogram showing the stone lying in the pelvis of the right kidney. The central part of the stone was composed of silica and the peripheral part consists of calcium oxalate. (By courtesy of the late Dr. Greta Hammarsten and Professor Ingermar Hessen)

of silica together with small amounts of calcium and fibrin. Calculi composed of silica were subsequently reported in three further patients who had also received Zeolite for the treatment of peptic ulcer, the inner part of one of the stones being composed of silica surrounded by a deposit of calcium oxalate [48] (Fig. 5.1). Larsen and Sigroth [75] reported that 5 among 40 patients with peptic ulcer treated with Zeolite had suffered from renal colic during their period of treatment; calculi were subsequently voided but they do not appear to have been analyzed. Holst [5] reported three proven cases of calculi composed of silica in patients similarly treated. Herman and Goldberg [56] recorded a male patient who had had long-standing epigastric pain associated with oesophagitis, which was readily controlled by tablets (30–35 daily for 2–3 years), each containing 0.5 g magnesium trisilicate and 0.25 g aluminium hydroxide; he ultimately voided a small silica calculus.

Lagergren [74] reported silica-containing calculi in 5 patients who had had treatment for peptic ulcer for 2–5 years with not especially large doses of magnesium trisilicate. Of the stones examined, one was composed of pure silica and three were composed of silica with either hydroxyapatite or calcium oxalate mono- or dihydrate. The silica when present was in fine crystalline form; with two calculi, weak but readily identifiable powder diffraction diagrams were obtained.

Hessen's [57] patient, a woman aged 31, who had had a long history of duodenal ulcer, had bilateral renal colic after only 5 weeks' treatment with Zeolite. Six years after beginning treatment, a calculus the size of a hazelnut was removed from the right kidney by pyelolithotomy, the interior of the stone being found on analysis to consist of silicates (shown crystallographically to be a double silicate) with a solid outer shell of calcium oxalate.

Lipworth et al. [80] reported a patient who had urinary calculi which contained silica. The patient reported by Joekes et al. [60], a 68-year-old man, had in the left pelvic ureter a stone which was shown after voiding to be composed mainly of silica. He had taken orally the equivalent of 2 g magnesium trisilicate after meals for many years. Other cases have been reported by Lunde [81] and by Ehrhart and McCullagh [29].

Since the oral administration of magnesium trisilicate in patients with peptic ulcer can give rise to renal calculi, its use should probably be avoided altogether. If a patient is reported to have voided (or had removed by operation) a silica-containing stone (the silica being present in considerable amount), unless he or she has had the kind of therapy referred to, the possibility of its being an artefact rather than a naturally occurring stone should be considered. Quartz pebbles composed of silica are known to have been occasionally introduced into the female bladder by patients who later claimed to have passed such stones spontaneously. The author has encountered one patient who had voided a doubtful stone spontaneously which, however, contained sufficient colloid as well as silica for it to seem quite certain that it had been formed naturally.

2. In Animals

Urinary silicate calculi in beef cattle were probably first recognized by Law [77] and by many subsequent observers. The stones usually also contain calcium oxalate when formed in an acid environment, or calcium carbonate in an alkaline environment [32, 33]. The calculi are hard in consistency and rather vitreous in appearance, the silica in them being in the form of opal $(SiO_2 \cdot n \cdot H_2O)$, a hydrated amorphous form of silica, often 4–7 mm in diameter [64], with numerous small black inclusions of organic matter. It has been suggested that the calculi result from gelation of silicic acid in the kidneys consequent upon an increased concentration of urine of low pH, the silica crystallizing out from the gel from a large number of small nuclei [32, 33]. The stones have a smooth to rough surface and may be amorphous or laminar in section and have an organic matrix which stains with mucicarmine and periodic acid Schiff reagent. The SiO_2 content varied from less than 50% to more than 70% of the stone; there was less than 10% of calcium and only small amounts of magnesium, sodium and potassium.

The stones tend to form in early life; thus calves from a ranch where obstructive urolithiasis had been a problem have been found to have no uroliths at 8 weeks old but an increasing proportion of the animals had calculi when examined up to 15 weeks old [33]. Sub-clinical urolithiasis in which the flow of urine is unimpeded may be almost a normal condition among some weaned calves on the ranges; but calculi recovered after autopsy have been found in 50% of some groups of animals [64]. Some of the uroliths become large enough to cause obstruction of the urethra followed by a fatal rupture of the bladder or a urinary extravasation.

The condition occurs sporadically in range and feedlot steers, especially between the months of October and March, in all parts of Saskatchewan and Alberta and to a lesser extent in the other provinces of Canada, where there is a high incidence of obstructive urolithiasis during the winter [18, 33].

The condition has presented serious economic problems in certain areas where as many as 4% of animals may be afflicted with urethral calculi [64]. Stones were present in 161 of 204 steers which were killed and examined by Connell et al. [18]; 130 of them had calculous material in the kidneys, commonly consisting of fine, gritty material in the calyces or in the ureters, though larger and more solid calculi were often found. The addition of calcium or

silica to a ration of native prairie hay and grain did not increase the incidence of stone. Range steers consume grasses and sedges which contain as much as 4%–8% dry weight of silicon [32, 64]. Only a small but variable part of the ingested silica is absorbed (after first being changed into an absorbable silicate) and excreted in the urine. A diet consisting of alfalfa may favour the formation of calcium-containing calculi.

Calculi composed largely of silica are frequently found in sheep in Western Australia [6]; in appearance they resemble the mineral opal, as in cattle, and they may have a silica content of over 70%. An outbreak in Western Australia of silica calculi (renal or vesical) in young sheep fed on dry pastures and mainly on cereals, was described by Bennets [7, 8]. The resulting loss of life among the animals sometimes reached 50%. The ash from the stones contained about 90% silica with very little organic matter; the uptake of silica from the gut was believed to have reached 200 mg/day. He also referred to calcium carbonate calculi (with varying amounts of magnesium) which have been found in sheep in the pastoral areas in Western Australia especially in seasons which favour lush pastures. Calculi were formed mostly in the bladder and the urethra, though small stones were found occasionally in the renal pelvis and ureters.

In areas in which silica stones are common, the addition of silica to the ration of sheep did not increase the incidence [6]; but in lambs an increased incidence of stones composed of magnesium phosphate followed the addition of 1% sodium silicate to their ration [25]. The addition of phosphorus, potassium and sugar beet pulp to the feedlot ration of male sheep has been found to result in an increased incidence of urolithiasis.

In experimental dietetic studies, Forman et al. [32] fed sheep with hay from Western Canada, which contained 8.28% silica (the urine of the animals having a pH of approximately 5.5) and compared the results with those found in a control group of sheep fed on hay from Eastern Canada containing 0.78% silica (the urine then having a pH of approximately 8.2). They considered that the polymerization of silicic acid in aqueous systems is dependent upon concentration and upon the pH, and the feeding of Western grass may have had an effect on these parameters, thereby producing the formation of silica calculi. The studies suggested that the low excretion of urine having a high pH (and controlled at such a figure by the administration of an appropriate salt mixture) may be more important than the actual content of silica in the diet in the formation of silica stones; and that the addition of suitable salts to the diet may reduce or prevent their incidence.

Experimental Siliceous Deposits in the Kidneys of Guinea Pigs. Settle and Sauer [107] were able to produce siliceous deposits in the kidneys of guinea pigs under experimental conditions. A solution of sodium metasilicate ($Na_2SiO_3 \cdot 5H_2O$) adjusted to pH 5 by the addition of hydrochloric acid, was given by intraperitoneal administration, or alternatively tetraethyl orthosilicate was administered orally to guinea pigs. The animals were killed after 24 h, when the kidneys, which were pale and enlarged, were shown to have tubular deposits of silica. Silicon administered orally to guinea pigs can be shown to be excreted in the urine and it seems probable that its concentration in the glomerular filtrate and ultimately in the urine, increases until polymerization occurs, when deposits of silica are formed.

II. The Sulphonamides

One of the several sulphonamides taken by mouth and excreted in crystalline form in the urine may be incorporated into a urinary calculus composed almost entirely of the sulphonamide. The subject of the sulphonamides has been reviewed by Goodman and Gilman [44].

When the sulphonamides came into general use for the treatment of infective conditions it was found that a few patients developed undesirable side-effects (cyanosis, skin rashes, granulocytopenia) and a few developed renal colic and obstructive anuria, later shown to be the result of the blockage of one or both ureters by tiny masses of crystalline concretions or actual calculi composed of the drug.

In a few reported fatal cases it was shown that crystals of the sulphonamide were also deposited in the distal (and occasionally the proximal) convoluted tubules, where they can be recognized by their characteristic shape; vacuolation with degeneration and epithelial necrosis of the cells of the proximal convoluted tubules has also been observed. There does not appear to be any well-defined relationship between the amount of the drug ingested and the severity of the renal damage. In some patients organs other than the kidney have been affected; thus interstitial cell granulomas and granulomas in the lungs and the bone marrow have been observed. In some reported cases it seems possible that sulphonamide therapy has given rise to vascular lesions simulating those of periarteritis nodosa, which may have been the result of hypersensitivity to the drugs.

Sulphapyridine, which is relatively insoluble in urine, is excreted in the urine partly unchanged, though a proportion of it is altered to the acetyl compound. Administration of the drug to rats, rabbits and monkeys has been followed in as short a time as 48 h following its administration by the formation of small urinary calculi, dilatation of the renal glomerular spaces and the collecting tubules (which may contain needle-like crystals). In 27 of the 39 rats fed with 1 g sulphapyridine/kg b. wt. for 2 weeks or less Gross et al. [46] observed urinary calculi which contained 6.4% sulphapyridine and 64.0% acetylsulphapyridine, some animals having haematuria and varying degrees of urinary obstruction, which was sometimes fatal. Following its use in humans, haematuria has occasionally been observed and sometimes masses of crystals or definitive calculi have been found in the lower ends of the ureters. The administration of alkalis to produce an alkaline urine goes far to prevent serious effects.

The thiazole derivatives of sulphanilamide (including sulphathiazole) were introduced in 1939 by Fosbinder and Walter [34]. Seventy-seven percent of mice given a diet containing 2% sulphathiazole died within 4 weeks; crystals of the drug were often found at autopsy in the renal pelves, ureters and renal tubules [99]. In the rat, feeding experiments have shown a considerable incidence of urinary calculi. The use of sulphathiazole in humans was attended with a greater margin of safety in the treatment of urinary infections than sulphapyridine, especially when given along with alkali, though there were a few early fatalities as a result of renal damage, the renal pelves and the lower ureters sometimes containing gritty crystalline material.

The use of sulphadiazine was accompanied at first by some renal complications. The intraperitoneal injection of sulphadiazine and acetylsulphadiazine into rats has been followed by blockage of the renal tubules. Blockage of the renal collecting tubules or of the ureters with crystals or concretions was occasionally observed in early cases following its use in humans, the symptoms being renal discomfort, haematuria and later oliguria and azotaemia or anuria. Helwig and Reed [55] reported a fatal case of anuria, where irrigation of the renal pelvis had been unsuccessful, autopsy showing degeneration of the renal convoluted tubules. The drug can usually be used with safety by achieving a sustained urinary

alkalinity, whereas crystalluria is often observed when the urine is acid in reaction.

Sulphonamides should not be given (or only with caution) to patients with renal impairment, or with marked dehydration. It used to be advised that the level of the drug in the blood (as a check against overdosage) and in the urine should be checked, though in practice this is rarely possible or necessary. The urine should be rendered alkaline by the administration of sodium bicarbonate and/or potassium citrate to achieve a pH 7.2.

If there is haematuria or if red cells are observed microscopically in the urine, the administration of the drug should be stopped. Tenderness over the kidneys on palpation, or renal pain are warnings of possible trouble. Oliguria is the most serious symptom and usually results from a blockage of the ureters with crystalline debris, which cannot usually be demonstrated radiologically.

If there is persistent oliguria or anuria the ureters should be catheterized, the catheters being left in situ, and lavage of the renal pelvis with warm saline carried out at 2-hourly intervals until normal drainage of urine has been re-established. Sodium bicarbonate is given orally to render the urine alkaline. If total suppression of urine persists, the patient should be given a low protein intake, alkalis (by the intravenous route if necessary), and minimal fluids until the flow of urine recommences. He or she should have daily electrolyte controls (with supplementation treatment as indicated), haemodialysis being used if necessary if urine still fails to drain down the ureters, the inference then being that the anuria is due to deposits of crystals in the renal parenchyma.

In an attempt to dislodge masses of crystalline debris in the pelvic ureters, massage per rectum of the ureteric openings into the bladder (0.75 in. above and to the outer side of the prostate) corresponding to the site at which the crystals of the drug are

Table 5.1. Causes of renal papillary necrosis

Diabetes:	Terminal renal infection
Obstruction of the lower urinary tract:	Bladder neck obstruction
	Simple or malignant enlargement of the prostate (terminal complication)
Following ureteric catheterization and retrograde pyelography:	Possibly result of infection
Non-diabetic pyelonephritis	
Cirrhosis of the liver:	In 11 of 102 patients, 6 of whom had diabetes
Trauma and shock	
Thrombosis of the renal vein:	Two cases in infants
Prolonged hypertension	
Rheumatoid arthritis:	Occasionally associated
Sickle-cell anaemia:	Occasionally associated
With renal calculi:	
Addiction to certain drugs:	Usually in women
Phenacetin	
Aspirin	
Acetophenetidin	
Organic mercurial diuretics	

deposited, has been recommended for periods of 2–3 min [31]; massage over the kidneys and ureters has also been advised. Short-wave diathermy to the renal areas has been followed by return of renal function following anuria [103]. Drainage of the kidneys or ureters by open operation is rarely if ever necessary, though ureterolithotomy for the removal of calculi may be required occasionally. In a few patients with anuria of intrarenal origin, decapsulation of the kidneys has been performed when other measures have failed to give relief [71].

III. Renal Papillary Necrosis: Phenacetin Addiction

Renal papillary necrosis, first described by von Friedrich in 1877 [40], refers to a non-specific necrotic lesion (usually bilateral) affecting the renal papillae and sometimes extending into the renal pyramids, which may be the result of or a complication of various diseased states, infective, toxic or circulatory (Table 5.1). The pathological changes are non-specific in the sense that

they seem to apply whatever the etiological factor. Renal calculi, however, are commonly found when the disorder has been initiated by phenacetin (or other drug) addiction, but not usually as a consequence of the other etiological factors.

Seen at autopsy, the kidneys, which may be smaller than normal in the chronic cases, have a granular surface with a diffusely demarcated cortico-medullary junction infiltrated by inflammatory cells. The papillary necrotic lesion, which does not necessarily involve the entire renal papilla, is found in two types: (1) In the papillary type small necrotic foci appear within the central portion of the papilla leading to the formation of cavities, which later communicate with the calyx. (2) In the medullary type the necrosis involves the entire papilla and may even extend into the renal medulla with a well-defined line of demarcation (with leucocytic infiltration) between the necrosed papilla and the unaffected tissue at the base of the pyramid (Fig. 5.2, see p. 102). The papillary collecting tubules may be filled with deposits of calcium salts, and inflammatory changes may extend into the renal pelvis and ureters.

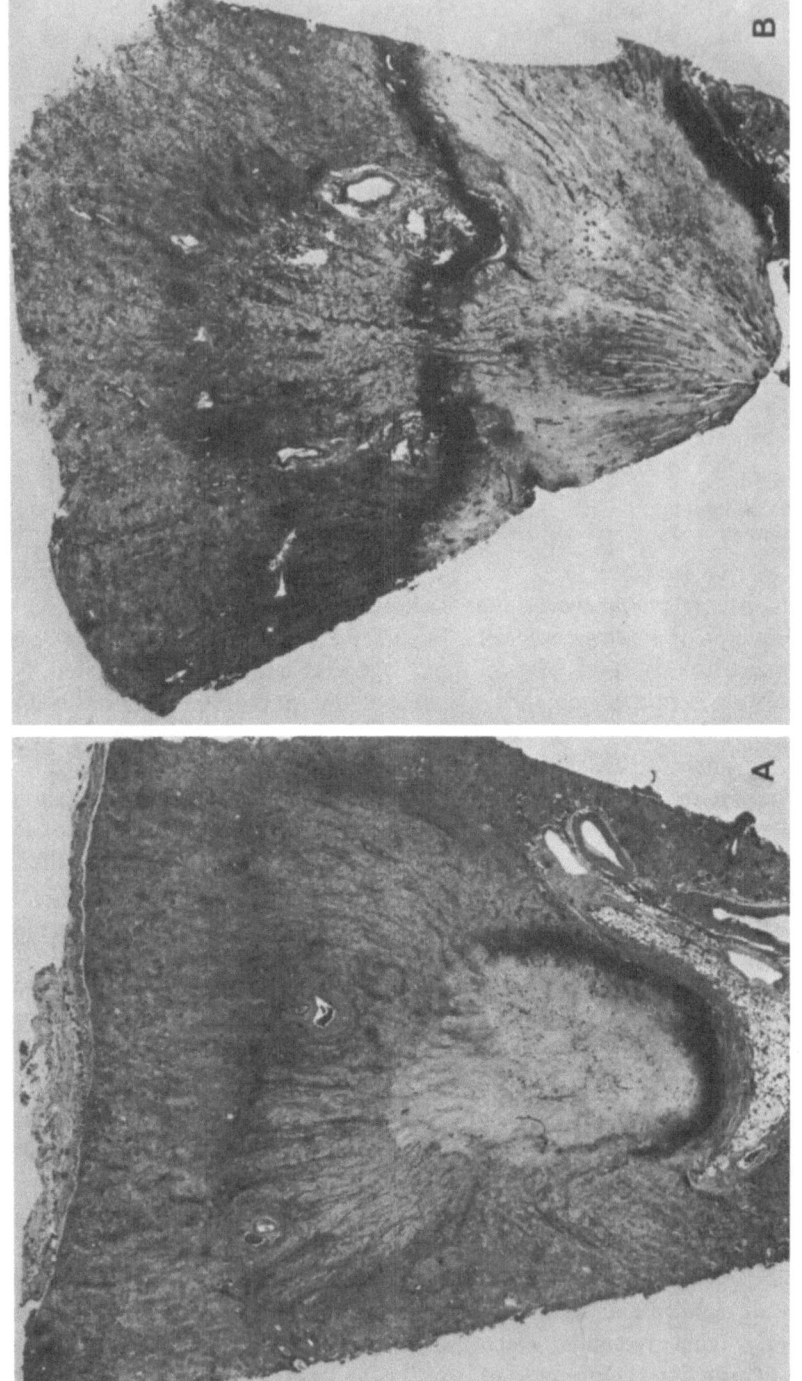

Fig. 5.2. Cross-section of a kidney recovered at autopsy from a patient who died from diabetes with chronic pyelonephritis. **A.** The necrosis involves an entire renal papilla shown as a pale pyramidal area in the middle of the picture; at the circumference of the papilla, around the apex and left lateral border is a zone of partly calcified tissue, showing black. **B.** Renal papillary necrosis showing the partial separation of the necrosed papilla from the renal medulla; a zone of dystrophic calcification is seen at the line of separation

When the papillae have sloughed away, re-epithelialization of the resulting cavity at the base of the papilla may take place, suggesting at least partial functional recovery. The kidneys in course of time usually undergo varying degrees of shrinkage though they are occasionally enlarged. Infection alone may not be the major cause and the evident susceptibility of the renal papillae to the toxic action of phenacetin is probably important. Local interference with the papillary circulation (thrombi or endarteritis obliterans) may contribute to the necrotic changes. The renal papilla has one blood supply by way of the efferent glomerular vessels, and a second by way of the tortuous arteries in the adventitia of the minor calyces, derived from the arcuate artery [4]. A plexus of thin-walled vessels at various levels of the renal medulla and at the tip of the papilla may render the local vessels vulnerable to thrombosis [97].

Blockage of the vasa recta seen sometimes in sickle-cell anaemia from aggregations of sickled cells may account for the papillary necrosis occasionally found in that condition, which then remains localized to the papillae. Papillary necrosis has been reported in association with medullary sponge kidney [26].

Renal calculi (or atypical calcific foci) form around a nucleus of necrotic renal papillary tissue in some patients. When such calculi are detached from the papilla from which they have originated, they may be voided spontaneously into the urine or may block one or both ureters, leading to acute calculous pyelonephritis or pyonephrosis, or to calculous anuria.

1. Experimental Renal Papillary Necrosis

The condition has been produced in rabbits by the administration of vinylamine [83]. Rats maintained on a fat-free diet (which can result in a nutritional deficiency of the unsaturated long-chain fatty acids) may develop a circumscribed renal papillary necrosis with calcification of the renal tubules [13]. In non-diabetic animals the condition has been produced experimentally by ligation of the ureter and the concomitant injection of *E. coli* [82]. Following the intravenous injection of staphylococci into mice Gorrill [45] found that many of the animals lost one kidney owing to loss of their single renal papilla. Phenacetin-induced renal disease in rats and rabbits has been produced experimentally [9]. Extensive renal papillary necrosis was produced in rats by the injection of human serum.

2. Clinical Picture

The clinical picture of renal papillary necrosis has to be seen against the background of the major disease or syndrome of which it is a complication or an iatrogenic overtone. It has often been unsuspected in diabetic patients. The age and sex groupings in pathological series have also changed over the years as the more recently recognized etiological factors have been allowed for. The condition is more common in women than in men and rare under the age of 40.

With improved radiographic techniques and a greater awareness of the frequency of phenacetin addiction and with the incidence of renal calculi in such cases, the condition began to be recognized clinically during life. Thus in Hultengren's [59] series of 103 cases (17 male, 86 female) the diagnosis had been made during life between the ages of 22 and 74, usually by radiography or histology; the period of time elapsing between the probable date of onset of the disease and its diagnosis ranged from 0 to 19 years. Almost one-fifth of diabetic subjects who died have been said to have a terminal acute renal infection and one-quarter of these have renal papillary necrosis, although often undiagnosed [47, 102].

In recent years it has often emerged when taking the clinical history that a patient with an infected renal stone has had persistent migrainous headaches, for which he, or generally she, has taken large doses of phenacetin and has gradually become addicted to it. Some such patients have given a history of recurrent attacks of pyelonephritis with rigors and fever, attacks of renal colic, haematuria (and occasionally massive haemorrhage), dysuria and the voiding of tissue fragments or small calculi in the urine (as in 13 of 103 cases in Hultengren's [59] series).

The condition can now often be recognized clinically as papillary necrosis with calculi, initiated by an addiction to phenacetin; an apparently unexplained pyonephrosis in a woman, who has earlier voided partly calcified solid necrotic masses in the urine and in whom radiography reveals small calcific masses in the kidney possibly thought to be atypical renal calculi, could be the result of a phenacetin addiction and renal papillary necrosis. As time passes the symptoms of urinary infection may be succeeded by those of hypertension, azotaemia, renal failure and fatal coma [112].

Phenacetin addicts may develop not only renal calculi but also chronic interstitial nephritis. Thus in 22 of 30 autopsies of patients who died from chronic interstitial nephritis, Spuhler and Zollinger [111] observed papillary necrosis, and in eight there had been a history of the abuse of phenacetin. However, phenacetin was shown to be only one of a range of drugs which may lead to addiction and serious consequences, others being aspirin, caffeine and pyramidon. The amount of phenacetin that will give rise to toxic symptoms was stated by Schweingruber [106] to be 0.9 g daily for at least 1 year. In Lindvall's [79] series of 155 patients with papillary necrosis 86 were shown to have had addiction

to phenacetin (10 males of mean age 46; 76 females of mean age 45) it being usually taken for the relief of intractable migraine-like headaches, neuralgia, headaches associated with sinusitis, a post-concussion syndrome or dysmenorrhoea.

The abuse of phenacetin, taken (especially by women) to relieve long-standing intractable migraine-like headache, was noted in 62 of 103 patients in Hultengren's [59] series, who were thought to have taken at least 1 kg phenacetin over a period of at least 1 year before the onset of subjective symptoms of renal disease. In his series, among other causes of renal papillary necrosis, 4 had diabetes and only a few had lower urinary tract obstruction.

The relationship between the intake of analgesics in general (including phenacetin) and renal calculus, at least in some groups of patients, may be closer than has formerly been thought, and there is room for further enquiry along these lines [15, 27].

In a useful survey by Blackman et al. [10] of 266 consecutive patients investigated for the presence of urinary calculi, 43 gave a history of a heavy consumption of analgesics, the type used being usually a mixture containing phenacetin, acetyl salicylic acid and caffeine [76], some of the patients taking up to 24 analgesic powders daily (4 g phenacetin). The diagnosis of calculus in their series was usually accepted on the basis of the radiological findings or the proved voiding of a stone, only 12 having been accepted on the basis of colic alone. However, not all women who are heavy consumers of analgesics develop renal calculi; thus in a control group of hospital patients (268 male and 221 female) who were known never to have voided a stone nor to have had one removed, it was found that 29 of the 221 female subjects against 28 of 103 patients in the group with renal calculi were classified as being heavy consumers of analgesics. Among the male stone-formers the consumption of analgesics was no more frequent than among the controls; the presence of urinary infection was greater in female patients [76]. The calculi as visualized radiologically were usually triangular, sometimes with a central lacuna. The effect of analgesics in general on the kidney not merely in respect of stone formation but to the kidney as a whole and also to renal function, has been studied extensively by Kincaid-Smith and her co-workers. Experiments designed to assess the effect of aspirin fed to the dehydrated experimental animal showed a considerable incidence of renal papillary necrosis when aspirin was fed over 8–30 weeks, the incidence being reduced by the simultaneous administration of caffeine, acetazolamide or sodium bicarbonate [67–69, 87–90].

3. Diagnosis

The diagnosis of renal papillary necrosis with stone formation may be made from the radiological examination of the affected kidney by the demonstration of small, rounded or oval cavities in the renal papillae. Lindvall [79] in a series based upon 155 cases (24 men, 131 women) and also Hultengren [59] have reported detailed urographic studies. Small cavities in one or more renal papillae may be seen in the first radiographs, and in later ones (or in retrograde pyelograms during and after ureteral compression) it may be possible to show the subsequent gradual increase in size and shape of the papillary cavities. It is not always easy to demonstrate the condition pyelographically in cases in which detachment of the papillae is just beginning or one in which a papilla has recently sloughed.

The diagnosis may be made from the clinical history and from the radiological examination of the affected kidney (Figs. 5.3 and 5.4, see p. 107) by the demonstration of small, rounded or oval cavities with or without calculi in the renal papillae [59, 79]. Small cavities in one or more renal papillae

may be seen in the first radiographs in a series to be followed by a gradual subsequent increase in their size and changes in shape. Retrograde pyelography (during and after ureteral compression) is often helpful; cases in which there is a commencing detachment of the papillae or those in which a papilla has sloughed may be difficult to interpret. Reflux of contrast medium from the calyx into the renal parenchyma may be a sign of commencing detachment.

Newly formed cavities have an irregular border but they become smoother in outline as they become epithelialized and may assume a clubbed appearance typical of pyelonephritis shrinkage. The so-called ring-shadows in the papillary region of the kidney, seen on the radiograph (observed in 92 kidneys in Lindvall's [79] series) which are pathognomonic of renal papillary necrosis, are caused by a detached papilla lying in the contrast-filled fully developed cavity. A filling defect in the shadow of the renal pelvis may be the result of a detached necrotic papilla which lies loose in the cavity of the renal pelvis. Of the 173 kidneys examined by Lindvall [79] calcified concretions or calculi were present in 55. Some had a calcareous shell and presented as an annular calcified shadow surrounding a more or less radiolucent nucleus, while in others the appearances were atypical (18 cases). The concretions were mostly found in cases in which there was more limited papillary necrosis (32 cases) but sometimes in kidneys with the more gross type of medullary necrosis (9 cases). It was considered that the interval between the time of the formation of a 'ring' shadow seen on the radiograph and that in which the detached papilla was first seen to have become calcified was between 2 and 16 months. Shrinkage of the papilla is often accompanied by calcification. Concretions from 15 patients were composed chiefly of struvite (when examined crystallographically), only two being pure calcium oxalate stones. Infection with various micro-

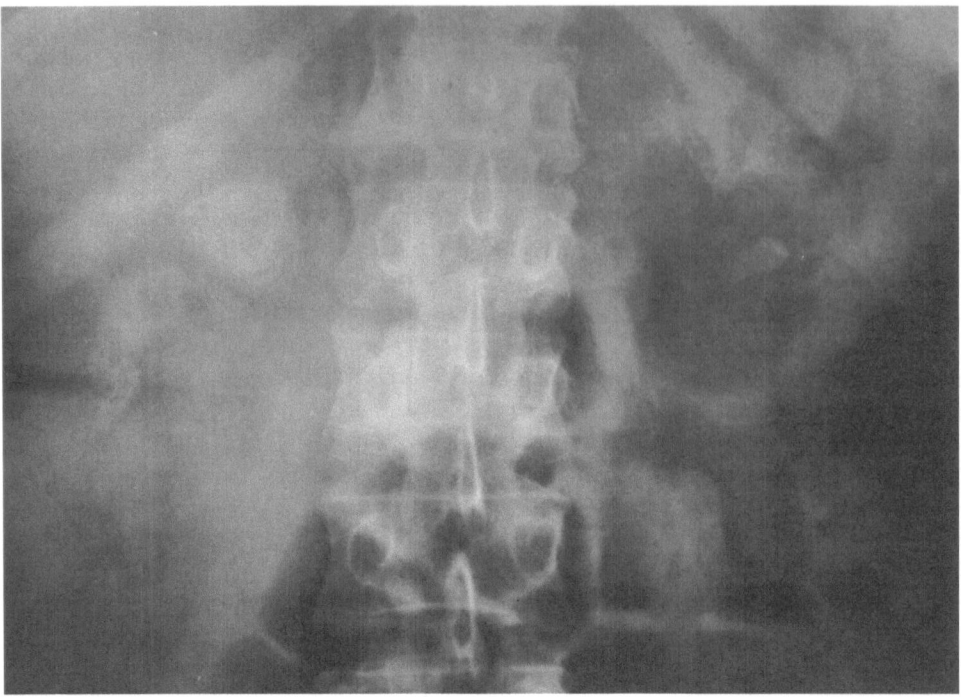

Fig. 5.3. Calculi in a patient with renal papillary necrosis. H.B., female, aged 52. Patient had had recurrent symptoms suggestive of pyelonephritis for 5 years; she admitted to having taken about 10 tablets containing phenacetin per day for at least 10 years. The straight radiograph showed bilateral calculi; those in the right kidney were laminated and showed central lacunae, surrounding which was calcific material of only moderate radio-opacity. The calculi were removed from the right kidney and a right lower-polar partial nephrectomy was done. The removed segment of the kidney was devoid of any of the normal renal papillae, and in view of the clinical and pathological findings the final diagnosis was renal papillary necrosis with secondary calcification of the sloughed papillae. The analysis of the stones revealed calcium phosphate and calcium carbonate. (By courtesy of Mr. Splatt of Brisbane)

organisms (especially *B. proteus*) aided the calcifying process in many cases, the necrotic papilla and clumps of bacteria acting as the nucleus.

In 27 of Hultengren's [59] 103 cases there was radiological evidence of renal calculus (unilateral in 16, bilateral in 11), which he grouped as: calcification within necrotic papillae; small to moderate-sized calculous deposits in the calyces, renal pelvis or ureter; and coral concretions.

Clinical Differential Diagnosis. On the plain radiograph small annular or irregularly shaped shadows of calculi often with a radiolucent centre should be readily dif-

ferentiated from the more solid calculi or nephrocalcinosis seen in some patients with primary hyperparathyroidism.

In renal tuberculosis there are more irregular calcific changes and pyramidal ulceration or destruction with irregular cavitation, and all the papillae are not equally involved in the destructive process. The radiological appearances in healed renal tuberculosis with calcification may possibly resemble those seen in papillary necrosis with calculi in which only a few papillae have been involved [79].

In renal dysplasia some calyces seen radiographically may lack the protruding papillary tips and the cortex may be thinner

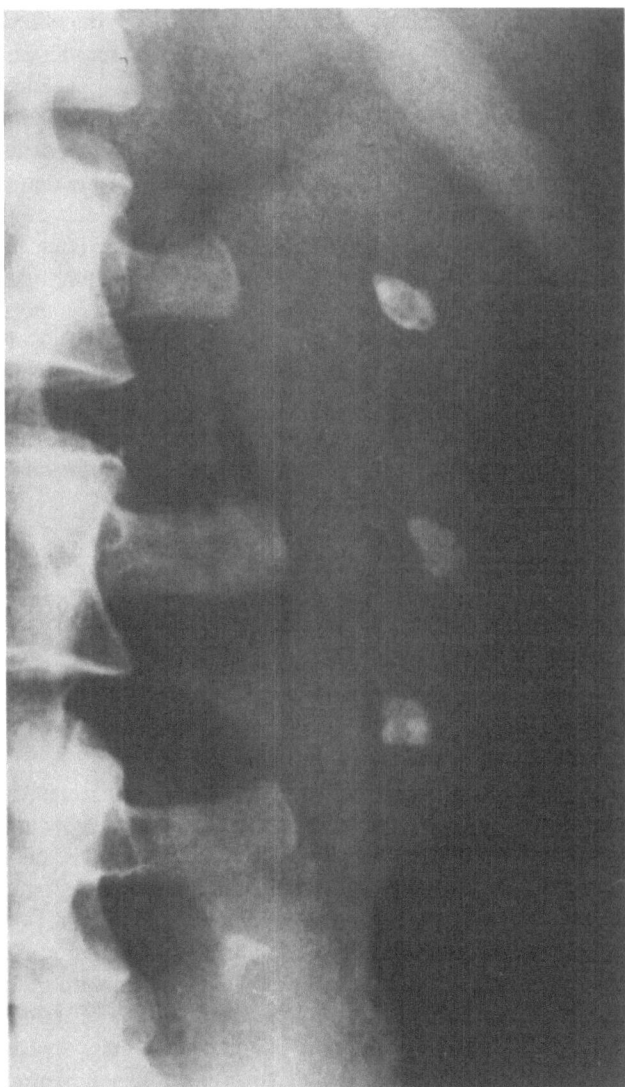

Fig. 5.4. Plain radiograph of the left kidney showing the typical appearance of medium-sized calcific foci in a patient with renal papillary necrosis. The centres of the stones are radiolucent. The radiograph is from a 45-year-old woman who admitted to a heavy intake of analgesics. (By courtesy of Mr. J.R. Blackman of Sydney, Australia, and the Editor of the British Medical Journal)

than normal, the calyx seeming to extend into the renal parenchyma almost to the outer surface.

Medullary sponge kidney can be recognized by the dilated ducts of Bellini in one or more pyramids (which usually contain clusters of concrements or smallish calculi) usually lying in several enlarged splayed-out calyces.

Pyelonephritis without papillary necrosis may show flattened pyramids or sometimes rounded or club-shaped calyces, and the entire kidney may be contracted, the cor-

tical part being narrower than normal with the calyces extending to the cortical surface.

4. Treatment

Prophylactic treatment of renal papillary necrosis consists in the adequate control of the initiating disorder. The modern treatment of diabetes (which in recent years has probably also reduced the incidence of infection of the urinary tract) and the early treatment of prostatic obstruction must have reduced its incidence. Patients who have taken excessive quantities of phenacetin must be advised to avoid the drug permanently, when their acute urological symptoms have been relieved and their calculi removed if necessary, if further renal damage is to be avoided.

Even in advanced cases analgesic nephropathy may be, with appropriate treatment, a recoverable form of renal failure. In 52 patients with that condition followed for a mean period of 41.2 months, Kincaid-Smith [70] found that renal function improved in 25 patients and remained unchanged in 19, no patient in the group needing to have either maintenance dialysis or renal transplantation. Treatment consisted of total withdrawal of all analgesic compounds, control of hypertension and of infection in the urinary tract and correction of the sodium-losing lesion by the administration of salt.

Surgical intervention for the relief of the renal calculi has been done with success in recent years in phenacetin addicts with quite advanced urological symptoms. In Hultengren's [59] series 12 patients had calculi removed surgically (pyelolithotomy, nephrolithotomy or ureterolithotomy) and nephrectomy was done in five (two having a non-functioning shrunken kidney). Partial nephrectomy in one patient, in whom changes seemed to have been restricted to the upper pole of the kidney, was followed later by the changes of papillary necrosis in other parts of the kidney. Meatotomy of the ureteric orifice may be appropriate for a stone at or near the ureterovesical opening. The stones after removal all had a nucleus of renal tissue, 11 being infected phosphatic stones and one (non-infected) being composed of calcium oxalate. Any associated urinary infection (and any associated anaemia) must receive appropriate treatment.

When the diagnosis of papillary necrosis with calculi is probable in patients with a pyonephrosis, the passage of an indwelling ureteric catheter to the renal pelvis allows the drainage of infected urine to take place to allow a planned operation (rather than a simple drainage procedure) for the removal of the detached necrotic calcified papilla to be successfully carried out at an appropriate later time and under antibiotic cover. Renal papillary necrosis has carried a heavy mortality in earlier years. In Hultengren's [56] series of 103 cases 12 patients died during the period of observation, from renal failure or from complicating diseases. In the other 91 the course of the disease was marked by alternative periods of clinical symptoms or relief ranging from weeks to years. Cases of complete recovery have been reported by Edmondson et al. [28].

IV. Nephrolithiasis and Chronic Peptic Ulcer

The ingestion of absorbable alkalis and of milk by patients with chronic peptic ulcer, prescribed as part of their medical treatment, may induce in some patients a temporary alkalosis and create conditions within the kidney which provide the formation of foci of calcification.

In a more advanced stage, the patient may develop pyloric stenosis, if operative treatment of the ulcer has been delayed; severe symptoms of alkalosis may then occur, which sometimes lead to coma and death. In the kidneys of such patients there may be changes in the renal tubular cells, associated with severe and widespread microscopic renal calcification (seen at autopsy), resulting either from the precipitation of calcium phosphate consequent on the alkalosis, or from dystrophic changes affecting the necrotic renal cells. The hazards, therefore, of the normal medical treatment of peptic ulcer by alkalis may give rise to local renal tubular calcific deposits similar to those which we have found in many patients with renal calcium-containing calculi, and with similar consequences (Chap. 2).

It is reasonable therefore to find in patients with peptic ulcer these twofold renal abnormalities: (1) interference with renal function (temporary or permanent but sometimes dramatic) expressed pathologically by renal cellular changes often with calcification; (2) insidious calcific changes promoting an incidence of calcium-containing renal calculi. Such clinical symptoms are sometimes found together.

In the extreme cases in this group, namely those who develop the milk-drinker's syndrome, a condition resulting from an actual addiction by the patient to milk and absorbable alkali, there may be severe impairment of renal function, nephrocalcinosis and renal calculi; there is in fact a graded series.

A few patients with a pre-existing chronic glomerulonephritis, who also have such an addiction to milk and alkali, provide a variant of these findings. The relationship between primary hyperparathyroidism, renal calculi and chronic duodenal ulcer has a bearing on these problems and is referred to in Chapter 4.

1. Alkalosis from Ingestion of Excess Alkali

Treatment of peptic ulcer with alkalis (often using the Sippy regime) may be followed in some patients by clinical symptoms resulting from an alkalosis associated with temporary impairment of renal function. Many examples have been recorded in the literature including a few fatal cases, in which the kidneys have shown histological abnormalities, including foci of calcification [50].

Symptoms may appear from as early as the fourth day (with large doses of alkali) after beginning the treatment until as late as the fourth week. The complaints include nervousness and irritability, a distaste for milk, severe and persistent temporal headaches, and eventually nausea followed by persistent vomiting, dizziness, vertigo and even mental changes. Later there is discomfort in the muscles and joints, twitchings, brisk reflexes and occasionally tetany with carpopedal spasms, followed sometimes by growing muscular weakness, drowsiness, apathy and coma. If the ingestion of alkali is stopped following the onset of nausea and vomiting, and 2-hourly feeds of milk, cereals, eggs and broth substituted, the symptoms usually disappear.

The biochemical changes in the blood include an increased CO_2-combining power, in association with low blood chlorides (a hypochloraemic alkalosis) [19, 20]. The pH of the blood may be 7.6 or higher instead of the normal 7.4; the low plasma chloride level accounts for the almost complete absence of chloride from the urine; and there is a reduced excretion of ammonia. A loss of sodium chloride in the vomitus may encourage a fall in the serum sodium level which, however, is counteracted by the absorption of ingested alkali.

Very few autopsies have been reported. In one fatal case the kidneys showed sclerosis of the intrarenal arteries, interstitial focal and lymphatic infiltration and glomerular sclerosis [50]. In another case, a man aged 64, there was slight reduction of the renal cortex, occasional arteriosclerotic changes, and calcareous renal deposits [93].

Dent [22] suggested that the renal damage in these cases is due not to the ingested alkali but to the calcium present in the milk, which is usually also given, and which is readily absorbable. The alkaline urine allows of the precipitation of calcium phosphate in the kidneys; he advocated a low calcium intake when alkali is given. The withdrawal of alkalis usually leads to clinical improvement with cessation of vomiting. If the alkalosis is severe ammonium chloride or acid sodium phosphate should be given until the alkali reserve has returned to normal.

2. Alkalosis from Simple or Malignant Pyloric Stenosis

Vomiting associated with pyloric obstruction resulting from peptic ulcer with stenosis, or from pyloric carcinoma may lead to severe extrarenal loss of water and electrolytes (chloride, sodium and potassium), followed by dehydration and severe biochemical imbalance leading to an alkalosis. The greatly increased secretion of sodium from the gastric mucosa, due to the associated gastritis and excessive secretion of mucus leads to a total body deficiency of sodium, a change which largely determines the extent of the dehydration. The loss of chloride in the vomitus is still, however, in excess of that of sodium. That there may be an associated renal lesion is evidenced by the presence of casts in the urine, a rising blood urea and proteinuria. Alkalotic tetany (not resulting from a reduced serum calcium level) may develop and if uncorrected may be followed by coma consequent upon the biochemical imbalance of the internal environment, and ultimately to fatal renal failure.

Histological changes in the renal tubules have included deposits of calcific material in the convoluted tubules in patients who had died as a result of pyloric obstruction associated with tetany [91] and in patients who died with regurgitant vomiting following gastroenterostomy for pyloric ulcer [116]. Many other cases were subsequently reported in the literature.

The author has observed four patients suffering from pyloric stenosis caused by a peptic ulcer, who died following a period of coma and a relatively short history. Histologically, the kidney showed degenerative changes in the tubular cells and moderate to severe microscopic parenchymal calcification in the cells of the cortex and the medullary rays.

More advanced renal histological changes were seen in the kidney of a man aged 41 who was admitted to hospital in coma and was subsequently shown to have had a long history of duodenal ulcer with intermittent attacks of pyloric obstruction, which had now led to his grave condition. He had severe hypochloraemic alkalosis, hypokalaemia and azotaemia, from which he was rescued by appropriate management of his blood electrolytes. He subsequently had a gastroenterostomy to relieve the pyloric stenosis, at a later date a partial gastrectomy for the relief of haemorrhage from an anastomotic peptic ulcer, and still later a nephrectomy for a renal carcinoma.

Sufficient residual renal tissue was available in the excised kidney for a histological examination to be made of the striking changes consequent upon the earlier pyloric stenosis with its grave alkalotic incidents, which were more far-reaching than those seen in the more 'acute' cases referred to above. Calcific deposits were found not only in the cells of the ascending limb of Henle's loop and the distal convoluted tubule but also in those of the proximal convoluted tubules and in the collecting tubules and in some glomeruli. There were also extensive extratubular calcific deposits. Calcification extended through a considerable portion of the lengths of individual nephrons. The distribution of the calcific changes was patchy, some areas showing extensive involvement alternating with other areas of normal-appearing renal tissue and tracts of gross parenchymal atrophy and interstitial fibrosis without calcification. Many of the affected tubules were denuded of lining cells, exposing the basement membrane, which itself was sometimes calcified; in many instances this membrane had disappeared and the calcium salts had spread outside the confines of the tubule to form irregular deposits in the tissue spaces between the tubules and in the interstitial connective tissue. Dilatation of some medullary renal tubules was accompanied by the formation of small or medium-sized cysts sometimes containing deposits of calcium salts and other debris. A varying degree of parenchymal atrophy was produced by glomerular hyalinization and tubular obliteration.

In spite of the fact that his remaining kidney must have been similarly severely damaged by cellular changes and calcification, the patient was still alive, well and symptom-free in 1975 and had worked at a garage for 10 years, though with a raised blood urea.

Many of the calcific deposits in the larger tubules were similar to those in stone-bearing kidneys (Chap. 2) and could well have led to calculus formation [95].

Experimental Work. Experimentation, chiefly on the cat, has demonstrated that renal changes including the presence of multiple calcific foci similar to those found in the kidneys of humans dying from pyloric stenosis, can be induced by ligating the pylorus. Following such a procedure, if life is being sustained for a time by administration of subcutaneous injections of 10% glucose solution, renal changes consisting of tubular degeneration or necrosis with calcific deposits, first in the spiral and the terminal straight part of the convoluted tubules and later in those portions of the tubules adjacent to the glomeruli have been found at autopsy [120].

The author carried out similar experiments on cats: thick silk ligatures were placed round the pylorus sufficiently tightly to occlude the lumen, but not to cause a risk of perforation of the gut from acute necrosis, the animals living thereafter from 3 to 6 days. Foci of renal calcification were found in the kidneys at autopsy in five of eight cases operated on (none being found in the control animals) either in the cortical or the medullary part of the kidney, being seen as large masses either in the cells or in the lumina of the convoluted tubules [98].

3. Nephrolithiasis and Peptic Ulcer in the Same Patient

It is believed by some observers that the incidence of nephrolithiasis in patients suffering from ulcer of the stomach and duodenum is higher than that in the normal population. Such an increased incidence, if true, may be a consequence of incidents during the treatment or clinical course of the ulcer just referred to. An alkaline urine of a high specific gravity over varying periods of time may be a favourable setting for the precipitation of stone-forming calcium salts in the renal tubules, possibly therefore promoting stone formation.

In recent years, however, it has been shown that both renal stone and chronic peptic ulcer are common complications of primary hyperparathyroidism, the co-existence of which as a renal stone-promoting disease must therefore always be suspected when these conditions are found simultaneously in one patient (Chap. 4).

Figures quoted below illustrate the possible association between the two diseases (renal stone and peptic ulcer). They were mostly published before the possible relationship with hyperparathyroidism was widely recognized and must now be read in that context. Cabot [16] stated that some patients, whose diet is planned in such a way as to require a high alkaline intake such as is indulged in by patients with gastric and duodenal ulcers, do tend to develop stone. Kretschmer and Brown [72] investigated the incidence of urinary calculus in 680 patients who had had medical treatment for peptic ulcer. Of these, 21 patients (3.1%) gave a history of urinary calculus before they presented themselves for treatment for ulcer; 33 (4.9%) gave a history of urinary calculus which had occurred as long as 10–20 years after medical treatment for peptic ulcer had been instituted. Conversely, in a series of 1260 cases of renal and ureteric calculi only 26 (2.06%) gave a history of peptic ulcer and only 15 had received alkali for the treatment of the ulcer, in 3 of which the stones had developed many years after the treatment for ulcer had been discontinued. No clear etiological relationship could be traced between the ulcer and the renal calculi in this series.

Eisele [30] found that of 505 patients suffering from renal or ureteric stone, 44 also had peptic ulcer (8.5%), the duration of the ulcer symptoms before the onset of stone averaging 8.3 years. In addition to the 43 patients who had received alkali treatment for peptic ulcer, there were 13 (2.5%) who had taken alkalis for a considerable time for gastro-intestinal distress and who had also developed stones. Thus, 56 patients (11.1%) of the stone series were known to have had prolonged treatment by alkalis, suggesting a relationship.

Becker et al. [5] compared the incidence of parenchymal renal calcification in 99 patients in whom an active or healed duodenal ulcer was found at autopsy, with that in a control group of 99 non-ulcer patients of the same age and sex. From both series cases were excluded in which any obvious cause of calcification existed (hyperparathyroidism, hypervitaminosis D, upper intestinal obstruction and destructive bone disease). In 36 cases (36.4%) with duodenal ulcer there was some degree of renal parenchymal calcification which was of moderate or severe degree in 21 (21.12%). In only 13 (13.1%) of the controls was there calcification which was of moderate or severe degree in 6 (6.0%); these differences are statistically significant.

In the cases with renal parenchymal calcification there had been a significantly higher incidence of ulcer (with a history of therapy with absorbable alkalis, or of complications requiring surgical treatment) than in those without renal parenchymal calcification; of the ulcer cases 11 had nephrolithiasis. The investigation seemed to show, however, that, in the cases examined, the incidence of renal calcification in the ulcer series lay somewhere between that found in a series of non-stone-bearing kidneys and that in a series of stone-bearing kidneys (Chap. 2).

Frame and Haubrich [35] during an examination of 300 patients with peptic ulcer found a history of urinary calculus in 17 (5.7%), in 7 of whom the symptoms of peptic ulcer had antedated those of urinary calculus, while in 7 the reverse was true; 2 of the patients were shown to have a proven parathyroid adenoma.

Blagg [11] carried out a survey of patients with peptic ulcer and renal stone in the author's hospital and department to determine if there was any possible association between the two diseases. During the period 1930–1949 in the Leeds General Infirmary there were 15,310 deaths, autopsy being done on 13,314 (88%). Peptic ulcers were found in 2214 cases (16.63%), and renal or ureteric calculi in 114 (0.86%). Assuming this distribution, one would expect to find 19 ulcer patients with stone, whereas in fact there were 25 cases, a figure which is not statistically significant ($\chi^2 = 1.89$, $p = $ approximately 1.15).

In a further investigation on inpatients, the incidence of peptic ulcer and renal and ureteric stone was obtained from the clinical diagnoses of patients discharged from the hospital during 1953 and 1954. Of 38,939 patients there were 1383 with peptic ulcer (3.55%) and 149 with renal or ureteric stone (0.38%). Unselected groups of ulcer and of stone patients were written to in 1955 to enquire as to whether they had had stone or ulcer. Of the 308 stone patients who replied, 14 had had ulcer; on the normal incidence given above one would have expected 10 cases, a figure which is not statistically significant ($\chi^2 = 1.67$, $p = 0.2$). Of the 495 ulcer patients who replied, 10 had had renal stones; in 2 of these stones were present before the ulcer developed and in the other 8 stone had developed later, figures which are statistically significant ($\chi^2 = 19.9$, $p < 0.01$). An association between peptic ulcer and stone was suggested.

4. Milk-drinker's Syndrome

Following the prolonged and excessive intake of large amounts of milk and of absorbable alkali, some patients suffering from long-standing chronic duodenal or gastric ulcer have developed symptoms of renal insufficiency with azotaemia, nephrocalcinosis or renal calculi and (in fatal cases) microscopic renal calcification, and often widespread metastatic calcification in the periarticular regions, in the lungs, the conjunctivae and sclerae, the costal cartilages, the blood vessels and the dura mater, falx and tentorium. The condition has been called milk-drinker's syndrome or calcium gout [14].

The reported cases have been mostly in men of middle or late-middle life between the ages of 36 and 65. Having found that the ingestion of milk and alkalis has relieved the pain, they have gradually acquired the habit (which has gradually become an addiction) of taking large quantities of milk (often 2–4 quarts or more in 24 h), and of excessive doses of alkalis or antacids, often combined with calcium and magnesium carbonate, or proprietary antacid powders, usually with a high calcium content. Although the kidneys under such circumstances suffer gradually increasing damage, high intakes of calcium and alkali may be tolerated by the body for years; the length of history in reported cases has varied from 3 to 28 years, though it is not always clear if the habit has been continuous over long periods.

In the pre-critical stage the patients complain of increasing general weakness, vague muscular pains, loss of interest in work, irritability, depression, loss of appetite and weight, general malaise. Thirst, polyuria, frequency of micturition and nocturia are indicative of increasing renal impairment when there may be hypertension and associated headache. Later the symptoms include insomnia, mental confusion and impairment of memory. A few patients have experienced renal colic or haematuria, and renal stones have been voided spontaneously [23, 24, 105].

In the early stages general nutrition is maintained, but later there is loss of weight and also anaemia, which is secondary to renal failure. Eye changes (as in many patients with hypercalcaemia) have been observed. Radiography frequently shows calcification in the walls of the aorta, the iliac vessels and the radial artery, and also demonstrates the irregular calcified periarticular masses of varied density. Changes in the bones are observed only rarely but extensive periosteal new bone formation in the long bones has been reported [14], as have been narrowing and sclerosis of the terminal interphalangeal joints of several fingers, and localized punched-out areas of bone destruction in the metacarpals and the phalanges. Osteosclerosis of the ribs, femora, lumbar spine and metacarpals has been observed [100].

At a still more advanced stage some of the joints become painful on movement, and swellings (firm or soft and semi-fluctuant and non-tender) may develop in the subcutaneous or periarticular regions of the hips, shoulders, elbows, ankles and metatarso-phalangeal joints, in the pulp of the fingers or in the penis.

Sooner or later a crisis occurs, often during an exacerbation of the ulcer symptoms (when even larger amounts than usual of milk and alkalis are being taken) or during a phase of persistent vomiting, intensifying the symptoms of alkalosis and leading to dehydration, drowsiness and even collapse with hypotension.

If untreated the clinical course is that of progressive renal failure with loss of weight or even emaciation, increasing weakness, apathy or mental disorientation, attacks of drowsiness or fainting and finally death from anuria or in uraemic coma. In fatal cases, the kidneys are seen to have become progressively contracted and show advanced granular changes; the cortex is reduced in thickness and there are zones of glomerular hyalinization, tubular atrophy and increase of the interstitial connective tissue. Extensive calcification in the convoluted and the collecting tubules with calcific masses in the tubular lumina are observed; there may be renal calculi; and there is often a secondary enlargement of the parathyroid glands.

Biochemical and Renal Changes. The serum calcium is elevated if the blood is examined when the patient is taking large amounts of milk and alkali, recorded figures having varied from 11.0 to 15.6 mg/100 ml blood; when milk and alkalis are withdrawn the serum calcium returns, often quite rapidly, to its normal level. When renal function has become seriously impaired, the serum calcium is normal or low. The serum phosphate level may be normal, but with the onset of renal failure it rises to values of 5.0–11.0 mg; the level may fall if milk and alkali are withdrawn from the diet. The alkaline phosphatase is usually normal. The daily urinary output of calcium may be normal for a long time but is low in the stage of renal failure.

Whereas during the advanced stages of renal insufficiency from other causes there is often an acidosis, in these patients there is usually a mild alkalosis, the persisting levels of the CO_2-combining power of the serum being 30–36 mEq/litre; acidosis may develop as a terminal finding. The serum sodium level is low with dehydration and there may be a hypokalaemia. There may also be hyperproteinaemia [14]. Azotaemia, which has usually been found, together with low urea clearance (blood urea of 150–300 mg/100 ml being not uncommon) diminishes following treatment. The urinary specific gravity becomes low (1006–1010) during the period of polyuria, and there is inability to concentrate as estimated by the water-deprivation test. Occasionally hyaline and granular casts are present in the urine.

Renal Calculi and Nephrocalcinosis. Of 29 cases from the literature referred to in Table 5.2 (see p. 116), stones in the renal calyces, pelvis or ureter were reported in 6 cases and nephrocalcinosis in a further 5, and often gave rise to clinical symptoms.

A female patient aged 42, under the care of the author, had had a long-standing duodenal ulcer. For this she took a milk diet (during a 4-year period) together with 8–15 tablets daily, each tablet containing about 250 mg calcium (mainly as carbonate); her daily intake of calcium was therefore 3–4 g in addition to that in the milk. She developed diffuse bilateral nephrocalcinosis affecting the pericalyceal parts of both kidneys (Fig. 5.5). The urine was infected and this was thought to have contributed to the condition.

A somewhat similar case was reported in a male patient aged 66 [97] who had had a duodenal ulcer for 30 years and had had treatment with various antacids and diets as well as proprietary 'indigestion' tablets, having become habituated to them. Each tablet contained about 5 mg bismuth aluminate, 25 mg trisilicate, 10 mg aluminium hydroxide gel, 80 mg heavy magnesium carbonate and 400 mg calcium carbonate; he had therefore taken approximately 8 g calcium carbonate daily for 30 years, together with calcium in milk and diet. He had hypercalcaemia; clinical improvement followed withdrawal of the tablets and the calcium from the diet, the high level of serum calcium falling to normal.

Other cases of milk-alkali syndrome have been published by Texter [114] and Soliani [109].

Differential Diagnosis. Hypercalcaemia has been reported in patients with gastric ulcer and with no previous renal disease who were being treated conservatively, the serum calcium level returning to normal when milk and alkali were withdrawn from the diet. The syndrome has to be differentiated from other conditions which are associated with hypercalcaemia accompanied by renal insufficiency.

Primary hyperparathyroidism with bone disease leads to hypercalcaemia (sometimes with eye changes), frequently hypophosphataemia and often a high urinary calcium, nephrocalcinosis and renal calculi; there is no alkalosis. Whereas a mild alkalosis is usually found in the milk-alkali syndrome, an acidosis was present in Kyle's case [73], probably resulting from the advanced stage of renal failure. Clinical improvement and a reversal of the abnor-

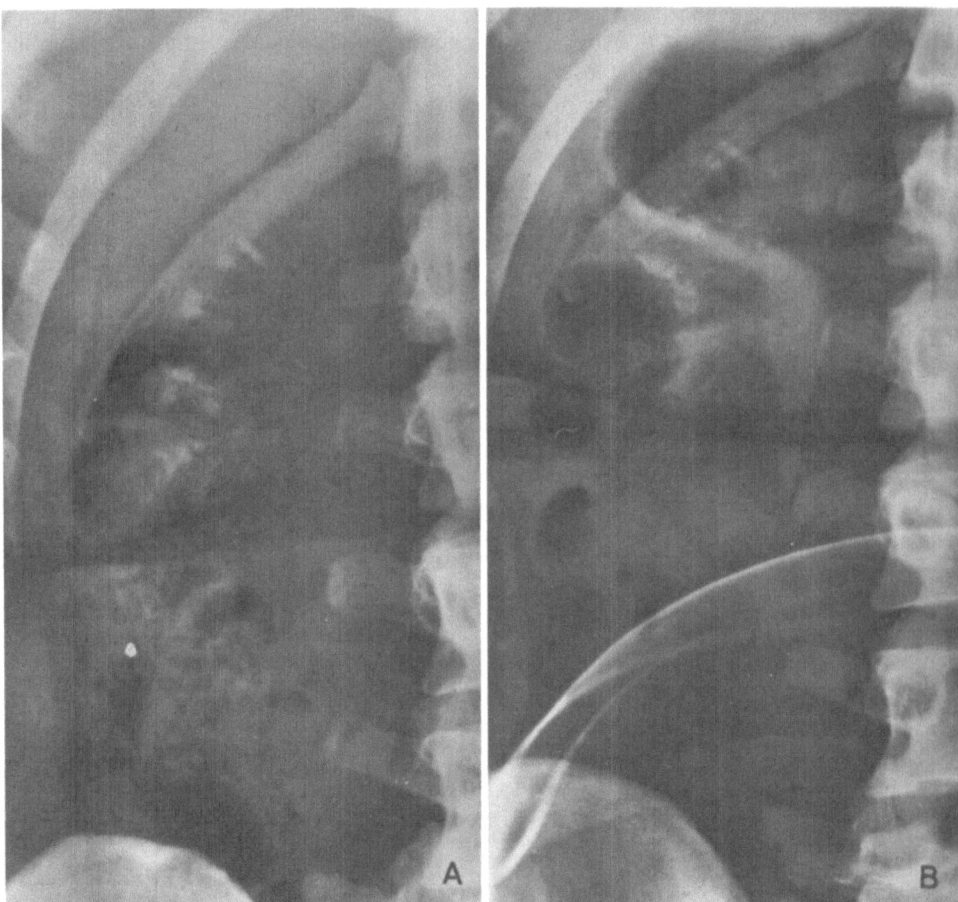

Fig. 5.5. Case of chronic duodenal ulcer; bilateral nephrocalcinosis; pyelonephritis; excessive ingestion of calcium. E.W., female, aged 42. In 1941 the patient suffered from acute pyelitis with bilateral renal pain, fever, and blood and pus in the urine. In 1942 she had a haematemesis and subsequently had typical post-prandial ulcer pain relieved by alkalis. Symptoms from the ulcer (proved radiologically) persisted for the whole of the subsequent 13 years with only short periods of relief. She had a very high intake of calcium tablets for many years (for details, see text). The radiograph shows bilateral diffuse nephrocalcinosis. A. Plain radiograph shows the pyramidal character of the nephrocalcinosis in the right kidney. The picture of the left kidney was similar. B. Intravenous pyelograms show that renal function is fairly well maintained.

mal biochemical findings may follow the administration of a diet low in calcium and absorbable alkalis and enable the two conditions to be differentiated during the more advanced stages of the diseases. In a few doubtful cases a surgical exploration of the neck in order to examine the para-thyroid tissue has been done [14]. Some patients with hyperparathyroidism have a chronic duodenal ulcer when the differen-

tial diagnosis may be difficult, especially if the patient has taken large amounts of milk [17].

Treatment. Patients who arrive in hospital critically ill and dehydrated must be given intravenous fluids with appropriate sup-plementation of electrolytes if needed. In the most severe cases no alkalis or calcium or milk products must be given orally; a

Table 5.2. Short summaries of some reported cases from the literature of the milk-alkali syndrome. Table gives sample figures in active stage and does not convey the variations of treatment, nor the terminal blood chemistry

Author and year	Age and sex	Ulcer	Length of history (years)	Amount of milk ingested per day (quarts)	Amount of alkalis ingested per day	Serum calcium mg/100 cc blood	Serum phosphorus mg/100 cc blood	Urine calcium mg/24 h	CO₂-combining power Vol% or mEq/litre
Burnett et al. (1949)	1. M 44	Gastric	3	Several	Large amounts	12.0–14.6	4.0–4.7	87	27.4–31 mEq/l
	2. M 75		2.5			12.0–12.8			23.3–30.2 mEq/l
	3. M 44	Duodenal	25			12.4–12.8	5.5–6.6		30.0–35.0 mEq/l
	4. M 38	Duodenal	3	2–3	6 or more teaspn. sod. bicarb.	12.5–12.7	6.5–7.3		26.8 mEq/l
	5. M 55	?Duodenal	16	4–5	Large amounts of sod. bicarb.	11.0–14.0	4.1–5.9	77	
	6. M 54	Duodenal	30	Several	Large amounts of sod. bicarb.	11.5	4.6		33.0 mEq/l
Miller et al. (1952)[a]	M 41	Duodenal	7	1–2	2 teaspn. sod. bicarb.	9.2–11.5	4.8		44 vol%
McQueen (1952)	M 56	Duodenal	6	4	Alkaline powders	11.3–13.5	3.2–4.3		35.0–66.0 vol%
Wermer et al. (1953)[b]	M 67	Duodenal	13	2–3	Sippy powders, alkalis, antacids	10.8–11.8	3.0–5.0	156	14.0–38.0 vol%
Dworetzky (1954)	M 50	Duodenal	28	2–8 or more	Up to 13 g CaCO₃ and 40 g sod. bicarb.	9.0–9.9	3.5–4.6	70 reduced later to 46	23–20 vol%
Snapper et al. (1954)[c]	1. M 62	Peptic	10	3	Large amounts of alkali (proprietary preparation)	9.3	11.0	Low	33 vol%
	2. F 65	Peptic	16	800 mg calcium	High intake of alkalis	10.3–12.0	5.5–5.9	148–202 (low calcium diet)	
Dufault and Tobias (1954)	1. M 57	Peptic	8	1	2 g Ca carb. + sod. bicarb.	12.8	3.4		
	2. M 52	Peptic	Longer than 2	1–3	12–100 g sod. bicarb.	16.0	4.2		40 mEq/l
	3. M 52	Peptic	20	2	6–16 g sod. bicarb.	14.5	5.6	Low	39 mEq/l
	4. M 50	Peptic	20	4	8–36 g sod. bicarb. and CaCO₃	11.5	6.0		37 mEq/l
Foltz (1954)[d]	M 54	Duodenal	25	2	Large amounts CaCO₃	12.2–12.4	1.8	30–60 daily	Normal
Kyle (1954)	M 49	Duodenal		2–3 l	Average of 226 g sod. bicarb.	(1) 12.1 (2) with renal failure 7.5	11.4 / 23.0	38–110	32 mEq/l / 20 mEq/l
Rodnan and Johnson (1954)[e]	M 52	Duodenal	17	Moderate amounts	Large amount sod. bicarb. also proprietary antacid powders containing 3.6–4.8 g calcium	9.8–10.3	3.5–7.9	Less than 20 mg	36–39 mEq/l

[a] Miller, J.M., Freeman, L., Heath, W.H.: Calcinosis due to treatment of duodenal ulcer. J. Amer. Med. Assoc. *148*, 198 (1952)

[b] Wermer, P., Kuschner, M., Riley, E.A.: Reversible metastatic calcification associated with excessive milk and alkali intake. Amer. J. Med. *14*, 108 (1963)

[c] Snapper, I., Bradley, W.G., Wilson, V.E.: Metastatic calcification and nephrocalcinosis from medical treatment of peptic ulcer. Arch. Intern. Med. *93*, 807 (1954)

Blood urea nitrogen	Renal function (sp. grav. of urine)	Alkaline phosphatase Bodansky units per 100 cc or King-Armstrong units	Hypertension	Eye calcification	Nephrocalcinosis or calculi	Metastatic calcification	Result
80 NPN	Albuminuria sp.g. 1012	5.3 BU	140/80	Positive	Had passed calculi Nephrocalcinosis	Dura, vessels, tendons, costal cartilage	Died
85 NPN	Albuminuria sp.g. 1008	2.8–6.8 BU		Positive		Tentorium, dura, bronchi	Died
198 NPN	Albuminuria sp.g. 1111	7.2 BU	175/105		Nephrocalcinosis	Aorta, iliac arteries	Improved
78 NPN	No albumen		150/100	Positive			Died
89–100 NPN	Albumn. 1011 poor renal function	3.2–5.9 BU	150/80	Positive		Falx cerebri, knees, elbows, hands, lungs	Died
131 NPN	No albumen sp.g. 1016	4.4 BU	130/70				Improved
232 NPN	Albuminuria impaired renal funct.			Positive		Lungs, lumbar region	Relieved
140–320 NPN	Urea clearance 16% sp.g. 1010	8–12 KA	140/100	Positive		Hands, pulp of fingers, elbow, hip; radial and iliac arteries	Metastatic calctn. resolved. Improved
58–61 NPN	Albuminuria impaired function sp.g. 1007–1018	3–5 BU	Normal	Positive		Inferior angle of scapulae, shoulder, wrist, fingers (interphalangeal joints)	Temporary improvement but died from uraemia
57–35	Urea clearance 24.3% of normal	4.5–5.2 BU	Intermittently raised	Positive	Stone R. renal pelvis and R. ureter. Had also had renal colic and passed calculi	Shoulders, wrists, fingers, elbows, feet. Intermittent claudication. Calcf. of aorta and iliac artery	Great reduction in periarticular calc. after treatment. Persistent renal insufficiency. Fairly good health
53–120	Impaired Albuminuria sp.g. 1010–1016	12.0 KA	115/80	Positive	Widespread nephrocalcinosis	Index finger, elbow, shoulder, hips, arm, penis. Arteries calcfd.	Died from anuria
31.7 NPN	Impaired sp.g. 1010	12.0 KA	130/80	Positive	Bilateral nephrocalcinosis	Subcutaneous, hips, shoulder, neck, aorta and femoral arteries	
51	Impaired Albumin Granular casts	2.6			Had had ureteric calculi		
60	Albuminuria sp.g. 1010			Positive			
	Albuminuria	4.0		Positive	Nephrocalcinosis (autopsy)	Metastatic calcification (autopsy)	Died of uraemia
	Albuminuria			Positive			
60 BUN	Impaired Albuminuria sp.g. 1008	Normal	Hypertension	Positive		Calcification of pelvic arteries	
132 NPN	Albuminuria sp.g. 1005–1011	4.4 BU		Positive	Nil on X rays		
291 NPN		22.0 BU		Positive	Very severe nephrocalcinosis at autopsy	Dura, lungs, orbits (autopsy)	Died
125–130 NPN	Albuminuria sp.g. 1005–1006	4.5 BU	140/90	Positive	Bilateral nephrocalcinosis (radiologically) (also renal colic)	Proximal to nail base of one finger	Improved

[d] Foltz, E.E.: Calcinosis complicating peptic ulcer therapy. Gastroenterology 27, 50 (1954)
[e] Rodnan, G., Johnson, H.: Chronic renal failure in association with excessive intake of calcium and alkali; report of case and review of pathogenesis. Gastroenterology 27, 584 (1954)

Table 5.2.—*Continued*

Author and year	Age and sex	Ulcer	Length of history (years)	Amount of milk ingested per day (quarts)	Amount of alkalis ingested per day	Serum calcium mg/100 cc blood	Serum phosphorus mg/100 cc blood	Urine calcium mg/24 h	CO₂-combining power Vol% or mEq/litre
Scholz and Keating (1955)	1. M 43	Duodenal	20	1.5–2	Large amounts of alkali and antacids (CaCO₃, MgCO₃, and Mag. Trisilicate, 4–6 teaspn.)	13.7	2.6	96–259 mg (on low calcium diet)	22 mEq/l
	2. M 52	Duodenal	22	1–2	1 lb alkaline powder weekly (CaCO₃, MgCO₃)	12.1	2.8		
	3. M 49	Peptic ulcer	25	1–2 glasses	2.5 lb Sippy powder weekly (CaCO₃, MgCO₃)	12.9	4.8		41.2 mEq/l
	4. M 39	Duodenal	7	0.5–1	Large amounts antacid; sod. bicarb. 3–4 teaspn.	11.8	3.2	126 (on low calcium diet)	
	5. M 49	Duodenal	6	1–4	'Virtually living on milk and alkaline powders.' 10–12 teaspn.	15.6	3.8		22 mEq/l
	6. M 47	Duodenal	2	1–2	Sod. bicarb. 1 lb weekly	11.2	3.4		39.4 mEq/l
	7. F 51	Duodenal	20	1 + 1 pt.: 0.5 milk 0.5 cream	Sippy powders (CaCO₃, MgO) 3–6 daily; sod. bicarb. 0.5 lb monthly; proprietary antacid 1 package every other day	13.6	6.2		29 mEq/l
	8. M 36	Duodenal	3	2–3	Proprietary antacid 4–6 tabs daily	12.8	3.8		23 mEq/l
Holten and Lundbaek (1955)[f]	M 49	Prepyloric	20	3 l milk, and 0.5 l cream	8–10 g sod. bicarb. daily for many years; admitted an addiction to 'baking powder'	10.9–8.5	6.3–9.0	55–79	38 mEq/l
Rifkind et al. (1960)	F 48	Gastric	12	1 pt. or less	Average of 20 g calcium (as carbonate), with very small amount calcium phosphate (taken as Rennie tablets)	9.3	6.1	78	20 mEq/l

[f] Holten, C., Lundbaek, K.: Renal insufficiency and severe calcinosis due to excessive alkali. Acta Med. Scand. *151*, 182 (1955)

rapid subjective and objective response often follows such treatment.

Aluminium hydroxide (aludrox, hyalgel), which precipitates ingested phosphate as insoluble aluminium phosphate in the intestine and also acts as an antacid, is useful [24]. The serum calcium may then rapidly return to normal, the blood urea level may be reduced and renal function may improve. The painful periarticular and ocular calcific deposits tend to diminish in size and may even disappear, but reappear unless the patient remains on a low-milk and low-alkali regime [82, 118]. Permanent medical supervision is subsequently needed to prevent relapse. If the patient can be made fit and if his renal function will allow, a radical operation for the removal of the ulcer (primarily to relieve pain) may offer the best hope of a long-term cure. Of the

cases noted in Table 5.2 eight died from uraemia.

Beneficial results followed treatment in the eight cases reported by Scholz and Keating [105]. The associated renal and ureteric calculi as well as the ulcer require treatment on established lines; nephrocalcinosis if present will not disappear though it may not increase.

V. Chronic Glomerulonephritis and Excessive Ingestion of Milk

Patients with chronic nephritis never suffer from renal stone; a patient may, in theory, develop a renal stone and in later life develop chronic nephritis but the coincidence of the two conditions is very rare. Microscopic renal calcification is unusual in

Blood urea nitrogen	Renal function (sp. grav. of urine)	Alkaline phosphatase Bodansky units per 100 cc or King-Armstrong units	Hyper-tension	Eye calcifi-cation	Nephrocalcinosis or calculi	Metastatic calcification	Result
120 BU	Albuminuria sp.g. 1014	2.7	140/90	Negative	Nil		Recovery
94 BU	No albuminuria sp.g. 1006		154/96	Negative	Nil		Recovery
234 BU	Albuminuria sp.g. 1013	3.2	80/60 (dehydration)	Negative	Renal calculi voided naturally 5 yr before		Recovery
116 BU	Albuminuria sp.g. 1009	2.7	150/105	Negative	Stone in right kidney		Recovery
102 BU	No albuminuria sp.g. 1008	3.5 KA	168/100	Negative	Nil		Recovery
100 BU	No albuminuria sp.g. 1012	4.2 BU	164/106		Bilateral renal calculi		Recovery
126 BU	Albuminuria sp.g. 1008	11.5 KA	180/160	Negative	Renal colic (passed a stone); focal and tubular calcifi-cation on renal biopsy		Recovery
85.4 BU	Albuminuria sp.g. 1008	11 KA	150/115	Negative	Nil		Recovery
334 BU	Grossly impaired. Albuminuria	86 (normal)	Variable to 160/120	Negative	No gross nephro-calcinosis. Microscopic calcification + + at autopsy	Shoulders, skin, hip, elbow	Died of uraemia
180 BU	Albuminuria sp.g. 1004–1008	9 KA	115/75	Positive	Bilateral nephrocalcinosis (radiologically)	Osteosclerosis of femur, meta-carpals, vertebrae. Calcification of aorta	Improved

chronic glomerulonephritis though a few cases have been reported in the literature [96]. A few patients with chronic glomerulonephritis have been reported who have taken large quantities of milk for long periods of time on medical advice and who have then developed widespread bilateral nephrocalcinosis of a peculiar and characteristic type. The first case of this syndrome was described by Vaughan et al. [117], and others were reported later [1, 42] (Fig. 5.6, see p. 120).

The condition is primarily a renal disease. The kidneys at autopsy have a granular surface, may be slightly smaller than normal, the cortex being thinner than normal, the medulla retaining its normal thickness. There is diffuse, finely nodular calcification throughout the entire cortex, easily detected as the examining finger is passed across the cut surface, the diffuse calcific foci being small granules 1–2 mm in diameter lying in tiny, smooth-walled cavities. The medulla is free from calcification though the boundary zone between the pyramids and the cortex may be the seat of a linear calcific deposit. Microscopically the cellular changes are those of glomerulonephritis. The principal lesions appear to be in the proximal tubules and in the glomeruli, many of which are almost obliterated by collagenous connective tissue, some being completely hyalinized, others atrophic and avascular. The glomerular capsular epithelium may show proliferation or thickening, 'crescent' formation and obliteration of the capsular space with occlusion of the capillaries and shrinkage of the glomerular tufts. Some of the cortical tubules are completely lost and

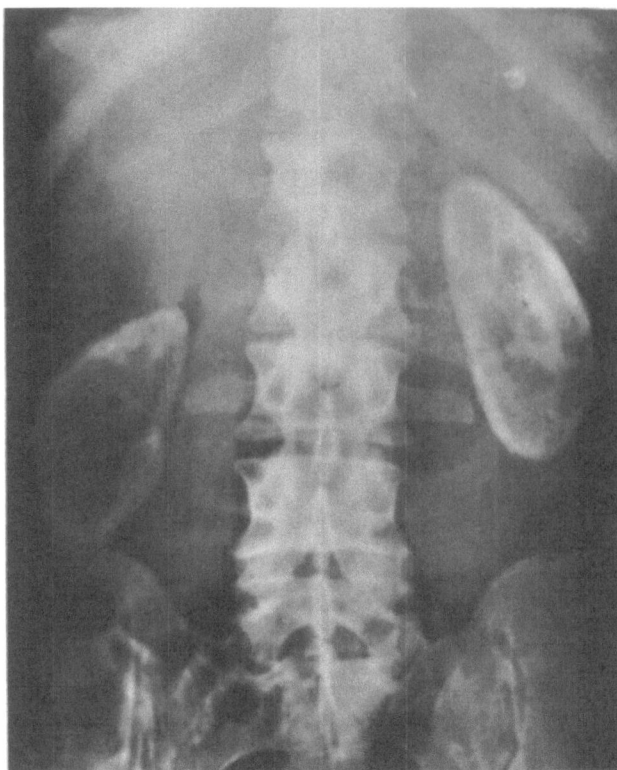

Fig. 5.6. Plain radiograph of the abdomen showing diffuse calcification of both kidneys in a patient with milk addiction and advanced glomerular nephritis. Tiny calcific deposits were found throughout both kidneys at subsequent autopsy. The radiograph shows the calcification to be maximal in the cortical regions of the kidney. (By courtesy of the late Dr. Sosman, Massachusetts General Hospital)

in many of the dilated tubular lumina (especially those of the loops of Henle, the distal convoluted tubules and the collecting tubules) are found masses of dark-blue-staining calcium granules or casts. Sometimes granular calcific deposits are found within and even beneath the tubular epithelial cells, suggesting that the epithelium had regenerated over the calcified material. The intima and the media of many of the small and medium-sized arterioles are thickened from cellular proliferation and may be partly calcified. Calcinosis of the skin associated with downgrowth of the cutaneous squamous epithelium may be found. The skeletal system shows no abnormality.

The reported patients (five male, one female in the papers referred to), whose ages varied from 27 to 54, have usually had in early life typical acute nephritis with swelling of the face and feet, sore throat with temperature, fatigue and vague ill-health, albuminuria and sometimes casts in the urine.

It is difficult to say with any precision how many years have elapsed after the onset of the condition before the kidneys have become radio-opaque, but it may well be 5 or 6 depending on the daily amount of calcium ingested; in the interval the patient may have enjoyed reasonably good health. The other important clinical feature has been the daily ingestion of 2 or 3 quarts of milk for many years.

Most of the cases have presented for investigation with symptoms of hypertension (headaches, cardiac embarrassment), of early renal failure (fatigue, loss of weight, polyuria and anaemia), or of advanced renal failure (acidosis, air-hunger, mental deterioration, coma). Some patients have

Table 5.3. Six cases of chronic glomerulonephritis with nephrocalcinosis, showing some chemical and biochemical details

Cases	Sex	Age at diagnosis	History of nephritis	Quantity of milk ingested	Urine			
					Albumin	Specific gravity	Casts	pH
Vaughan et al., 1947	Male	26	6 yr before	1–2 qt skim milk daily	+	1010–1017	Granular and fatty casts	5.5–6.0
Geraci et al., 1950 (Case 2)	Male	52	3 yr or more	1 qt daily + much butter and cheese	+	1000–1010	Occasional granular casts	
Arons et al., 1955	1. Female	27	Albuminuria at 18 yr	2 qt daily for many yr	+	1007–1017	Rare granular casts	5.5
	2. Male	33	12 yr	1–2 qt daily for many yr	+	1003–1007	Occasional granular casts	5.5–6.0
	3. Male	44		1–3 qt daily	+	1007–1015		
	4. Male	24	Since age of 5 yr		+	1006–1010	Hyaline and granular casts	6.0

Table 5.3—*continued*

Cases	Blood pressure	Red blood cells (millions)	Blood chemistry					
			Blood urea nitrogen or non-protein nitrogen (mg/100 cc)	CO_2 combining power (vol%)	Chloride (mEq/litre)	Calcium (mEq/litre)	Phosphorus mM/litre	
Vaughan et al., 1947	196/120	4,750,000	BUN 30–177 mg	22.9–17.8	108–96	4.6–4.3	1.5–5.6	
Geraci et al., 1950 (Case 2)	240/130	3,150,000	NPN 82 mg	12.6	103.7	5.5	18.1	
Arons et al., 1955	230/140	3,700,000	BUN 32 mg	18.2	103	5.3	1.5	
	170/98	2,600,000	BUN 72 mg	17.3	107	4.3	1.0	
	180/100	3,650,000	NPN 62 mg	21.1	95.9	4.0	1.3	
	140/90		BUN 67–135 mg	21.6–16.0	94–105	7.5–5.1	1.7, 2.2 and 4.2	

had pruritus with a papular skin eruption which ulcerates and heals, forming pigmented scars. Pericarditis or cerebral haemorrhage may precede death.

The urine is abundant and of low specific gravity, acid in reaction and sterile on culture; it contains albumin, usually an excess of leucocytes and red cells, and occasionally granular or hyaline casts. The blood urea is raised moderately during the intermediate stages and considerably towards the end of the illness. By the time the patient has presented clinically there may be a moderate to severe acidosis and often a hyperchloraemia, and the blood potassium may be elevated before the end. The serum calcium level may be normal but may fall during the late changes; the serum phosphorus level rises in keeping with the degree of renal failure; the urinary calcium may be normal or low. A secondary anaemia is usual. The plain radiograph of the kidneys is unique and diagnostic and shows a bilateral diffuse stippled or finely granular deposit of calcific material affecting virtually the entire cortices of the kidneys, the medullary portions being relatively unaffected. By the time the diagnosis has been made, renal function is usually so poor that an intravenous pyelogram shows no excretion of the medium. Calculi in the calyces were found in one reported case (Table 5.3).

The condition can be differentiated from hyperparathyroidism by the blood chemistry (especially by the absence of hypercalcaemia). In the nephrocalcinosis found occasionally in association with hyperparathyroidism, the calcific masses are in the renal pyramids and the boundary zone and not in the cortical part of the kidney. The symmetrical distribution of the calcification affecting the whole of both kidneys is quite different from the patchy renal calcification resulting from bilateral tuberculosis, tumours or infarcts.

No radical treatment for the condition is known and there is no evidence that the process of calcification can be reversed. Treatment for renal failure and the withholding of calcium from the diet may prolong life. Of the cases referred to, five of six proved fatal.

VI. Beryllium Poisoning

Beryllium poisoning is rare in Britain though more than 500 cases have been reported in the United States [51–54]. Renal calculi are commonly found as a complication. The characteristic pathological lesion is a granuloma, subsequently replaced by fibrous tissue, at the affected sites; the pathological manifestations bear a close relationship to those seen in sarcoidosis [41].

In the acute form of the disease, which has been largely eliminated by the improved methods of protection of workers, there is irritation of the skin, eyes, nose and throat, and bronchitis and pneumonitis have been reported following harmful exposure to the fumes of beryllium metal or its oxide. Miliary shadows in the lung fields have been demonstrated radiologically, somewhat similar to those seen in sarcoidosis [53].

In the chronic form, varied clinical syndromes have been recorded, the disease usually being systemic rather than merely local in the lungs; some patients have had cutaneous lesions on the face and the chest wall, and febrile episodes and arthritic pains [110]. Lesions in the liver, spleen, kidneys, heart muscle, lungs and lymph nodes have been observed. In both sarcoidosis and beryllium poisoning patients may experience fatigue, weakness, anorexia and loss of weight as well as pulmonary symptoms, though ocular, tonsillar, parotid and skeletal lesions appear to be absent in berylliosis. In chronic beryllium poisoning the mortality may be as high as 25%, and some patients who survive sometimes become completely disabled but may still live for years. Cortisone and corticotropin have been shown to have a beneficial effect on the clinical course of the disease by Hardy [51, 52], who reported metabolic studies; the radiological pulmonary changes may resolve and the enlarged liver, spleen and hilar lymph nodes may return to normal.

Renal Calculi. Renal calculi, which may give rise to clinical symptoms, occur in about 20% of all patients with the disease [51–53]; there may or may not be associated hypercalcaemia or hypercalciuria. Hyperuricaemia was reported in a series of 6 of 15 patients with the syndrome though clinical symptoms of gout appear to be rare [65]. Three patients in the group had renal calculi, 2 being hyperuricaemic and 1 being normouricaemic.

VII. Cadmium Poisoning

Cadmium is said to present more lethal hazards to man than any other metal [104]. Chronic cadmium poisoning, in which renal damage is one of the consequences, occasionally affects workmen employed in the construction of accumulators and batteries, for which cadmium alloyed with nickel or other elements is used; in a few such patients renal calculi have been reported.

In patients so affected the general health is impaired; there is a loss of the normal sense of smell, dryness of the mouth, chronic cough (resulting from pulmonary emphysema), anaemia, gastrointestinal disturbances and occasionally eczematous skin changes. A yellow circle on the gums round the neck of the teeth, referred to as an 'alarm sign' [3] has been observed in some patients. Cadmium is found in the urine in the fully developed cases of poisoning in industrial workers, its level falling rapidly when exposure of the subject to the metal has ceased; and 1.0–3.2 g protein/litre is excreted in the urine daily, first as α- and β-globulins, then as albumin [108]. The protein has been held to be non-specific and of a type seen in any renal tubular disorder [21]; or it may arise by way of the glomerular filtrate, the route by which cadmium is excreted, possibly with some resulting glomerular damage [108]. The urinary proteins in patients with cadmium poisoning, however, have different molecular weights from those usually associated with conditions of abnormal glomerular function; alternatively they may belong to the group known as minial-bumins [66, 78], reaching the urine only when renal tubular absorption has become impaired. The relation of these urinary proteins to the occasional renal stone which has been found is not known.

Kazantzis et al. [63] have shown the renal tubular dysfunction of cadmium workers to be characterized by a proteinuria, abnormal aminoaciduria, renal glycosuria, hypercalciuria, an increased clearance of phosphate and urate, an impaired ability to excrete an acid load, and an impaired ability to concentrate the urine; the serum calcium level is normal. These subjects in fact seem to develop the equivalent of Fanconi's syndrome. Skeletal demineralization in industrial workers has been described [92].

In Japan the disease known as *itai itai* has been attributed to environmental pollution resulting from a high cadmium intake derived from rice which was the staple diet of the affected community [113]. The average dietary intake of calcium by the rural Japanese workers may be lower than that of workers in the United Kingdom, who rarely show skeletal decalcification, presumably since the absorption of calcium from the gut adequately compensates for the urinary loss of calcium [62].

Using radioactive cadmium, Friberg [38], who examined the distribution of the element after administration experimentally to the rabbit, found a relatively low urinary excretion of cadmium during the first 4 weeks, rising rapidly by 50–100 times the average amount during the succeeding week. A relationship was shown to exist between the occurrence of proteinuria and the high level of the urinary cadmium; at autopsy cadmium (as well as cellular changes) has been found in the liver, pancreas, kidneys and spleen, and the whole blood had a relatively high content of cadmium [12, 36, 37, 39].

Renal Calculi. Friberg [36, 37] reported the presence of renal stones in seven workers in a factory in which accumulators were being made; in three, proteinuria had been observed. Axelsson [2] reported that 44% of a group of cadmium workers who had been exposed to cadmium dust for more than 15 years had a history of formation of renal stones, which were composed mainly of basic calcium phosphate. Two patients reported by Kazantzis [61] had bilateral renal calculi and a third had nephrocalcinosis; a renal calculus from one of his patients was composed of calcium phosphate and calcium carbonate. He considered that the renal calculi observed in some patients with cadmium poisoning are the result of the associated hypercalciuria [62]. It is not known if cadmium is a constituent of the stones. Kench [66] stated that in his experience, renal calculi were not a noteworthy feature of chronically poisoned cadmium workers and he had never observed them in his experimental animals; even if renal calculi occurred in workers in cadmium, he would not expect cadmium to be present in such stones.

VIII. Food Emulsifiers

It has been shown that hamsters and rats fed with the emulsifier polyoxyethylene stearic acid (MYRJ 45) at various strengths in the food developed vesical calculi and sometimes vesical tumours. We have not found any reference to stone formation in humans which could be attributed to this substance.

References

1. Arons,W.L., Christensen,W.H., Sosman, M.C.: Nephrocalcinosis visible by X-ray associated with chronic glomerulonephritis. Ann. Int. Med. *42*, 260 (1955)

2. Axelsson,B., Friberg,L.: On the tolerable limits of mercury in the atmosphere and biologic milieus. Occup. Health. Rev. *15*, 18 (1963)

3. Baader,E.: Chronic cadmium poisoning. Ind. Med. *21*, 427 (1952)

4. Baker,S.B.deC.: The blood supply of the renal papilla. Br. J. Urol. *31*, 53 (1959)

5. Becker,DL., Baggenstoss,A.H., Weir,J.F.: Parenchymal calcification of kidneys in patients with duodenal ulcer. Am. J. Clin. Pathol. *22*, 843 (1952)

6. Beeson,W.M., Prence,J.W., Holm,J.C.: Urinary calculi in sheep. Am. J. Vet. Res. *4*, 120 (1943)

7. Bennets,H.W.: Urinary calculi of sheep in Western Australia. J. Dept. Agric. West. Aust. *27*, 129 (1950)

8. Bennets,H.W.: In: Urinary calculi in sheep. Sutherland,A.K. (ed.). Aust. Vet. J. *34*, 44 (1958)

9. Beswick,I.P., Schatzki,P.F.: Experimental renal papillary necrosis. Arch. Pathol. *69*, 733 (1960)

10. Blackman,J.E., Gibson,G.R., Lavan,J.N., Learoyd,H.M., Rosen,S.: Urinary calculi and the consumption of analgesics. Br. Med. J. *2*, 800 (1967)

11. Blagg,C.: Personal communication (1955)

12. Bonnell,J.A.: Emphysema and proteinuria in men casting copper-cadmium alloys. Br. J. Ind. Med. *12*, 181 (1955)

13. Borland,V.G., Jackson,C.M.: Effects of fat-free diet on structure of kidney of rats. Arch. Pathol. *11*, 687 (1931)

14. Burnett,C., Commons,R.R., Albright,F., Howard,J.E.: Hypercalcaemia without hypercalciuria or hypophosphatemia, calcinosis and renal insufficiency. N. Engl. J. Med. *240*, 787 (1949)

15. Burry,A.F., Axelson,R.A.: Analgesic nephropathy. Med. J. Aust. *2*, 266 (1974)

16. Cabot,H.: Recent advances in our knowledge of pathogenesis of renal calculus. Mississippi Doctor *16*, 1 (1938)

17. Carpenter,H.M., Pautler,E.E.: Hyperparathyroidism with renal insufficiency. Report of a case confused with the Burnett syndrome. N. Engl. J. Med. *250*, 453 (1954)

18. Connell,R., Whiting,F., Forman,S.A.: Silica urolithiasis in beef cattle. 1. Observations on its occurrence. Can. J. Comp. Med. *23*, 41 (1959)

19. Cooke,A.M.: Alkalosis occurring in the alkaline treatment of peptic ulcer. Q. J. Med. *1*, 527 (1932)

20. Cooke,A.M.: Calcification of the kidneys in pyloric stenosis. Q. J. Med. *2*, 539 (1933)

21. Creeth,J.M., Kekwick,R.A., Flynn,F.V., Harris,H., Robson,E.B.: An ultracentrifuge study of urine proteins with particular reference to the proteinuria of renal tubular disorders. Clin. Chim. Acta *8*, 406 (1963)

22. Dent,C.E.: The kidney. Ciba Foundation Symposium. Lewis,A.A.G., Wolstenholme,G.E.W. (eds.). London: Churchill 1954

23. Dufault,F.X., Tobias,C.J.: Potentially reversible renal failure following excessive calcium and alkali intake in peptic ulcer therapy. Am. J. Med. *16*, 231 (1954)

24. Dworetzky,M.: Reversible metastatic calcification (Milk-drinker's syndrome). J. Am. Med. Assoc. *155*, 830 (1954)

25. Earle,I.P., Lyndahl,I.L.: Some observations on effects of fattening lambs of high vitamin D and dietary silication factors associated with formation of urinary calculi. J. Anim. Sci. *10*, 1046 (1951)

26. Eckstrom,T., Engfeldt,B., Lagergren,C., Lindvall,N.: Medullary sponge kidney. Stockholm: Almquist and Wickwell 1959

27. Editorial: Aspirin and the kidneys. Can. Med. Assoc. J. *111*, 629 (1974)

28. Edmondson,H.A., Reynolds,T.B., Jacobson,H.G.: Renal papillary necrosis with special reference to chronic alcoholism. A report of 20 cases. Arch. Int. Med. *118*, 255 (1966)

29. Ehrhart,L.A., McCullagh,K.G.: Silica urolithiasis in dogs fed on atherogenic diet. Proc. Soc. Exp. Biol. Med. *143*, 131 (1973)

30. Eisele,C.W.: Role of alkali therapy for peptic ulcer in the formation of renal calculi. J. Am. Med. Assoc. *114*, 2363 (1940)

31. Flynn,W.A.: Sulphapyridine anuria and its treatment. Lancet *I*, 646 (1943)

32. Forman,S.A., Sauer,F., Laughland,D.H., Davidson,W.M.: Volume and acidity of urine of sheep fed hay rich in silica and effect of dietary salt additions. Nature (London) *182*, 1385 (1958)

33. Forman,S.A., Whiting,F., Connell,R.: Silica urolithiasis in beef cattle: 3. Chemical and physical composition of the uroliths. Can. J. Comp. Med. *23*, 157 (1959)

34. Fosbinder,R.J., Walter,L.A.: Sulfanilamide derivatives of heterocyclic amines. J. Am. Chem. Soc. *61*, 2032 (1939)

35. Frame,B., Haubrich,E.: Peptic ulcer and hyperparathyroidism: a survey of 300 ulcer patients. Arch. Int. Med. *105*, 536 (1960)

36. Friberg,L.: Health hazards in the manufacture of alkaline accumulators with special reference to chronic cadmium poisoning. Acta Med. Scand. (Suppl. 240) *138*, 1 (1950a)

37. Friberg,L.: Injuries following continued administration of cadmium: preliminary report of a clinical and experimental study. Arch. Ind. Hyg. Occupt. Med. *1*, 458 (1950b)

38. Friberg,L.: Further investigations on chronic cadmium poisoning: a study on rabbits with radioactive cadmium. Arch. Ind. Hyg. Occup. Med. *5*, 30 (1952)

39. Friberg,L.: Ion and liver administration in chronic cadmium poisoning and studies of the distribution and excretion of cadmium: experimental investigations in rabbits. Acta Pharmacol. Toxicol. *11*, 168 (1955)

40. Friedreich,N,von: Über Nekrose der Nieren papillen bei Hydronephrose. Virchows Arch. *69*, 308 (1877)

41. Frieman,D.G., Hardy,H.L.: Beryllium disease: the relation of pulmonary pathology to clinical course and prognosis based on a study of 163 cases from the U.S. Beryllium Case Registry. Human Pathol. *1* (1970)

42. Geraci,J.E., Harris,H.W., Keith,N.M.: Bilateral diffuse nephrocalcinosis: report of two cases. Proc. Mayo Clin. *25*, 305 (1950)

43. Gilligan,D.R., Garb,S., Wheeler,C., Plummer,N.: Adjuvant alkali therapy in the prevention of renal complications from sulphadiazine. J. Am. Med. Assoc. *122*, 1160 (1943)

44. Goodman,L.S., Gilman,A.: The pharmacological basis of therapeutics. 4th ed. New York, London: Macmillan 1970

45. Gorrill,R.H.: The establishment of staphylococcal abscesses in the mouse kidney. Br. J. Exp. Pathol. *39*, 203 (1958)

46. Gross,P., Cooper,F.B., Lewis,M.: Urinary calculi caused by sulfapyridine. Urol. Cutan. Rev. *43*, 299 (1939)

47. Gunther,G.W.: Die Pallennekrosen der Niere bei Diabetes. Münch. Med Wochenschr. *84*, 1695 (1937)

48. Hammarsten,G.: Personal communication (1961)

49. Hammarsten,G., Helldorff,I., Magnusson,W., Rilton,T.: Dubbelsidiga njurstener av Kiselsyra efter bruk av silikathaltige antacidum. Sven. Lakartidning *50*, 1242 (1953)

50. Hardt,L., Rivers,A.B.: Toxic manifestations following the alkaline treatment of peptic ulcer. Arch. Intern. Med. *31*, 171 (1923)

51. Hardy,H.L.: Epidemiology, clinical character and treatment of beryllium poisoning. A.M.A. Arch. Ind. Health *11*, 273 (1955a)

52. Hardy,H.L.: The disability found in persons exposed to certain beryllium compounds. A.M.A. Arch. Ind. Health *12*, 174 (1955b)

53. Hardy,H.L.: Differential diagnosis between beryllium poisoning and sarcoidosis. Am. Rev. Tuberc. *74*, 885 (1956)

54. Hardy,H.L., Bartter,F.C., Jaffin,A.E.: Metabolic study of a case of chronic beryllium poisoning treated with ACTH. A.M.A. Arch. Ind. Hyg. Occup. Med. *3*. 579 (1951)

55. Helwig,C.A., Reed,H.L.: Fatal anuria following sulphadiazine therapy. J. Am. Med. Assoc. *119*, 561 (1942)

56. Herman,J.R., Goldberg,A.S.: New type of urinary calculus caused by antacid therapy. J. Am. Med. Assoc. *174*, 1206 (1960)

57. Hessen,I.: Njursten av Kiselsyra efter silikat som antacidum. Nord. Med. *69*, 424 (1963)

58. Holst,S.: Norsk Magazine for Laege-videnskaben. Silicate calculi in the urinary tract. Nord. Med. *60*, 1169 (1958)

59. Hultengren,N.: Renal papillary necrosis. Acta Chir. Scand. *277*, 1 (1961)

60. Joekes,A.M., Rose,G.A., Sutor,J.: Multiple renal silica calculi. Br. Med. J. *1*, 146 (1973)

61. Kazantzis,G.: Mercury and the kidney. Trans. Soc. Occup. Med. *20*, 54 (1970)

62. Kazantzis,G.: Chromium and nickel. Ann. Occup. Hyg. *15*, 25 (1972)

63. Kazantzis,G., Flynn,F.V., Spowage,J.S., Trott,D.G.: Renal tubular malfunction and pulmonary emphysema in cadmium pigment workers. Q. J. Med. *32*, 165 (1963)

64. Keeler,R.F.: Silicon metabolism and silica–protein matrix interrelationship in bovine urolithiasis, Am. J. N.Y. Acad. Sci. *104*, 592 (1963)

65. Kelley,W.N., Goldfinger,S.E., Hardy, H.L.: Hyperuricaemia in chronic beryllium disease. Ann. Intern. Med. *70*, 977 (1969)

66. Kench,J.E., Gain,A.C., Sutherland,E.M.: A biochemical study of urine of man and animals poisoned by cadmium. S. Afr. Med. J. *39*, 1191 (1965)

67. Kincaid-Smith,P.: Pathogenesis of the renal lesion associated with the abuse of analgesics. Lancet *I*, 859 (1967a)

68. Kincaid-Smith,P.: Analgesic nephropathy in perspective. Med. J. Aust. *2*, 320 (1967b)

69. Kincaid-Smith,P.: Analgesic nephropathy and papillary necrosis. Postgrad. Med. J. *44*, 807 (1968)

70. Kincaid-Smith,P., Fairley,K.F.: Renal infection and renal scarring. Melbourne: Mercedes 1971

71. Kleiman,A.H.: Sulphathiazole anuria with recovery following renal decapsulation. J. Urol. *56*, 598 (1946)

72. Kretschmer,H.L., Brown,R.C.: Do alkalis used in the treatment of peptic ulcer cause renal stones? Study of 1940 cases. J. Am. Med. Assoc. *113*, 1471 (1949)

73. Kyle,L.H.: Differentiation of hyperparathyroidism and the milk-alkali (Burnett) syndrome. N. Engl. J. Med. *251*, 1035 (1954)

74. Lagergren,C.: Development of silica calculi after oral administration of magnesium trisilicate J. Urol. *87*, 994 (1962)

75. Larson,A., Sigroth,K.: Sven. Lak-Tidn *52*, 2751 (1955)

76. Lavan,J.N., Benson,W.J., Gatenby,A.H.: The consumption of analgesics by Australian hospital patients. Med. J. Aust. *2*, 694 (1966)

77. Law,J.: In: Special report on diseases of cattle. Revised edition, p. 113. U.S.D.A. Washington, 1912

78. Leading Article: Cadmium and metabolism of albumen. Lancet *I*, 133 (1968)

79. Lindvall,N.: Renal papillary necrosis—a roentgenographic study of 155 cases. Acta Radiol. (Suppl. 192). (1960)

80. Lipworth,E., Bloomberg,B.M., Reid,F.P.: Urinary calculi containing silica: a case report. S. Afr. Med. J. *38*, 50 (1964)

81. Lunde,I.: Silicates and renal calculi. Tidsskr. Nor. Laegeforen *91*, 257 (1971)

82. Mallory,G.K., Crane,A.R., Edwards,J.E.: Pathology of acute and of healed experimental pyelonephritis. Arch. Pathol. *30*, 330 (1940)

83. Mandel,E.E., Popper,H.: Experimental medullary necrosis of the kidney. Arch. Pathol. *52*, 1 (1951)

84. McQueen,E.G.: 'Milk poisoning' and 'calcium gout'. Lancet *II*, 67 (1952)

85. Merrill,R.C.: Activated sols in water treatment. Ind. Eng. Chem. *40*, 1355 (1948)

86. Mutch,N.: Synthetic magnesium trisilicate; its action on the alimentary tract. Br. Med. J. *I*, 205 (1936)

87. Nanra,R.S., Kincaid-Smith,P.: Papillary necrosis in rats caused by aspirin and aspirin-containing mixtures. Br. Med. J. *III*, 559 (1970)

88. Nanra,R.S., Hicks,J.D., McNamara, J.N., Lie,J.T., Leslie,D.W., Jackson,B., Kincaid-Smith,P.: Seasonal variations in the postmortem incidence of renal papillary necrosis. Med. J. Aust. *1*, 293 (1970a)

89. Nanra,R.S., Fairley,K.F., Kincaid-Smith, P.: Recovery of function in patients with analgesic nephropathy. Aust. Ann. Med. *19*, 195 (1970b)

90. Nanra,R.S., Chirawong,P., Kincaid-Smith,P.: Renal papillary necrosis in rats produced by aspirin, A.P.C. and other analgesics. In: Renal infection and renal scarring. Kincaid-Smith,P., Fairley,K.F. (eds.), p. 347. Melbourne; Mercedes 1971

91. Nazzari,A.: Heterazioni renali nella tetania gastrica. Policlinica, Roma. *11*, 146 (1904)

92. Nicaud,P., Lafitte,A., Gros,S.: Les troubles de l'intoxication chronique par le

cadmium. Arch. Med. Prof. *5–6*, 192 (1942)

93. Oakley,W.: Alkalosis arising in treatment of peptic ulcer. Lancet *II*, 187 (1935)

94. Page,R.C., Heffner,R.R., Frey,A.: Urinary excretion of silica in humans following oral administration of magnesium trisilicate. Am. J. Dig. Dis. *8*, 13 (1941)

95. Parsons,F.M., Watkinson,G.: The treatment of pyloric stenosis in peptic ulceration. Postgrad. Med. J. *30*, 145 (1954)

96. Patrassi,G.: Calcificazioni renali e mobbo di Bright. Arch. Pathol. Clin. Med. *10*, 104 (1930)

97. Plakke,R.K., Pfeiffer,E.W.: Blood vessels of the mammalian renal medulla. Science *146*, 1683 (1964)

98. Pyrah,L.N., Bonser,G.M.: Personal communication (1942)

99. Rake,G., van Dyke,H.B., Corwin,W.C.: Pathological changes following prolonged administration of sulphathiazole and sulphapyridine. Am. J. Sci. *200*, 353 (1940)

100. Rifkind,B.M., Chazin,B.I., Aitchison,J.D.: Chronic milk-alkali syndrome with generalized osteosclerosis after prolonged excessive intake of 'Rennie's' tablets. Br. Med. J. *I*, 317 (1960)

101. Riley,C.J.: Chronic milk-alkali syndrome associated with prolonged excessive intake of 'Moorland' tablets. Practitioner *205*, 657 (1970)

102. Robbins,S.L., Mallory,G.K., Kinney, T.D.: Necrotizing renal papillitis: a form of acute pyelonephritis. N. Engl. J. Med. *235*, 885 (1946)

103. Rogan,J.M., Cruickshank,E.K.: Inductotherm treatment of sulphapyridine anuria. Br. Med. J. *I*, 757 (1942)

104. Rutherford-Johnstone: Quoted by E. Baader (1952). Chronic cadmium poisoning. Ind. Med. *21*, 427 (1948)

105. Scholz,D.A., Keating,F.R.: Milk-alkali syndrome. Arch. Int. Med. *95*, 460 (1955)

106. Schweingruber,R.: Probleme bei chronischen Vergiftung mit Kombinierten

Phenacetin-präparaten. Schweiz. Med. Wochenschr. *85*, 1162 (1955)

107. Settle,W.R., Sauer,F.: Demonstration of siliceous deposits in the kidneys of the guinea pig. Am. J. Vet. Res. *21*, 709 (1960)

108. Smith,J.C., Kench,J.E., Lane,R.E.: Determination of cadmium in urine and observations on urinary cadmium and protein excretion in men exposed to cadmium oxide dust. Biochem. J. *61*, 4864 (1955)

109. Soliani,F.: Burnett's syndrome. Minerva Med. *62*, 4864 (1971)

110. Sprague,H.B., Hardy,H.L.: An unusual case of joint pains and fever. Circulation *10*, 129 (1954)

111. Spuhler,O., Zollinger,H.U.: Die chronisch-interstitielle Nephritis. Z. Clin. Med. *151*, 1 (1953)

112. Strimer,R.M. et al.: Phenacetin induced renal papillary necrosis: pyonephrosis, anuria and bilateral ureteral obstruction. Urology *5*, 780 (1975)

113. Takeuchi,J.: Kidney injury in *itai-itai* disease. Naika *21*, 876 (1969)

114. Texter,E.C.Jr., Lauretta,H.C.: The milk-alkali syndrome. Am. J. Dig. Dis. *11*, 413 (1966)

115. Thomas,W.C.: Inhibition of mineralization and renal stones. In: Renal Stone Research Symposium. Hodgkinson,A., Nordin,B.E.C. (eds.). London: Churchill 1969

116. Tucker,W.J.: Uraemia following gastroenterostomy: eight cases. Wis. Med. J. *20*, 528 (1922)

117. Vaughan,J.H., Sosman,M.C., Kinney, T.D.: Nephrocalcinosis. Am. J. Roentgenol. *58*, 33 (1947)

118. Werner,P., Kushner,M., Riley,E.A.: Reversible metastatic calcification associated with excessive milk and alkali intake. Am. J. Med. *14*, 108 (1953)

119. Whiting,F., Connell,R., Forman,S.A.: Silica urolithiasis in beef cattle: the incidence on different rations and on range. Can. J. Comp. Med. *22*, 332 (1958)

120. Zeman,F.D., Friedman,W., Mann,L.: Kidney changes in pyloric obstruction. Proc. N.Y. Pathol. Soc. *24*, 41 (1924)

Chapter 6

Levels of the Principal Crystalloids in the Urine of Patients with Calcium-Containing Calculi

I. Urinary Calcium

When investigations were begun about 30 years ago concerning the urinary calcium level in stone-formers it was found that many patients who had no recognizable associated disease had unexplained high urinary calcium levels.

Flocks [11] in a study of 35 patients with renal calculi who had normal serum calcium and serum phosphorus levels (22 male, 13 female) found that 21 (60%) excreted more than 200 mg calcium/day when on a moderately low daily dietary intake of 300 mg calcium; he introduced the term 'idiopathic high urinary calcium' to denote the abnormality of calcium excretion. Albright and his co-workers [1] reported some patients with renal calculi and hypercalciuria whom they considered fell into a definite syndrome which they designated 'idiopathic hypercalciuria'. Sutherland [32] found that 15 of 26 patients (58%) with renal stone placed on a low-calcium diet excreted more than 200 mg/day.

Cottet and Vittu [6] found that the average daily urinary excretion of calcium in 73% of 52 patients with calcium-containing renal stone on a normal diet exceeded 200 mg compared with 31% of 56 normal individuals. The level of the urinary calcium, which is itself variable, is partly dependent upon the dietary intake of calcium, which is also variable: hence the difficulty of defining hypercalciuria with precision.

In order to arrive at a practical working figure for the normal urinary calcium level, as well as the levels found in patients with

renal calculus, without the necessity of making a precise examination of the dietary calcium, the distribution of the urinary calcium level in a series of normal healthy male and female subjects on a normal hospital ward diet (800 ± 200 mg calcium/day) in the author's department was compared with that of a representative sample of 344 patients (220 male, 124 female) with renal urolithiasis presenting at the clinic (Fig. 6.1). It was decided that the upper normal limit under such conditions of the daily urinary calcium level was 300 mg/24 h in males and 250 mg in females, and that any subject or patient in whom that limit was exceeded had hypercalciuria [14]. There was a considerable spread of values of the urinary calcium level, but using these guide-lines it was found that among normal non-calculous subjects so investigated, 8% had hypercalciuria, and that the incidence of high urinary calcium values was greater in normal men than in normal women. Of the 344 patients with renal calculi it was found that 108 (31%) had hypercalciuria as defined above, compared with an incidence of 8% in their normal subjects, the urinary calcium level in the other stone-formers being within the normal range.

Some subsequent observers have considered that the figure of 400 mg in males is a more appropriate upper normal figure for practical use [28]. In patients with calculi who had some impairment of renal function (as measured by the urea clearance test) the level of the urinary calcium tended to be reduced (Fig. 6.2). Flocks [11] had also observed that marked pathological changes in the kidneys of stone-formers were usually

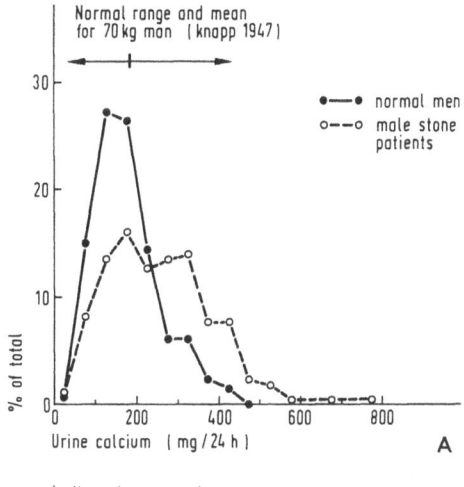

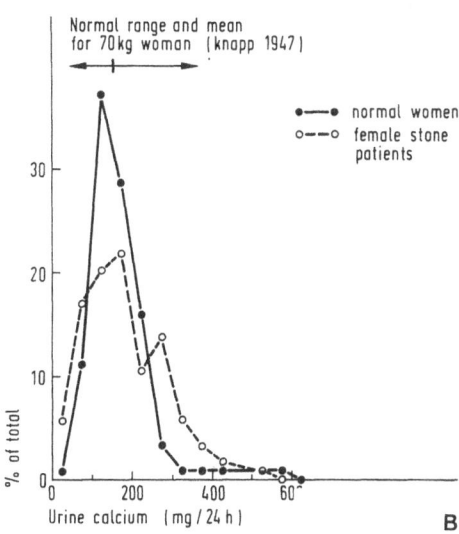

Fig. 6.1. **A.** Distribution of the urinary calcium levels in a series of 220 *male* patients with renal calculi compared with those in a series of normal *male* subjects on a normal diet. **B.** Distribution of the urinary calcium levels in a series of 124 *female* patients with renal calculi compared with those in a series of normal *female* subjects. (From A. Hodgkinson and L.N. Pyrah, British Journal of Surgery, 1958, *46*, 195; by courtesy of the Editor)

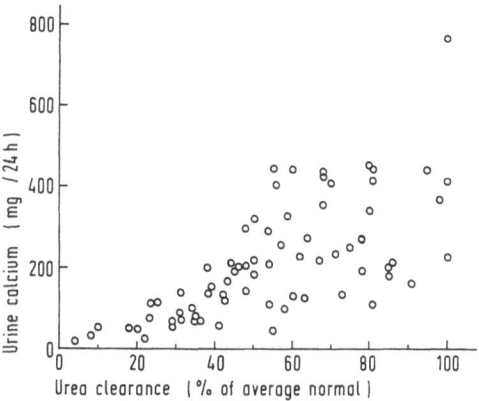

Fig. 6.2. Relationship between the urinary excretion of calcium by patients having a normal diet, and the clearance of urea in 72 patients. (From A. Hodgkinson and L.N. Pyrah, British Journal of Surgery, 1958, *46*, 195; by courtesy of the Editor)

associated with a relatively low urinary calcium level.

McGeown and Bull [20] found that while in normal individuals having a diet containing 154 mg calcium/day the urinary excretion of calcium was within the range

48–148 mg/day (mean, 83 mg; S.D., 32 mg), in a series of 73 stone patients on the same diet 30% had values for daily urinary calcium excretion greater than the mean plus twice the standard deviation (mean, 83 mg; S.D., 32 mg).

Hypercalciuria has been found by other observers in approximately one-third of patients with renal calculus [13, 17, 22, 27]. Jackson and Dancaster [15], who found that some 7% of otherwise 'normal' non-stone-bearing subjects had hypercalciuria, designated these individuals 'healthy hypercalciurics'.

A small minority in any series of patients with hypercalciuria have a metabolic or other type of general disease. Litin et al. [19] in an examination of 119 patients with urolithiasis on a standard diet with a normal calcium content, found that 7.6% had hypercalciuria for which there was some significant metabolic cause (hyperparathyroidism, 5; Wilson's disease, 1; reticulum cell sarcoma, 1; sarcoidosis, 1; Paget's disease, 1). There was idiopathic hypercalciuria in 36 (23 men, 13 women; 21.8%).

In a group of 48 children with urolithiasis (13 with recurrent and 35 with nonrecurrent stone), some observers found hypercalciuria in 8 (61%) of the recurrent cases and in 20 (57.1%) of the non-recurrent cases [26, 35].

The significance of hypercalciuria in the 7% or 8% of individuals who are otherwise 'normal' is not clear; it may be that such people are part of the population of potential stone-formers and that they are at risk in that sense, though it has so far been impossible to follow up such patients to see if they develop urolithiasis in later life. It is not known if the hypercalciuria in such subjects is a temporary phase or a life-long metabolic anomaly.

Since hypercalciuria is found occasionally in some patients who have diseases not associated with urolithiasis (thyrotoxicosis, Fanconi's syndrome and metabolic acidosis), it may be that the so-called healthy hypercalciuric has some built-in protection against stone formation which is not yet understood. Studies on normal subjects by several workers have suggested that the urinary calcium excretion increases rapidly during periods of growth, that it reaches a maximum between the ages of 20 and 40 (when the incidence of renal stone is high) and decreases thereafter, the changes being more marked in males than in females [7, 18, 25].

Relation to Type of Stone

When the incidence of hypercalciuria was considered in relation to the chemical composition and the topographical type of stone, it was found in our departmental enquiries that in patients with calculi composed of pure calcium phosphate (excluding those who had primary hyperparathyroidism), or of calcium phosphate (apatite) mixed with magnesium ammonium phosphate, the incidence of hypercalciuria was no higher than that found in normal healthy subjects. In such cases we considered that hypercalciuria is not an important contributory factor to the formation of stones of that particular composition.

We found that the incidence of hypercalciuria in a group of 28 patients who had formed stones of the 'nodular' or 'pisolitic' type was 32%, the incidence in a group of normal subjects (with the criteria used for the enquiry) being 26%. We considered that hypercalciuria did not appear to be a contributory cause of stone formation in that group of nodular calculi (which may have been pre-formed in colloidal nuclei). But in a group of 42 patients who had formed a 'crystalline' type of stone (patients who had some impairment of renal function being excluded from the test), the incidence of hypercalciuria was 71%, and it appeared to be an important contributory cause to the stone formation [14]. Cottet and Vittu [6] found similar results.

II. Urinary Phosphate

The daily normal urinary excretion of inorganic phosphate by healthy adults is about 800 mg. The daily intake of phosphorus on our normal (departmental) hospital ward diet was within the range 1100 ± 300 mg, which corresponds to a variation in the urinary excretion of inorganic phosphate of plus or minus 11%. The distribution of the urine-phosphate values for 92 normal men and 118 normal women (which differ significantly in the two sexes), and for 198 male and 108 female patients with renal calculus from our departmental series, on intakes of phosphate within the range 1100 ± 400 mg/day are given in Figure 6.3 [14].

The distribution of the urinary phosphate value for normal men differed significantly from that for normal women; in the male patients no significant difference was observed between the normal and the calculous patients, but the daily urinary phosphate values were greater than 900 mg in 17 calculous female patients (15.7%) compared with only 3.4% of normal women. In

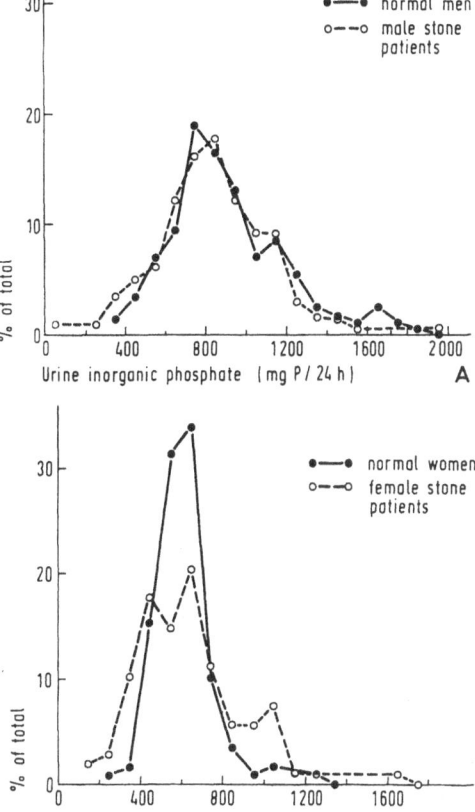

Fig. 6.3. **A.** Distribution of the urinary phosphate levels for *normal men* and 198 male renal-stone patients having a normal diet. **B.** Distribution of the urinary phosphate levels for *normal women* and 108 female stone patients having a normal diet. (From A. Hodgkinson and L.N. Pyrah, British Journal of Surgery, 1958, *46*, 195; by courtesy of the Editor)

11 of these 17 patients the high phosphate excretion was associated with a high urinary calcium excretion; four had a high or moderately high serum calcium level (one of whom had a proven parathyroid adenoma), the other three being regarded as possible cases of primary hyperparathyroidism.

The relation between the incidence of high urinary inorganic phosphate values in normal individuals and in patients with different types of stone is shown in Figure 6.3. While hyperphosphaturia does not

appear to be an important factor in the initiation or promotion of renal stone formation, phosphate is not a passive partner to calcium in this respect; thus the administration of Aludrox (aluminium hydroxide) may bring about a considerable reduction in the urinary phosphate and may even reduce the size of a predominantly phosphate calculus (Chap. 14).

III. Urinary Oxalate

In the great majority of patients with renal calculi composed of calcium oxalate, with or without an admixture of calcium phosphate, the level of the urinary oxalate is normal, namely between 12.5 and 40 mg/24 h; in only a few patients is the upper normal level reached or exceeded. The range of values of the urinary oxalic acid in 80 patients with calcium oxalate nephrolithiasis (from the department) was usually within the normal range; excluding one patient with primary hyperoxaluria the highest level was 47.1 mg. In a few patients with pure calcium oxalate calculi the urinary oxalic acid level exceeded our top normal level [14] (Fig. 6.4).

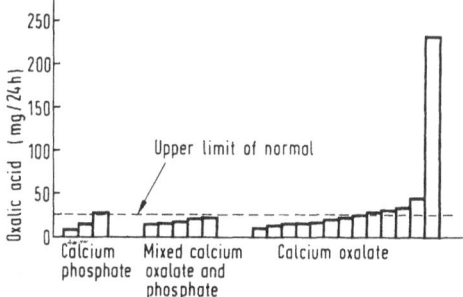

Fig. 6.4. Relationship between the urinary oxalic acid excretion in 21 patients with renal calculi and the composition of the calculi. *Broken line* shows the upper limit of the normal level of urinary oxalate and it is seen that a few patients with pure calcium oxalate calculi had a urinary oxalate level above the upper limit of normal; the single patient whose urinary oxalate level was 240 mg/24 h had primary hyperoxaluria.

McIntosh and Read [21] found that the urinary oxalic acid excretion in 11 patients with urolithiasis (10 having calcium oxalate calculi) varied between 21 and 48 mg/24 h (average 30.1 mg). Dempsey and co-workers [8, 9] found the oxalate urinary excretion in 35 patients with calcium oxalate renal calculi to be within the range of 15–50 mg/24 h. The urinary oxalate increased to 50–55 mg/day if the patients were given a diet rich in oxalate-containing food. The varied oxalate levels may result either from an increased synthesis of oxalate in the body in some patients or from abnormal renal handling of oxalate. However, Nordin and Robertson [23] found that the concentration of oxalate in the urine did not necessarily differ significantly from that in the normal group because of the somewhat larger volume of urine excreted by patients with calculus.

IV. Urinary Crystalluria

Crystals deposited in the urine of normal subjects are frequently observed either on routine microscopic examination of the urine or macroscopically, and give rise to no clinical symptoms, but they have clinical and etiological importance.

1. Oxaluria

Crystals of calcium oxalate in the urine, first identified by Donné [10] (the term 'oxaluria' designating their presence), cannot be regarded as an abnormality. The conditions under which such crystals are deposited involve a consideration of the urinary pH, the urinary concentration of oxalate and of calcium ions. The oxalate crystals are those of weddellite (calcium oxalate dihydrate) even when found in the urine passed by patients who had previously had whewellite calculi (calcium oxalate monohydrate). Tovborg Jensen [33]

calculated that weddellite is 2.8 times more soluble than whewellite in urine. The term 'oxalic acid diathesis' came into use many years ago to describe a wide range of gastrointestinal, nervous and skeletal symptoms, many of which would not now be linked with the presence of oxalate crystals in the urine; these were discussed by Jeghers and Murphy [16].

The true renal manifestations of oxaluria are, however, on firmer ground and are manifested clinically by unilateral or occasionally bilateral renal pain or even colic, cystalgia, occasionally frequency and burning pain on micturition and macroscopic or microscopic haematuria. In addition to red blood corpuscles, the urine contains abundant isolated or clustered oxalate crystals. The symptoms, which recur in some individuals during spring and early summer, have been associated with the ingestion of certain fruits and vegetables (rhubarb, spinach, strawberries, gooseberries and tomatoes) which have a comparatively high oxalate content. Oxaluria may persist intermittently for years without the culminating sequence of an obvious calcium oxalate stone, though the syndrome, which has been called oxaluria, may really be the result of the voiding of recurrent microcalculi undetectable radiologically.

Black [3] investigated 43 cases of oxaluria in British soldiers in India; the men had complained of renal colic and haematuria, other causes of the symptoms having been excluded by radiography, urinary cytology and cystoscopy, before a diagnosis of oxaluria was accepted. In some of the cases it was suggested that epididymitis, which was common among soldiers in hot countries during the wars, might occasionally have been caused by oxaluria.

In 24 patients (19 male and 5 female) with recurrent or bilateral calcium oxalate renal lithiasis observed by Albuquerque and Tuma [2], oxalate crystalluria was found to be readily demonstrable on microscopic examination of freshly voided urine. The average daily urinary oxalate levels were 26.97 mg in males and 44.57 in females; after 14 days treatment with 0.15 g magnesium oxide thrice daily, the crystalluria was eliminated in almost all the cases and the level of the urinary oxalate was significantly reduced.

2. Phosphaturia

If urine is rendered sufficiently alkaline, insoluble calcium and magnesium phosphates will be precipitated. In the condition known as phosphaturia there is a precipitate of magnesium ammonium phosphate (triple phosphate) resulting from decreased urinary acidity and not from an increase in its phosphate content. Cifuentes et al. [5], using the electron microscope, found that the phosphaturic precipitate contained spherulite-like elements either separate or in clusters, having a diameter of 0.2–0.5 μm, similar to those found in the carbonate apatites by Carlstrom [4]. Occasionally they tended to show a hexagonal crystalline arrangement; when studied by X-ray diffraction techniques the pattern was that of an amorphous material, but with some indication of an apatite-like crystalline structure.

Fraser et al. [12] tried to prevent the precipitation of calcium oxalate in urine in the experimental animal, using the technique of implantation of zinc pellets into the bladders of rats given various diets [34] to induce stone formation of varied composition. They examined the effect on the size and composition of stones so induced, of disodium ethane-1-hydroxy-1,1-diphosphonate (or EHDP), given in the drinking water at concentrations of 0.0025%, 0.05% and 0.5%. They found that the weight of the experimental calcium oxalate calculi was decreased at all the concentrations of EHDP used, that only the highest concentration of EHDP inhibited calcium hydrogen phosphate stone formation, and that the formation of stones composed of magnesium ammonium phosphate was unaffected. The results were consistent with the finding that EHDP inhibited the precipitation of crystallization of calcium oxalate from solution in vitro and that it might be of use in the prevention of some types of urinary calculi in man.

When EHDP is given to humans, the average size of urinary calcium oxalate crystals is reduced, though the total urinary oxalate excretion and the total volume of the crystals excreted are increased, to some extent therefore nullifying its effectiveness [24, 31].

It has been suggested that an inhibitor of urinary crystal formation may be an (as yet) undefined acid mucopolysaccharide [30].

In studies on urinary crystal formation in oxalate stone-formers, Robertson and Nordin [28] showed that active recurrent idiopathic stone-formers pass more calcium-containing crystals than do normal subjects. They devised methods to count the crystals in freshly voided urine within a size range of 3.8–48.6 μm diameter; between a urinary pH of 4.9 and 6.2, crystals were composed of calcium oxalate, while above pH 6.2 the deposits consisted predominantly of calcium phosphate, often with small amounts of calcium oxalate.

There were two groups of recurrent calcium stone-formers: those with high urinary calcium and oxalate excretions and high calcium oxalate activity products whose stones are composed predominantly of calcium oxalate; and those with high urinary calcium and oxalate excretions, a high urinary pH, a high calcium oxalate and octocalcium phosphate (OCP) activity products, whose stones are composed of mixed calcium-oxalate–calcium-phosphate. These two groups of 'recurrent idiopathic stone-formers' differ from the main group of idiopathic stone-formers in that they have another lesion additional to the hypercalciuria common to all three groups.

Hypercalciuria per se is not sufficient to cause the persistent precipitation of calcium salts in urine, but must be accompanied by an increase in either urinary oxalate excretion or urinary pH, or both, before spontaneous precipitation takes place [28].

Dietary supplements of calcium, sufficient to produce a 7.0% increase in the urinary calcium, do not cause a significant increase in the urinary supersaturation of hypercalciuric stone-formers; whereas dietary supplements of oxalate and bicarbonate produce significant increases in calcium oxalate and OCP activity products respectively [29].

References

1. Albright,F., Henneman,P., Benedict,P.H., Forbes,A.P.: Idiopathic hypercalciuria. Proc. R. Soc. Med. 46, 1077 (1953)
2. Albuquerque,P.F., Tuma,M.: Investigations on urolithiasis. II. Studies on oxalate. J. Urol. 87, 504 (1962)
3. Black,J.M.: Oxaluria in British troops in India. Br. Med. J. 1, 590 (1945)
4. Carlstrom,D.: Acta Radiol. (Suppl. 121) (1955)
5. Cifuentes,L., Catalina,F., Garcia-Vincente, J.: Electron-microscopy and X-ray diffraction of precipitated urinary calcium phosphate. Br. J. Urol. 39, 450 (1967).
6. Cottet,J., Vittu,C.: Calcium urinaire et lithiases urinaires. Presse Méd. 63, 878 (1955)
7. Cottet,J., Vittu,C., Canarelli,G.: Calciuries et lithiases urinaires. Int. Symp. on Calcium Lithiasis, Vittel, France 1962
8. Dempsey,E.F.: Urinary oxalate excretion in relation to renal stone formation. J. Clin. Invest. 36, 882 (1957)
9. Dempsey,E.F., Forbes,A.O., Melick,R.A., Henneman,P.H.: Urinary oxalate excretion. Metabolism 9, 52 (1960)
10. Donné,M.A.: Tableau de différents depôts de matières salines et de substance organisés qui se font dans les urines, presentant les caractères propre à les distinguer entre eux et à reconnaître leur natute. C.R. Acad. Sci. (Paris) 1, 419 (1838)
11. Flocks,R.H.: Calcium and phosphorus excretion in the urine of patients with renal or ureteric calculi. J. Amer. Med. Assoc. 113, 1466 (1939)
12. Fraser,D., Russell,R.G., Pohler, P., Robertson,W.G., Fleisch,H.: The influence of disodium ethane-1-hydroxy-1,1-diphosphonate (EHDP) on the development of experimentally-induced urinary stones in rats. Clin. Sci. 42, 197 (1972)
13. Harrison,A.H.: Some results of metabolic investigation in cases of renal stone. Br. J. Urol. 31, 398 (1959)
14. Hodgkinson,A., Pyrah, L.N.: The urinary excretion of calcium and inorganic phosphate in 344 patients with calcium stone of renal origin. Br. J. Surg. 46, 10 (1958)
15. Jackson,W.P.U., Dancaster,C.: A consideration of the hypercalciuria, sarcoidosis, idiopathic hypercalciuria and that produced by vitamin D: a new suggestion. J. Clin. Endocrinol. 19, 658 (1959)
16. Jeghers,H., Murphy,R.: Practical aspects of oxalate metabolism. N. Engl. J. Med. 233, 208 (1945)
17. Jorgensen,F.S.: Hypercalciuria and stone formation. N. Engl. J. Med. 292, 756 (1975)
18. Knapp,L.: Facteurs influençant la calciurie. J. Clin. Invest. 26, 182 (1947)
19. Litin,R.B., Diessner,G.R., Keating,F.R.: Urinary excretion of calcium in patients with renal lithiasis. J. Urol. 68, 17 (1961)
20. McGeown,M.G., Bull,G.M.: The pathogenesis of urinary calculus formation. Br. Med. Bull. 13, 53 (1957)
21. McIntosh,J.F., Read,M.K.: Oxalic acid excretion in oxalate urolithiasis. J. Urol. 80, 272 (1958)
22. Melick,R.A., Henneman,P.H.: Clinical and laboratory studies of 207 consecutive patients in a kidney stone clinic. N. Engl. J. Med. 259, 307 (1958)
23. Nordin,B.E.C., Robertson,W.G.: Calcium phosphate and oxalate ion products in normal and stone-forming urines. Br. Med. J. 54, 85 (1966)
24. Oata,M., Pak,C.Y.: Preliminary studies of the treatment of nephrolithiasis (calcium stone) with diphosphonate. Metabolism 23, 1167 (1974)
25. Ohlson,M.A., Brewer,W.D., Jackson,L., Swanson,P.P., Roberts,P.H., Mangel,M., Leverton,R.M., Chaloupka,S., Gram,M.R., Reynolds,M.S., Ludz,R.: Intakes and retentions of nitrogen, calcium and phosphorus by 136 women between 30 and 85 years of age. Fed. Proc. 11, 775 (1952)
26. Revusova,V., Zara,V.: Dynamika hyperkalkurie u detis Urolitiazou. Vysledky Olhodobeho Sledovania Deti Cest Pediatr. 24, 683 (1969)

27. Robertson,W.G., Morgan,D.B.: The distribution of urinary calcium excretion in normal persons and stone-formers. Clin. Chim Acta *37*, 503 (1972)

28. Robertson,W.G., Nordin, B.E.C.: Physicochemical factors governing stone formation. In: Scientific foundation of urology. Vol. 1, p. 254. London: Heinemann 1976

29. Robertson,W.G., Peacock,M., Nordin, B.E.C.: Urolithiasis—Physical aspects. Finlayson,B., Hench,L.L., Smith,L.H. (eds.), p. 79. Washington D.C.: National Academy of Sciences 1972

30. Robertson,W.G., Peacock,M., Knowles,F.: Calcium oxalate crystalluria and inhibitors of crystallization in recurrent renal stone-formers. In: Urinary calculi. Delatte,L.C., Rapado,A., Hodgkinson,A. (eds.), p. 302. Proceedings of International Symposium on Renal Stone Research, Madrid 1972. Basel: S. Karger 1973

31. Robertson,W.G., Peacock,M., Marshall, R.W., Knowles,F.: The effect of ethane-1-hydroxy-1,1-diphosphonate (EHDP) on calcium oxalate crystalluria in recurrent renal stone-formers. Clin. Sci. *47*, 13 (1974)

32. Sutherland,J.W.: Recurrence following operation for upper urinary tract stone. Br. J. Urol. *26*, 22 (1954)

33. Tovborg Jensen,A.: On concrements from the urinary tract. Acta Chir. Scand. *84*, 207 (1941)

34. Vermeulen,C.W., Grove,W.J., Goetz,R., Raggins,D.H., Carroll,N.O.: Experimental lithiasis. I. Development of calculi upon foreign bodies introduced into the bladders of rats. J. Urol. *64*, 541 (1950)

35. Zvara,V., Revusova,V.: Hyperkalkuria a jej vztah k tvorbe mocovych kankrementov u deti. Bratisl. Lek Listy *46*, 604 (1966)

Chapter 7

Primary Hyperoxaluria and Related Conditions

I. Primary Hyperoxaluria

Primary hyperoxaluria is the name at present given to a genetically determined disorder of oxalate metabolism, the clinical manifestations of which are recurrent calcium oxalate nephrolithiasis and later in the disease radiologically demonstrable nephrocalcinosis, with a continuously high output of oxalic acid and usually of glycollic acid and glyoxylic acid in the urine and progressive renal damage leading to death in uraemia. At autopsy, though not demonstrable clinically, extrarenal crystalline deposits of calcium oxalate are found in many organs as well as in the kidney, the syndrome then being called 'oxalosis'.

The basic defect is believed to be the impairment of glyoxylate metabolism, leading to a secondary increase in the synthesis and urinary excretion of oxalic acid. The disorder is found most commonly in subjects younger than 30, most patients having their first symptoms between the ages of 2 and 10 years.

Primary hyperoxaluria should be suspected in any child who has recurrent unilateral or bilateral calcium oxalate nephrolithiasis, especially if there are no recognized anatomical defects in the urinary tract, and if there is a family history of nephrolithiasis. A similar and possibly identical disease has been observed in older subjects who have recurrent unilateral or bilateral calcium oxalate calculi. In 'typical cases' collected by Hockaday et al. [44] there were 36 males and 27 females and in his 'atypical cases' 27 males and 20 females.

Early Cases. Some of the early recorded cases of recurrent oxalate nephrolithiasis

associated with oxalate crystals in the kidney and generalized oxalosis, must be accepted as cases of primary hyperoxaluria, even though the urinary oxalate level had not been measured [18, 54]. Chou and Donohue [14] reported as a case of oxalosis a boy aged 2 who had recurrent renal calculi composed of calcium oxalate and who died from renal failure at the age of 7. Sparkling crystalline masses of calcium oxalate were found in the renal parenchyma and also in the vertebrae, sternum, ribs, heart muscle, thymus, lungs, spleen and pituitary; the urinary oxalate was not estimated.

Newnes and Black [64], who were the first to diagnose the condition during life in a child (aged 2), showed the association of recurrent renal calculi with a high urinary excretion of oxalate; the brother of the child had died at the age of 8 from recurrent calcium oxalate renal stones and renal failure. Aponte and Fetter [5] observed three brothers (two being identical twins), aged 12, 12 and 7, all of whom had calcium oxalate nephrocalcinosis demonstrable radiologically and who died from renal failure 2 and 4 years after having been first seen. At autopsy calculi were found in the kidneys and oxalate crystals in the renal parenchyma and in the bones. The daily urinary oxalate levels in the first two cases were 200 and 180 mg respectively, and all three had high normal or raised serum uric acid levels, which may have been contributed to by their impaired renal function. Godwin et al. [41] collected reports of 24 cases from the literature.

Symptoms. The presenting symptoms in young patients have been renal colic, haematuria, urinary infection, and sooner or later (in virtually all the cases) unilateral or more commonly bilateral renal or ureteric calculi often recurring over many years, have been demonstrated radiologically; crystals or small calculi occasionally block the urethra. Some patients have voided one, two, or large numbers of calculi spontaneously; instrumental or operative removal of ureteric calculi has often been necessary. The stones do not differ in their radiological appearance from those of any other calcium-containing stone.

The rate of progress of the disease has varied considerably, depending to some extent upon the presence or absence of renal infection. In the early stages there are no notable physical signs. Cardiac irregularities including complete heart-block have been observed clinically and have possibly resulted from crystalline oxalate deposits in the conducting musculature of the myocardium [4, 78]. Hypertension has been observed during the late stages. Arthritic symptoms resembling those of gout, resulting from inflammation of synovial membranes in which there may be a deposit of crystals, have been reported [13, 60].

In the late stages of the disease, which may not be very prolonged and which usually occur in late adolescence or early adult life, there are the symptoms of renal failure (the immediate cause of death). The blood urea is raised at this stage often to high levels, electrolyte imbalance is usual and the urinary excretion of oxalate may fall from a high to a near-normal level [6, 7].

Nephrocalcinosis (demonstrable radiologically) with finely distributed stippling of the calcific foci (a late development) implies that the intrarenal crystalline deposits have reached a considerable size and are occasionally widely spread throughout the cortex [44]. In a patient of the author's the nephrocalcinosis was noted radiologically only a few months before death, though medium-sized calculi had been present inter-mittently for several years [70]. Bone marrow biopsies have not usually led to the discovery of skeletal oxalate crystals though they were found in a case reported by Lagrue et al. [52].

In a review of 19 cases it was found that the mean duration of the illness from its clinical onset to the time of death was 4 years [32]. In a review of the clinical course of 63 patients Hockaday et al. [44] found that symptoms had always begun before the age of 30 and that 28 had died before reaching that age, only one patient living beyond the age of 40. In other studies, an occasional patient has survived the sixth decade.

In general, the presence of oxalate crystals in the renal parenchyma (for example, in the kidney following partial nephrectomy) is indicative of an advanced stage of the syndrome and possibly the point of no return; from then on the renal tubules gradually suffer from mechanical blockage with crystals, accelerating the inevitable fatal ending [60]. However, in a patient with a history of 20 years recurrent stone formation reported by Scowen et al. [71] no oxalate crystals were found microscopically in a section of kidney tissue removed 6 years before death. Since the late widespread oxalosis gives rise to no diagnostic symptoms it is difficult to say precisely at what stage in the disease it has occurred; so long as the kidneys are able to excrete large amounts of oxalate, possibly little or none passes into the organs of the body.

Biochemical Changes. The diagnosis depends on the discovery of a higher than normal urinary oxalate excretion. The upper limit of the daily urinary excretion of oxalic acid in normal subjects in the author's department has been about 40 mg; in a series of 21 calculous patients the highest recorded level (47.1 mg/24 h) was found in a patient with pure calcium oxalate stones. It may not be easy to distinguish biochemically between a patient with a high normal urinary oxalate excretion and one with late primary hyperoxaluria who has a urinary oxalate lower than usual for that condition, though the clinical history should help. In patients with primary hyperoxaluria, the amount of oxalic acid in the urine varies widely from 70 to as much as 300 mg/24 h if renal function is still good; when renal function is impaired as the disease advances the urinary oxalic acid may be much reduced.

The serum oxalic acid level was found by Zarembski and Hodgkinson [84] to be within the normal limits (344–687 μg/100 ml) in eight patients with primary hyperoxaluria. The estimation of the renal clearance of oxalate has been beset with technical difficulties and does not appear to have been as yet completely resolved [47]. Hyperuricaemia has been observed occasionally [5, 70, 86]. Similar symptoms are found in the less common adult type of the disease when possibly the stones only began to form at a later age [56, 66].

Adult Type. A few patients who are later shown to have primary hyperoxaluria do not develop the clinical symptoms of calcium oxalate stone until middle life or later, nor do they when young develop the high levels of urinary oxalate excretion seen in the infantile or adolescent type. In some late cases the diagnosis has only been made at autopsy, the urinary oxalic acid not having been examined. Cases in the adult group have been reported by various observers [23, 51, 53, 62, 87].

It is possible that some patients in this group have a milder form in which there is an abnormally high urinary excretion of oxalate from infancy, yet one with which the kidneys can cope without developing the more serious complications of nephrolithiasis. Not all of the adult cases have a discoverable family history of the disease. Of the four cases of primary hyperoxaluria reported by McLaurin et al. [60], one

patient, who had lived until the age of 51, had a calcium oxalate stone at the age of 16, several ureterolithotomies being needed later, and the urinary oxalic acid excretion had varied between 200 and 654 mg daily. Another patient, now aged 36, had voided the first stone 5 years earlier, the daily urinary oxalate excretion being 72 mg.

Chisholm and Heard [13] reported a male patient, aged 52, who had had recurrent lithiasis when first seen and who died following renal failure for which dialysis had been performed. Autopsy showed the typical renal changes associated with primary hyperoxaluria, and oxalate crystals were found to be widely distributed in various organs, which is characteristic of generalized oxalosis. The urinary oxalate does not appear to have been measured.

In a report by Cochran et al. [15] of five cases of primary hyperoxaluria, all of whom survived until the third decade or later, the apparent age of onset in one patient was 39 (she died at age 43). Another patient, aged 30, was still living; the centre of the calculi in these patients consisted of apatite and was surrounded by an outer shell containing calcium oxalate, a finding which suggested that the hyperoxaluria may not have been present from birth. One of the patients had a normal urinary excretion of oxalate during the early period of observation but had high values 6 months later. Only one had a family history of renal disease. The serum oxalic acid level was higher than normal in four of the patients all of whom had impaired renal function. In three the daily urinary oxalate excretion exceeded 100 mg/1.75 m², the remaining patients excreting 40–80 mg and 60–80 mg/24 h/1.75 m² respectively. All three patients excreted increased quantities of glycollic acid in the urine, but the urinary excretion of glyoxylic acid appeared to be within normal limits.

Of three patients with primary hyperoxaluria reported by Walls et al. [78] one, in whom stones were not detected until the age of 29, was still alive (having had operative treatment and haemodialysis) at the age of 40.

Genetic Considerations. Frederick et al. [32] pointed out that in most human diseases which have a genetic basis the metabolic abnormality, when elucidated, has resulted from the loss of a single enzymatic activity, and that no human disorder has been demonstrated which resulted from a genetically determined primary excess of enzymatic activity with the possible exception of an elevated leucocyte alkaline phosphatase in mongolism.

The accumulation of a metabolic endproduct such as oxalate, in a disorder assumed to be genetic, suggests the existence of an enzymatic block in an alternate pathway of one of its precursors. The five cases which they described included brother and sister in two separate families. Other patients with siblings who had probable oxalosis or primary hyperoxaluria have been recorded by several observers [5, 30, 42, 64].

Hockaday et al. [44] stated that in at least 16 families, two or more siblings with primary hyperoxaluria have been described without clinical evidence of the disorder in their parents; and that in '13 families in which data were sufficiently complete, 30 to 59 siblings had hyperoxaluria', findings which deviate from the 1:3 ratio classically expected with transmission of recessive traits, but in fact never found because of bias in selecting cases.

There are some reports of increased urinary oxalate excretion by parents of patients with primary hyperoxaluria [25, 52]. The occurrence of renal calculi in the forbears of a patient with hyperoxaluria, does not necessarily imply that those forbears also had the disease.

Thus the mother of three sisters with primary hyperoxaluria who had bilateral nephrolithiasis herself had a normal urinary excretion of oxalate, as did her two brothers [17]. Hockaday et al. [44] pointed out that it cannot be assumed that all the cases reported as primary hyperoxaluria necessarily suffer from the same disease. In most familial cases the available data have suggested an autosomal recessive pattern of inheritance [47, 83].

Renal Changes. Histological examination of sections of parts of the kidneys removed at operation (partial nephrectomy) for stone in early cases show surprisingly little cellular damage apart from the masses of oxalate crystals in the renal tubules; in more advanced cases infection may complicate the picture [70]. The histological changes in the fully developed case are similar to those found in oxalate poisoning in the experimental animal [29].

In an early case the kidney may not differ in size or external appearance from a normal kidney, nor in texture when cut with a scalpel. Later in the disease it may be smaller than normal, the convex surface being granular, scarred and pitted from the changes of pyelonephritis; when sectioned it is gritty from the presence of crystalline masses. The calyces and the renal pelvis (and sometimes the parenchyma) usually contain brown calculi, the cortex and the medulla are reduced in depth, and show white or yellowish flecks of oxalate crystals, most marked in the renal pyramids. The heavy intrarenal deposit of crystalline material composed of calcium oxalate has been known to be as much as 5% of the weight of the kidney [71].

When sections are stained with haematoxylin, the parts impregnated with calcium oxalate (which do not take this stain) are seen histologically as dull, structureless zones, suggesting deposits of colloid, but with the Von Kossa stain, the crystals in these areas are stained black. Under the polarizing microscope, circumscribed zones of crystals may be seen mostly arranged in rosettes or sheaves (characteristic of calcium oxalate monohydrate), usually in the grossly dilated lumina of the proximal and distal convoluted tubules, the cells of which may show some degree of desquamation and even disintegration from the pressure of the crystals, which may then migrate to the interstitial tissue (Fig. 7.1). Deposits of calcium oxalate may be seen in the interstitial tissue in the collecting tubules of the medulla or in the ducts of Bellini.

In some long-standing cases the amount of crystalline material visible in the renal parenchyma may be relatively small and there may be little in the way of inflammatory response. Crystals are sometimes seen within the glomerular tufts. The late changes seen at autopsy are those of tubular destruction, interstitial fibrosis, scarring of the tissue between the crystal masses, and infiltration by chronic inflammatory cells, the picture being that of severe renal damage with associated infection. The widespread deposition of the renal calcific masses can be shown by radiography of the isolated kidney after autopsy.

Oxalosis. In cases seen at autopsy, deposits of oxalate crystals are found in many organs: notably in the middle coats of the large, medium and small arteries, including the aorta and the coronary arteries [71]; the pulmonary alveoli, the splenic pulp, the parathyroid glands, voluntary muscles, bladder, seminal vesicles, liver, salivary glands, thymus, pancreas, and the interstitial tissue of the thyroid gland, cerebrum, hypothalamus and cerebellum [44]; and in the cells of the seminiferous tubules of the testis and in the ducts of the rete testis. Sometimes there is extensive myocardial fibrosis which may contribute to clinical episodes of congestive cardiac failure [78].

Crystals may be attached to the trabeculae of the medullary part of the bone (where they may occupy pits on the surface), in the Haversian systems in younger patients [28], and in the bone marrow. It is impossible from the relative

paucity of autopsy material to say with certainty whether all patients who die from renal failure from primary hyperoxaluria ultimately develop disseminated oxalosis, though this seems probable. Since these patients usually die from gradual renal failure, the changes of secondary hyperparathyroidism as shown by enlargement of the parathyroid glands, demineralization of bone and new periosteal bone formation may be observed [78]. Radiolucent zones in the long bones may signify the deposition of calcium oxalate crystals [58].

Metabolism. The urinary oxalate in normal subjects is derived during the course of endogenous metabolism from three main sources: ascorbic acid (35% to 44% of the total urinary oxalate); glycine by way of glyoxylate (40%); and glycollate (in a varying percentage from 6% to 33%). Only a very small proportion seems to be derived from direct exogenous dietary sources. The interrelationships of the three principal substances acting as the precursors are shown in Figure 7.2 (see p. 142). It is believed that the fundamental lesion in primary hyperoxaluria is a failure to metabolize glyoxylate at a normal rate rather than an excessive metabolism of glycine by way of glyoxylate (Table 7.1, see p. 142).

Metabolic Types of the Disease. Two distinct types of primary hyperoxaluria are known which are biochemically different but clinically appear to be the same disease: primary hyperoxaluria with urinary glycollic aciduria (type I), and primary hyperoxaluria with urinary L-glyceric aciduria (type II).

Patients with the type I disorder (the first to be described) excrete excessive amounts of oxalic and glycollic acid and usually glyoxylic acid, and they incorporate excessive amounts of glyoxylate-1-C^{14} into urinary glycollate. They manifest a deficiency of the enzyme 2-oxo-glutarate;

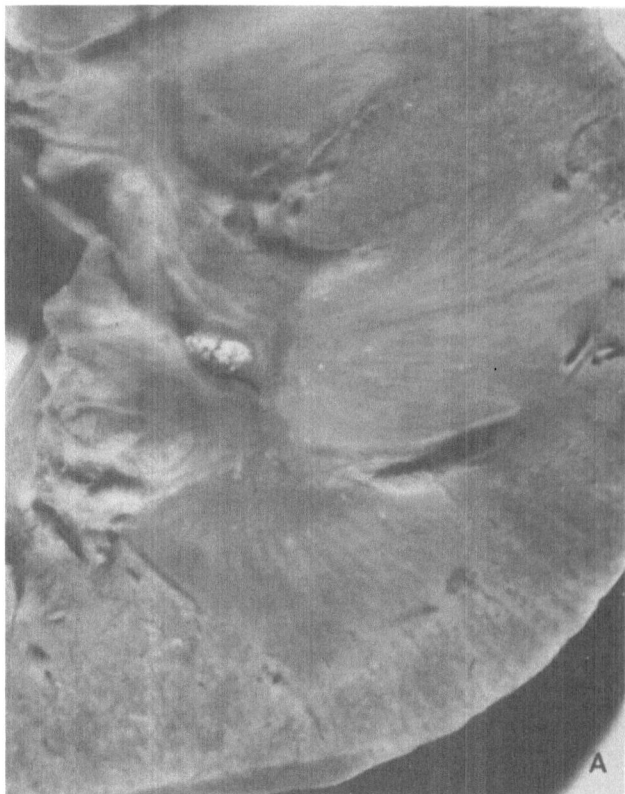

Fig. 7.1. Case of primary hyperoxaluria. **A.** Section of a partial
nephrectomy specimen removed
at operation. There is an ellipsoidal crystalline stone in a
lower calyx and many spotty
calcific foci (*white*) in the
medulla; the kidney as a whole
appears at this stage to be
fairly well preserved. **B.** Microscopic section of medullary part
of the kidney showing heavy
crystalline deposits of calcium
oxalate in some major tubules;
there is round cell infiltration
(*polarized light*)

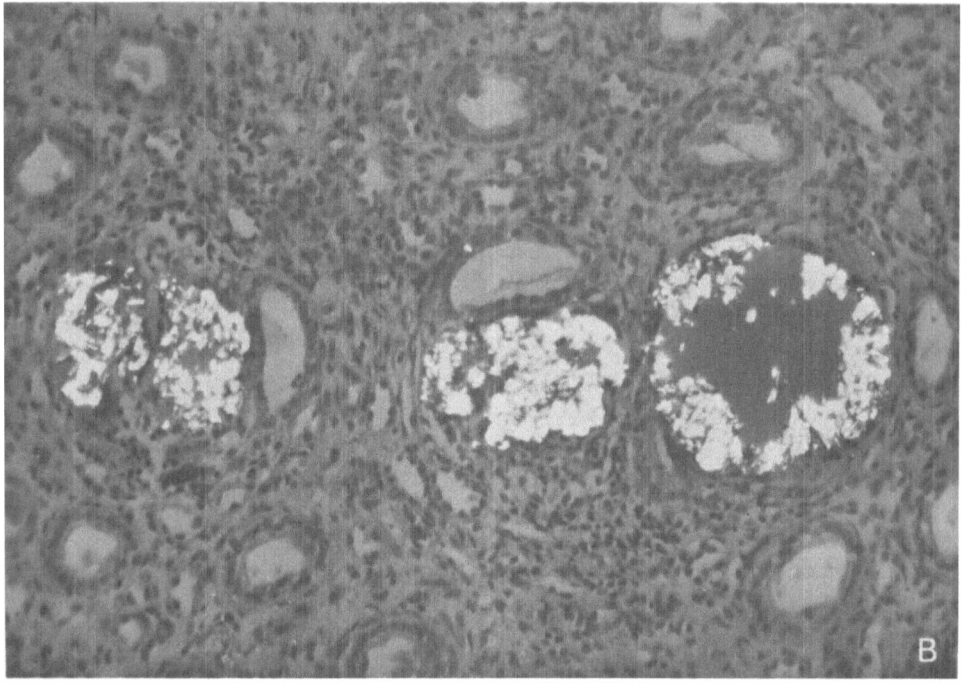

Table 7.1. Urinary oxalate

Origin	In normal subjects		In primary hyperoxaluria	
	% of total	Absolute amount (mg/24 h)	% of total	Absolute amount (mg/24 h)
Ascorbic acid	35–44	15	5	15
Glycine by way of glyoxylate	40	15	32–50	60–120
Glycollate 'other reactions forming glyoxylate'	6–33	7	50–55	90–170
Total		37		165–305

These approximations were first made by Hockaday et al. (1964).

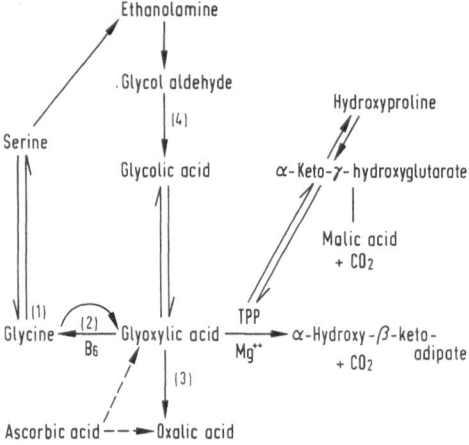

Fig. 7.2. The pathways of oxalate synthesis in primary hyperoxaluria. (By permission of Dr. A. Hodgkinson)

and glyoxylate carboligase can be demonstrated in the liver, kidney and spleen [50].

Patients with the type II disorder described by Williams and Smith [80–82] excrete normal amounts of glycollic acid but an excessive urinary excretion of L-glyceric acid. The incorporation of glyoxylate-1-C[14] into urinary glycollate is reduced and there is a deficiency in the activity of leucocyte D-glyceric hydrogenase, an enzyme which catalyses the interconversion of hydroxypyruvate and D-glycerate. The first four patients described by them (three children and one male adult now aged 33, in whom stones had not been observed until the age of 24), had recurrent

calcium oxalate nephrolithiasis, recurrent urinary infection but no renal impairment. The L-glyceric acid (which is not found in the urine of normal subjects nor in patients with renal calculi from other causes) varied in three patients between 196 and 638 mg/24 h. There was no history of nephrolithiasis in other members of the families of their patients and an autosomal recessive mode of inheritance seems most likely.

Zarembski et al. [86] found that eight patients with primary hyperoxaluria fell into two groups: in six patients the urinary glyoxylic and pyruvic acid excretion was normal or slightly raised, the excretion of urinary glycollic and lactic acid excretion was usually appreciably raised and the levels of serum uric acid and lactic acid were raised. In two patients the urinary excretion of glycollic and lactic acids was normal but the excretion of glyceric acid was raised. One patient exhibited at different times both glycollic and glyceric aciduria, suggesting that these abnormalities are manifestations of a single genetic defect; their results supported the conclusions of Williams and Smith [80, 81] that there are at least two biochemical variants of primary hyperoxaluria.

Treatment. In patients with the common oxalate stone, the urinary oxalate levels are within the well-defined normal range (or sometimes at the upper limit of the normal range). Dietetic measures are, however, desirable to assist in the prevention of further calculi.

In patients with primary hyperoxaluria, medicinal measures so far used have not provided an effective remedy which will reduce to normal the high level of urinary oxalate. Attempts to give relief, such as those referred to below, will, however, usually be tried.

Dietary Measures. The patient should be put on a low-oxalate diet (probably in association with a low-calcium diet) on the lines of that given in detail by Hodgkinson [47], though such a measure may not help materially to reduce the level of the urinary oxalate. In order to reduce the intake of glycine (a precursor of oxalate) and of the oxalate-containing foods a restriction of the dietary protein has been advised, but such a measure does not appear to have any recognizable effect. Since the daily turnover of glycine is 0.5–10 g/kg [79], less than 0.5% of which is converted to oxalate, even in patients with hyperoxaluria, protein restriction therefore cannot be expected to succeed [44]. The search must go on for some substance which can be tolerated by the patient and which will inhibit the enzymatic synthesis of oxalate.

Suggested Medicinal Measures. *Sodium benzoate* which 'traps' glycine and consequently increases the level of urinary hippurate, has been used in an attempt to reduce the level of urinary oxalate in patients with primary hyperoxaluria [8]. In a patient with primary hyperoxaluria under the care of the author, the administration of sodium benzoate resulted in only a temporary reduction of the urine oxalate; after 4 weeks the high level of urinary oxalate returned, together with further attacks of renal colic and haematuria [70]. Several observers have reported only temporary or indifferent results from the use of sodium benzoate [17, 59, 60].

Magnesium salts have been given to try to reduce the urinary oxalate, on the basis of the work of Hammarsten, but have not been successful [15, 24, 46, 70]. A high phosphate and high magnesium diet (a measure which should reduce the level of the urinary calcium and increase the urinary magnesium–calcium ratio) was used for the treatment of two patients with primary hyperoxaluria by Frederick et al. [32]; in one, the stone disappeared though there was no reduction in the level of the urinary excretion of oxalate.

The administration of magnesium along with phosphates and sodium phytate may possibly bring some beneficial results. Dent and Stamp [21] have reported some clinical improvement in the incidence of nephrocalcinosis and calculi in patients in this group by the use of these remedies but have not observed a reduction of the urinary oxalate. In the treatment of four patients with primary hyperoxaluria Silver and Brendler [72] found that though the administration of magnesium was not followed by any reduction of the urinary oxalate level, further calculus formation was prevented in three of four cases during a 4-year follow-up.

Calcium carbimide inhibits the enzyme aldehyde dehydrogenase, which by promoting the oxidation of glycaldehyde forms glycollic acid. The administration of this substance was reported to have reduced the excretion of oxalic acid in the urine of two patients with primary hyperoxaluria [74]. However, in three patients with primary hyperoxaluria treated by Zarembski et al. [85], the administration of this substance did not reduce the level of urinary oxalate nor that of oxalic acid in the blood. The treatment was also unsuccessful in a patient treated by Giertz [40].

Isocarboxazid, which is a monoamine oxidase, has been reported by Bourke et al. [10] to reduce the urinary oxalate excretion; other workers have not been able to confirm its efficacy.

Allopurinol, which inhibits xanthine oxidase, might be expected to bring about a reduction of glyoxylate to oxalic acid; it appears, however, to have no effect in the treatment of primary hyperoxaluria [39].

Pyridoxine (vitamin B_6), when administered to patients with true primary hyperoxaluria has usually resulted in only a slight reduction in the urinary oxalate excretion [45]; though in a small number of patients with hyperoxaluria (but with not a very high level of urinary oxalate), the administration of pyridoxine has resulted in a reduction of the urinary oxalate excretion to normal level, suggesting that the pyridoxine deficiency may have been a contributory cause of stone formation [55].

Smith and Williams [73], who treated five patients with primary hyperoxaluria with pyridoxine and phosphate, found the combination to be beneficial with some reduction of the level of the urinary oxalate excretion in four; in two cases stone formation was brought under control, the stones being possibly reduced in size. In a few patients there has been a gradual decrease and relative relief from attacks of colic when it was continued for many months [17, 31, 38, 60, 75].

Haemodialysis and Renal Transplantation. When the patient reaches the advanced stage of renal failure the question may arise as to whether attempts should be made to prolong life by haemodialysis or peritoneal dialysis, and renal transplantation. Since oxalate in the plasma is largely unbound to peptides or proteins, it is to be expected that haemodialysis would be more efficient than peritoneal dialysis for the removal of oxalate.

Zarembski et al. [86] showed that haemodialysis will reduce the raised plasma oxalate levels in renal failure due to causes other than the primary hyperoxaluria. They used peritoneal dialysis for the treatment of renal failure in a woman aged 27, with primary hyperoxaluria, bilateral renal calculi and nephrocalcinosis. It was shown that although the dialysis removed 43 mg oxalic acid per day from the body fluids, this rate was less than the rate of endogenous production of oxalic acid and it was not therefore found to be possible to lower the concentration of the plasma oxalate by this means. Walls et al. [78] reported one patient aged 27 who was kept alive for 18 months by haemodialysis using the Scribner shunt technique. Another patient aged 23 with a staghorn calculus has been well for a considerable time since having haemodialysis and a third patient now aged 31, who had had various calculous episodes for 20 years had been kept alive by intermittent haemodialysis for 9 months.

Bilateral renal transplantation with or without bilateral nephrectomy has been done for some advanced cases of this condition. Since, however, such a procedure could not cure the basic enzymatic defect which causes the hyperoxaluria a radical cure could not be expected, as the disease would appear in the transplanted kidneys in due course. There may, however, be an appreciable prolongation of life. Klauwers et al. [49] reported a patient aged 22 who had had calculi since the age of 3 and had developed renal failure, which was treated first by peritoneal dialysis and later by bilateral nephrectomy, splenectomy and renal transplantation. Autopsy 3 weeks later showed histological deposits of oxalate crystals in the transplanted kidney as well as in many organs. Deodhar et al. [22] reported renal transplantation in a patient with primary hyperoxaluria. Giertz [40] referred to one patient with primary hyperoxaluria, bilateral renal calculi and renal failure, who did not respond to renal transplantation. Solomons et al. [74] reported a good result in a patient with primary oxalosis, who was treated by renal transplantation in combination with calcium carbimide.

II. Related Conditions

1. Vitamin B₆ Deficiency

It has been shown in the experimental animal that a deficiency of pyridoxine (vitamin B_6) in the diet may lead to an increase of urinary oxalates and sometimes to the formation of oxalate calculi. Such a vitamin B_6 deficiency may occasionally be present in the human diet, when it could be a contributory cause to the formation of oxalate-containing stones.

Vitamin B_6 (pyridoxine) is the co-enzyme required in several important reactions of amino acid metabolism. The increased urinary oxalate excretion may be due to reduced transamination of glyoxylate to glycine, when glyoxylate would accumulate and be oxidized to oxalate. When pyridoxine is absent from the diet of the rat there is cessation of growth, a specific symmetrical dermatitis (ears, nose, mouth, tail, paws), demyelination and nerve-cell changes (in the pig), atrophy of the accessory organs of reproduction, changes in the adrenals and lymphoid tissues, deposits of haemosiderin in the liver and ultimately convulsions.

Gershoff and his co-workers fed weaning rats with a casein diet deficient in vitamin B_6. The level of the urinary oxalate was sometimes more than double that of the controls and the animals ultimately developed renal calculi, which sometimes descended to the ureter, urethra or bladder. When a vitamin B_6-deficient diet was supplemented with glycine there was a further increase in the level of the urinary oxalate excretion and an acceleration in the process of calculus formation. Crystalline material found at the apex of the papillae at autopsy sometimes resembled Randall's plaques histologically (type I), and was sometimes seen to extend into the collecting ducts. In animals which survived for 3–6 months the kidneys seen at autopsy had deep irregular or linear scars extending into the medulla, some cortical tubules were

destroyed, others were dilated (with a partial or complete loss of the basement membrane). Birefringent oxalate crystals (needles, rods, rosettes, sheaves or plates) mostly restricted to the apex of the renal papilla were seen in the distal collecting tubules and in the scars; concretions appeared later on the papilla.

Kittens fed with a vitamin B_6-low diet and sacrificed after 3–6 months showed a gradual failure of growth, anaemia, hyperoxaluria and sometimes convulsions. Oxalate crystals (and sometimes nephrocalcinosis) were found in the renal cortex and medulla; if the intake of magnesium was sufficiently raised in the diet, protection was afforded against renal stone formation [3, 35–38].

In rats fed with a pyridoxine-deficient diet Vermeulen and his co-workers [57, 77], using their techniques of an implanted foreign body in the bladder [76] showed that calcium oxalate calculi were formed around the foreign body in the bladder as well as on the renal papilla. When the diet was supplemented with a threefold increase in the calcium, the stone formation was aggravated; but when the diet was supplemented with a high magnesium intake, no renal papillary tip stones were observed, though stones composed of newberyite ($MgHPO_4 \cdot 3H_2O$) with a small admixture of apatite, were formed around the foreign body in the bladder. When the magnesium intake was low, brushite ($CaHPO_4 \cdot 2H_2O$) stones were formed. The high-magnesium diet had apparently completely prevented the oxalate lithiasis but had provided conditions favourable for the development of another type of stone. When rats were fed with a diet deficient in vitamin B_6 but with glycine supplementation, renal papillary calculosis was observed, but not when the diet contained magnesium to a final concentration of 0.49–100 g [57].

There is some evidence that there may be a small number of vitamin B_6-dependent cases of hyperoxaluria among those usually classified as cases of primary hyper-oxaluria. Thus, Ludwig [55] described a patient with what he called 'the adult or milder form of hyperoxaluria' in a woman aged 41 who had bilateral infected renal calculi and a daily urinary oxalate excretion of 72–75 mg. An estimation of the amount of urinary xanthenuric acid before and after the administration of an oral loading dose of 10 g tryptophane, suggested the presence of a relative pyridoxine deficiency. The right kidney was removed; following treatment by daily oral and parenteral pyridoxine for 2 months, a fall in the basal daily excretion of urinary xanthenuric acid from 47 to 14.5 mg (after the loading dose of 10 g trypto-phane) was thought to indicate a return of the level of pyridoxine in the body to normal. There was a gradual decrease in urinary oxalate excretion which, however, increased after the patient had left hospital, possibly because she reverted from a low to a normal protein diet.

Prien and Gershoff [69] treated 39 patients who had passed at least two calculi a year (some had passed as many as five), for a minimum of 2 years on a mixed diet with adequate fluid, 10 mg pyridoxine hydrochloride (vitamin B_6) and two to four tablets of milk of magnesia daily for a minimum period of 4.5 years. Of 15 of the author's own cases in the series, 9 remained entirely free from stone, 4 have had one or two stones, while 1 was not improved. In 24 patients from the practices of co-operating urologists, 16 have had no further stone or only an occasional stone, and 5 have shown no improvement. It was considered that the treatment was encouraging and was worthy of an extended trial, though it is not clear what part the administration of magnesium played in achieving these results.

Giertz [40] reported a patient who had a daily urinary oxalate excretion of 200 mg with 500 mg/day pyridoxine (vitamin B_6); the urinary excretion of oxalic and glycollic acid returned nearly to normal for a period of 10 months; possibly this case was an example of the so-called B_6-dependent type of hyperoxaluria.

2. Hyperoxaluria from Other Causes

A high urinary excretion of oxalates, not accounted for by the presence of the disease primary hyperoxaluria, has been found in some patients with hepatic cirrhosis. A similar increase was noted in two of six patients who had Klinefelter's syndrome in association with renal calculi [19].

Resection of the Ileum. In some patients with regional enteritis, and following sur-gical resection of portions of ileum for various diseases of the small intestine, some patients have developed calcium oxalate stones and hyperoxaluria, the daily urinary oxalate being as high as 90–200 mg. It has been suggested that in such patients glycine which would normally have been absorbed in the intestine is converted into glyoxylate in the large intestine, which is then absorbed and converted into oxalic acid by the liver, which in turn is excreted into the urine [11, 12, 27, 48]; alternatively it may be caused by excessive absorption of dietary oxalate [12].

The hyperoxaluria may be abolished by the use of a low-oxalate diet (a discipline which is not always easy for the patient to accept) or by the use of cholestyranine (4 g given three or four times daily) which is an anion-exchange resin. The subject was reviewed by Harrison [43]. Renal calculi sometimes complicate ulcerative colitis [63]. Hyperoxaluria and calcium oxalate renal calculi may complicate various kinds of ileal dysfunction possibly because of bile-salt malabsorption; the hyperoxaluria can be corrected by the administration of taurine [1, 27].

Oxalic Acid Poisoning. While small amounts of the salts of oxalic acid are non-toxic, large doses of oxalic acid or soluble oxalate may give rise to serious illness or death from poisoning preceded by anuria and renal failure. There is hyperoxaluria in the early stages and birefringent oxalate crystals are found in the renal tubules. The effects of poisoning in the experimental animal have been studied [29].

Methoxyflurane Poisoning. This anaesthetic agent is partly metabolized to oxalic acid in the body, giving rise to hyperoxaluria, which could be dangerous [59, 67].

Ethylene Glycol Poisoning. A number of cases of poisoning with ethylene glycol ($HO \cdot CH_2 \cdot CH_2 \cdot OH$; anti-freeze) which had been taken by mouth as a substitute for alcohol because of its intoxicating effects, have been reported. Ethylene glycol is believed to be metabolized to oxalate by way of glycol aldehyde, glycollic acid and glyoxylic acid, probably only 3%–10% being converted into oxalic acid [9, 33]. The approximate lethal dose is thought to be between 90 and 100 ml but survival has followed the ingestion of larger amounts. Some 40–60 deaths each year have been reported from the United States.

Following an initial period of stimulation there is persistent vomiting, excitation simulating that of alcoholic intoxication, convulsions, pulmonary oedema and shock; there is a metabolic acidosis and an excess of urinary oxalates. In severe cases death may occur within 48 h [68].

At autopsy the kidneys are enlarged and may harbour calculi and histologically show the changes of acute renal tubular necrosis. The changes are most marked in the proximal convoluted tubules, the epithelium of which is flattened, and the lumina usually dilated and containing a deposit of birefringent crystals of calcium oxalate, presenting as sheaves, prisms or rhomboids. Allen [2] recorded 76 deaths which had followed the ingestion of 2–4.5 oz of an elixir of sulphonilamide which also contained 72% diethylene glycol. Oxalate

lithiasis has been induced experimentally in rats by the administration of ethylene glycol [61].

3. Glycinuria; Hyperglycinaemia; Calcium Oxalate Calculi

Two pathological conditions possibly related metabolically to primary hyperoxaluria have been described: De Vries et al. [26] found excessive urinary glycine excretion in four members of a family, associated with nephrolithiasis in three. They showed that the glycinuria was due to a renal mechanism and the failure to reabsorb glycine was not associated with defective reabsorption of other amino acids or of phosphate or glucose. A renal stone from one of the patients was composed mainly of calcium oxalate and contained a small amount of glycine present in the non-protein non-peptide form.

Cusworth and Dent [16] reported two patients with osteomalacia who had an increased urinary excretion of glycine and also a decreased renal tubular reabsorption; they suggested that the condition was the result of a selective interference with renal tubular function possibly related to the renal phosphate leak found in some patients with osteomalacia. Dent and Friedman [20] reported a further patient with hypophosphataemic osteomalacia which had begun at the age of 16, and who had remained well following treatment with calciferol. She was found 8 years later to have a large urinary excretion of glycine, believed to be due to a defective renal tubular reabsorption of glycine.

Gerritsen et al. [34] reported a mentally retarded child who was observed to have hyperglycinaemia, hyperglycinuria and a urinary excretion of oxalate which was reduced to about one-tenth of that excreted by two controls, but which was increased to normal by feeding glyoxylic acid in amounts of 100 to 250 mg. The condition was believed to have resulted from an absence or decreased activity of the enzyme glycine oxidase. Nyhan [65] discussed the metabolic abnormalities related to hypoglycinaemia.

References

1. Admirand,W.H., Earnest,D., Williams,H.: Hyperoxaluria and bowel disease. Clin. Res. *19*, 562 (Abstr.) (1971)
2. Allen,A.C.: The kidney: medical and surgical disease. London: Churchill 1952
3. Andrus,S.B., Gershoff,S.N., Faragalla,F.F., Prien,E.L.: Production of calcium oxalate renal calculi in vitamin B6 deficient rats. Lab. Invest. *9*, 7 (1960)
4. Antoine,B., Slama,R., Josso,F., Montera, H.de, Habib,R., Richet,G.: The destruction of renal parenchyma by invasion by calcium oxalate crystals. Two new cases of 'renal oxalosis'. Presse Med. *68*, 803 (1960)
5. Aponte,G.E., Fetter,T.B.: Familial idiopathic oxalate nephrocalcinosis. Am. J. Clin. Pathol. *24*, 1363 (1954)
6. Archer,H.E., Dormer,A.E., Scowen,E.F., Watts,R.W.E.: Primary hyperoxaluria. Lancet *II*, 320 (1957a)
7. Archer,H.E., Dormer,A.E., Scowen,E.F., Watts,R.W.E.: Studies on the urinary excretion of oxalate by normal subjects. Clin. Sci. *16*, 405 (1957b)
8. Archer,H.E., Dormer,A.E., Scowen,E.F., Watts,R.W.E.: The etiology of primary hyperoxaluria. Br. Med. J. *1*, 175 (1958)
9. Berman,L.B., Schiemer,G.E., Feys,J.: The nephrotoxic lesion of ethylene glycol. Ann. Int. Med. *46*, 611 (1962)
10. Bourke,E., Frindt,G., Flynn,P., Schreiner, G.E.: Primary hyperoxaluria with normal alpha-ketoglutarate: glyoxylate carboligase activity. Ann. Int. Med. *76*, 279 (1972)
11. Chadwick,V.S., Modha,K., Dowling,R.H.: Mechanism for hyperoxaluria in patients with ileal dysfunction. N. Engl. J. Med. *289*, 172 (1973)
12. Chikos,P.M., McDonald,G.B.: Regional enteritis complicated by nephrocalcinosis and nephrolithiasis. Case report. Radiology *121*, 75 (1976)
13. Chisholm,G.D., Heard,E.G.: Oxalosis. Br. J. Surg. *50*, 78 (1962)
14. Chou,L.Y., Donohue,W.L.: Oxalosis: possible 'inborn error of metabolism' with nephrolithiasis and nephrocalcinosis due to calcium oxalate as the predominating features. Pediatrics *10*, 660 (1952)
15. Cochran,M., Hodgkinson,A., Zarembski, P.M.: Hyperoxaluria in adults. Br. J. Surg. *55*, 121 (1968)
16. Cusworth,D.C., Dent,C.E.: Renal clearance in normal subjects and in patients with aminoaciduria. Biochem. J. *74*, 550 (1960)
17. Daniels,R.A., Michels,R., Aisen,P., Goldstein,G.: Familial hyperoxaluria: report of a family, review of the literature. Am. J. Med. *29*, 820 (1960)
18. Davis,J.S., Klineberg,W.G., Stowell,R.E.: Nephrolithiasis and nephrocalcinosis with calcium oxalate crystals in kidneys and bones. J. Pediat. *36*, 323 (1950)
19. Dempsey,E.F., Forbes,A.P., Melick,R.A., Henneman,P.H.: Urinary oxalate excretion. Metabolism *9*, 52 (1960)
20. Dent,C.E., Friedman,M.: Hypophosphaturic osteomalacia with complete recovery. Br. Med. J. *1*, 1676 (1964)
21. Dent,C.E., Stamp,T.C.B.: Treatment of primary hyperoxaluria. Arch. Dis. Child. *45*, 244 (1970)
22. Deodhar,S.D., Tung,K.S.K., Zuhlke,V., Nakatoto,S.: Renal transplantation in a patient with primary familial oxalosis. Arch. Pathol. *87*, 118 (1969)
23. Derot,M., Legrain,M., Prunier,P., Quenu, L.: Two cases of familial oxalosis in adults. J. Urol. Nephrol. *68*, 589 (1962)
24. Desgrez,P., Thomas,J., Thomas,E., Rabussier,P.: Facteurs influençant l'équilibre urinaire dans la lithiase calcique. Rein Foie *4*, 189 (1962)
25. De Toni,G., Durand,P., Rosso,C.: L'asslosi una nuova malattia del ricambio a carattere tessurismico. Minerva Pediatr. *2*, 623 (1967)
26. De Vries,A., Kochwa,S., Lazebnick,J.: Glycinuria, hereditary disorder associated with nephrolithiasis. Am. J. Med. *23*, 408 (1957)
27. Dowling,R.H., Rose,G.A., Sutor,J.S.: Hyperoxaluria and renal calculi in ileal disease. Lancet *I*, 1103 (1971)
28. Dunn,H.G.: Oxalosis. Am. J. Dis. Child. *90*, 58 (1955)
29. Dunn,H.G., Haworth,A., Jones,N.A.: The pathology of oxalate nephritis. J. Pathol. Bacteriol. *27*, 299 (1924)
30. Elder,T.D., Wyngaarden,J.B.: The biosynthesis and turnover of oxalate in normal and hyperoxaluric subjects. J. Clin. Invest. *39*, 1337 (1960)

31. Faber,S.R., Feitler,W.W., Bleiler,R.E., Ohlson,M.A., Hodges,R.E.: The effects of an induced pyridoxine and pentothenic acid deficiency on excretion of oxalic and xanthurenic acids in the urine. Am. J. Clin. Nutr. *12*, 406 (1963)

32. Frederick,E.W., Rabkin,M.T., Ritchie, R.H.Jr., Smith,L.E.Jr.: Studies on primary hyperoxaluria. I. In vivo demonstrations of a defect in glyoxylate metabolism. N. Engl. J. Med. *269*, 821 (1963)

33. Friedman,E.A., Greenberg,J.B., Merrill, J.P., Dammin,G.J.: Consequences of ethylene glycol poisoning. Am. J. Med. *32*, 811 (1962)

34. Gerritsen,T., Kaveggia,E., Waisman,H.A.: A new type of idiopathic hyperglycinemia with hypo-oxaluria. Pediatrics *36*, 882 (1965)

35. Gershoff,S.N., Andrus,S.B.: Effect of vitamin B_6 and magnesium on renal deposition of calcium oxalate induced by ethylene glycol administration. Proc. Soc. Exp. Biol. Med. *109*, 99 (1962)

36. Gershoff,S.N., Faragalla,F.F.: Endogenous oxalate synthesis and glycine, serine, desoxypyridoxine interrelationships in vitamin B_6 deficient rats. J. Biol. Chem. *234*, 2391 (1959)

37. Gershoff,S.N., Prien,E.L.: Excretion of urinary metabolites in calcium oxalate urolithiasis. Effect of tryptophan and vitamin B_6 administration. Am. J. Clin. Nutr. *8*, 812 (1960)

38. Gershoff,S.N., Faragalla,F.F., Nelson, D.A., Andrus,S.B.: Vitamin B_6 deficiency and oxalate nephrocalcinosis in the cat. Am. J. Med. *27*, 72 (1959)

39. Gibbs,A., Watts,R.W.E.: Biochemical studies on treatment of primary hyperoxaluria. Arch. Dis. Child. *42*, 505 (1967)

40. Giertz,G.: Hyperoxaluria. Urologists' Correspondents Club 2nd Jan. 1970

41. Godwin,J.T., Fowler,M.R., Dempsey,E.F., Henneman,P.H.: Primary hyperoxaluria and oxalosis; Report of a case and review of the literature. N. Engl. J. Med. *259*, 1099 (1958)

42. Hall,E.G., Scowen,E.F., Watts,R.W.E.: Clinical manifestations of primary hyperoxaluria. Arch. Dis. Child. *35*, 108 (1960)

43. Harrison,A.R.: Urinary calculi in bowel disorders. In: Scientific foundations of urology. Williams,D.I., Chisholm,G.D. (eds.), Vol. I, p. 315. Heinemann: London 1976

44. Hockaday,T.D.R., Clayton,J.E., Frederick, E.W., Smith,L.H.Jr.: Primary hyperoxaluria. Medicine *43*, 315 (1964)

45. Hockaday,T.D.R., Frederick,E.W., Clayton,J.E., Smith,L.H.Jr.: Studies on primary hyperoxaluria. II. Urinary oxalate, glycolate and glyoxylate measurement by isotope dilution methods. J. Lab. Clin. Med. *65*, 677 (1965)

46. Hodgkinson,A.: The urinary excretion of oxalic acid in nephrolithiasis. Proc. R. Soc. Med. *51*, 970 (1958)

47. Hodgkinson,A.: Oxalate metabolism and hyperoxaluria. In: Scientific foundations of urology. Williams,D.I., Chisholm,G.D. (eds.), Vol. I, p. 289. Heinemann: London 1976

48. Hofmann,A.F., Thomas,P.J., Smith,L.H., McCall,J.T.: Pathogenesis of secondary hyperoxaluria in patients with ileal resection. Gastroenterology *58*, 960 (1970)

49. Klauwers,J., Wolf,P.L., Cohn,R.: Failure of renal transplantation in primary oxalosis. J. Am. Med. Assoc. *209*, 551 (1969)

50. Koch,J., Stokstad,E.L.R., Williams,H.E., Smith,L.H.Jr.: Deficiency of 2-oxo-glutarate, glyoxylate carboligase activity in primary hyperoxaluria. Proc. Natl. Acad. Sci. USA. *57*, 1123 (1967)

51. Koten,J.W., Gastel,C.van, Mees,E.J.: Two cases of primary oxalosis. J. Clin. Pathol. *18*, 223 (1965)

52. Lagrue,G., Laudat,M.H., Meyer,P., Sapil, M., Milliez,P.: Oxalose familiale avec acidose hyperchloremique secondaire. Semaine Hopital de Paris *35*, 2023 (1959)

53. Largiader,F., Zollinger,H.U.: Oxalosis. Part I. Empirical studies. Virchows Arch. *333*, 368 (1960)

54. Lapoutre,C.: Calculs multiples chez un enfant: infiltration du parenchyme renal par des depots cristallins. J. Urol. *20*, 424 (1925)

55. Ludwig,G.D.: Renal calculi associated with hyperoxaluria. Ann. N.Y. Acad. Sci. *104*, 621 (1963)

56. Lund,T., Reske-Nielsen,E.: Nephrolithiasis and nephrocalcinosis with calcium oxalate crystals in the kidneys and other organs. Report on two cases. Acta Pathol. Microbiol. Scand. *38*, 353 (1956)

57. Lyon,E.S., Borden,T.A., Ellis,J.E., Vermeulen,C.W.: Calcium oxalate lithiasis produced by pyridoxine deficiency and inhibition with high magnesium diets. Invest. Urol. *4*, 133 (1966)

58. Marshall,V.F., Horwith,M.: Oxalosis. J. Urol. *82*, 278 (1959)

59. Mazze,R.I. et al.: Methoxyflurane anaesthesia. Arch. Pathol. *92*, 484 (1971)

60. McLaurin,A.W., Beisel,W.R., McCormick, G.J., Scaletter,R., Herman,R.H.: Primary hyperoxaluria. Ann. Int. Med. *55*, 70 (1961)

61. Melon,J.M. et al.: Experimental oxalic lithiasis induced with ethylene glycol in rats. Its value in trial hypoxaluria treatment. Therapie *26*, 991 (1971)

62. Milne,M.D.: Oxalosis in an adult. Br. Med. J. *II*, 637 (1961)

63. Modlin,M.: Hyperoxaluria urinary calculi and ulcerative colitis. Br. Med. J. *III*, 292 (1972)

64. Newnes,G.H., Black,J.A.: Calcium oxalate nephrocalcinosis. Gt. Ormond St. J. *5*, 40 (1953)

65. Nyhan,W.L.: Non-ketoic hyperglycinemia. In: The metabolic basis of inherited disease Stanbury,J.B., Wyngaarden,J.B., Fredrickson,D.G. (eds.). 3rd ed. New York: McGraw-Hill 1972

66. Olgaard,H., Soderkjelm,L.: Familial oxalosis. Acta Soc. Med. Upsal. *62*, 176 (1957)

67. Paddock,R.B., Parker,J.W., Guadagni, N.P.: The effects of methoxyflurane on renal function. Anesthesiology *25*, 707 (1964)

68. Pons,C.A., Custer,R.P.: Acute ethylene glycol poisoning: clinicopathologic report of 18 fatal cases. Am. J. Med. Sci. *211*, 544 (1946)

69. Prien,E.L., Gershoff,S.N.: Newton-Wellesley Med. Bull. *18*, 28 (1966)

70. Pyrah,L.N., Anderson,C.K., Hodgkinson, A., Zarembski,P.M.: A case of oxalate nephrocalcinosis and primary hyperoxaluria. Br. J. Urol. *31*, 235 (1959)

71. Scowen,E.F.,Stansfield,A.G.,Watts,R.W.E.: Oxalosis and primary hyperoxaluria. J. Pathol. Bacteriol. *77*, 195 (1959)

72. Silver,L., Brendler,H.: The use of magnesium oxide in the management of familial hyperoxaluria. J. Urol. *106*, 274 (1971)

73. Smith,L.H.Jr., Williams,H.E.: Treatment of primary hyperoxaluria. Mod. Treat. *4*, 522 (1969)

74. Solomons,C.C., Goodman,S.I., Riley,C.M.: Calcium carbimide in the treatment of primary hyperoxaluria. N. Engl. J Med. *276*, 207 (1964)

75. Swartz,D., Israels,S.: Primary hyperoxaluria. J. Urol. *90*, 94 (1963)

76. Vermeulen,C.W., Grove,W.J., Goetz,R., Raggins,H.D., Carroll,N.O.: Experimental lithiasis. I. Development of calculi upon foreign bodies introduced into the bladders of rats. J. Urol. *64*, 541 (1950)

77. Vermeulen,C.W., Lyon,E.S., Gill,W.B., Chapman,W.H.: Prevention of phosphate stones by phytate, phosphate and hexametaphosphate: experimental urolithiasis. J. Urol. *82*, 249 (1959)

78. Walls,J., Morley,A.R., Kerr,D.N.: Primary hyperoxaluria in adult siblings: with some observations on the role of regular haemodialysis therapy. Br. J. Urol. *41*, 546 (1969)

79. Watts,R.W.E., Crawhall,J.C.: The first glycine metabolic pool in man. Biochem. J. *73*, 277 (1959)

80. Williams,H.E., Smith,L.H.Jr.: Disorders of oxalate metabolism. Am. J. Med. *45*, 713 (1968a)

81. Williams,H.E., Smith,L.H.Jr.: L-glyceric aciduria: a new genetic variant of primary hyperoxaluria. N. Eng. J. Med. *278*, 233 (1968b)

82. Williams,H.E., Smith,L.H.: L-glyceric aciduria. In: Renal Stone Research Symposium. Hodgkinson,A., Nordin,B.E.C. (eds.), p. 309. London: Churchill 1969

83. Wyngaarden,J.B., Elder,T.D.: Primary hyperoxaluria and oxalosis. In: The metabolic basis of inherited disease Stanbury,J.B., Wyngaarden,J., Fredrickson, D.S. (eds.). New York: McGraw-Hill 1966

84. Zarembski,P.M., Hodgkinson,A.: The renal clearance of oxalic acid in normal subjects and in patients with primary hyperoxaluria. Invest. Urol. *1*, 87 (1963)

85. Zarembski,P.M., Hodgkinson,A., Cochran, M.: Treatment of primary hyperoxaluria with calcium carbimide. N. Engl. J. Med. *277*, 1000 (1967)

86. Zarembski,P.M., Hodgkinson,A., Cochran, M.: Urinary excretion of lactic acid and other organic acids in patients with primary hyperoxaluria. In: Renal Stone Research Symposium. Hodgkinson,A., Nordin,B.E.C. (eds.), p. 319. London: Churchill 1969

87. Zollinger,H.U., Rosenmund,H.: Uramie bei androgen bedingter subakuter und chronischen Calciumoxalatniere (calciumoxalatnephritis und calcium oxalatschrumpfniere). Schweiz. Med. Wochnschr. *82*, 1261 (1952)

Chapter 8

Idiopathic Hypercalciuria

Hypercalciuria is found in some subjects in whom there is no clinical evidence of disease. Various terms have been used to try to define etiological variants relating to hypercalciuria. The term 'relative hypercalciuria' was introduced [40] to indicate the variable levels of the urinary calcium following alterations in the concentration of urinary solutes. The terms 'relative' and 'absolute' hypercalciuria have been used [9] to refer to subdivisions of hypercalciuric patients selected by special techniques designed to estimate the urinary calcium level during a 24 h period. Dietary hypercalciuria depends upon a high intake of calcium. Absorptive hypercalciuria depends upon a higher than normal amount of calcium being absorbed from the intestine. Resorptive hypercalciuria refers to the degree of hypercalciuria representing the difference between the net loss of calcium from the bone into the bloodstream and hence into the urine (resulting from certain skeletal diseases), and the rate of bone mineralization.

Hypercalcaemia from any cause may be associated with hypercalciuria as in primary hyperparathyroidism and sarcoidosis; conversely, however, hypercalciuria is not always associated with hypercalcaemia. The various factors which contribute to hypercalciuria do not necessarily move in step one with another. It seems that many stone-formers with hypercalciuria do not in fact ingest large amounts of calcium with the food [61]. While simple hyperexcretion of the principal stone-forming substances (such as cystine), given the appropriate pH in the urine, may be an adequate explanation for the formation of some kinds of stone, it does not fully explain the formation of most calcium oxalate stones (either those composed of calcium oxalate alone or those which have a varying content of apatite). In the search for an explanation of the formation of such stones, more complex physico-chemical principles concerning the condition of saturation of the urine with the stone-forming substances must be involved.

I. Clinical Features and Diagnosis

By a process of exclusion the term idiopathic hypercalciuria is now used to describe a syndrome found in a group of patients with calcium-oxalate-containing renal calculi (sometimes also with an admixture of apatite), in whom the 24-hourly urinary excretion of calcium when the patient is on a normal hospital diet is persistently above normal, the faecal calcium is low, the serum calcium level is normal, the serum phosphate level is frequently low, and from whom all the known causes of hypercalciuria have been excluded.

Since there are as yet no generally accepted morbid anatomical or histological changes in the kidney or elsewhere in the body whereby to identify idiopathic hypercalciuria with the precision associated with most diseases, an explanation (or more than one explanation) has to be sought in terms of altered function rather than of organic change.

The syndrome was characterized as 'idiopathic hypercalciuria' by Albright and his co-workers [2, 28]. In their cases the biochemical findings were so similar to those of patients with primary hyperparathyroidism, and especially in those in whom the serum calcium levels were slightly above normal, that in 11 patients in their series the neck was explored because of doubt concerning the diagnosis, no parathyroid tumours, however, being found. Normal biopsies of all four parathyroid glands were reported in four of these patients. They postulated (from histological evidence from the kidneys) that the primary lesion was probably a pyelonephritis which resulted in damage to the normal tubular resorption of calcium.

The condition is common and occurs mostly but not exclusively in males in the first decades of life, at which age renal calculi tend to form; the term is somewhat imprecise, since the upper normal level of the daily urinary calcium excretion is only as yet approximately agreed, and varies with the calcium content of the diet.

The clinical features of patients with idiopathic hypercalciuria and the radiological appearance of the stones are similar to those of any non-hypercalciuric group of patients with calcium-containing renal stone. There are no radiological changes in the bones indicative of skeletal demineralization, though even a considerable loss of skeletal calcium would not necessarily be reflected in such changes [28, 47]. There is probably therefore no net loss of calcium from the body over long periods of time. Balance studies have shown that the patients are usually in normal calcium balance on a normal diet.

1. Biochemical Findings

The most important finding is the higher than normal level of the urinary calcium, which has been already referred to. In a departmental investigation it was found that in seven patients with idiopathic hypercalciuria the nocturnal level of calcium excretion was higher than that in normal patients. The ingestion of 1 pt milk resulted in a more pronounced quantitative increase in the urinary excretion of calcium (but a

similar percentage increase) in the hypercalciurics than in normal subjects [26].

Edwards and Hodgkinson [17, 18] found that the level of the daily urinary magnesium and that of urinary phosphate in patients with idiopathic hypercalciuria was in the same range as that in normal subjects, and that the serum calcium levels were within the normal range for the laboratory (9.6–10.7 mg/100 ml).

In a proportion of patients with idiopathic hypercalciuria and calculi the serum phosphate level has been found to be low [2, 28], while other observers have found that it is more often normal [24, 34, 48]. It has been suggested that patients could be divided in this respect into two groups, namely those with normophosphataemia and those with hypophosphataemia, the latter type being designated 'hypercalciuria with hypophosphataemia' [43, 53].

Edwards and Hodgkinson [17, 18] in a departmental study showed that hypophosphataemia is also found not uncommonly in patients with renal calculus who have a normal urinary excretion of calcium. They found that the mean value of the serum phosphate in 73 patients with idiopathic hypercalciuria was 3.0 mg/100 ml, which was significantly lower than the normal mean value (3.5 mg/100 ml); 13 patients in this group (18%) had values which were below the normal range. The mean value of the renal clearance of phosphate (Cp) in 23 patients with idiopathic hypercalciuria was found to be 15.2 ml/min, which was also significantly higher than the normal mean. The plasma alkaline phosphatase level was within normal limits.

The administration of ammonium chloride (or an acid-ash diet) to patients with idiopathic hypercalciuria gives rise to an increased urinary excretion of calcium (and of magnesium) and a negative calcium balance [30, 65]; such patients are able to acidify the urine in a normal manner [17, 18, 59]. There is a reduced urinary excretion of citrate. The administration of alkali to patients with idiopathic hyper-calciuria has resulted in a fall in the level of urinary calcium [59, 65] but not in normal subjects [17, 18].

Edwards and Hodgkinson [17] observed that cortisone (100 mg/day) produces a rise in the level of the urinary excretion of calcium in normocalciuric subjects and in patients with idiopathic hypercalciuria. Vitamin D (Calciferol) given in moderate doses to patients with idiopathic hyper-calciuria gives rise to an increase in the urinary excretion of calcium, but not of magnesium or phosphate, but following the administration of cortisone there was no reversal of the hypercalciuric effect. In most patients with idiopathic hypercalciuria, the renal function is normal, as judged by the ordinary tests, though impairment in water concentration by the kidney has been found in some patients, possibly as a result of renal tubular damage [23, 59].

2. Diagnosis

Idiopathic hypercalciuria has to be differen-tiated from other conditions in which hyper-calciuria is usually (or sometimes) present; in most such cases there are easily recogniz-able clinical findings which point to the diagnosis.

Primary hyperparathyroidism is the syn-drome most likely to be confused with idio-pathic hypercalciuria. The biochemical find-ings in the two conditions are in some respects similar: the urinary calcium, which is increased in patients with idiopathic hypercalciuria, is often increased in those with primary hyperparathyroidism. In both conditions the plasma phosphorus level tends to be low, as does the renal tubular reabsorption of phosphate; while the serum calcium level is normal in patients with idio-pathic hypercalciuria, in some it tends to be near the upper limit of normal [68]. The faecal calcium is low and the capacity to absorb calcium from the gut is increased in both idiopathic hypercalciuria and primary hyperparathyroidism.

The difficulty of diagnosis in some cases has been enhanced somewhat by some recent reports which have shown that at least some patients who appear to have had what has been called idiopathic hyper-calciuria have in fact had 'hyperpara-thyroidism' of the type which conforms either to one of the clearly recognized pathological types (adenoma; hyperplasia), or to a type perhaps not yet clearly defined. Conversely, some patients subsequently shown to have proven primary hyperpara-thyroidism of a well-recognized patho-logical type (adenoma or hyperplasia) have had normocalcaemia, and at least some of these will have had hypercalciuria and might well have been diagnosed as having idiopathic hypercalciuria, if the neck had not been explored.

In a group of patients believed to have had idiopathic hypercalciuria, an attempt was made by Adams et al. to promote increased parathyroid activity by demon-strating the presence of hypercalcaemia following some 'challenge' tests [1]. A group of 19 patients (14 male, 5 female) between the ages of 16 and 66 years was investigated. All patients had had at least one renal stone and none showed radio-logical evidence of skeletal primary hyper-parathyroidism nor evidence of renal failure. They were given a low-calcium diet (160 mg calcium, 700 mg phosphorus daily) and, after 5 days, aluminium hydroxide to secure a reduction of urinary phosphate, and (between days nine and twelve) 1 g chlorothiazide twice daily to reduce the level of the urinary calcium without altering its level of intestinal absorption. After the phosphate deprivation 5 patients developed hypercalcaemia (which tended to increase still further following the administration of chlorothiazide, and also to appear in 3 others). Following the chlorothiazide the urinary calcium became normal in all the patients. When the neck was explored for a possible parathyroid adenoma in 6 male patients (5 of whom had developed hypercalcaemia, and 1 of whom had a family history of primary hyperparathyroidism), 3 were found to have chief-cell parathyroid adenomata and the patient without hypercalcaemia was found to have primary chief-cell hyperplasia. Another patient in the group had parathyroid glands of normal size, but a subtotal parathyroidectomy revealed that two of the glands (after microscopy) contained small chief-cell adenomata. All 6 patients postoperatively had a normal urinary calcium (on a normal diet) for more than 1 year and none formed renal calculi. The patients who developed hypercalcaemia following the challenge test, and also the patient with proven hyperparathyroidism (who did not) had on average significantly high normal levels of serum calcium and of urinary calcium and also significantly low serum inorganic phosphate levels.

The difficulty confronting the urologist in the assessment of supposedly high normal serum calcium levels has been referred to (Chap. 4). The findings just quoted suggest the possibility that overactivity of the parathyroids (not always or necessarily resulting from true parathyroid adenomata) may be related to idiopathic hypercalciuria, in some kind of graded series of cases.

II. Pathogenesis

The cause of all cases of idiopathic hypercalciuria is not yet completely agreed, and not all the reported experimental findings appear to lead to the same conclusion; there may be more than one cause. It was earlier thought that the condition was the result of a primary renal tubular defect which interfered with the normal reabsorption of the calcium passed down the renal tubules from the glomerular filtrate, thereby leading to an excess of calcium in the urine. Many observers now consider that an abnormally high level of absorption of dietary calcium is the principal reason for the hypercalciuria. Still more recently a number of reports have appeared to link idiopathic hypercalciuria with overactivity of one or more parathyroid glands (adenoma or hyperplasia), in a manner not easy to explain.

1. Renal Tubular Defect

The hypothesis suggested by Albright and his co-workers [2, 28], that the initiating lesion of idiopathic hypercalciuria is a pyelonephritis of infective origin which led to a renal tubular defect, which in turn interfered with the normal tubular reabsorption of calcium, has already been referred to. In our own numerous patients with idiopathic hypercalciuria we have found no consistent evidence of any such regular urinary infection, though infected urine is found in a few patients with calcium-containing renal calculi; other workers have reported similar experience [24, 46–48].

In spite of the fact that the infective origin is no longer the chief accepted explanation of the cause, the view that a renal tubular defect is the primary cause of the condition has been supported by much evidence. The principal finding has been that the urinary calcium in many patients has remained at a higher than normal level (instead of falling to near normal) when the patient has been given a low-calcium diet.

The observations of Chen and Neuman [10], which suggested the presence of a renal tubular defect, found a marked increase in the urinary calcium excretion following the intravenous injection of certain renal tubular inhibitors (phloridzin, dinitrophenol and para-amino-hippurate/ PAH), the excretion of sodium and potassium being relatively unaffected and it was concluded that these agents inhibited an active transport mechanism for calcium. In the author's department [30] it was shown that when PAH was administered intravenously at tubular maximum ('Tm') levels to subjects with a normal daily urinary excretion of calcium, there was an increase of 2.0–2.5 times in the clearance of ultrafiltrable calcium, a marked increase in the clearance of phosphate and to a lesser extent in that of potassium, but the clearance of inulin and urea was unaffected. In subjects with idiopathic hypercalciuria the administration of PAH had little or no effect on the calcium clearance; it was concluded that the mechanism for the renal tubular transport of calcium is impaired in at least some cases of idiopathic hypercalciuria.

Jackson and Dancaster [41] in balance studies on a patient with bilateral renal calculi and idiopathic hypercalciuria, found that with an intake of 800–1000 mg calcium/day, the patient was in normal calcium balance, and the faecal calcium was low. They suggested that the sequence of events was: (1) decreased renal tubular resorption of calcium, (2) increased urinary calcium, (3) increased intestinal absorption of calcium, (4) reduced faecal calcium. It was thought that the increased absorption of calcium from the gut was in some way compensatory for the loss sustained in consequence of the renal tubular defect.

It is generally assumed that the calcium which is reabsorbed from the urine in the renal tubules is in the ionic form, and that poorly ionized calcium is reabsorbed less readily, a view supported by the finding that the intravenous injection of chelating compounds (such as EDTA) which bind calcium in the plasma, results in a marked increase in urinary calcium in both animals and in man. It has therefore been suggested that at least some cases of idiopathic hypercalciuria are due to the presence of increased amounts of filterable complexed calcium in the blood, of which there is normally 0.5 mg/100 ml, mainly as a calcium citrate complex. Isocitric acid,

which is present in the plasma, may be another possible complexing agent. Following a detailed study described in his papers, Hodgkinson [31, 32] concluded that the increased level of urinary calcium excretion was not the result of an abnormal amount of calcium complexed with citrate.

Investigations designed to establish whether the urinary calcium excretion in normal and in hypercalciuric renal stone-formers was attributable to a decreased renal tubular reabsorption of calcium or only to an increase in filtered load, were carried out by Nordin et al. in normal subjects and in hypercalciuric renal stone patients, using direct measurements of the renal tubular resorption and the urinary calcium excretion. It was concluded that there was no significant difference in the renal tubular absorption of calcium in the normocalciuric or in the hypercalciuric subjects when there was an increase in the filtered load of calcium, which, in fact, determined the presence of hypercalciuria [49, 56].

2. Intestinal Absorption of Dietary Calcium

In normal subjects a reduction in the dietary intake of calcium brings about a reduction to a varying extent in the level of the urinary calcium. If in patients with idiopathic hypercalciuria there is a proportionate increase above the normal level in the absorption of dietary calcium from the gut, the administration of a low-calcium diet would also be expected to be accompanied by a marked fall in the urinary excretion of calcium (since less would then be absorbed from the gut). Such a sequence has been recorded by some observers, though others have found that such a reduction does not occur in all cases [17, 23, 24, 28, 34, 41, 70].

Many observers have noted a reduced faecal excretion of calcium in patients with

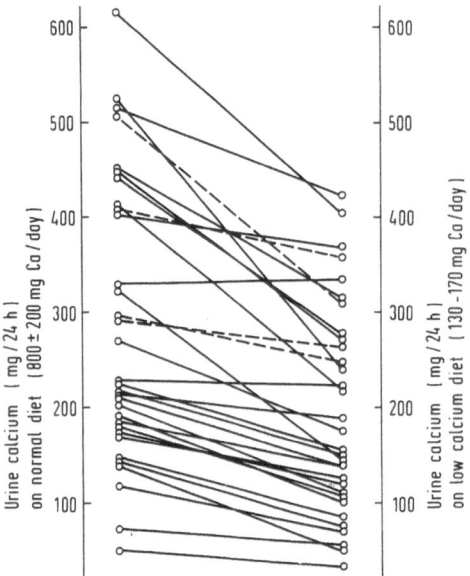

Fig. 8.1. Urinary excretion of calcium for 24 h by 32 patients with renal calculus on normal and on low-calcium diet. (From A. Hodgkinson and L.N. Pyrah, British Journal of Surgery, 1958, *46*, 195; by courtesy of the Editor)

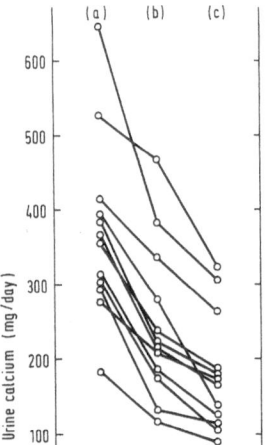

Fig. 8.2. Effect of calcium deprivation on the urinary excretion of calcium in 12 patients with renal calculus. The experimental points indicate the mean daily excretion of calcium during 10 days on (*a*) normal diet, (*b*) low-calcium diet and (*c*) low-calcium diet + 4.5 g EDTA daily. (By courtesy of N.A. Edwards and A. Hodgkinson and the Editor of Clinical Science)

idiopathic hypercalciuria when the patient is given a normal or a high calcium diet [24, 30, 65], a finding which has suggested that the primary phenomenon in the production of the hypercalciuria may be an excessive absorption of calcium from the gut.

In the author's department [34] the urinary excretion of calcium was examined in 32 patients with renal calculi (14 of whom had abnormally high urinary calcium values) having a normal ward diet (800 ± 200 mg calcium/day), and later having a low-calcium diet (130–170 mg calcium/day). The findings showed that in many patients (but not in all) in whom the urinary calcium was high there was a considerable fall in its excretion when the daily amount of calcium in the diet was reduced; in others, the urinary calcium level fell somewhat, but not to normal. In patients in whom the urinary calcium was low, a reduction of the calcium dietary intake resulted in only a small fall in the urinary calcium excretion (Figs. 8.1 and 8.2). The findings were interpreted as suggesting that in more than half the cases in which the urinary calcium did not fall very much if at all, with the low-calcium diet, there was a failure of the normal renal tubular reabsorption of calcium, and as a consequence there was hypercalciuria. In the remainder, in which the urinary calcium fell with the low-calcium diet, it was thought that there may have been an increased intestinal absorption of calcium.

Nordin and his co-workers investigated the relationship between the serum calcium and the urinary calcium levels in normal and in hypercalciuric subjects (with renal calculi) under various conditions of high- and low-calcium diet, and also during loading by the intravenous infusion of calcium. The subjects were given diets with a low calcium intake of 2–5 mg/kg/day and a high intake of 15–20 mg/kg/day, for periods of not less than 5 days, the average calcium excretion of the last 3 days of the particular regimen being used for comparison. In the majority of the male stone-formers given a low-calcium diet, the urinary calcium fell within the normal range. The patients could be classified into three categories: firstly those (who represented the majority) in whom the urinary calcium was high on a high intake of calcium, falling to within the normal range on a low intake. Secondly, there were subjects in whom the urinary calcium was high on a high dietary intake, but remained high when the dietary calcium was low (in the absence of hypercalcaemia this sequence may have probably denoted a reduced renal tubular reabsorption of calcium). Thirdly, there were those patients whose levels of urinary calcium fell within the normal range during high and low calcium intakes and who were entirely normal from this point of view. The close relationship between the levels of dietary and urinary calcium suggested that the hypercalciuria was usually the result of increased absorption of calcium.

The relationship between the amount of calcium ingested in the food, and the levels of the plasma and the urinary calcium was further examined in a group of hyper-calciuric male stone-formers and a group of healthy male non-hypercalciuric subjects [67]. The calcium and the creatinine levels in the blood and in the urine were measured first in the non-fasting state and later after 24 h of fasting. The mean fasting serum calcium level and that of the urinary calcium was found to be significantly higher in the hypercalciuric patients than in the controls; fasting overnight significantly reduced the non-fasting serum calcium and the urinary calcium levels in the stone-formers. Fasting for a further 6–8 h almost invariably reduced the mean serum and urinary calcium values to levels which were not significantly higher than the normal fasting values, the urinary calcium level in fact being brought to within the normal range except in one patient. The results showed that in idiopathic stone-formers with hypercalciuria, the urinary calcium excretion was increased in the non-fasting state, but usually fell to normal after an overnight fast, which in some patients had to be prolonged even for a further period. They believed that the differences in the length of the period of the calcium deprivation in carrying out similar tests, which were used by different workers, may partly have explained the conflicting results obtained by other observers. The results and especially the response to the oral load of calcium, suggested that this form of hyper-calciuria is usually due to hyperabsorption.

Using direct methods of measurement (with calcium radio-kinetic techniques) various observers have shown that the absorption of calcium from the intestine is significantly greater in patients with idiopathic hypercalciuria than that in normal controls [4, 45, 80]. Such patients with idiopathic hypercalciuria are in normal or only in slightly negative calcium balance when on a normal diet. Calcium absorption as measured by radio-isotope techniques was found to be increased in about 50% of male calcium-stone-formers [55]. The cases included all those with absolute hyper-calciuria, and about 40% of cases with a normal urinary calcium excretion on a free diet. In addition to an increased absorption of calcium, they showed that the absorption of phosphate as well as that of calcium may be increased in calculous patients with idiopathic hypercalciuria. There is no evidence of resorptive hypercalciuria in idiopathic stone cases without hypercalciuria [67].

3. Hyperfunction of Parathyroid Glands

Calcitonin, the hormone which is produced in most mammals by certain specialized cells of the thyroid gland, has the effect of depressing a raised serum calcium level [12, 13]. Calcium homeostasis in man appears to be subject to a dual hormonal control, parathormone and calcitonin being continuously secreted at normal concentrations of blood calcium. If the serum calcium level rises, the secretion of parathyroid hormone is decreased, and that of calcitonin is proportionately increased, while the converse happens when the serum calcium level falls [3].

On the basis of an assessment of the known laboratory and radiocalcium kinetic studies in patients with idiopathic hypercalciuria and with primary hyperparathyroidism, Liberman and de Vries [44] have suggested that in some patients with idiopathic hypercalciuria there is a primary hypersecretion of parathormone with a compensatory increase in the secretion of calcitonin. Such a combined action might explain the increased rates of urinary and skeletal calcium turnover (which they found), and the increased intestinal absorption of calcium. This hypothesis could explain the findings in patients thought to have idiopathic hypercalciuria and who also had normocalcaemia, but who were also shown to have hyperparathyroidism; they suggested for these patients the term 'compensated hyperparathyroidism' rather than 'normocalcaemic hyperparathyroidism'. The proof of the hypothesis would require the demonstration of elevated levels of parathormone and of calcitonin at appropriate times in patients with so-called idiopathic hypercalciuria.

Shieber et al. [73] examined 10 hypercalciuric patients with recurrent renal calculi who had persistently normal serum calcium levels and normal or low serum phosphorus levels. Each patient in addition, however, had a reduced tubular reabsorption of phosphorus in the presence of normal renal function, which was consistent with a diagnosis of hyperparathyroidism and the neck was explored. Although four apparently normal parathyroid glands were identified in each patient, three (and sometimes three and a half of the parathyroids) were removed. In 6 patients, examination of the excised tissue by electron-microscopic techniques, using the criteria of

Black [7] showed the presence of hyperfunctioning parathyroid tissue. The changes included a decrease in the number and size of the intracellular deposits of fat, an increase in the interdigitations and complexity of the cytoplasmic membrane, an increase in the size and number of the Golgi apparatus, and conspicuous intracellular organelles with prominent endoplasmic reticulum which had rough surfaces. Subsequent follow-up showed that there had been a prompt and sustained fall in the level of the urinary calcium, and a significant fall in the serum calcium level with a rise in the tubular reabsorption of phosphorus with no evidence of postoperative hypoparathyroidism. These findings together with a dramatic reduction in the frequency of renal stone formation, both soon after the operation and during a follow-up period extending to 3.5 years, led to the conclusion that these patients, who had appeared to have idiopathic hypercalciuria, in reality had hyperfunction of the parathyroid glands.

4. Summary

In summary, it would seem that the causes of idiopathic hypercalciuria are probably multifactorial. An increased absorption of calcium from the gut is probably the immediate explanation for most cases of idiopathic hypercalciuria associated with renal calculous disease. It still remains to be discovered why the intestinal mucosa in some members of the population should absorb larger than normal amounts of calcium. Is it possible that only a variable length of the ileal mucosa in different individuals has the capacity to absorb calcium to such a degree as to account quantitatively for the different amounts absorbed? There could be a variable response to (or a sensitivity to) vitamin D in respect of the absorption of calcium in some people. Alternatively the cause may lie elsewhere in the body as, for example, a hormonal factor which may influence the intestine. There is growing evidence that some patients formerly classified as having idiopathic hyper-calciuria, in fact have primary hyperpara-thyroidism.

There is support for the view that in some patients a renal tubular defect is the cause, the chief evidence for which is the fact that in some patients the change from a high- to a low-calcium diet does not result in the expected fall in the level of the urinary calcium to normal, even when time is allowed for such a fall to take place.

The evidence is suggestive that idio-pathic hypercalciuria in some patients is the result of an over-activity of the para-thyroid glands resulting from either hyper-plasia of the glands or a tumour of one gland, which has escaped detection by the usual tests. It is possible that over-activity of the parathyroid glands is one of the causes of idiopathic hypercalciuria, and is thus an even more important promoting cause of renal stone formation than has hitherto been thought. It is possible that in addition to primary, secondary and ter-tiary hyperparathyroidism, there is a quaternary hyperparathyroidism in which the parathyroids appear to be normal to the naked eye (and perhaps histologically ex-cept under the electron microscope) but are in fact hyperfunctioning to a degree that can cause hypercalciuria, high normal hypercalcaemia and a low faecal calcium.

The investigations into the causes of idio-pathic hypercalciuria carried out in recent years have increased our knowledge of the conditions without finally defining the entire cause.

III. Treatment Measures to Reduce Urinary Calcium

1. Diet

Since a reduction in the urinary calcium (achieved, for example, by dietetic measures) may be accompanied by an increase in the urinary oxalate level, which could render such treatment ineffective for the prevention of further stone formation [60], a low-calcium, low-oxalate diet should help to reduce the levels of the urinary calcium and oxalate [56]. Details of such a diet, which is not always easy for the patient to accept, are given by Hodgkinson [33].

The average amount of calcium taken daily in the food (usually 800 ± 200 mg) should be reduced to a level of 200–300 mg by giving a low-calcium diet, mainly by reducing the intake of milk and milk pro-ducts [22]. Since milk contains phosphate, perhaps a slight disadvantage in such a dietary change is that there will be a decreased intake of orthophosphate, which if present in the diet in adequate amounts, itself assists in the prevention of stone formation when absorbed. The timing of the intake of calcium-containing foods during the day can cause variations in the amount of calcium excreted in the urine; an amount of milk given in six divided feeds produces a greater 24-h urinary excretion of calcium than the same amount of milk given in a single daily feed [69]. Possibly there exists a mechanism for the gastrointestinal ab-sorption of calcium which is more likely to be saturated by a single large feed than by small frequent feeds.

While the carbohydrate and fat in the diet have no effect upon the amount of calcium absorbed, some observers have stated that a high level of protein in the diet (and hence of amino acid in the gut; Chap. 9) renders the calcium more soluble and hence more readily available for absorption. If such be the case more calcium would then be excreted in the urine; a reduction of protein in the food should therefore reduce the amount of urinary calcium [51, 72].

2. Intake of Fluids

A high daily intake of fluid of 2–3 litres, taken evenly throughout the 24 h, should maintain a dilute urine and reduce the tendency for the precipitation of calcium salts. The calcium content of 'hard' water may, however, add considerably to a patient's daily calcium intake.

In a patient with recurrent renal calculi and hypercalciuria in whom it was desired to reduce the urinary calcium level, a low-calcium diet had not produced the desired effect [16]. It was then found that the patient was drinking 4–5 litres of tap-water daily, which was shown to contain 500 mg calcium. The substitution of distilled water for the hard tap water to reduce the calcium intake controlled further stone formation.

In a similar context Thomas [75] observed a paraplegic male patient in whom an indwelling urethral catheter became necessary because of urinary incontinence. Following difficulty with recurrent encrustation and obstruction of the catheter by deposits of calcium phosphate, it was ultimately found that if the patient's daily intake of water was from his own deep well or from the public water supply, the catheter became obstructed every 3 and 5 days respectively; but that if he took distilled water the catheter remained unobstructed. The incidence of renal calculi is said to be low among the inhabitants of some of the islands of the West Indies where distilled sea water (containing therefore no calcium) constitutes the entire supply of drinking water [84].

3. Specific Measures

Alkalis. The administration of alkalis helps to reduce the urinary calcium in patients with idiopathic hypercalciuria [17].

Phosphate. If sodium phosphate is administered by mouth, more phosphate than normal is absorbed, the urinary phosphate level is increased and that of the urinary calcium is reduced [54, 65]. Conversely, the administration of aluminium hydroxide (which forms insoluble aluminium phosphate in the gut) reduces the amount of phosphate absorbed from the gut, which results in a rise in the urinary calcium. This principle has been applied to the treatment of recumbency calculi [14].

Good results with the treatment of repeated stone-formers with neutral sodium phosphate have been reported by Howard and other observers, the formation of further stones in such patients being frequently prevented [5, 36, 39]. In later communications Howard [37, 38] stated that during the past 10 years he had used orthophosphate for the treatment of recurrent calcium-containing calculi in about 50 patients, some of whom had been followed up for as long as 8 years. The amount of orthophosphate needed to arrest stone formation varied from one patient to another, being sometimes as much as 2 g phosphorus daily, though a more usual daily dose was 1.3–1.5 g, the presence of diarrhoea sometimes necessitating a restriction in the daily dosage. When amounts of orthophosphate yielding 1500–2000 mg urinary phosphorus daily were given, it was found that almost all the patients had ceased to form calculi [39, 75]. As a result of treatment there was a twofold increase in the urinary pyrophosphate (Chap. 9) and some reduction of the urinary calcium.

It was found in departmental studies that while the urinary citrates are increased in patients who are given alkaline dibasic phosphate, the administration of acid or neutral orthophosphate does not result in such an increase. No significant changes were observed in the levels of urinary aluminium, silicate or manganese, which may also have been possible factors in inhibiting mineralization; the percentage of ionic calcium in the urine was unchanged by the phosphate therapy. Supplements of oral orthophosphate given to patients with renal calculi for periods ranging up to 2 years were well tolerated except for occasional complaints of indigestion. The urinary calcium remained at a reduced level during the period of treatment, but returned to 'control' level if treatment was suspended. There was no further recurrence of stone nor any increase in the size of existing stones in 18 patients, though in 2, pre-existing stones increased in size [17, 18].

The results warrant further experience with this form of therapy. Calcification in the corticomedullary boundary zone in the kidney of the rat, fed with large doses of orthophosphate, has been shown to occur fairly readily [35]; such a change, if it occurs in the human, shows the need for caution in long-term treatment. Other observers have also summarized the use of phosphate therapy [20, 21, 76].

Phytic Acid and Sodium Phytate. Sodium phytate, a constituent of wheat and oats, and the sodium salt of phytic acid (which is approximately inositol hexaphosphate) have been used to reduce the urinary calcium level in patients with idiopathic hypercalciuria. Between 40% and 90% of the total phosphorus content of cereals is accounted for by phytic acid, which is found in the outer cover of the grain and which is extracted during the preparation of white flour.

Mellanby [57] first demonstrated the anticalcific effect of oatmeal on growing puppies, resulting from its content of phytic acid. During the last war the 'national loaf', which had a high content of phytate (and hence of phosphate), was enriched by the addition of calcium [50]. When given orally, part of the sodium phytate forms insoluble complexes of calcium and magnesium phytate in the intestine, thus reducing the proportion of ingested calcium available for absorption; 30%–40% of it is hydrolyzed in the intestine by the enzyme phytase forming inorganic phosphate and inositol.

Because of its considerable content of phosphate the administration of sodium phytate in appropriate doses is comparable to that of orthophosphate. If ingested by humans, more phosphate is available for absorption from the gut; the urinary phosphate level is therefore increased substantially [65], and the urinary calcium can be reduced [59, 65]. Too large an increase in the urinary phosphate excretion may be detrimental by encouraging the precipitation of calcium phosphate; in cases in which there is a renal tubular defect, the continued use of sodium phytate could theoretically lead to appreciable demineralization of the skeleton. When given orally, the faecal calcium and magnesium levels are increased.

The administration of sodium phytate (with a moderate reduction of dietary calcium) has resulted in a marked reduction of the urinary calcium and magnesium in patients with idiopathic hypercalciuria and renal calculi with no further growth of renal stones in several patients [8, 27, 28]. The results of treatment by sodium phytate could be duplicated by the administration of inorganic phosphate in correspondingly similar quantities.

The Vermeulen technique to produce vesical calculi by implanting pieces of magnesium ribbon into the bladder of rats [77] has been used to compare the effects of sodium phytate and neutral sodium phosphate in respect of their power to bring about either complete dissolution or reduction in size of the stones. Similar favourable results were obtained with both substances [52]. In similar experiments by Vermeulen et al. [78] with doses of sodium phytate equivalent to 7.5% of the food, there was a fall in the urinary calcium and magnesium level to less than 40% of that in the control animals, while the urinary phosphate rose steadily.

Magnesium. In another section (Chap. 9) it has been shown that there is evidence that in the urine of patients with calcium-containing renal stone taken as a whole, there is an increased magnesium-to-calcium ratio compared with that in non-calculous subjects. A magnesium deficiency in the experimental animal may be associated with renal calcification or stone formation. It has therefore been suggested that a high oral intake of magnesium may give favourable results in preventing recurrent stone formation, and some urologists have used it. Promising results from the administration of magnesium salts to stone-forming patients have been achieved by some observers [58] though others report less satisfactory results [8].

Chlorothiazide and Its Derivatives. Hydrochlorothiazide synthesized by Novello and Sprague [62], was first used as an oral diuretic by Beyer [6], who showed that it increases the urinary excretion of water, sodium, chloride and to a lesser extent, potassium and bicarbonate. Its administration also reduces the urinary excretion of calcium in normal subjects and in hypercalciuric patients [42, 47].

In further studies Yendt and co-workers [73, 82–84, 86] reported that thiazides were effective in reducing the urinary calcium excretion and in increasing that of magnesium, therefore giving an increase in the Mg/Ca ratio, which may possibly have partly accounted for the reported good results. The excretion of calcium in the faeces was reduced and the calcium balance became strongly positive in at least 90% of normal subjects, in patients with idiopathic hypercalciuria and in those with primary hyperparathyroidism. In 7 patients with idiopathic hypercalciuria given 50 mg hydrochlorothiazide twice daily, the urinary calcium excretion was reduced maximally from the third day of treatment and was sustained thereafter. Side-effects (important only occasionally) were noted in 25 patients; a feeling of weakness and fatigue was the most common complaint, beginning usually during the first week of treatment and becoming gradually less noticeable. The mean serum potassium level fell during the treatment (average 3.2 mEq/litre).

A series of 67 patients with calcium-containing renal stone were treated with hydrochlorothiazide for long periods of time. Patients in the first group [38], who had no evidence of urinary calculi when treatment was begun, before treatment had had a total of 194 episodes (83 stones voided spontaneously; 30 major operations), but during and after thiazide treatment there were only 2 episodes, in both of which calculi were voided spontaneously. Patients in the second group [39] had calculi when the treatment was begun; in these there was a marked reduction in the number of incidents, and only in four patients was there considered to be evidence of new stone formation or an increase in size of existing stones.

The use of hydrochlorothiazide would appear to be the most valuable remedy so far suggested in the treatment of calculous patients with hypercalciuria. The mode of action of chlorothiazide may be related either to a change in the filtered load of calcium, to changes in its tubular reabsorption or to a combination of both, since the intestinal absorption of calcium remains unchanged [25]. Other observers have summarized their experiences with chlorothiazide [19, 64, 81, 87].

Bendrofluazide, a derivative of chlorothiazide, in doses of 5–7.5 mg daily, has been found to reduce the level of the urinary calcium by between 35% and 50% [29, 59], the maximum fall being delayed for 3 or 4 days; there was a small rise in that of the urinary magnesium. Bendrofluazide has also been found to be effective in reducing a high level of urinary calcium artificially induced by the administration of large doses of vitamin D, by prolonged immobilization, or by an acidosis induced by the administration of mandelamine (3 g/day) or ammonium chloride (5 g/day).

Cellulose Phosphate. Cellulose phosphate has been developed as a laboratory ion exchange substance with a particular affinity for divalent cations. When given orally (in tablet form with water in a dosage of 12–15 g daily with meals) it combines with the calcium in the intestine, resulting in an increased faecal calcium, less calcium being then absorbed. There is a consequent decrease in the urinary calcium, with only a small increase in the urinary phosphate excretion [15, 59, 65]; no side-effects have been observed. Further trials are needed to establish its possible use for the treatment of patients with renal calculi [11, 65, 71, 74, 79].

References

1. Adams,P., Chalmers,T.M., Hill, L.F., Truscott,C.McN.: Idiopathic hypercalciuria and hyperparathyroidism. Br. Med. J. *IV*, 582 (1970)
2. Albright,F., Henneman,P., Benedict,P.H., Forbes,A.P.: Idiopathic hypercalciuria. J. Clin. Endocrinol. *13*, 860 (1953)
3. Arnaud,C.D., Littledike,T., Tsao,H.S.: Calcium homeostasis and the simultaneous measurement of calcitonin and parathyroid hormone in the pig. In: Calcitonin. Proc. Second Int. Symp. London: Heinemann 1970
4. Avioli,L.V., McDonald,J.E., Singer,R.A., Henneman,P.H. A new oral isotope test of calcium absorption. J. Clin. Invest. *44*, 128 (1965)
5. Bernstein,D.S., Newton,R.: The effect of sodium phosphate on the formation of renal calculi and on idiopathic hypercalciuria. Lancet *II*, 1105 (1966)
6. Beyer,K.H.: The mechanism of action of chlorothiazide. Ann. N.Y. Acad. Sci. *71*, 363 (1958)
7. Black,W.C.: III. Correlative light and electron microscopy in primary hyperparathyroidism. Arch. Pathol. *88*, 225 (1969)
8. Boyce,W.H., Garvey,F.K., Govan,C.E.: Abnormalities of calcium metabolism in patients with idiopathic urinary calculi. J. Am. Med. Ass. *166*, 1577 (1958)
9. Chambers,R.M., Dormandy,T.L.: Hypercalciuria, relative and absolute. In: Renal Stone Research Symposium, Hodgkinson, A., Nordin,B.E.C. (eds.), p. 233. London: Churchill 1969
10. Chen,P.S., Neuman,W.F.: Renal excretion

11. Cook,D.A.: Treatment of renal stones: cellulose phosphate or magnesium? N. Eng. J. Med. *291*, 1034 (1974)
12. Copp,D.H., Cameron,E.C., Cheney,B.A., Davidson,A.G.F., Henze,K.G.: Evidence for calcitonin, a new hormone from the parathyroid that lowers blood calcium. Endocrinology *70*, 638 (1962)
13. Copp,D.H., Davidson,A.G.F., Cheney, B.A.: Evidence for a new parathyroid hormone which lowers blood calcium. Proc. Can. Fed. Biol. Soc. *4*, 17 (1961).
14. Cordonnier,J.J., Talbot,B.S.: Effect of ingestion of sodium and phosphate on urinary calcium in recumbency. J. Urol. *60*, 316 (1948)
15. Dent,C.E., Harper,C.M., Parfitt,A.M.: The effect of cellulose phosphate on calcium metabolism in patients with hypercalciuria. Clin. Sci. *27*, 417 (1964)
16. Dent,C.E., Watson,L.: Metabolic studies in a patient with idiopathic hypercalciuria. Br. Med. J. *II*, 449 (1965)
17. Edwards,N., Hodgkinson,A.: Metabolic studies in patients with idiopathic hypercalciuria. Clin. Sci. *29*, 147 (1965a)
18. Edwards,N., Hodgkinson,A.: Studies of renal function in patients with idiopathic hypercalciuria. Clin. Sci. *29*, 327 (1965b)
19. Ehrig,U., Harrison,J.E., Wilson,J.R.: Effect of long-term thiazide therapy on intestinal calcium absorption in patients with recurrent renal calculi. Metabolism *23*, 139 (1974)
20. Ettinger,B.: Recurrent nephrolithiasis: natural history and effect of phosphate therapy. A double-blind controlled study. Am. J. Med. *61*, 200 (1976)
21. Ettinger,B., Kolb,F.O.: Inorganic phosphate treatment of nephrolithiasis. Am. J. Med. *55*, 32 (1973)
22. Gibbon,N.: Calcium-fortified flour and renal stone. Letter. Lancet *II*, 616 (1975)
23. Gill,J.R., Bartter,F.C.: On the impairment of renal concentrating ability in prolonged hypercalcaemia and hypercalciuria in man. J. Clin. Invest. *40*, 716 (1961)
24. Harrison,A.R.: Some results of metabolic investigations in cases of renal stone. Br. J. Urol. *31*, 398 (1959)
25. Harrison,A.R., Rose,G.A.: The effect of bendrofluazide on urinary and faecal calcium and phosphate. Clin. Sci. *34*, 343 (1968)
26. Heaton,F.W., Hodgkinson,A.: External

of calcium by the dog. Am. J. Physiol. *180*, 623 (1955)

factors affecting diurnal variation in electrolyte excretion with particular reference to calcium and magnesium. Clin. Chim. Acta 8, 246 (1963)

27. Henneman,P.H., Dempsey,E.F., Carroll, E.W., Albright,F.: The cause of hypercalciuria in sarcoid and its treatment with cortisone and sodium phytate. J. Clin. Invest. 35, 1229 (1956)

28. Henneman,P.H., Benedict,P.H., Forbes, A.P., Dudley,H.R.: Idiopathic hypercalciuria. N. Engl. J. Med. 259, 802 (1958)

29. Higgins,B.A., Nassim,J.R. Collins,J., Hilt, A.: The effect of bendrofluazide on urine calcium. Clin. Sci. 27, 457 (1964)

30. Hodgkinson,A.: Idiopathic hypercalciuria. Proc. Assoc. Clin. Biochem. 1, 52 (1961)

31. Hodgkinson,A.: Citric acid excretion in normal adults and in patients with renal calculus. Clin. Sci. 23, 203 (1963a)

32. Hodgkinson,A.: The relation between citric acid and calcium metabolism with particular reference to primary hyperparathyroidism and idiopathic hypercalciuria. Clin. Sci. 24, 167 (1963b)

33. Hodgkinson,A.: Oxalate metabolism and hyperoxaluria. In: Scientific foundations of urology. Williams,D.I., Chisholm,G.D. (eds.). Vol. 1, p. 289. London: Heinemann (1976)

34. Hodgkinson,A., Pyrah,L.N.: The urinary excretion of calcium and inorganic phosphate in 344 patients with calcium stone of renal origin. Br. J. Surg. 46, 10 (1958)

35. Holdsworth,M.J., Hodgkinson,A.: The hexosamine content of the kidney in experimental renal calcification. Br. J. Exp. Pathol. 42, 331 (1961)

36. Howard,J.E.: Urinary stone. Can. Med. Assoc. J. 86, 22 (1962)

37. Howard,J.E.: Reflections on calcium habits. Can. Med. Assoc. J. 99, 41 (1968)

38. Howard,J.E.: Serendipity in clinical investigation. J. Am. Med. Assoc. 207, 736 (1969)

39. Howard,J.E., Thomas,W.C.: Control of crystallization in urine. Am. J. Med. 45, 693 (1968)

40. Isaacson,L.C.: Relative hypercalciuria in nephrolithiasis. Br. Med. J. II, 558 (1966)

41. Jackson,W.P.U., Dancaster,C.: A consideration of the hypercalciuria in sarcoidosis, idiopathic hypercalciuria and that produced by vitamin D. A new suggestion. J. Clin. Endocrinol. 19, 658 (1959)

42. Lamberg,B.A., Kuhlback,B.: Effect of chlorothiazide and hydrochlorothiazide on the excretion of calcium in urine. Scand. J. Clin. Lab. Invest. 11, 357 (1959)

43. Leading article: Calcium requirements. Br. Med. J. 1, 671 (1963)

44. Liberman,U.A., De Vries,A.: Idiopathic hypercalciuria. A state of compensated hyperparathyroidism? Rev. Fr. Clin. Biol. 16, 860 (1971)

45. Liberman,U.A., Sperling,O., Atsmon,A., Frank,M., Modan,M., DeVries,A.: Metabolic and calcium kinetic studies in idiopathic hypercalciuria. J. Clin. Invest. 47, 2580 (1968)

46. Lichtwitz,A., Seze,S.de, Hioco,D., Parlier,R., Lanham,C., Miramet,L.: Physiopathologie et traitement des formes rénales et entero-rénales du diabète calcique. Sem. Hôp. Paris 37, 674 (1961)

47. Lichtwitz,A., Seze,S.de, Hioco,D., Miramet,L., Lanham,C., Parlier,R.: I. Double syndrome d'hyperabsorption intestinale du ca et d'insuffisance de la réabsorption tubulaire. II. Physiopathologie et traitment. Présse Med. 71, 107 and 165 (1963)

48. Litin,R.B., Diessner,G.R., Keating,F.R.: Urinary excretion of calcium in patients with renal lithiasis. J. Urol. 68, 17 (1961)

49. MacFadyen,I.J., Nordin,B.E.C., Smith, D.A., Wayne,D.J., Rae,S.L.: Effect of variations in dietary calcium on plasma concentration and urinary excretion of calcium. Br. Med. J. 1, 161 (1963)

50. McCance,R.A.: Bread (Finlayson Memorial Lecture). Lancet 1, 77 (1946)

51. McCance,R.A., Widdowson,E.M., Lehman,H.: The effect of protein intake on the absorption of calcium and magnesium. Biochem. J. 36, 686 (1942)

52. McDonald,D.F., Orallo,M.D.: Dissolution of experimentally induced vesical calculi in rats by sodium phytate and sodium neutral phosphate treatment. J. Urol. 81, 534 (1959)

53. McGeown,M.G.: The causes of kidney stones. Ir. J. Med. Sci. 451, 301 (1963)

54. Malm,O.J.: Calcium requirements and adaptation in adult men. Scand. J. Clin. Lab. Invest. (Suppl. 36) 10, (1958)

55. Marshall,D.H., Nordin,B.E.C.: Kinetic analysis of plasma radioactivity after oral ingestion of radiocalcium. Nature (London) 222, 797 (1969)

56. Marshall,R.W., Cochran,M., Robertson, W.G., Hodgkinson,A., Nordin,B.E.C.: The relation between the concentration of calcium salts in the urine and renal stone composition in patients with calcium-containing renal stones. Clin. Sci. 43, 433 (1972)

57. Mellanby,E.: Special Report Series. Med. Res. Council, London. No. 93 (1925)

58. Moore,C.A., Bunce,G.E.: Reduction in frequency of renal calculus formation by oral magnesium administration. A preliminary report. Invest. Urol. *2*, 7 (1964)

59. Nassim,J.R., Higgins,B.A.: Control of idiopathic hypercalciuria. Br. Med. J. *I*, 675 (1965)

60. Nordin,B.E.C., Hodgkinson,A., Peacock, M., Robertson,W.G.: The medical treatment of renal stone disease. In: Xth Congres International de Therapeutique, p. 191 Paris: Doin 1971

61. Nordin,B.E.C., Peacock,M., Wilkinson,R.: Hypercalciuria and calcium stone disease. Clin. Endocrinol. Metab. *1*, 169 (1972)

62. Novello,F.C., Sprague,J.M.: Benzothiadiazine dioxides as novel diuretics. J. Am. Chem. Soc. *79*, 2028 (1957)

63. Oliver,I., Weinberger,A., Bar-Meir,S.: Orthophosphate treatment of calcium lithiasis associated with idiopathic hypercalciuria. Urol. Int. *29*, 414 (1974)

64. Pak,Y.C., Delea,C.S., Bartter,F.O.: Successful treatment of recurrent nephrolithiasis (calcium stone) with cellulose phosphate. N.Engl. J. Med. *290*, 175 (1974)

65. Parfitt,A.M., Higgins,B.A., Nassim,J.R., Collins,J.A., Hilb, A.: Metabolic studies in patients with hypercalciuria. Clin. Sci. *27*, 463 (1964)

66. Peacock,M., Nordin,B.E.C.: Tubular reabsorption of calcium in normal and hypercalciuric subjects. J. Clin. Pathol. *21*, 353 (1968)

67. Peacock,M., Hodgkinson,A., Nordin, B.E.C.: Importance of dietary calcium in the definition of idiopathic hypercalciuria. Br. Med. J. *II*, 469 (1967)

68. Peacock,M., Knowles,F., Nordin,B.E.C.: Effect of calcium administration and deprivation on serum and urine calcium in stone-forming and control subjects. Br. Med. J. *II*, 729 (1968)

69. Phang,J.M., Kales,A.N., Harn,T.J.: Effect of divided calcium intake on urinary calcium excretion. Lancet *II*, 84 (1968)

70. Phillips,M.J., Cooke,M.J.C.: Relation between urinary calcium and sodium in patients with idiopathic hypercalciuria. Lancet *I*, 1354 (1967)

71. Pietrek,J., Kokof,F.: Treatment of patients with calcium containing renal stones with cellulose phosphate. Br. J. Urol. *45*, 136 (1973)

72. Pittman,M.S., Kunerth,B.L.: Long-term study of nitrogen, calcium and phosphorus metabolism on medium-protein diet. J. Nutr. *17*, 175 (1939)

73. Shieber,W., Birge,S.J., Avioli,L., Teitelbaum,S.L.: Normocalcemic hyperparathyroidism with 'normal' parathyroid glands. Arch. Surg. *103*, 259 (1971)

74. Teotia,M., Singh,R.K.: Treatment of idiopathic hypercalciuria and nephrolithiasis with sodium cellulose phosphates. J. Assoc. Phys. India. *22*, 709 (1974)

75. Thomas,W.C.: Quoted by Howard,J.E.: Urinary stone. Can. Med. Ass. J. *86*, 22 (1968)

76. Thomas,W.C.jr.: Effectiveness and mode of action of orthophosphates in patients with calcareous renal calculi. Trans. Am. Clin. Assoc. *83*, 113 (1972)

77. Vermeulen,C.W., Grove,W.J., Goetz,R., Raggins,H.D., Carroll,N.O.: Experimental lithiasis I. Development of calculi upon foreign bodies introduced into bladders of rats. J. Urol. *64*, 541 (1950)

78. Vermeulen,C.W., Lyon,E.S., Gill,W.B., Chapman,W.H.: Prevention of phosphate stone by phytate, phosphate and hexametaphosphate: experimental urolithiasis XV. J. Urol. *82*, 249 (1959)

79. Williams,H.E.: Editorial. Calcium nephrolithiasis and cellulose phosphate. N. Engl. J. Med. *290*, 224 (1974)

80. Wills,M.R., Zisman,E., Wortsman,J., Evens,R.G., Pak,C.Y.C., Bartter,F.C.: The measurement of intestinal calcium absorption by external radio-isotopic counting: application to the study of nephrolithiasis. Clin. Sci. *39*, 95 (1970)

81. Wilson,D.R., Siddiqui,A.A., Eheig,U.: The effect of thiazide diuretics on carbohydrate-induced calciuria in patients with recurrent renal calculi. J. Lab. Clin. Med. *86*, 118 (1975)

82. Yendt,E.R.: Drugs used in the management of renal calculi. Can. Med. Ass. J. *93*, 315 (1965a)

83. Yendt,E.R.: The effect of thiazides in idiopathic hypercalciuria. Trans. Am. Clin. Climatol. Assoc. *77*, 96 (1965b)

84. Yendt,E.R.: Renal calculi. Can. Med. Assoc. J. *102*, 479 (1970)

85. Yendt,E.R., Gagne,R.J.A., Cohanim,M.: The effects of thiazides in idiopathic hypercalciuria. Am. J. Med. Sci. *251*, 449 (1966)

86. Yendt,E.R., Guay,G.R., Garcia,D.A.: The use of thiazides in the prevention of renal calculi. Can. Med. Assoc. J. *102*, 614 (1970)

87. Yendt,E.R. et al.: Ten-year experience with the use of thiazides in the prevention of kidney stones. Trans. Am. Clin. Climatol. Assoc. *85*, 65 (1973)

Chapter 9

Chemical Substances in Urine Promoting or Preventing Renal Stone

In some patients with renal stone there are easily recognizable predisposing factors, some of which have already been referred to (primary hyperparathyroidism, hydronephrosis, a 'communicating' cyst of the kidney). Not all patients in whom such predisposing causes are present do, in fact, develop renal calculi; and conversely many patients without such an obvious predisposing factor do develop calcium-containing calculi.

Many workers have sought to define the physicochemical environment in the urine in terms of the behaviour of crystalloid substances in such a complex solution, under which urinary stone formation can be initiated. Other observers have sought to identify chemical substances in the urine, the absence of which in a certain concentration may allow crystallization to begin and stone formation to follow, and the presence of which may prevent such crystallization and stone formation. Urinary magnesium, citrates and sodium have been thought to be concerned with the prevention or promotion of urinary stone formation. Substances which have been suggested as being possible inhibitors of urinary stone formation include: amino acids, pyrophosphate, certain metallic ions and certain peptides.

I. Some Chemical Substances and Their Relation to Renal Stone Formation

1. Citric Acid and Citrates

It has long been believed that the citric acid in urine plays some part in the prevention of renal stone, a view based upon the fact that citrate is able to bind calcium ions, forming a soluble and only slightly ionizable complex, which could only with difficulty be precipitated. Opinion has moved in recent years, however, from an emphasis upon a positive role which it was thought to play, to the feeling that its function in respect of the prevention of human stone formation is slight. If a poorly soluble calcium salt is placed in water, some calcium ions are freed; any added citrate would combine with them to form a soluble and only slightly ionized complex, when still more calcium ions would be freed [85]. The application of this principle enabled Albright et al. [1] to cause a vesical calculus to go into solution by instilling citrate solution into the bladder.

The serum citric acid in 29 healthy subjects in the author's department (15 male, 14 female) has ranged from 1.7 to 3.1 mg/100 ml (mean value 2.6 mg) with no significant differences between the sexes; the level rose by 0.4–0.9 mg/100 ml after a meal. Variations in the level of serum citric acid appear to depend upon the level of the serum calcium rather than on the type of disease; hypocalcaemia and hypercalcaemia are associated respectively with hypocitricaemia and hypercitricaemia [31, 32].

Citrate is excreted in the urine by the mechanism of glomerular filtration and tubular reabsorption, without active tubular secretion. The normal daily level of citrate in the urine in subjects on a normal diet has been reported in different series as being between 140 and 1500 mg. The urinary citrate excretion is increased after each meal and by the administration of vitamin D; it is decreased during the acidotic phase of uraemia in chronic nephritis, in diabetic coma (presumably because of impaired renal function), when the urine is acid, during the administration of acetazolamide in humans and in rats and after parathyroid adenomectomy. In those patients with radiologically demonstrable nephrocalcinosis who have impairment of renal function or infection the urinary citric acid level is reduced [31, 32]. There is a relationship between the urinary excretion of citric acid and that of calcium in normal subjects taken as a group.

Kissin and Locke [41] found that in 15 of 16 patients with urolithiasis, the concentration of citric acid in the urine was below 20 mg/100 ml (average 13 mg) compared with 61 mg in their control group. It has been suggested that the low levels of urinary citrate found in some patients with renal calculus appeared to be the result of a postrenal destruction of citric acid by organisms infecting the urinary tract, and not to a deficiency of the renal excretion of citric acid [10]. Some organisms such as *B. proteus* and *B. lactis aerogenes* are, in fact, able to reduce the concentration of citric acid in a substrate when the conditions would possibly be more favourable for the formation of renal stones quite irrespective of the urinary concentration of citrate.

Hodgkinson [31] in the author's department found that the average daily urinary excretion of citric acid in male patients with renal calculi and sterile urine and with good renal function, and also in those with infected urine, was significantly lower than the average daily excretion in normal subjects. A fall in the level of the urinary citrate excretion was found in 32 patients with renal calculi when there was evidence of impairment of renal function, suggesting that impairment of renal function was an important cause of decreased urinary citrate excretion (Fig. 9.1). Hypocitricuria did

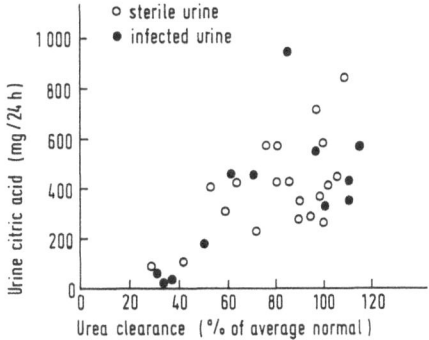

Fig. 9.1. The relationship between the urinary citric acid and the urea clearance in 32 patients with calcium-containing renal stones. (By courtesy of A. Hodgkinson, 1962, and the Editors of Clinical Science)

not appear to be as frequent or as marked as was found by other observers. It was tentatively defined as an average daily excretion of citric acid of less than 200 mg in males and 400 mg in females, on a normal balanced diet. In eight of nine patients with hypocitricuria there was appreciable evidence of impaired renal function and hypocitricaemia was found in the other patient, who had primary hyperoxaluria, also probably as a consequence of impaired renal function, the urea clearance being only 37% of average normal [68] (Table 9.1, see p. 168).

The evidence as a whole suggests that urinary citrate plays little part in maintaining calcium phosphate in solution [19, 97] though it may play a minor part in maintaining calcium oxalate in solution. Efforts to increase the level of the urinary citrate by medicinal measures are therefore unlikely to be of significant value in the prevention of calcium-containing renal calculi.

2. Urinary Magnesium

Magnesium is a major component of struvite calculi, found in infected urine, and a minor component of many stones com-

Table 9.1. Urinary excretion of citric acid on a normal diet in normal adults and in patients with calculi

Author	Normal adults (mg/24 h)			Patients with renal calculi (mg/24 h)		
	No.	Range	Mean	No.	Range	Mean
Ostberg, 1931	300	140–1340	540			
Sherman et al., 1936a,b	7	356–1180				
Kissin and Locke, 1941	16	180–1260	627	16	30–342	165
Scott et al., 1943	8	30–120 (mg%)	Average 72.2	8	31–130 (mg%)	Average 47
Shorr, 1945		400–1500				
Conway et al., 1949	14	310–742	496			
1. Sterile urine				17	204–670	416
2. Infected urine				17	42–289	144
Hodgkinson, 1962, 1963	29	242–1315	636			
1. Sterile urine				33	90–842	437
2. Infected urine				15	27–949	348

posed chiefly of calcium oxalate. Quite apart from its participation in the composition of calculi, the quantitative amount of urinary magnesium relative to that of calcium has a bearing upon renal stone formation and prevention; thus a relatively higher level of urinary magnesium discourages or sometimes prevents renal stone formation, whereas a deficiency of magnesium in the body generally (in animals and in man), or a low level of urinary magnesium encourages renal stone formation or nephrocalcinosis.

The histological changes in the kidneys of the experimental animal (usually the rat) in states of dietary magnesium deficiency have been reported by several observers including Heaton and Anderson [30] in the author's department. There were degenerative lesions in the glomeruli; the cells of the proximal convoluted tubules in the outer part of the renal cortex were swollen, vacuolated and desquamated, and there was focal necrosis. In the thin portion of Henle's loop at the cortico-medullary junction some cells had undergone necrosis and there was intracellular precipitation of calcium salts. Calcific granules were occasionally observed in the cells and the basement membranes of the distal convoluted tubules and the collecting tubules, and calcium casts were observed within the tubular lamina.

Urinary Calcium/Magnesium Ratio. As long ago as 1902 Klemperer and Tritschler [42] showed that with a calcium oxalate/magnesium oxalate ratio of 120:80 the calcium oxalate in the urine remained in solution. More recent findings have also suggested that the ratio of calcium to magnesium in the urine of many stone-formers is higher than that in normal subjects. Even allowing for such a situation in the hypercalciuric stone-formers the urinary magnesium level may still be within the normal range; but in the normocalciuric stone-formers the urinary magnesium level may be lower than the normal range.

Desgrez et al. [15, 16] found an average urinary calcium/magnesium ratio of 215:116 (range 1.83 ± 0.7) in a group of normal subjects compared with a ratio of 317:122 in a group of patients with calcium oxalate lithiasis. In 54 male patients with calcium-containing calculi, of whom 37 had hypercalciuria, and 83 control subjects, the mean daily urinary magnesium excretion of the 'normocalciuric' renal stone-formers was significantly lower than that of the normocalciuric controls, 4 of whom had very low 24-h urinary magnesium outputs. The results supported the view that a low urinary magnesium excretion may be a factor in the formation of renal calculi in some patients. King et al. [40] reported similar findings.

Oreopoulos et al. [62–64] found that the urinary magnesium/calcium ratio in 54 stone-formers had a mean value of 44.8%, and in 20 normal subjects, 89.3%, the difference being highly significant ($p < 0.001$). They also found that the magnesium/calcium ratios (calculated from the magnesium and calcium concentrations) of the 'evil' urines reported by Mukai and Howard]58] which calcified the cartilage of the rachitic rat, and of the 'good' urines which did not, showed a similar distribution with approximately the same mean levels. Sutton and Watson [87] considered that a relatively low urinary magnesium may be a contributory factor to the formation of urinary calculi in some patients with hyperparathyroidism.

Magnesium Intake. In experimental animals, calculi resulting from the ingestion of acetazolamide [93] or ethylene glycol [24, 25], or from pyridoxine deficiency [26] can be inhibited by the addition of magnesium to the diet. However, if a foreign body is present in the bladder as a local stimulus to stone formation, a high intake of magnesium has resulted in stones composed of newberyite ($MgHPO_4 \cdot 3H_2O$), while a low intake of magnesium has resulted in stones composed of brushite ($CaHPO_4 \cdot 2H_2O$), magnesium then being absent from the stones.

In illustrating the diverse factors which can influence the composition of renal stone formation in the experimental animal, Vermeulen et al. [96, 97], using their previously described technique [95] to induce vesical calculi in rats, found that the genetic strain

and the sex of the animals influenced the composition of the experimental stone. Thus in Harlan male rats (with a sterile urine of pH 6.7) magnesium-containing stones were formed, which could be prevented or even caused to go into solution by a planned reduction in the urinary excretion of magnesium. In Hotzman female rats given the same dietary and other conditions, calcium-containing stones were formed. After infection of the urine with urea-splitting organisms, both strains formed magnesium-containing stones. The fact that the magnesium intake and its urinary excretion in the rat was proportionately considerably higher than that in man, may have been partially responsible for the findings.

3. Urinary Sodium and Total Solutes

It has been suggested that there is a relationship between the urinary sodium (and/or total solutes) and renal stone formation and prevention; possibly, however, the total urinary solutes (of which sodium is one) are of greater importance.

Neuman and Neuman [61] have shown that sodium can increase the apparent solubility of hydroxyapatite by a process of the substitition of sodium for calcium ions in the crystal lattice of the hydroxyapatite by competitive binding [45, 55–57]. Infusion experiments in the dog have shown that a correlation exists between the reabsorption of calcium and of sodium ions by the renal tubules. Udall et al. [94] reported that a high intake of sodium chloride inhibited the formation of stones in lambs on a calculogenic diet. When salt had been added to the diet of 48 lambs before slaughter, it was found at autopsy that none had detectable stones, but that 20 lambs which were not given additional salt had formed stones. Bailey [3] demonstrated that the addition of a 4% sodium chloride to the

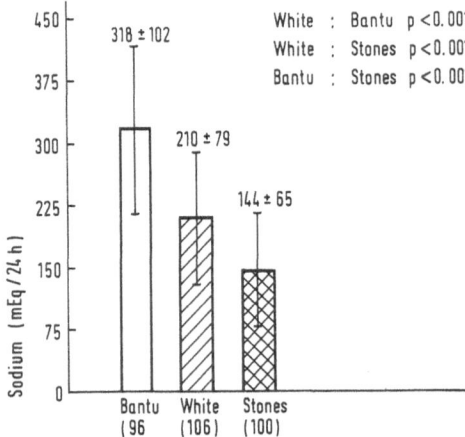

White : Bantu p < 0.001
White : Stones p < 0.001
Bantu : Stones p < 0.001

Fig. 9.2. Urinary sodium and renal stone: 24-h urinary sodium in normal white and Bantu subjects and patients with renal stone; mean values (the number of subjects in each group is shown in parentheses). (By courtesy of M. Modlin and the Editors of Renal Stone Research Symposium, published by Churchill, London, 1969)

ration prevented the formation of siliceous calculi in calves.

Modlin [55–57] studied the relative 24-h urinary concentrations of sodium and calcium in normal white subjects, in white stone-formers and in normal Bantu subjects in South Africa (who rarely form stones). He found that the daily urinary sodium/calcium ratio differed in each group, the highest values in the white patients with stone just reaching the lowest values in the Bantu, with very little overlap. The ratio was significantly higher in the normal white subjects than in the white stone-formers; there was therefore an inverse relationship between the daily urinary sodium/calcium ratio and the liability to renal stone formation. He suggested that renal stone formation is influenced by the amount of sodium in relation to that of calcium in the urine (Fig. 9.2). Modlin assembled evidence to support his contention concerning the influence of sodium from enquiries concerning the urinary content of sodium in patients suffering from various diseases who were known to have developed renal

calculi. In stone-formers in certain hot countries the excessive loss of fluid from the skin (the sweat contains sodium) may be responsible for the reduced urinary sodium level. The salt content of certain foods (soya sauce, miso and pickles) consumed by the inhabitants of the Hokkaido region in the north of Japan averaged 18.3 g daily (the average daily intake of salt in western countries being approximately 10 g), the incidence of renal stone patients (calculated as a percentage of all urological patients in the hospitals) being 1.8%. The daily dietary salt intake in the Chugoko region in the south averaged 14.5 g [78], the incidence of renal stone patients being 8%. The incidence of renal calculus in Kuwait is high, and the urinary excretion level of sodium (but not of calcium) was found to be lower in patients with renal stones than that in normal subjects [77].

The Eskimos have a low incidence of renal stone and a low average daily intake of salt; the average 24-h urinary sodium/calcium ratio in 75 adult Eskimos was found to be approximately equal to that in the Bantu (in whom renal stone formation is equally rare [11]). Patients with Cushing's disease and those under treatment with glucocorticoids (in whom there is a reduced excretion of sodium) not uncommonly have renal calculi [39]. In some patients with Cushing's disease there is hypercalciuria, which could lead to a lowering of the urinary sodium/calcium. When acetazolamide (Diamox) was given to normal adults (some of whom had developed renal stone) the mean urinary calcium rose significantly in every instance whereas the mean urinary sodium either rose or fell slightly, though not significantly.

Robertson et al. [69] in an assessment of Modlin's data considered that the differences in the sodium/calcium ratio to which he drew attention could be attributed more logically to differences in the urinary calcium levels in his groups of subjects than to differences in the urinary sodium levels.

They deduced from his data that the urines of the Bantu subjects investigated (non-calculous subjects) were very much more undersaturated relative to calcium phosphate than are the urines of white people, circumstances which would probably themselves much reduce the tendency to stone formation in the Bantu. They considered that a possible beneficial effect of the high urinary level of the sodium would be offset by the calciuric effect of the increased sodium intake. They pointed out that the stone-free Eskimo subjects referred to by Modlin excreted not only less urinary sodium but also much less calcium than the stone-formers, which would militate against stone formation. In 60 male idiopathic stone-formers and 60 age-matched control subjects they had found no difference in the concentration of the urinary sodium in the two groups, though there was a somewhat greater mean urine volume and greater total daily output of sodium in the stone-formers so that in those groups a reduced excretion of sodium in stone-formers could not be a contributory factor to their disease.

In an investigation of the relationship between sodium and calcium excretion in 14 patients with renal stone and idiopathic hypercalciuria, and 10 healthy control subjects, Phillips and Cooke [66] found a highly significant relationship which held good throughout alterations of the dietary intake of calcium and sodium, high levels of urinary calcium excretion being found in association with high levels of sodium excretion. They considered the possibility that idiopathic hypercalciuria was the result of a high-sodium diet; they found, however, that the urinary calcium excretion in patients with idiopathic hypercalciuria was always higher than that found in controls throughout all the variations in diet studied.

Isaacson and his co-workers [36, 37] carried out studies to determine which is the primary feature in the stone-forming patients: hypercalciuria relative to all the urinary solutes (of which sodium chloride is one), or hypercalciuria relative essentially to the sodium alone. When the urines of a group of non-calculous patients suffering from a variety of diseases were compared with those of patients with calcium-containing renal stones, they found that hypercalciuria relative to the total solutes, rather than to sodium alone, was the primary feature which characterized the urine of their patients with nephrolithiasis.

4. Urinary Amino Acids

It has been suggested following studies in vitro that the urinary amino acids may act as chelating agents to increase the solubility of calcium salts [52, 53]. The evidence as a whole suggests that urinary amino acids may help to inhibit crystallization in urine and that their quantitative reduction there may be a factor in promoting stone formation.

The total concentration of the 20 or so amino acids in the plasma is 3–6 mg/100 ml, whence they pass through the glomerular filtrate, and are almost completely reabsorbed by the renal tubules. Studies in vitro have shown that hydroxyapatite is more soluble in solutions of glycine and alanine than in water. It was shown by Lehmann and Pollak [47] and confirmed by McGeown [53] in in vitro experiments, that the presence of some amino acids in solution increases the solubility of calcium and magnesium phosphate, the most active in this respect being cysteine, glycine, glutamic acid, arginine, citrulline, alanine, ornithine, lysine, leucine and thiolactic acid. They suggested, however, that cystine might form an insoluble complex with calcium. On the other hand Elliot and Eusebio [18] showed that at average concentrations, the urinary amino acids (including glycine) had no effect upon calcium oxalate solubility.

The possible effect of amino acids present in the gut upon the absorption of calcium has relevance to the question of stone formation. It was reported many years ago by Mellanby [54] that casein had an antirachitic effect in excess of that due to its calcium content. It was also recorded that very little calcium is absorbed from the intestine if the diet contains no meat [27, 51]. It was suggested that meat in the diet, because of its content of protein (and hence a source of amino acids), though itself relatively poor in calcium, may promote the absorption of the available calcium [51] and even be the equivalent of a food rich in calcium [54]; in other words the presence of amino acids in the gut is desirable for the adequate absorption of calcium.

Dent [13], however, using balance experiments, was unable to confirm that the presence of protein in the diet led to an increased absorption of calcium. Pathological deposits of calcium in the excretory channels are most commonly found in the liver and the kidney, organs which are particularly rich in amino acid oxidases [44, 46].

In the experimental field McGeown [52] feeding rats with a vitamin-A-free diet, induced calculus formation which was prevented by the administration of glutamic acid but not by the administration of glycine together with sodium benzoate. Glutamic acid also significantly reduced the incidence of calculi in mice given a vitamin-A-free diet together with acetazolamide (Diamox), which had been shown by Harrison and Harrison [28] to induce calculus formation and renal calcification. No difference was found in the pH of the urine of the animals given glutamic acid and that from the controls; it was suggested that glutamic acid may form a soluble compound with calcium, thereby helping to prevent precipitation of calcium salts.

At the clinical level, it is known that in Fanconi's syndrome, in which there is an excess of urinary calcium and amino acids,

urinary calculi are not found [14], a fact which might possibly suggest that the presence of amino acids has some influence on the prevention of stone.

McGeown [53] found that the mean daily urinary amino acid nitrogen in 29 healthy control subjects was 322.9 mg, while in 100 patients with calcium-containing renal stones, the mean daily level was 235.0 mg, a figure which did not appear to be related to impairment of renal function. Of the patients with renal stone, 31% had an unexplained higher urinary excretion of cystine than had the controls, a circumstance which may have been the result of renal tubular damage (though many had no evidence of this) or to a specific renal tubular defect in the handling of that amino acid [44]. Possibly patients with an abnormally high urinary calcium excretion (which many stone patients have) and a normal urinary excretion of amino acids may be more likely to form calculi, because the balance between the urinary calcium and the amino acids had been upset, thereby creating a relative deficiency of chelating substance in the urine.

During the course of an investigation of over 100 patients with bilateral and recurrent urinary calculi Murphy [59, 60] found two patients (both aged 20) with bilateral renal calculi who were found on routine chromatography to have an abnormally high urinary excretion of many amino acids, together with a history of long-continued ingestion of excessive amounts of Worcestershire sauce; no other factor which may have helped to promote the recurrent renal stones was observed. There was no further increase in the size of the calculi following the withdrawal from the diet of the Worcestershire sauce, which, it was suggested, had been the source of a nephrotoxic agent which had encouraged the formation of renal stones, possibly by a mechanism similar to that postulated for the stones found in association with the habitual excessive use of certain analgesics.

The local Worcestershire sauce (the patients lived in Australia) contained a high concentration of acetic acid which can cause renal damage [49] as well as garlic and spices which contain volatile oils and are potential nephrotoxins.

5. Urinary Pyrophosphates and Orthophosphates

The possibility that pyrophosphate in urine may be a crystal inhibitor [20, 21] which could prevent the initiation of stone formation and also the relationship in this respect of pyrophosphate to orthophosphate, has received attention in recent years. It seems that while pyrophosphate is not of great importance in the field of prevention, the administration of orthophosphate has a place in the treatment of stone (Chap. 12).

In view of the findings of Thomas and Howard [92] that the mineralization of rachitic rat cartilage can be inhibited by a substance found in normal urine, Fleisch and Neuman [22] carried out experiments in which urine adjusted to pH 7.4 was added to their collagen-catalyzed solution, the minimal ion product needed for calcification being then greatly exceeded. They suggested that the presence of a nucleating collagen (and also the presence of phosphatase for the local destruction of an inhibitor or inhibitors present in the plasma) was necessary for mineralization; and also that collagen (or some moiety associated with it) might possess the specific nucleating property which could induce the formation of crystal nuclei in solutions of calcium phosphate (in vitro and under standard conditions) which are otherwise metastable. They determined quantitatively the minimum ion product (Ca $\times$ P) needed to allow the formation of calcium phosphate crystals: plasma ultrafiltrate was found to contain one or more substances which increased this minimum ion product (and which, therefore, inhibited calcium phosphate nucleation), and which were inactivated by alkaline phosphatase.

They concluded that the substance which had inhibited the collagen-induced precipitation of calcium phosphate present in the plasma was probably excreted in the urine, and they showed it to be inorganic pyrophosphate [20, 21]. It was suggested that the pyrophosphate in the plasma inhibits the precipitation of hydroxyapatite, which could, however, take place if the pyrophosphatase in growing bone (which is known to be present) could destroy the inhibitor locally.

It has long been known that some of the longer-chain compounds containing P—O—P bonds often in minute amounts (such as polysodium metaphosphate) have the property (as a chelating agent) of being able to reduce or prevent the scaling in water pipes and boilers by calcium carbonate [29, 75]. In the experimental animal, following the introduction of foreign bodies into the bladders of rats as seeds to produce stone formation, Care and Wilson [18] found that the oral administration of hexametaphosphate arrested calculus formation.

Fleisch and Neuman [22] found that the mean daily urinary excretion of pyrophosphate in healthy males was of the order of 2.16 mg (expressed as phosphorus), that in young women it was below 1 mg, and that it increased with age. Its concentration in urine was high enough to inhibit strongly the precipitation of calcium salts in vitro, and seemed to offer a possible explanation of the high supersaturation of normal urine with calcium salts [23].

It was thought that the inhibition of the precipitation of calcium phosphate by pyrophosphate results from its adsorption onto the nuclei of crystals, thus impeding their growth, especially at the amorphous stage of crystal nucleus formation. It was necessary to know if the level of urinary pyrophosphate which (based on in vitro evidence) was theoretically necessary to prevent crystal and stone formation, did in fact exist in human urine; and if it did not exist, if it could be increased by suitable measures in order possibly to assist in the prevention of urolithiasis. Some observers reported that the daily amount excreted in stone-formers was less than that found in normal subjects [23, 76], while others have found little difference in the two values. Pyrophosphate given orally in daily doses of 70 mg is not excreted in the urine to any significant extent and larger doses may give rise to abdominal discomfort and diarrhoea.

Fleisch et al. [23] showed that the addition of orthophosphate to the food in rats resulted in an immediate increase of the urinary excretion of pyrophosphate, which in turn was reduced when the dietary orthophosphate was reduced; similarly the oral administration of orthophosphate in man causes a prompt, marked and proportionate increase in the renal output of orthophosphate and also of pyrophosphate [75]. When oral aluminium hydroxide is given, to precipitate phosphate in the gut (thereby reducing its availability for absorption), a decrease of both orthophosphate and pyrophosphate has been found.

Russell, Hodgkinson and their co-workers [74, 76] found that the administration of oral disodium hydrogen phosphate to a group of male patients with recurrent renal calculi, resulted in a prompt increase in the urinary excretion of orthophosphate and pyrophosphate, a decrease in that of calcium and magnesium, and usually a significant increase in the mean daily excretion of citrate. They found that the distribution of the urinary pyrophosphate levels was comparable in normal subjects and in patients with urolithiasis, a few individuals in each group having high values. The excretion of pyrophosphate was reduced in patients in whom renal function was impaired. They concluded that a diminished urinary excretion of pyrophosphate is not an important factor in most patients with urinary calculi; the administration of orthophosphate probably produces its beneficial results in the treatment of urolithiasis largely because it effects a reduction in the urinary excretion of calcium. Lewis et al. [48] similarly considered that the amount of pyrophosphate present in normal urine was inadequate to be a major determinant of its mineralizing potential, and that the reduced content of pyrophosphate found in the urine of some patients with calculi is unlikely to have been an important factor in their development.

If a non-toxic polyphosphate can be found which can be shown to be a crystal inhibitor, and which can be administered orally and excreted in the urine, the result may be rewarding.

6. Vitamin D (Calciferol)

An excess of vitamin D in the human diet and in that of the experimental animal has been shown to be a cause of toxic symptoms (usually known as hypervitaminosis D), hypercalcaemia, renal calcification and sometimes of renal calculi.

Young rats fed on a standard diet and given daily overdoses of vitamin D show diminished activity, alteration of their coat, retarded growth and herpes on the snout. Changes are visible after a few days and many animals die within 1 month; a high dietary calcium content probably exacerbated the symptoms.

In a series of rats fed in this way by the author calcific foci in the renal tubules were demonstrated microscopically in about 4 days after the commencement of the experiment. In animals allowed to survive for 3 or 4 weeks, a crescentic calcific deposit could sometimes be demonstrated radiologically (and when the kidney was cut with a knife) in the boundary zone between the renal cortex and the medulla. Microscopically there was cellular destruction of the calcified part of the kidney and the animals had apparently died from renal failure. The renal changes (described by many observers) have been associated with focal and sometimes widespread degeneration (with calcification) of the aorta, the cardiac muscle and the mucosa and muscularis of the stomach, as well as calcareous casts in the renal tubules [17]. The essential lesion of vitamin D sclerosis is believed to be a degeneration followed by calcification in the media of the arteries.

Nephrocalcinosis induced in rats by large doses of vitamin D is not prevented by the administration of cortisone, which in that situation therefore does not completely antagonize the results of overdosage with vitamin D [99].

The clinical symptoms of hypervitaminosis D in infants include loss of appetite, fatigue and pallor, thirst, nausea, vomiting. dry tongue, epigastric discomfort, diarrhoea, headache, muscular weakness and polyuria, and in fatal cases apathy, dehydration, drowsiness and coma. In suspected cases the discovery of hypercalcaemia leads to the diagnosis, though the possibility of idiopathic hypercalcaemia of infancy has to be considered.

In fatal cases metastatic calcification affecting various organs, including the kidney, has been observed, as well as calcific masses around joints if the patient has survived for a long time. If the patient ceases to take vitamin D before the impaired renal function has become irreversible, some of the metastatic deposits may be partly resolved. Fatal cases in infants have been described by Malmberg [50], Thatcher [89, 90], and Ross and Williams [73].

In adults, clinical symptoms may be present for relatively long periods, before important renal symptoms are detected. Patients who have had a high dietary intake of calcium, those whose treatment has needed immobilization (and who may have had impairment of renal function) and those with sarcoidosis seem to be predisposed to

vitamin D intoxication, which, when it occurs, may be unsuspected until the patient is clinically very ill.

Fatal cases in adults have been reported by Kerr [38], and by Bauer and Freyberg [5]. Calciferol has been used as a therapeutic measure in the treatment of rheumatoid arthritis and some skin diseases and toxic symptoms have been reported [2, 9]. In some cases there were radiologically demonstrable calcific deposits around various joints (shoulders, sternoclavicular region and ischium), and in one case, a male aged 29 'innumerable fine calculi' were seen radiographically in the right renal calyces and several larger calculi in the left renal pelvis. After withdrawal of the vitamin D there was usually partial resolution of the calcific periarticular masses. David et al. [12] referred to a patient (a female, aged 69) who had had a stone removed from the right kidney. She then developed weakness, loss of appetite, confusion, loss of memory, disorientation, polyuria, dehydration and later vomiting, and was found to have a mild hypokalaemic alkalosis with azotaemia, the serum calcium level being 14.4 mg. Only after the neck had been explored for a possible parathyroid adenoma with negative results was it found that she had been taking unprescribed doses of vitamin D for over 3 years before admission to hospital. A young adult male with clear evidence of overdosage of vitamin D resulting in nephrocalcinosis and renal calculi was shown at a meeting by Mr. D. Poole-Wilson [67].

In an investigation of 104 patients with renal calculi, Taylor [88] found that 42% gave a history of previous self-medication with tablets containing vitamin D, compared with 37% of a control group of 51 patients without renal calculi; this difference is not statistically significant. The highest mean supplemented intake of vitamin D occurred among those patients in whom no metabolic or other cause for renal stone formation could be found. The results suggested that self-medication with vitamin D should be included among the acknowledged factors promoting the formation of renal calculi.

II. Inhibitors of Calcification

1. Experimental Calcification of Rachitic Rat Cartilage and of Isolated Tendon Bundles

Robison [72] showed that rickets can be induced in weanling rats by feeding a low-phosphorus high-calcium diet for 21 to 34 days. Studies on the use of rachitic rat cartilage as a tool for the investigation of the problems of calcification have been made by Shipley, Kramer and their co-workers [43, 82, 83]. Sterile preparations of the cartilaginous matrix taken, for example, from the tibial epiphysis of rachitic rats, can be mineralized in vitro if incubated in a fluid substrate of appropriate pH (for example, of normal serum or of urine incubated at 37°C) and containing suitable concentrations of calcium and phosphorus which are normal for the baby rat [34]. The calcium-phosphorus product (expressed as milligrams per 100 ml) must be approximately 20 or more, before such mineralization will occur.

Similar results may be obtained by incubation of the preparation of cartilage in solutions of inorganic salts equivalent in composition to that of serum, but which had been freed from organic substances, provided that the calcium and phosphorus concentrations and the pH of the solution were adequately controlled. A pH of between 7.25 and 7.35 is necessary to obtain calcification in vitro.

Calcification occurred most readily in the absence of magnesium ions, was partially inhibited with a magnesium concentration of 1.8 mg/100 ml of solution, and completely inhibited with a concentration of 3.0 mg/100 ml (especially when the concentration of inorganic phosphate

was increased). Sodium chloride was also found to exercise an inhibitory effect [83]. Mineralization will be prevented by substances which interfere either with the availability of calcium ions or with the enzymatic activity of the cartilage [92]. Patients with renal insufficiency nearly always have combined concentrations of calcium and phosphorus in their serum higher than those in healthy subjects, but they may still develop their special type of rickets; rachitic rat cartilage failed to calcify when placed in most sera (or in their ultrafiltrates) from uraemic patients, a fact which suggests that uraemic serum contains an inhibitor to calcification [100].

Preparations of fresh bovine Achilles tendon are suitable for providing what seems to be an enzyme-independent heat-stable test tissue which will mineralize in vitro under conditions similar (as regards the requirements of calcium and phosphorus) to those of the preparation of rachitic cartilage, hydroxyapatite crystals being deposited in an unorganized way within the collagen fibres instead of on the surface. Similarly the preparation will respond to the various crystal inhibitors such as magnesium, pyrophosphate or chelators of calcium (except zinc).

The tendon taken from the animal is divided into bundles, cleaned of fat, washed, cut into pieces 1 cm long, placed in a flask with 20 ml 3% Na_2HPO_4/g tendon, shaken for 72 h, subsequently washed with distilled water, lyophilized, and stored at 4°C for subsequent use; it can be cut as required into sections 1 mm thick parallel to the grain of the collagen fibres [93].

'Good' and 'Evil' Urine. The conditions which had been found to apply regarding calcification of rachitic rat cartilage in respect of serum have been examined with reference to urine, and have been reported in a series of papers by Howard, Thomas and their co-workers and summarized by Barker et al. [4], who also give the references in the literature.

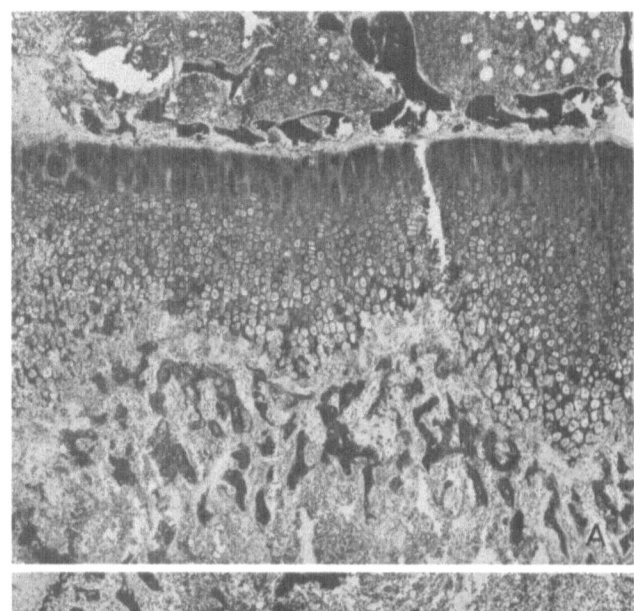

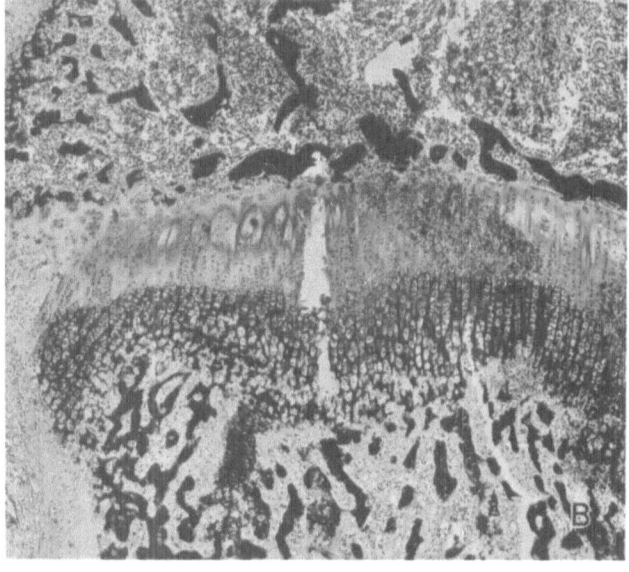

Fig. 9.3. Section of the proximal end of the tibia in a rachitic rat. **A.** Control section before incubation in a mineralizing medium. **B.** Section after incubation in the mineralizing medium: mineralization of the cartilage matrix is indicated by the black silver stain in the distal half of the zone of proliferative cartilage. (By courtesy of Dr. W.C. Thomas, University of Florida; and of Editors and Publishers of Renal Stone Research Symposium, Drs. A. Hodgkinson and B.E.C. Nordin, Churchill, London 1969)

Thomas and Howard [92] showed that the preparation of rachitic rat cartilage in vitro was not mineralized by immersion in urine from normal individuals (save exceptionally), even though it contained an apparent excess of calcium and of phosphate, but that urine from patients with urolithiasis, having apparently similar concentrations of calcium, magnesium and phosphorus often did mineralize. In urine from normal subjects and in that from calculous patients, the calcium–phosphate product was 5–25 times greater than that which was needed for mineralization of the preparation of rachitic cartilage to take place in vitro, using inorganic solutions (Fig. 9.3). Urine which did not calcify the rachitic rat cartilage came to be called 'good' urine and that which did calcify was called 'evil' urine [34]. Experiments and circumstances were then devised to identify the substance or substances which were present in the urine of the patients with renal calculi but were absent from that from normal subjects, and which enabled or encouraged the mineralization of the cartilage to take place.

Urines from a few non-calculous patients were found not to mineralize the cartilage, but the urine of a few in this group did mineralize cartilage following 6 months' residence in Florida, where the incidence of renal stone is high. Not every single sample of urine voided by a given subject was either always good or always evil. To determine the nature or the properties of the factors affecting the mineralizing propensity, separate sterilized specimens of urine were adjusted to pH 7.4 and diluted to a specific gravity of 1011 and submitted to various procedures. Dilution or concentration of the urine, freezing or thawing, boiling, acidification to pH 1, alkalinization with sodium hydroxide to pH 12, passage of the urine through activated charcoal (the latter having been freed of calcium and magnesium), exposure to the action of enzymes (such as papain or hyaluronidase), incubation for 1 h at 37°C with intestinal alkaline phosphatase, or changes in the specific gravity of the urine, did not alter the property of the urine in respect of its ability or otherwise to mineralize rachitic cartilage [34].

Evil urines accepted more calcium at pH 7.4 without forming a calcium phosphate precipitate, than did good urines. When neutral phosphate was added to evil urine it remained evil and precipitation did not occur. When good urine, which had been acid when it was voided, was brought to pH 7.4 by the addition of ammonium hydroxide (and not sodium hydroxide in this context) the resulting precipitate contained nearly all the magnesium from the original urine but left behind much of the calcium; the supernatant fluid after filtration became evil urine.

An evil urine could be made into good urine by the addition of a few milligrams percent of magnesium chloride. When all the calcium and magnesium was precipitated from urine by bringing it to pH 12 with sodium hydroxide, and 6 mg% of calcium was then added to the supernatant, the solution would then calcify cartilage (that is, it was evil urine), though the addition of small moieties of magnesium would block this process.

When all the cations were removed from the urine of normal subjects (which did not mineralize cartilage) by passage through an ion exchange resin, and the original concentration of calcium was then restored, the partially reconstituted urine mineralized cartilage with regularity [58]. If magnesium was then added to the modified urine in gradually increasing amounts so as to achieve a concentration at which mineralization failed to occur, it was found that much more magnesium was needed to inhibit mineralization by urine from calculous patients than from that by normal subjects [91]. Manganese, zinc and other cations inhibited calcification in the standard preparation, though none of these elements, however, is present in human urine in amounts which are sufficient to account for its usual inhibitory property [6].

The mineralizing property of urine from patients with urolithiasis was inhibited by the addition of citrate to the calculous urine (100 mg/100 ml). Somewhat different concentrations of calcium and magnesium in the urine (and the product of the two) were required for the mineralization of collagen; inhibition of mineralization by magnesium could be overcome by increasing the concentration of calcium or phosphorus. When urine which would calcify the test cartilage was mixed in equal proportions with urine which would not calcify cartilage, calcification followed. If more than half the mixture consisted of urine which was capable of calcifying cartilage, calcification occurred [35].

An artificial urine which included the known urinary constituents in their normal concentrations caused vigorous calcification of the test cartilage [48]. When evil urine was dialyzed and the dialyzate was evaporated to obtain a filtrate of specific gravity 1011 it remained evil. It was concluded that the substance (or substances) responsible for the property of the urine in this context is a small molecule which can pass through the pores of the cellophane membrane, and smaller therefore than a protein molecule [34]. It was deduced that there must be in the urine of normal subjects (good urine) anions which can inhibit the mineralization of the experimental cartilage, and which are quantitatively reduced in the urine of patients with urolithiasis [91]; and that in those urines which do not mineralize the cartilaginous preparation, there are one or more inhibitors to calcification which are ultrafiltrable, heat-labile in an acid medium, destructible by certain bacteria and precipitated at least in part by the addition of large amounts of calcium. The addition of inorganic metaphosphate to evil urines changed them to good urines in 6 of 10 specimens so treated. No difference was found in the amount of the urinary ionic calcium in normal and in calculous patients [91]. Pyrophosphate added to the calcifying urine would block calcification but often only when much more was added to the substrate than occurs in vivo [48].

Howard, Thomas and their co-workers postulated that urine contained, perhaps in very small concentrations, some substances which had the property of inhibiting not only the mineralization of cartilage and collagen in their experimental preparation, but also of inhibiting crystallization and stone formation in urine if present in sufficient concentration.

2. Urinary Peptides and Crystallization Inhibitors

Howard and his co-workers, during the fractionation of anionic compounds, considered that they had isolated two ultra-

filtrable ninhydrin-negative peptides from urine and from plasma which powerfully inhibited the mineralization of cartilage or collagen in an assay system, when they were present in amounts of the order of 12–60 $\mu g/100$ ml of the substrate solution. When these substances in similar concentrations were added to metastable solutions containing calcium and phosphorus they inhibited the formation of hydroxyapatite crystals. By means of electron microscopy techniques they showed that the inhibitor peptide was able to delay crystal formation for periods of from 30 s to 96 h [35, 92, 93].

Smith and McCall [86] have described the complicated process of the isolation, purification and assay of these peptides. It was found that the daily amount excreted in the urine in five normal subjects was approximately 4 mg and that it was less than that amount by 20% to 60% in the urine of six patients with calcium-containing stones. They isolated from pooled urine a third ninhydrin-negative acidic peptide which was also able to prevent mineralization in a collagen assay system. The three peptides shared a common amino acid residue or grouping, the amino acids, aspartic acid, glutamic acid, serine and glycine being common components of the three peptides. The origin of the peptides is not known but there was some evidence that they are widely distributed in biological fluids and tissues. An acidic ninhydrin-negative peptide having the same characteristics as those in urine has been found in extracts from liver mitochondria [98].

In a recent communication it was reported that hydrolysis in 6 N · HCl for 72 h at 115° of whole urine which had been ultrafiltered at pH 4 produced little or no reduction of the inhibitory potency of evil urine. When the same extracts were subjected to alkaline hydrolysis in a boiling methanol solution of sodium hydroxide, there was similarly no significant loss of inhibitor potency; these observations cast doubt upon the suggestion that the most potent crystal inhibitor in urine is of a peptide nature [4].

In studies of the peptide inhibitors of calcium phosphate precipitation in eight normal subjects and eight renal-stone-forming male patients, Robertson et al. [71] isolated peptide fractions from the urines by ion-exchange and gel-filtration, and examined their ability to inhibit the homogeneous nucleation of calcium phosphate from aqueous solution. Comparison between the various urines revealed a lower mean inhibitory activity in the stone-forming urines than in normal urine, but there was considerable overlap, the difference being significant only at the 5% level. When calcium oxalate was substituted for calcium phosphate in the precipitation test, no inhibitory activity could be demonstrated in normal or stone-forming urine. They concluded that the absence of peptide inhibitors of homogeneous nucleation was not a primary cause of stone formation in these patients. It has been shown that when the various soluble complexes formed between the ionizable constituents of urine are taken into account, urine is usually in a metastable rather than an oversaturated state, hence it may not be necessary to invoke the presence of such inhibitors in urine, to account for the stability of calcium salts, even though their presence can be demonstrated [33, 70].

3. Metallic Inhibitors of Crystallization

Certain metallic ions have the property of inhibiting the mineralization of experimental rachitic rat cartilage; the question arises as to the possible place of such ions in the formation or prevention of renal calculi.

The mineralization of rachitic rat cartilage can be prevented by the presence in the incubating solution of beryllium, copper, magnesium and strontium, and also of zinc, manganese, cadmium, cobalt and chromium if the incubating solution does not contain magnesium [6]. A greater concentration of the respective element was needed to inhibit mineralization than when magnesium was present. Much higher concentrations of copper, strontium and molybdenum than of the above-mentioned metals were needed.

Zinc was the most potent inhibitor of mineralization, and was the only metallic ion present in plasma to be examined, which completely inhibited mineralization at the concentrations which could be detected. In a concentration of 0.001 mM, in an incubating solution which contained magnesium, zinc enhanced the inhibitory effect of other metallic ions on mineralization, and in a concentration of 0.01 mM, in the presence of magnesium, detectable mineralization was prevented. Most of the elements referred to are present in plasma at concentrations which range from 0.001 to 0.01 mM, and appear to be protein bound. It is possible that these various elements may act additively in the production of their effect upon mineralization, hence the total concentration of the various inhibitory ions may be more relevant than that of several single inhibitory ions. It is not yet known which, if any, of these metallic inhibitors which are effective in the experimental animal against the formation of apatite, are relevant to the problem of human stone formation.

The possibility has been considered that aluminium derived from cooking utensils in regions where the water is 'hard' (which becomes alkaline on heating), may have a relation to the high incidence of renal stone in the south-eastern part of the United States and in other regions where hard water preponderates. It has been shown that the use of hard water with aluminium cooking utensils may lead to an increase in the urinary and faecal aluminium of several milligrams per day, which is more than would be present if the food had been prepared in suitable glassware and with the use of distilled water [7, 91]. So far it has not been shown that aluminium modified the inhibitor action of urinary peptides or of pyrophosphate; the urine of patients fed with diets prepared with hard water in aluminium utensils did not mineralize collagen, so that it would appear that more aluminium than is ingested by individuals in this way would be needed to have a demonstrable effect on mineralization [91].

References

1. Albright,F., Sulkowitch,H.W., Chute,R.: Non-surgical aspects of the kidney stone problem. J. Am. Med. Assoc. *113*, 2049 (1939)
2. Anning,S.T., Dawson,J., Dolby, D.E., Ingram,J.T.: Toxic effects of calcification. Q. J. Med. *17*, 203 (1948)
3. Bailey,C.R.: Siliceous urinary calculi in calves: prevention by addition of sodium chloride to the diet. Science *155*, 696 (1967)
4. Barker,L.M., McPhillips,J.J., Lawrence, G.D., Doty,S.T., Pallante,S.L., Bills,C.E., Scott,W.W.Jr., Howard,J.E.: Studies on mechanisms of calcification. I. Properties of urinary derivatives which inhibit cartilage calcification. II. Electron microscopic observations of the effect of inhibitors on crystal formation. Bull. Johns Hopkins Hosp. *127*, 2 (1970)
5. Bauer,J.M., Freyberg,R.H.: Vitamin D intoxication and metastatic calcification. J. Am. Med. Assoc. *130*, 1208 (1946)
6. Bird,E.D., Thomas,W.C.: Effect of various metals on mineralization in vitro. Proc. Soc. Exp. Biol. *112*, 640 (1963)
7. Campbell,I.R., Cass,J.S., Cholak,J., Kehoe,R.A.: Aluminium in the environment of man. Arch. Ind. Health *15*, 359 (1957)
8. Care,A.D., Wilson,G.: The prevention of vesical calculi in rats by the oral administration of polysodium metaphosphate. Clin. Sci. *15*, 183 (1956)
9. Christensen,W.R., Liebman,C., Sosman, M.C.: Skeletal and periarticular manifestations of hypervitaminosis D. Am. J. Roentgenol. *65*, 27 (1951)
10. Conway,N.S., Maitland,A.I.L., Rennie, J.B.: Urinary citrate excretion in patients with renal calculi. Br. J. Urol. *21*, 30 (1949)
11. Dahl,L.K.: Possible role of salt intake in the development of essential hypertension. In: Essential hypertension: an International Symposium sponsored by Ciba. Bock,K.D., Cottier,P.J. (eds.). Berlin, Göttingen, Heidelberg: Springer 1960
12. David,N.J., Verner,J.V., Engel,F.L.: The first diagnostic spectrum of hypercalcaemia. Am. J. Med. *33*, 88 (1962)
13. Dent,C.E.: Personal communication (1971)
14. Dent,C.E., Harris,H.: Hereditary forms of rickets and osteomalacia. J. Bone Joint Surg. *38b*, 204 (1956)
15. Desgrez,P., Thomas,J., Thomas,E., Rabussier,H.: Calcium et magnésium urinaire chez le sujet sain et le sujet atteint de lithiase rénale. Ann. Biol. clin. *15*, 5 (1957)
16. Desgrez,P., Thomas,J., Thomas,E., Rabussier,H.: Elinnation urinaire calcique et magnésienne chez le sujet sain et le sujet atteint de lithiase rénale; étude comparative. Sem. Hop. Paris. *34*, 2995 (1958)
17. Duguid,J.B., Duggan,M.M., Gough,J.: The toxicity of irradiated ergosterol. I. J. Pathol. Bacteriol. *33*, 353 (1930)
18. Elliot,J.S., Eusebio,S.: The effect of urinary amino acids upon the solubility of calcium oxalate. Invest. Urol. *2*, 428 (1965)
19. Elliot,J.S., Todd,H.E., Lewis,L.: Some aspects of calcium phosphate solubility. J. Urol. *85*, 428 (1961)
20. Fleisch,H., Bisaz,S.: Isolation from urine of pyrophosphate. A calcification inhibitor. Am. J. Physiol. *203*, 671 (1962a)
21. Fleisch,H., Bisaz,S.: Mechanism of calcification: inhibitory role of pyrophosphate. Nature (London) *195*, 911 (1962b)
22. Fleisch,H., Neuman,W.F.: Mechanisms of calcification: role of collagen, polyphosphates and phosphates. Am. J. Physiol. *200*, 1296 (1961)
23. Fleisch,H., Bisaz,S., Care,A.D.: Effect of orthophosphate on urinary pyrophosphate excretion and the prevention of urolithiasis. Lancet *I*, 1065 (1964)
24. Gershoff,S.N., Andrus,S.B.: Dietary magnesium, calcium, vitamin B6 and experimental nephropathies in rats: calcium oxalate calculi, apatite nephrocalcinosis. J. Nutr. *73*, 308 (1961)

25. Gershoff,S.N., Andrus,S.B.: Effect of vitamin B6 and magnesium on renal deposition of calcium oxalate induced by ethylene glycol administration. Proc. Soc. Exp. Biol. Med. *109*, 102 (1962)

26. Gershoff,S.N., Farangella,F.F., Nelson, D.A., Andrus,S.B.: Vitamin B6 deficiency and oxalate nephrocalcinosis in the cat. Am. J. Med. *27*, 72 (1959)

27. Hall,T.C., Lehmann,H.: Experiments in practicability of increasing calcium absorption with protein derivatives. Biochem. J. *38*, 117 (1944)

28. Harrison,H.E., Harrison,H.C.: Inhibition of urine citrate excretion and the production of renal calcinosis in the rat by acetazolamide (Diamox) administration. J. Clin. Invest. *34*, 1662 (1955)

29. Hatch,G.B., Rice,O.: Surface-active properties of hexametaphosphate. Ind. Eng. Chem. *31*, 51 (1939)

30. Heaton,F.W., Anderson,C.K.: The mechanism of renal calcification induced by magnesium deficiency in the rat. Clin. Sci. *28*, 106 (1965)

31. Hodgkinson,A.: Citric acid excretion in normal adults and in patients with renal stone. Clin. Sci, *23*, 203 (1962)

32. Hodgkinson,A.: The relation between citric acid and calcium metabolism with particular reference to primary hyperparathyroidism and idiopathic hypercalciuria. Clin. Sci. *24*, 167 (1963)

33. Hodgkinson,A., Peacock,M., Nicholson, M.: Quantitative analysis of calcium-containing urinary calculi. Invest. Urol. *6*, 549 (1969)

34. Howard,J.E.: Urinary stone. Can. Med. Assoc. J. *86*, 22 (1962)

35. Howard,J.E., Thomas,W.C.: Control of crystallization in urine. Am. J. Med. *45*, 693 (1968)

36. Isaacson,L.C.: Hypercalciuria relative to total solutes in nephrolithiasis. Br. Med. J. *II*, 668 (1968)

37. Isaacson,L.C., Modlin,M., Jackson, W.P.U.: Relative hypercalciuria in nephrolithiasis. Br. Med. J. *II*, 558 (1966)

38. Kerr,W.: In: Discussion of paper by Freyberg,R.H., Grant,R.L., Robb,M.A. (eds.). Hypoparathyroidism: the treatment of chronic cases. J. Am. Med. Assoc. *107*, 1769 (1936)

39. King,J.S., Jackson,R., Ashe,B.: Relation of sodium intake to urinary calcium excretion. Invest. Urol. *1*, 555 (1964)

40. King,J.S., O'Connor,F.J., Smith,M.J.V., Chouse, L.: The urinary calcium/ magnesium ratio in calcareous stone formers. Invest. Urol. *6*, 60 (1968)

41. Kissin,B., Locke,M.O.: Urinary citrates in calcium urolithiasis. Proc. Soc. Exp. Biol. N.Y. *46*, 216 (1941)

42. Klemperer,G., Tritschler,F.: Untersuchungen über Herkunft und Löslichkeit der im Urin ausgeschiedenen Oxalsäure. Z. Clin. Med. *44*, 337 (1902)

43. Kramer,B., Shelling,D.H., Orant,E.R.: Studies upon calcification in vitro. II. On the inhibiting effect of the magnesium ion. Bull. Johns Hopkins Hosp. *41*, 428 (1927)

44. Leading Article: Lancet *II*, 657 (1959)

45. Leading Article: Renal stones and sodium. Lancet *I*, 889 (1967)

46. Lehmann,H.: Biochem. Soc. Symp. No. 1 (1948)

47. Lehmann,H., Pollak,L.: The influence of amino acids on transfer of phosphate in muscle extracts and on the solubility of magnesium and calcium salts. J. Physiol. *100*, 17 (1942)

48. Lewis,A.M., Thomas,W.C.Jr., Tomita,A.: Pyrophosphate and the mineralizing potential of urine. Clin. Sci. *30*, 389 (1966)

49. Locket,S.: Clin. Toxicol. London (1959)

50. Malmberg,N.: Some histologic organic changes after cod liver oil medication. Acta Paediatr. *8*, 364 (1928)

51. McCance,R.A., Widdowson,E.M., Lehmann,H.: Effect of protein intake on absorption of calcium and magnesium. Biochem. J. *36*, 686 (1942)

52. McGeown,M.G.: The urinary amino acids in relation to calculus disease. J. Urol. *78*, 318 (1957)

53. McGeown,M.G.: The urinary excretion of amino acids in calculous patients. Clin. Sci. *18*, 185 (1959)

54. Mellanby,E.: Special Report Series. Med. Res. Council. London. No. 93 (1928)

55. Modlin,M.: Renal stones and sodium. Lancet *I*, 1162 (1967a)

56. Modlin,M.: The aetiology of renal stone: a new concept arising from studies of a stone-free population. Ann. Roy. Coll. Surg. Engl. *40*, 155 (1967b)

57. Modlin,M.: Urinary sodium and renal disease. In: Renal Stone Research Symposium. Hodgkinson,A., Nordin,B.E.C. (eds.). London: Churchill 1969

58. Mukai,T., Howard,J.E.: Some observations on the calcification of rachitic cartilage by urine; the difference between 'good' and 'evil' urines dependent upon

content of magnesium. Bull. Johns Hopkins Hosp. *112*, 279 (1963)

59. Murphy,K.J.: Bilateral renal calculi and amino aciduria after excessive intake of Worcestershire sauce. Lancet *II*, 401 (1967)

60. Murphy,K.J.: Sauce, spices and the kidney. Br. Med. J. *III*, 770 (1971)

61. Neuman,W.F., Neuman,M.W.: Chem. Rev. *53*, 1 (1953)

62. Oreopoulos,D.A.: Hypomagnesaemia in nephrosis. Lancet *I*, 1092 (1968)

63. Oreopoulos,D.A., Soyannwo,M.A.O., McGeown,M.G.: The influence of gluconate and glucogalactogluconate on the fluormetric estimation of magnesium with *O,O*-dihydroxyazobenzene. Clin. Chim. Acta *20*, 349 (1968)

64. Oreopoulos,D.A., Soyannwo,M.A.O., McGeown,M.G.: Magnesium excretion after calcium infusion and the significance of the Mg/Ca ratio in patients with renal stones. In: Renal Stone Research Symposium. Hodgkinson,A., Nordin,B.E.C. (eds.). London: Churchill 1969

65. Ostberg,O.: Studien über die Zitronensäureausscheidung der Menschenniere in normalen und pathologischen Zustanden. Scand. Arch. Physiol. *62*, 81 (1931)

66. Phillips,M.J., Cooke,J.N.C.: Relation between urinary calcium and sodium in patients with idiopathic hypercalciuria. Lancet *I*, 1354 (1967)

67. Poole-Wilson,D.S.: Personal communication (1969)

68. Pyrah,L.N., Anderson,C.K., Hodgkinson,A., Zarembski,P.M.: A case of oxalate nephrocalcinosis and primary hyperoxaluria. Br. J. Urol. *31*, 235 (1959)

69. Robertson,W.G., Peacock,M., Nordin,B.E.C.: Renal stones and sodium. Lancet *I*, 1008 (1967)

70. Robertson,W.G., Peacock,M., Nordin,B.E.C.: Activity products in stone-forming and non-stone-forming urine. Clin. Sci. *34*, 579 (1968)

71. Robertson,W.G., Hambleton,J., Hodgkinson,A.: Peptide inhibitors of calcium phosphate precipitation in the urine of normal and stone-forming men. Clin. Chim. Acta *25*, 247 (1969)

72. Robison,R.: The possible significance of hexose phosphoric esters in ossification. Biochem. J. *17*, 286 (1923)

73. Ross,S.G., Williams,W.E.: Vitamin D intoxication in infancy. Am. J. Dis. Child. *58*, 1142 (1939)

74. Russell,R.G.G., Edwards,N.A., Hodgkinson,A.: Urinary pyrophosphate and urolithiasis. Lancet *I*, 1446 (1964)

75. Russell,R.G.G., Fleisch,H.: Pyrophosphate and stone formation. In: Renal Stone Research Symposium. Hodgkinson, A., Nordin,B.E.C. (eds.). London: Churchill 1969

76. Russell,R.G.G., Hodgkinson,A.: The urinary excretion of inorganic pyrophosphates by normal subjects and patients with renal calculus. Clin. Sci. *31*, 51 (1966)

77. Salem,S.N.: Letter—in Lancet *I*, 1223 (1967)

78. Sasaki,N.: The relationship of salt intake to hypertension in the Japanese. Geriatrics *19*, 735 (1964)

79. Scott,W.W., Huggins,C., Selman,B.C.: Metabolism of citric acid in urolithiasis. J. Urol. *50*, 202 (1943)

80. Sherman,C.C., Mendel,L.B., Smith,A.H.: The citric acid formed in animal metabolism. J. Biol. Chem. *113*, 247 (1936a)

81. Sherman,C.C., Mendel,L.B., Smith,A.H.: The metabolism of orally administered citric acid. J. Biol. Chem. *113*, 265 (1936b)

82. Shipley,P.G.: The healing of rickety bones in vitro. Bull. Johns Hopkins Hosp. *41*, 437 (1924)

83. Shipley,P.G., Holt,L.E.Jr.: Studies on calcification in vitro. IV. The effect of inorganic salts. Bull. Johns Hopkins Hosp. *41*, 437 (1927)

84. Shorr,E.: Possible usefulness of estrogens and aluminium hydroxide gels in the management of renal stone. J. Urol. *53*, 507 (1945)

85. Shorr,E., Almy,T.P., Sloan,M.H., Taussky,H., Toscani,V.: The relation between the urinary excretion of citric acid and calcium; its implications for urinary calcium stone formation. Science *96*, 587 (1942)

86. Smith,L.H., McCall,J.T.: Chemical nature of peptide inhibitors isolated from urine. In: Renal Stone Research Symposium. Hodgkinson,A., Nordin,B.E.C. (eds.), p. 153. London: Churchill 1969

87. Sutton,R.A., Watson,L.: Urinary excretion of calcium and magnesium in primary hyperparathyroidism. Lancet *I*, 1000 (1969)

88. Taylor,W.H.: Renal calculi and self-medication with multivitamin preparations containing vitamin D. Clin. Sci. *42*, 515 (1972)

89. Thatcher,L.: Hypervitaminosis D with report of a fatal case in a child. Edinburgh Med. J. 38, 457 (1931)

90. Thatcher,L.: Hypervitaminosis D. Lancet I, 20 (1936)

91. Thomas,W.C.Jr.: Inhibitors of mineralization and renal stone. In: Renal Stone Research Symposium. Hodgkinson,A., Nordin,B.E.C. (eds.), p. 141. London: Churchill 1969

92. Thomas,W.C.Jr., Howard,J.E.: Studies on the mineralizing propensity of urine from patients with and without renal calculi. Trans. Assoc. Am. Physiol. 72, 181 (1959)

93. Thomas,W.C.Jr., Tomita,A.: Mineralization of human and bovine tissue in vitro. Am. J. Pathol. 51, 621 (1967)

94. Udall,R.H., Seger,C.L., Fu-Ho Chen Chow: Studies on urolithiasis. VI. The mechanism of action of sodium chloride on the control of urinary calculi. Cornell Vet. 55, 198 (1965)

95. Vermeulen,C.W., Grove,W.J., Goetz,R., Raggins,H.D., Carroll,N.O.: Experimental lithiasis. I. Development of calculi upon foreign bodies introduced into bladders of rats. J. Urol. 64, 541 (1950)

96. Vermeulen,C.W., Miller,G.H., Chapman, W.H.: Experimental urolithiasis. X. On the state of calcium in the urine. J. Urol. 75, 592 (1956)

97. Vermeulen,C.W., Lyon,E.S., Miller,G.H.: Calcium phosphate solubility in urine as measured by a precipitation test. Experimental urolithiasis. XIII. J. Urol. 79, 596 (1958)

98. Wadkins,G.L.: Quoted by Thomas,W.C. Jr. Inhibitors of mineralization and renal stones. In: Renal Stone Research Symposium. Hodgkinson,A., Nordin,B.E.C. (eds.), p. 141. London: Churchill 1969

99. Wilson, G., Care,A.D., Anderson,C.K.: The effect of cortisone on vitamin D_2-induced nephrocalcinosis in the rat. Clin. Sci. 16, 181 (1957)

100. Yendt,E.R., Connor,T.B., Howard,J.E.: In vitro calcification of rachitic rat cartilage in normal and pathological human serum with some observations on the pathogenesis of renal rickets. Bull. Johns Hopkins Hosp. 96, 1 (1955)

Chapter 10

Clinical Picture of Renal and Ureteric Calculus

I. Etiological Factors

1. Incidence of Calcium Oxalate Stone

Approximately two-thirds of all urinary calculi in man contain calcium oxalate as a major component. In the author's department, in a series of 504 urinary calculi analysed by X-ray diffraction, 68.7% contained calcium oxalate [41]. In an analysis of renal calculi from 3000 patients, calcium oxalate was present in significant quantities in 64% [17, 18]. Similarly, the incidence of calcium oxalate calculi among all stone cases in man in Western Europe and North America has been stated to be 65% [37].

The remaining one-third of renal calculi have one of the calcium phosphates or magnesium ammonium phosphate (in the badly infected cases) as their major component, uric acid and cystine stones (at least in the United Kingdom) accounting for less than 5%; uric acid calculi constitute a larger fraction of all calculi, however, seen in the United States, Australia and South Africa. In a series of approximately 25,000 autopsies the incidence of renal calculi was reported as 1.12%, 0.38% of the deaths being directly related to the presence of calculi [6].

2. Age and Sex

In the author's department, male patients with renal stone were mostly aged between 20 and 39 when first seen. In females the age distribution was evenly spread between the ages of 20 and 49 [33, 35]. A few cases are found in children and a few first present in elderly subjects. The sex incidence in various series shows a proportion of males to females of approximately two to one. The higher incidence of hypercalciuria, hyperphosphaturia and a higher than average urinary oxalate level in the male are probable contributory factors. Urinary alkalinity and the citrate content tend to be somewhat higher in women than in men and are possible factors which may help to reduce the incidence in women.

3. Familial Incidence

A family history is not uncommonly traceable among sufferers from calcium-containing renal calculi. Gram [29] reported a study of five generations in one family (15 people in all) many of whom (usually males) had had calcium oxalate stones. Goldstein [28] found a history of stone in one parent in 8%, in one sibling in 10% and in two siblings in 3% of patients. Melick and Henneman [39] reported a family history in 25 of 207 patients (12.5%) with renal stone.

McGeown [36] found a family history in over 20% of 300 patients with calcium-containing stones, an increased urinary excretion of phosphate being often associated; 48 had suffered from hyperparathyroidism in which there is also sometimes a family history. In a series of 538 patients in the author's department there was a family history in 21 [58]. Thomas et al. [55] found that 37.8% of calcium oxalate stone-formers had at least one stone-former among first-degree relatives, but only 9.5% of those with calcium phosphate stones had an affected relative. Pridgen et al. [48] found significantly more calcium oxalate stones among the fathers, mothers, brothers and sisters of propositi of stone-formers than among control relatives (being the relatives of the spouses of propositi).

Genetic considerations, therefore, would appear to play a part in the incidence of renal calculi, though these have not yet been sufficiently investigated in the human. Burch and his co-workers, from a mathematical analysis of the age distribution of various diseases including renal lithiasis, and from broad biological considerations, proposed that renal lithiasis belongs to a general class of disease which they described as 'autoaggressive', predisposition to which is determined by one or more specific genetic factors [11, 12].

4. Anatomical Position

Renal calculi are most commonly found in the lowest calyx, and less commonly in the middle and upper calyces. The lower incidence of stones in the upper calyces may be explained by the relative ease with which calcific particles can escape by downward drainage as a result of gravity when they are detached and free to move, and hence do not remain to develop into definitive calculi. Stones are commonly found in the renal pelvis, and sometimes in association with ureteric stones on the same or the opposite side. Renal stones are most often unilateral at first; they are sometimes bilateral when first seen, but frequently so after a variable interval of months or years.

Ureteric calculi are formed in the kidney but are often observed clinically as the sole manifestation of calculous disease in the upper urinary tract; they tend to come to rest at the narrow sites in the ureter, the internal diameter of which varies from 3.5 to 8.0 mm [46]. Probably two-thirds of ureteric stones are arrested at various sites in the lowest third of the ureter, namely, where it crosses the iliac vessels, near the spine of the ischium just outside the wall of the bladder and in the intramural part of the

ureter including the ureterovesical orifice. Approximately one-third of ureteric calculi are arrested in the upper two-thirds of the ureter, namely just below the pelviureteric junction or in the neighbourhood of the transverse process of the fourth lumbar vertebra.

5. Size of Stone

Stones nowadays tend to be dealt with when still small before they have reached an enormous size. Massive staghorn renal calculi (usually infected and bilateral) are still seen not infrequently, however, some having given rise to relatively few symptoms. Mylvagnan [44] removed at operation a renal stone which weighed 1440 g, the patient having had pain and a rapidly growing mass in the loin for only 6 months. Giant ureteric calculi (some occupying almost the entire length of the ureter, and usually multiple) have been reported in patients who have declined treatment for many years.

II. Clinical Course of Renal Stone Relative to Time

A portrayal of the clinical picture of stone in the upper urinary tract requires reference to the total period during the lifetime of the patient during which calculus formation is a problem. Is renal calculous disease a transient resolvable and curable disorder, or does it persist through life?

The individual incidents (including the spontaneous voiding of a stone and surgical operations) which make up the clinical picture are in fact parts of an on-going ailment which in three-quarters of the patients is probably lifelong (albeit often at a slow rate of progress), an assumption which has sometimes escaped the notice of urologists, partly because of the apparent successes of instrumental or operative

NAME	No.	YEAR	SIDE LEFT	RIGHT	SPON PASS.	X RAY	N	U	P	PN	FN	TIME 1st 2nd	BILAT.
J S	1	1945	+		+								
	2	1951	+						+			6	
	3	1955		+					+				10
	4	1960	+			K-RT							
A P	1	1949	+								+		
	2	1958		+	+							9	9
	3	1959		+	+								

Fig. 10.1. Schematic representation of the histories of two patients with renal calculi depicting the 'incidents' of calculi (for explanation of 'incidents' see text). Patient J.S. had stones, ultimately bilateral, over a 15-year period and the 'incidents' in his history are shown by the plus signs. Patient A.P. had bilateral stones during a 10-year period. (N, nephrolithotomy; U, ureterolithotomy; P, pyelolithotomy; PN, partial nephrectomy; FN, nephrectomy; K-RT, stone seen in kidney on X-ray—the patient refused treatment.) (By permission of Mr. R.E. Williams and the publishers of the British Journal of Urology)

treatment. Many have thought that if there was no recurrence of stone for 3, 4 or more years a permanent 'cure' had been achieved.

In recent years it has been realized that a far longer period of time must elapse before such an assumption can be made following surgical treatment or spontaneous voiding of a stone. A 10-year, or even a 20-year follow-up will show that late recurrence after the removal of a stone in the affected kidney is common. Furthermore, in one-third or even more of the patients a stone subsequently presents in the opposite kidney [54, 58]. Many patients therefore appear to have a lifelong tendency to form calculi.

In order to assess the long-term natural history of patients with renal calculi, a survey was undertaken in the author's department during 1963. Among the 20,000 patients who had attended the department during the years 1951 to 1961 were 1725 patients with calculi in the upper urinary tract. From this number the case histories of 538 patients (358 males, 180 females) who had had renal calculous disease for a minimum period of 10 years were surveyed in detail from the available records and radiographs, by enquiry from

their family doctors, and by personal interview with 309 patients [58].

In order to record accurately the time and the site of the recurrence of stone during a long period, the clinical history of each patient was broken down into separate units which we called 'incidents', each one representing the appearance of a new stone. Charts were prepared showing the history of each patient (right and left kidneys) during the follow-up period. The incidents were classified as: spontaneous passage of stone following ureteric colic; stone removed after diagnosis following instrumentation or by operation; stone diagnosed by radiography (but not removed surgically) (Fig. 10.1). The survey extended from the onset of the symptoms of the stone until the closing date of the enquiry (minimum 10 years). The mean length of history for all the patients in the group was 18.5 years; 20% of the patients had a history longer than 25 years.

1. Duration of Symptoms

The duration of symptoms prior to diagnosis was ascertained as far as possible.

It was found that the first calculus was voided spontaneously in 275 (51%), and that of 241 patients for whom the history was available, it was voided within 1 month of the onset of symptoms in 77%; 248 (46%) patients had their first recognized calculus removed by surgical operation. Of 176 patients in this group and for whom an accurate history was available clinical symptoms had been reported for at least 6 months in 28%, from 1 to 5 years in 56%, and for more than 5 years in 16%. The figures approximated closely to those of Sutherland [54].

The survey showed that the 538 patients had between them 1949 incidents of stone; there were 139 single-stone-formers who only formed one stone during the entire period of the enquiry; there were 339 recurrent stone-formers who continued to produce stones during the period.

Of the total number of incidents, spontaneous passage of stone accounted for 1209 (62%). In 51 instances the voiding of the stone had been assisted by some form of perureteral instrumentation. Operative removal of the stone had been performed on 554 occasions (28% of the total number of incidents); at least one surgical operation had been performed in 70% of all the patients during the period of the survey and 22% had had multiple operations. The presence of the stone was sometimes assessed by radio-diagnosis (when operation was not indicated or desirable) and represented 186 incidents (9.5%). In 125 of these cases the stones were small and had given rise to minimal symptoms, eight being in the ureter and the remainder in one kidney.

2. The Single-Stone-Former

Of the 139 patients (74 male, 65 female) who had formed during the period under survey one single calculus, it had been voided spontaneously in 36 (28%) and had

been removed by operation in 89 (69%), with no subsequent recurrence.

While the majority of such cases fall into the class of idiopathic stone-formers, no obvious initiating or promoting cause having been found, in some there has been a recognizable temporary or transient metabolic abnormality which has either been resolved spontaneously and which has not recurred, or in which the cause has been removed soon after the calculus-forming episode.

Thus, the patient who has had the surgical removal of an adenoma of a parathyroid gland, having already voided a single stone, will probably form no further stones. A period of residence in a tropical country say for 3 or 4 years, during which the patient experienced relative and continuous dehydration with the consequent voiding of highly concentrated urine (as with a Service soldier), is another etiological factor of a temporary character which may contribute to, or determine the formation of a single stone; when such a period is terminated there may be no further stone formation.

A period of enforced complete recumbency necessary for the treatment of a spinal or other skeletal injury may determine the formation of a stone which does not recur when the period of recumbency has been terminated. Possibly in some patients hypercalciuria (a factor in stone formation in some patients) may have been resolved as a result of treatment, following which stone formation may have ceased.

Some observers have recorded higher percentages of patients believed to have formed only one stone. Garvey and Boyce [23] stated that about 85% of calculous patients had one single small stone which was voided spontaneously; and Baker and Connelly [5] stated that 90% of patients who develop one renal calculus never develop another. Admittedly, an accurate figure is difficult to determine, since not all patients with a single attack of renal colic reach a hospital department (following which attack a stone may be voided) and such patients may never have a further stone.

3. Recurrence

If the cause of the stone formation cannot be eliminated even though some of its principal promoting factors, such as hypercalciuria, are known, the tendency to stone formation will probably persist for many years or through life. Of the 458 patients in our series who were followed up for a minimum of 10 years, 339 (male 249; female 90) proved to be recurrent stone-formers. In the patients in the recurrent group there were 1243 incidents (sometimes numbering two, three or four in one patient) of stone formation, often with long periods of freedom in between them. In 733 (59%) of the incidents stones were voided spontaneously; in 373 (30%) the stone was removed by operation.

There was a small group of patients who formed 8–20 more calculi in succession during several years; in such patients the problem is scarcely one of long-term recurrence but one of a continued high tendency to form renal stones. Chronic urinary infection affected only 4 of the 22 patients in this group; in some there may have been an initiating or promoting cause which had remained uncorrected as, for example, hypercalciuria. It is, of course, to be hoped that the incidence of recurrent stone formation will be changed into a higher incidence of single-stone-formers in future decades, not merely by an improvement in operative techniques, which is important, but by a more adequate correction of the causes of such calculi.

4. Bilateral Stones

The incidence of bilateral calculi, viewed as a long-term clinical event, was found to be much higher than had previously been thought. Stones are sometimes bilateral when the patient is first seen. In another group stones appear in sequence first in one kidney and months or even years later they appear in the opposite kidney; a large branched calculus in one kidney and a small calyceal stone in the other is then not an infrequent combination.

The true incidence of bilateral stones can only be assessed by a follow-up of patients extending over many years (probably 20 or more); there is room for such follow-ups in two or three large departments. Earlier figures in the literature giving the incidence of bilateral calculi as being of the order of 10% or 12% almost certainly ignore the long-term factor.

In the author's department in the series of 538 patients referred to above only 12% had bilateral stones when first seen but after follow-up, in some cases as long as 20 years, 301 patients (56.0%) had bilateral calculi. Sutherland [54] found that in at least one-third of the patients the same condition subsequently occurs in the opposite kidney.

III. Clinical Course of Renal Stone and Associated Factors

It has already been shown that renal calculus is often secondary to, or closely associated with an intrarenal, extrarenal or environmental pathological or metabolic condition (Chaps. 3–7). Such a condition must usually be looked for in order to complete the clinical picture. There are still many idiopathic calculi for which no obvious promoting cause is yet clear. In our departmental series of 538 cases of urolithiasis reported by Williams [58], a contributory factor for stone formation was observed in 60%, while no such factor was noted in 40%. Since the patient's records have not always referred specifically to the presence or absence of such causes, the figure probably underestimates rather than overestimates the number of idiopathic stones.

Hypercalciuria was observed in 107 of 268 patients for whom a report was available. In 451 cases for which reports on the presence or absence of urinary infection were available the figures were: no evidence of infection, 66% per cent; infection at some time, 17%; chronic infection, 17%. The occasional infection reported as being present in some patients usually cleared after the stone had been voided spontaneously or removed surgically.

Primary hyperparathyroidism was the etiological cause in several patients in the series though all the author's 68 reported patients with that condition [49] did not come within the scope of the enquiry here referred to.

Recumbency calculi accounted for 14 cases in the series resulting from fractures of the pelvis or the bones of the lower limbs in 9, and chronic skeletal or joint disease (tuberculosis, spondylitis and rheumatoid arthritis) in 5. Skeletal diseases including Paget's disease were present in 10 patients.

Various renal anatomical abnormalities were regarded as being contributory causes to stone formation: pelviureteric hydronephrosis, 13; polycystic disease, 3; horseshoe kidney, 3; bifid upper urinary tract, 3. There was a history of the prolonged ingestion of alkali for the treatment of peptic ulcer in 22 patients; Sutherland [54] noted a similar association in 3.7% of his cases. Prolonged residence in the tropics was thought to have been a promoting factor in 6 patients. In 13 patients the onset of the stone appeared to have been during pregnancy.

IV. Clinical Symptoms of Renal and Ureteric Calculi

1. Silent Renal Calculi

Renal calculi at the time of their formation in a calyx and for some time afterwards are symptomless. Such silent calculi may attain the size of 1 cm or more. Clinical symptoms may occur when the stone has reached a certain critical size, particularly if there is partial obstruction or when it changes its position. Some comparatively large stones are clinically silent.

2. Non-infected Calculi in the Upper Urinary Tract

Non-migrating Stone in Renal Pelvis or Calyx. While some retained calculi give rise to no symptoms, a fixed dull pain or discomfort in the loin, increased by movement or exercise, is characteristic of a renal stone resting in a calyx or in the renal pelvis [14]. The pain, which is most marked posteriorly, may radiate downwards and forwards; it may be intermittent, or may have a troublesome persistence, coming on with the onset of the day's activities and usually being relieved by rest. It is relatively mild if there is some associated hydronephrosis.

Probably about a third of patients with renal stone have recognizable haematuria at some time or other; on physical examination there is tenderness between the twelfth rib and the erector spinae on firm pressure by the examining finger; the kidney may be palpably enlarged (and even tense) if there is some associated hydronephrosis. Crepitation sensed by the palpating hand from the rubbing one over the other of multiple calculi in a dilated renal pelvis must nowadays be very rare.

Migrating Stone: Renal and Ureteric Colic. Movement of a stone from a calyx to the renal pelvis or from the pelvis to a ureter, may give rise to renal colic, which may be the first symptom of its presence. Renal colic is non-specific in the sense that a similar sequence of symptoms may occur if any solid renal mass (calculus, blood clot, tumour debris, necrotic papilla) starts to move down the ureter. Discomfort in the loin or even slight haematuria may precede the sudden onset of the acute pain (which is often precipitated by movement) and rapidly reaches an agonizing crisis, and may be accompanied by vomiting.

The pain, which is usually spasmodic in character and may cause the patient to writhe in agony, originates in the angle between the last rib and the erector spinae, radiates downwards and forwards along the line of the ureter in the direction of the anterior superior iliac spine, and still later to a position parallel to Poupart's ligament towards the external abdominal ring and to the testicle. In severe attacks the pain may radiate widely over the abdomen, which then may be tender on palpation and tympanitic.

Frequency of urine and strangury are common as the stone moves downwards. The attack usually lasts 2, 3 or 4 h and may cease spontaneously or be relieved by morphia; occasionally it lasts intermittently for 24–36 h. Little urine may be voided during the attack but much may be passed following the cessation of pain; small quantities of blood (or even clots) are occasionally passed, presumably resulting from trauma to the ureter.

Movement of the stone down the ureter usually provokes an attack of ureteric colic, sometimes much muted if the ureter is relatively dilated. The agonizing pain which is experienced in the loin or the iliac fossa at a level lower than that of renal colic radiates upwards to the region of the kidney and downwards to the testicle (which may become tender and retracted) or the labium major. As the stone moves downwards, so does the site of the pain during successive attacks of colic. Colic resulting from a stone in the intramural part of the ureter gives rise to pain of maximum intensity in the region of the external abdominal ring or sometimes over the symphysis pubis and at the tip of the penis at the end of micturition.

Frequency of micturition and strangury with the voiding of only a few drops of urine at each act, and sometimes tenesmus, often accompany movement of a stone down the lowest segment of the ureter; occasionally there is haematuria.

The patient with renal or ureteric colic is seen on examination to be in intense agony, is restless and even writhing, hoping that some change in position will bring relief (as distinct from the patient with peritonitis, who lies still). The temperature is normal in the absence of infection of the urinary tract. There is exquisite tenderness below the angle of the twelfth rib and the erector spinae, or downwards along the line of the ureter (depending upon the position of the stone) but true muscular rigidity is absent (thereby differentiating a colic from an acute inflammatory lesion or a perforated viscus, in which conditions the pain is also severe). Hyperaesthesia of the skin in the loin or the iliac fossa may indicate almost complete obstruction of the ureter. Following the attack of colic, the tenderness persists, becoming less severe after a few hours and disappearing entirely except on deep pressure.

Non-migrating Calculus in the Ureter. There is usually a history of a recent attack (or of past attacks) of ureteric colic. The complaint now is of aching discomfort or of intermittent fixed pain of moderate intensity (often increased by movement) situated in the abdominal parietes at a point along the line of the ureter, corresponding to the site of impaction of the stone:

1. in the back with a stone impacted just below the pelviureteric junction;

2. at a position 2 in. or so to the right or left of the umbilicus (or in the region of McBurney's point) for a stone in the middle zone of the ureter;

3. over the external abdominal ring or near to the symphysis pubis for a stone in the lowest inch of the ureter or at the uretero-vesical orifice. There may be pain in the testicle and along the course of the vas. Pain may sometimes be absent if the stone is stationary in the ureter and if urine is being voided into the bladder. Haematuria

(occasionally painless) is observed in probably one-third of the patients.

Frequency of micturition, pain at the end of the penis during micturition, strangury, painful nocturnal emissions, pain during intercourse, tenesmus and pain during defaecation are occasional symptoms associated with stones at or near the lower end of the ureter. Between the attacks of colic there may be tenderness at a point in the line of the ureter corresponding approximately to the position of the stone. In some long-standing cases of ureteric stone which have remained uninfected, an enlarged hydronephrotic kidney (which may be relatively symptomless) can occasionally be palpated; such a swelling may be flaccid and not easy to palpate, or tense during phases of ureteric spasm.

The rare massive stone in the ureter can occasionally be palpated through the abdominal wall as a fixed hard mass in the line of the ureter, not moving on respiration. Single medium-sized stones (or multiple stones, as in a ureterocele) can sometimes be palpated (especially in sparely built and co-operative patients or in children) through the postero-lateral wall of the rectum in the position corresponding to the forward sweep of the ureter towards the bladder. Similarly on vaginal examination a round or ovoid slightly movable swelling may be palpated in the lateral fornix.

3. Infected Calculi in the Upper Urinary Tract

In an Infected Kidney. The symptoms may be a replica of those described for non-infected calculi if infection is slight. With more established infection the attacks of colic may be more prolonged and extend over some days, and be associated with temperature, indicative of the presence of pyelonephritis. The gradual development of a pyonephrosis is suggested when the pain is severe and persists over several days with temperature.

Toxic absorption from such a grossly infected kidney may give rise to varying degrees of malaise, anorexia, loss of energy and nausea; in bilateral cases the general health may be impaired. The gradual deterioration of the kidney is revealed by the increasing severity of the symptoms. The kidney at this stage may be slightly or moderately enlarged, and tender on palpation from the presence of pyelonephritis or a small pyonephrosis associated with biggish calculi. Sometimes the kidney may be transformed into a large, tender, pyonephrotic sac which fills the loin and becomes immobile on respiration.

Impacted Ureteric Stone. The patient may give a history of earlier attacks of colic often with fever and malaise. Prolonged obstruction of the ureter from stone in a patient whose infected kidney may also contain calculi, results in serious back-pressure and chronic or acute renal suppuration. If the ureteric obstruction is incomplete and urine is able to drain down the ureter, the symptoms may be troublesome but not severe and the renal abnormality may be that of advancing pyelonephritis merging into chronic pyonephrosis. There may be toxic symptoms, inability to work normally, impairment of appetite and a varying degree of anaemia; pain and frequency of micturition may accompany the voiding of pus-laden urine. The kidney may be palpably enlarged and tender though sometimes it remains smaller than a normal kidney.

With a nearly complete ureteric obstruction there will be an intensification of the local pain, a persistently high temperature (perhaps ushered in by a rigor) and an elevated pulse rate and general malaise suggesting the development of a pyonephrosis. There is either oliguria or the urine is muddy if purulent urine seeps past the stone; a tender enlarged kidney of variable size and tenseness, moving little or not at all on respiration, may be palpable in the loin.

4. Less Common Symptoms of Renal Calculi

Hypertension. Since hypertension and renal calculous disease are both fairly common, the two diseases may be found in the same patient by coincidence. It is less easy to determine whether the hypertension may be the consequence of an infected stone-bearing kidney and perhaps this question has not been fully considered in a large series of cases.

A few patients with unilateral renal disease (usually of an inflammatory type) have been shown to develop hypertension as a result of such a disease. Goldblatt et al. [27] showed that ischaemia of the kidney in the experimental animal produced by a controlled partial constriction of one renal artery by the use of a silver clamp, resulted in an elevation of blood pressure and impairment of renal function; subsequent removal of the clamp or of the ischaemic kidney (after hypertension was shown to be present) resulted in a return of the blood pressure to normal. It has been thought that a substance (renin) which has been detected in renal tissue in such cases is chiefly responsible for the hypertension. A few reports are available of unilateral renal hypertension apparently resulting from the presence of a stone-bearing kidney (usually shrunken and infected), following the removal of which the blood pressure has returned to normal. Probably most patients with unilateral renal calculous disease develop calculous pyelonephritis or pyonephrosis which calls for surgical intervention on clinical grounds, long before they might have developed the very gradual impairment of the renal circulation believed to be responsible for the development of hypertension [51].

Spontaneous Rupture of Kidney or Ureter. This is an occasional clinical complication which may be sudden and dramatic, or gradual and slow. Extravasation of urine usually occurs at or near the pelviureteric junction, especially at a time when a calculus has reached the lower end of the ureter, the already damaged upper segment then giving way under back pressure. The leakage may occur from a dilated stone-bearing renal calyx, because of pressure on the thinned-out infected cortex. Abeshouse [1] collected 31 cases of traumatic and 26 of spontaneous rupture of the renal pelvis which 'were almost invariably secondary to nephrolithiasis or ureterolithiasis'; urgent treatment was usually needed [7, 10, 50, 53].

Perinephric Abscess. This condition has already been referred to (Chap. 2). A pyonephrosis can often reach enormous proportions without giving rise to a perinephric abscess, a consequence either of the strength and resistance of the renal capsule or of the protective reactive changes in the surroundings. Partial or complete ureteric obstruction by a stone will predispose to the formation of a perinephric abscess in such cases. When pus escapes in this way it may track downwards into the retroperitoneal tissues, it may go upwards into the pleural cavity, lungs or bronchus, or it may penetrate the parietal muscles giving rise to a subcutaneous abscess and, if not treated, to a renal sinus or a nephrocutaneous fistula.

With the development of a perinephric abscess there is an intensification of the local symptoms in the loin and a palpable tender swelling presents in the renal region which becomes red and angry when the pus has tracked through the parietal muscles. Some perinephric abscesses, for example, those in the subphrenic region, are impalpable clinically and are ultimately diagnosed by radiography; thus time may elapse before this severe complication can be recognized. Alternatively the radiograph may show evidence of a mass in the region of the kidney which is displaced towards the middle line (or upwards or downwards), its mobility on inspiration being impaired.

Renal and Ureteric Fistulae. The various fistulae which may complicate a badly infected calculous kidney have already been referred to (Chap. 2). A reno-pulmonary or broncho-renal fistula is accompanied by the expectoration of pus, urine and possibly calculi, the perinephric abscess diminishing in size as the condition progresses, though the pulmonary condition becomes gradually more grave. The diagnosis can be established by radiography and bronchoscopy. The treatment includes drainage of the principal abscess cavity and aspiration of intrabronchial pus and urine through a bronchoscope.

Nephrocolic Fistula (see Chap. 2). This results from a gradual extension of a calculous pyonephrosis with rupture of the abscess into the colon. The symptoms at first are those of the primary calculous disease, which may have been in existence for months or years (the kidney being grossly infected and sometimes almost functionless). The formation of the fistula is heralded by local exacerbation of the renal symptoms followed by the development of a tender swelling in the loin. At this stage there may be nausea, vomiting and general abdominal distension, the symptoms even suggesting intestinal obstruction. Later the local symptoms may undergo remission gradually or sometimes suddenly (pus from the kidney being voided through the fistula into the colon) and the abdominal swelling may disappear; diarrhoea with the passage of tarry stools may follow the disappearance of the swelling, and urine (or rarely the stone) may be voided per rectum. Alternatively gas, faeces, pus or food debris may be voided in the urine.

There may be the general symptoms of serious illness (if total renal function is grossly impaired), sometimes with disturbance of the blood electrolyte levels such as is commonly found in patients who have had a surgically constructed ureterocolic anastomosis.

Urography may now reveal a large calculus in a lower renal calyx or in the colon, and also a pneumopyelogram; the existence of the fistula may sometimes be demonstrated beyond doubt on retrograde pyelography, the opaque medium delineating the track leading from the renal calyx to the colon; methylene blue injected along the ureteric catheter may be observed later in the stools. If there is a co-existent cutaneous sinus (as there may be, resulting from an earlier operation on the kidney) injection along it of opaque medium may demonstrate the presence of a colonic fistula; a barium enema may also demonstrate the presence of a fistula.

Pyeloduodenal Fistula resulting from calculous disease (see Chap. 2) is usually only discovered after systematic investigation though the clinical symptoms may suggest its presence. There is usually a unidirectional flow of the visceral contents and in nearly all reported cases pus, with or without urine, has passed from the renal pelvis to the duodenum and only rarely in the opposite direction. The clinical symptoms include intermittent pain, attacks of nausea, vomiting, diarrhoea and loss of appetite; gastric debris and gas may be voided into the urine and a palpable mass in the renal region is commonly observed. The illness may be prolonged and tedious and be punctuated by periods of partial clinical recovery though there is usually loss of weight, anaemia and even cachexia.

The plain radiograph may show the presence of one or more calculi in the renal pelvis or in the duodenum. Intravenous pyelography usually reveals either a nonfunctioning kidney (or one with only poor function), and occasionally the fistulous connection can be demonstrated on the film. On cystoscopy there is a non-functioning kidney. Opaque medium injected along a ureteric catheter introduced into the renal pelvis may pass into the duodenum, when radiography may establish the diagnosis. Occasionally a barium meal had led to the demonstration of a fistula.

Renoperitoneal and Renovaginal Fistulae complicating calculous pyonephrosis or perinephric abscess have been reported [2].

Clinical Features of Bilateral Renal Calculi. Some patients presenting with their first attack of renal colic (and having sterile urine) are found on radiography to have a small or medium-sized stone in the painful kidney and a small or tiny symptomless stone in the opposite kidney. By contrast some patients with bilateral renal calculi often of medium size, have either no symptoms (or merely minimal discomfort) referable to the kidney for some years until the disease is advanced, while some have had bilateral symptoms. The presence of infection (especially if progressive) and of obstruction usually determines the onset of symptoms. Patients with bilateral calculi are at risk from the development of calculous anuria (Chap. 14).

V. Clinical Differential Diagnosis of Renal and Ureteric Calculi

Renal and ureteric colic resulting from a definitive calculus may have to be distinguished from symptoms resulting from the passage of clumps of oxalate crystals being voided down the ureter. Masses of sulphonamide crystals (given medicinally) may come to rest in the pelvic ureter following an attack of colic in patients who have not been given a protective alkaline medicine. Colic resulting from the voiding of blood clot or necrotic debris from a renal

tumour or as a late complication of a breaking down tuberculous kidney is clinically indistinguishable from colic due to calculus except after appropriate investigations (urine, radiography, cystoscopy). Renal colic clinically indistinguishable from that caused by a stone is often the first symptom resulting from a renal pelvic hydronephrosis caused by a stricture, achalasia or aberrant vessel at the pelviureteric junction.

1. Acute Pyelonephritis

Severe renal or ureteric pain somewhat similar to renal or ureteric colic produced by a calculus may usher in acute pyelonephritis, though the onset of the pain is usually more gradual and is associated with a greater feeling of tension in the renal region. There may be an early rigor and symptoms may persist for some days with fever and malaise unless relieved by treatment. The kidney is acutely tender on palpation and the urine contains pus cells, and organisms are grown on culture.

2. Embolism of the Renal Artery

Occasionally, in patients with auricular fibrillation or heart failure, an acute pain must suggest embolism of the renal artery; intravenous pyelography will reveal no renal function.

3. Extrarenal Syndrome

Several extrarenal syndromes may mimic renal and ureteric colic.

Acute appendicitis is ushered in with epigastric pain which radiates to the right iliac fossa and is commonly associated with vomiting and after some hours with slight elevation of the temperature and pulse rate. Clinically there is acute tenderness and rigidity at or near McBurney's point; the attack may subside after several hours or increase in severity until the patient is operated on.

Gall stone colic, which is ushered in by epigastric pain which radiates below the right costal margin and into the right scapular region, usually lasts for 8–12 h; it is not associated with fever, but there is acute tenderness on palpation below the ninth costal cartilage. If the condition is followed by acute cholecystitis, the painful symptoms may be prolonged for some days and are associated with fever and sometimes with slight jaundice. There is persistent abdominal tenderness in the region of the gall bladder.

Diverticulitis of the sigmoid colon may give rise to acute attacks of pain often said to simulate left-sided appendicitis, and which may mimic renal colic. There is usually a long history of chronic constipation and of recurrent attacks of aching pain; there may be a tender palpable mass in the iliac fossa or per rectum. The condition is diagnosed radiologically.

Prolapsed intervertebral disc affecting one of those between D11, D12 and L1 vertebrae sometimes gives rise to acute attacks of severe and persistent pain which closely simulate renal or ureteric colic. The diagnosis can be made radiologically.

Torsion of the pedicle of an ovarian cyst, which is not uncommon, typically gives rise to pain beginning acutely in the hypogastrium and which then radiates to the corresponding iliac fossa and to the region of the kidney and hence may mimic renal colic. The pain is quite as severe as renal or ureteric colic but usually more persistent, lasting for 2 or 3 days or until surgical interference. The diagnosis is made by the discovery of a tender cystic swelling palpable on abdominal examination or bimanually.

It is not proposed to discuss in detail the differential diagnosis of the many conditions which can give rise to the fixed pain in the renal region or in the line of the ureter resulting from calculi retained in those positions. Many vertebral, hepatic and abdominal disorders would be included in such a group, presenting usually not only with pain but also with other symptoms which would give a lead to the diagnosis.

VI. Investigation

1. Blood Tests

The serum calcium level is within the normal range (9.0–10.8 mg/100 ml) except in calculous patients with primary hyperparathyroidism, when it is usually elevated though occasionally normal (Chap. 4). The serum calcium level in patients with idiopathic hypercalciuria is discussed in Chapter 8; and the occasional raised serum calcium levels in some extrarenal diseases associated with stone (additional to primary hyperparathyroidism) is referred to in Chapter 4.

The serum phosphate level in 133 patients with renal calculus and a normal urinary calcium excretion was found by Edwards and Hodgkinson [21] to average 3.0 mg/100 ml (range between 2.0 and 5.0 mg/100 ml), a value which was significantly lower than the normal mean value ($p < 0.001$); 19 patients (14%) had serum phosphate levels which were considerably below 2.6 mg/100 ml. The mean phosphate clearance in 27 patients with renal stone and a normal urinary calcium excretion was 12.5 ml/min, a value which was significantly higher than the normal mean value.

In five calculous patients, phosphorus deprivation (induced, for example, by the administration of oral aluminium hydroxide 180 ml/day, which results in a marked fall in the urinary phosphorus and a small rise in the urinary calcium), caused a slight fall in the fasting serum phosphate level and a more marked fall in the non-fasting level; by contrast phosphorus supplementation (by the administration of disodium hydrogen phosphate dihydrate, 12 g/day, which caused a rapid increase in the urinary phosphate, a fall in the level of the urinary calcium and a positive phosphorus balance) resulted in a rise in the non-fasting serum phosphate level (but a slight fall in the fasting level) but no significant difference in the serum calcium levels. In some calculous patients with primary hyperparathyroidism (Chap. 4) and in some with idiopathic hypercalciuria (Chap. 8) the serum phosphate level is below normal. It is raised if renal function is impaired, sometimes reaching high levels. The serum phosphate level is less stable than that of the serum calcium.

The serum oxalate level in patients with renal calculi is normal, though it may be raised in the late stage of primary hyperoxaluria.

The blood urea or non-protein nitrogen must be routinely examined and urea or creatinine clearance or other renal function tests must be deployed as is necessary. The serum electrolytes (sodium, potassium, CO_2-combining power and chlorides) must be assessed in patients in whom the diagnosis of renal tubular acidosis is the question (Chap. 3) and in the more serious cases on the brink of renal failure.

2. Urine Tests

In many patients, following an attack of renal or ureteric colic red blood cells may be found microscopically in the centrifugalized sediment from the urine and occasionally frank blood or smoky urine is voided. A few leucocytes but usually no pus cells or organisms are found and the urine is sterile on culture; in the small proportion of infected cases, the urine contains pus and organisms and occasionally a trace of albumin. Of the three principal urinary constituents of the calcium oxalate stone, namely the calcium, the oxalate and the

phosphate, the first two have an especial bearing on the clinical category of calculous disease into which some of the cases fall and should be used as and when possible (Chap. 6). The recognition of idiopathic hypercalciuria (Chap. 8) and primary hyperoxaluria (Chap. 7) gives a guide as to eventual prognosis and appropriate treatment.

3. Radiodiagnosis

Renal Calculus. Calcium oxalate stones, most calcium phosphate stones and cystine stones are radio-opaque, while uric acid and matrix stones (unless admixed with calcium salts) are radiolucent. In the renal region, a rounded or ovoid shadow of the same density throughout, which lies within the renal outline is most likely to be that of a stone. The shadow of a stone in the renal pelvis bears a close relation to the inner border of the renal outline (which it may overlap) and that of a calyceal stone lies within the renal outline. The larger stones may be demonstrably laminated, coralliform, mulberry-shaped or pyramidal.

If the opaque shadow in a lateral radiograph lies superimposed over the body of a vertebra it is almost certainly that of a calculus, while a shadow lying some distance in front of the vertebral bodies is most likely to be that of a calcified tuberculous gland. The shadow of a stone has the same downward movement on inspiration as that of the renal outline (demonstrable on successive radiographs taken during full inspiration and expiration), to which it bears a constant relationship on the film. The shadow of a mobile stone within a cavity (as in a hydronephrotic renal pelvis) may not always bear a constant relationship to that of the renal outline. Multiple calculi may be in the renal pelvis or in one or more calyces or be crowded together in one dilated calyx. In the urogram the shadow of the opaque medium must be seen

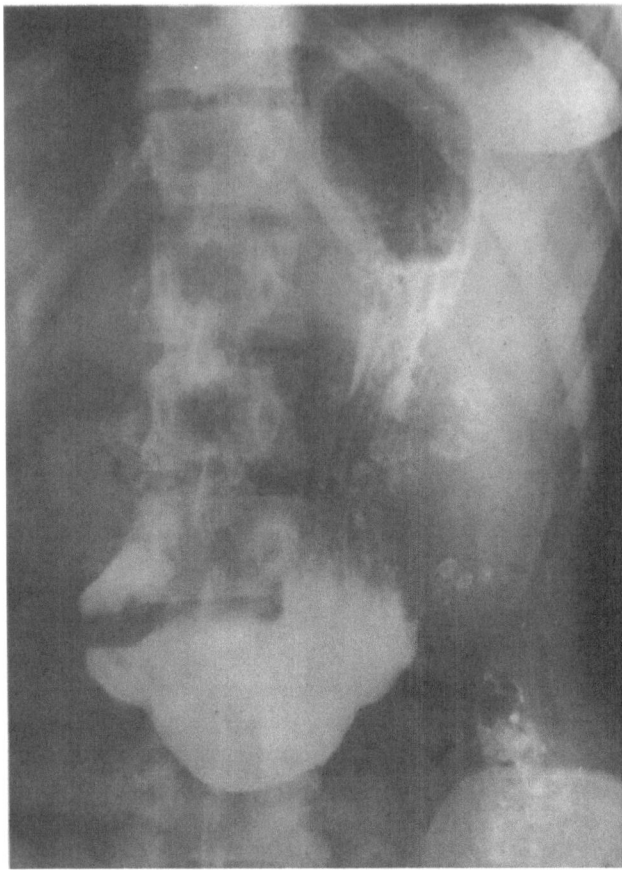

Fig. 10.2. Differential diagnosis of renal calculi: radiograph of the abdomen in a young girl suffering from indigestion; a barium meal shows a normal stomach. On the left side of the shadow of the stomach are a number of medium-sized and large stones of annular or signet-ring type overlying what appears to be the shadow of the kidney, and which could be mistaken for renal calculi. In fact the upper stones are in the pancreas while the lower group of five or six smaller stones lie in a pancreatic cyst into which they had dropped from the pancreatic duct. (By courtesy of Sir Rodney Smith, F.R.C.S.)

to overlap the shadow of the stone in order finally to establish the diagnosis.

Of the shadows in the radiograph which may mimic those of renal calculi are those of gallstones, which are usually multiple ring shadows, often laminated and faceted, and are usually outside the renal outline and on respiration move downwards and outwards. The cholecystogram and the urogram together confirm their extrarenal position. Calcification may be present in the wall of an old empyema of the gall bladder [22].

Other shadows which may mimic those of renal calculi include those of tuberculous mesenteric glands (multiple, of varying density, with fuzzy or irregular outlines, and often moving with coils of small intestine), calcified plaques in the abdominal aorta or of the renal or splenic vessels, calcified concrements in the pancreas and in the wall of a pancreatic cyst including the rare pancreatic calculi (Fig. 10.2), calcific foci in the adrenals which lie at the upper pole of the kidneys in Addison's disease, and which may almost delineate the glands on the radiograph and the incomplete or complete ring shadow characteristic of a calcified aneurysm of the renal or splenic artery.

A shadow believed to be that of a stone in the renal pelvis or the ureter can be identified with virtual certainty if an opaque catheter is passed up the ureter and is shown to be in contact with the stone in the two views (anteroposterior and lateral). The intravenous pyelogram covers the shadow of the stone and demonstrates the extent of any hydrocalycosis or hydronephrosis, and in advanced cases of calculous disease it may demonstrate the presence of some deterioration of renal function; and it also provides radiological evidence of some renal disorders with which the renal stone may be associated, including the various cysts and cystic diseases of the kidney (including polycystic kidney), horseshoe kidney, renal tuberculosis, the annular calcific deposits seen frequently in the radiographs of patients with malignant renal neoplasia and aneurysms of the intra-renal part of the renal artery. If doubt exists, a retrograde pyelogram with medium of a low density or an air-pyelogram should help to elucidate the diagnosis. Tomo-graphy can be useful in diagnosis [3, 52].

Intrarenal Calcification. The shadows of calcific foci found in renal tuberculosis, which can be mistaken for renal calculi, are usually multiple, of equal size and are disposed round an ulcerated calyx; more-over renal calculi and tuberculosis occasio-nally co-exist in the same kidney. The plain radiograph together with the intravenous pyelogram show the various types of nephrocalcinosis (really a collection of small or minute calcific foci, concrements or small calculi) in certain affected parts of the kidney, especially in the renal pyramids (in renal tubular acidosis and medullary sponge kidney) or in the cortical part of the kidney in the nephrocalcinosis occasionally seen in patients with glomerulonephritis who have had long-standing addiction to milk (Chap. 6).

Non-opaque Renal Calculi. Negative ovoid or circular shadows in the intravenous pyelograms and ureterogram may repre-sent non-opaque uric acid calculi (readily recognized by urologists in countries where that condition is fairly common), matrix calculi (which have a very low mineral

content), neoplasm of the renal pelvis or a calyx or a blood clot associated, for example, with a neoplasm, or even with a tiny calculus the shadow of which may have disappeared if a radiograph is taken 2 weeks later. Some 'non-opaque' shadows of possible stones may be of very low density and may be covered by intestinal gas so as almost to escape notice on the plain film; they can usually be diagnosed by the urogram. While uric acid stones and 'matrix' calculi may be completely radio-lucent and only diagnosed by their negative shadows, if they have a slight mineral content from admixture with calcium, their shadows come into the group of 'low density' shadows.

Pneumopyelography, or the injection of oxygen or carbon dioxide along a ureteric catheter, may assist in the identification of a small calculus of low density in the renal pelvis or a calyx.

By defining the blood supply to the stone-bearing kidney, renal angiography assists in determining the potential renal function and therefore helps to assess the desirability of conservation or ablation of a stone-bearing pole of a kidney and assists in determining the place for the line of section of the kidney or the level of the ligation of a branch of the renal artery during the operation of partial nephrectomy for lower calyceal calculi.

Ureteric Calculus. The course of the normal abdominal ureter follows a line connecting the transverse processes of the lumbar vertebrae; the upper extremity lies approxi-mately at the tip of the transverse process of the second lumbar vertebra and passes downwards and slightly inwards, crossing the transverse processes of the third and fourth lumbar vertebrae about their middle and thence to the base of the fifth lumbar vertebra. From here it passes almost verti-cally downwards across the lateral mass of the sacrum, crossing the brim of the true pelvis slightly medial to the lower end of the sacroiliac synchondrosis.

The pelvic ureter on the radiograph describes a curve with a lateral convexity, first passing downwards and outwards from the pelvic brim to a point 1 cm or more internal to the spine of the ischium and 1 in. or so from the brim of the pelvis; it then changes direction inwards to terminate 0.5 in. lateral to the tip of the coccyx.

An ellipsoidal opaque shadow of almost uniform density (and occasionally laminated or spiculated) with a fairly sharp outline and with its long axis seen in the anteroposterior radiograph along the line of the ureter, is very likely to be that of a ureteric stone; the nucleus of the stone may be observed nearer to the pointed lower extremity than to the broader upper extremity.

The shadow of a large ureteric stone may resemble that of a date stone or may assume the shape of the normal curve of the pelvic ureter. Multiple shadows are occasionally seen (two or more) as a chain of shadows in the lower part of the ureter like the beads of a rosary. The shadow of the kidney can usually be seen on the plain radiograph in a well-prepared patient and helps to differentiate a shadow of a stone in the lowest renal calyx, which lies within the renal outline, from that of a ureteric stone at or below the pelviureteric junction, which lies outside the shadow of the renal outline. The intravenous pyelogram helps to define such findings.

The ellipsoidal shadow of a stone in the intramural ureter (or just outside the bladder wall) has an almost horizontal axis and lies nearly 0.5 in. from the middle line and may lie in front of the shadow of the bladder. It can be distinguished from a stone in a vesical diverticulum situated close to the line of the ureter by the use of the intravenous pyelogram, cystogram or the indwelling opaque ureteric catheter. Stones in a ureterocele (which may be single or multiple and faceted and may lie in a dilated lower ureter), can be diagnosed by the use of the intravenous pyelo-

gram/cystogram and from the cystoscopic findings.

A stone in the upper end of the ureter of a horseshoe kidney may lie in a more lateral position than expected. The shadow of a stone in a ureter which is dilated and tortuous may lie outside the line of the normal ureter. A ureter containing a stone may be displaced from its normal position by an abdominal or pelvic tumour.

Various shadows seen on the plain radiograph, representing those of many pathological conditions, can be confused with those of ureteric calculi but can be differentiated by the use of the intravenous pyelogram or of the opaque ureteric catheter: the shadows of phleboliths (which are very common in adults) are usually multiple, well defined, spheroidal or ovoid, of a diameter rarely larger than 2–4 mm, often homogeneous but commonly fenestrated, due to a central core of organic material, and located in the pelvis (being derived from the walls of the veins of the male vesico-prostatic venous plexus or the female pampiniform plexus) and located usually in groups below and to the outer side of the line of the lower ureter below the level of the ischial spine. The shadows of calcified ileocaecal mesenteric or retroperitoneal para-aortic glands (which usually lie opposite the upper two-thirds of the ureter) are often multiple, are usually larger than ureteric calculi, of varying size and density and of irregular outline and (with the exception of retroperitoneal glands) are seen in successive radiographs to have changed their position following deep inspiration or expiration.

The shadow of a gland may overlie that of the ureter (or the ureteric catheter) and stereoscopic pictures may give the diagnosis in a doubtful case. The shadows of calcified intestinal contents include those of ingested pills, bismuth from an opaque enema examination, concretions in the vermiform appendix (which usually lie close to each other disposed in a linear fashion),

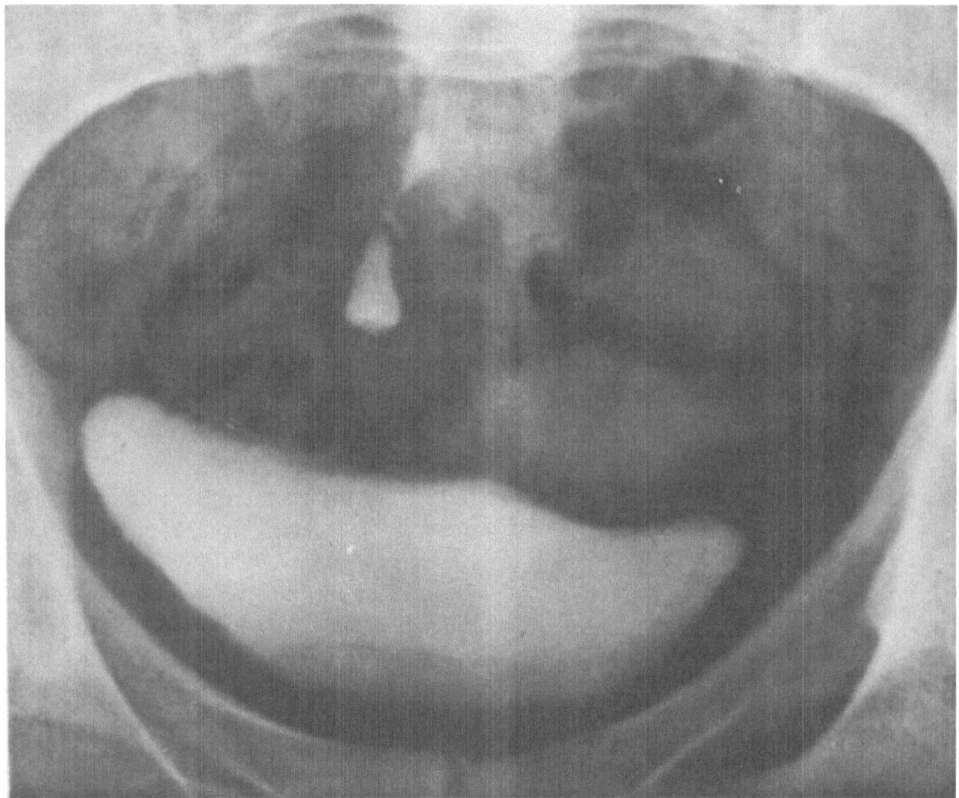

Fig. 10.3. Differential diagnosis of ureteric calculi: radiograph of a female patient aged 60, who had complained of long-standing frequency of micturition. The intravenous pyelogram was normal; on the straight radiograph there was the shadow of a well-formed tooth near the middle line of the pelvis and an imperfectly developed one at a higher level. At operation a cystic ovarian teratoma (dermoid) was removed which contained two teeth with a dental papilla, enamel organ, cartilage and smooth muscle

or the appendices epiploicae or even small hard faecal masses in the colon.

The shadows of concretions in the seminal vesicles or the vasa deferentia are small, multiple, irregular, calcified masses running obliquely upwards and outwards from above the pubic ramus and lying fairly close to the wall of the bony pelvis, but readily differentiated by the passage of an opaque ureteric catheter. The shadows of calcified foci in pelvic tumours (such as uterine fibroids), are usually seen as one or more rounded or ovoid shadows of varied density, 1 or 2 in. in diameter, and can be diagnosed by intravenous pyelography. The shadows of bone or teeth in ovarian der-

moids (which are usually palpable bimanually) may need an intravenous pyelogram for diagnosis (Fig. 10.3). The shadows of calcified atheromatous plaques in the large arteries of the pelvis are seen singly or multiply as linear, curved or tubular plaques of irregular density delineating the course of the vessels. A localized increase in the density of the tip of a lumbar transverse process or near the upper margin of the sacrum may be mistaken for a ureteric stone, the diagnosis usually being decided by the urogram.

The intravenous pyelogram demonstrates not only the stones within the ureteric lumen but also the degree of dilatation of

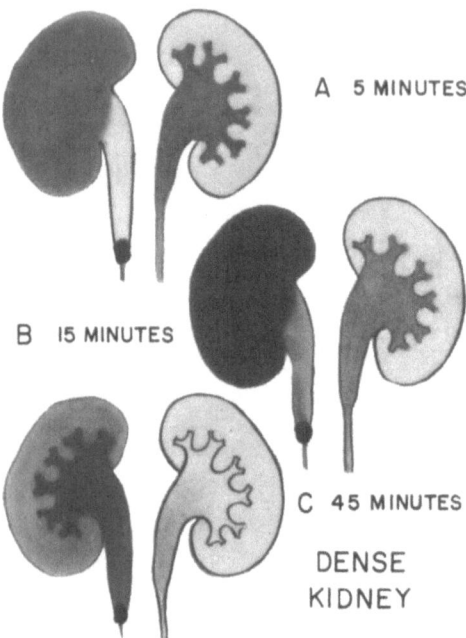

A 5 MINUTES

B 15 MINUTES

C 45 MINUTES

DENSE
KIDNEY

Fig. 10.4. Schematic drawing to show the mode of production of the 'dense kidney' in a case of a ureteric stone causing a moderate degree of obstruction. **A.** The pyelogram after 5 min shows normal filling with opaque medium of the left renal pelvis, calyces and ureter; the medium is dammed back in the right kidney to give a nephrogram effect. **B.** Pyelogram after 15 min; in the normal left kidney the medium is now less dense than at 5 min; the nephrogram effect in the right kidney now shows maximum density; the renal pelvis is still not filled with medium. **C.** 45 min: the opaque medium is now almost completely absent from the left kidney; there is still a partial nephrogram effect in the right kidney but a moderately dense filling of the pelvis and calyces with medium above the stone

the ureter above the stone (and hence the severity of the obstruction) and the state of the corresponding kidney. There may be a moderate degree of dilatation of the ureter limited to 1 in. or so above the shadow of the stone when the pyelographic medium in the kidney is of average density. Or there may be moderate dilatation of the entire ureter with early dilatation of the renal pelvis and calyces, sometimes associated with a 'nephrogram' effect with a dense

renal shadow, commonly seen in the 'acute intravenous pyelogram' referred to below.

Acute Intravenous Pyelogram. This pyelogram is taken either during or immediately following an attack of ureteric colic when the stone is probably still gripped firmly by the muscular wall of the ureter, at a time when urine is only seeping past the stone into the bladder in small amounts and is largely held up in the renal tubules and renal passages. It assists materially in the diagnosis of a small ureteric stone which is casting a doubtful shadow in the line of the ureter on the plain radiograph, when there is almost complete ureteric obstruction from a calculus. The radiograph taken 5 min after the injection of the opaque medium shows it to be largely retained in the parenchyma of the kidney on the affected side, resulting in a moderately dense shadow of the whole kidney, or a nephrogram (being more dense, the greater the degree of obstruction). There is then no opaque medium in the renal calyces and pelvis. In the opposite normal unobstructed kidney the excretion of opaque medium results in a normal radiograph of the calyces and pelvis (Fig. 10.4).

The 15-min radiograph may show that the shadow of the renal parenchyma on the side of the stone has become still more dense from the increasing concentration of opaque medium within it, but with the pelvis and calyces still not outlined by urine containing opaque medium. The opposite normal kidney now shows a complete filling of the calyces and pelvis with urine containing a high concentration of opaque medium.

The 45-min radiograph may show that the opaque medium has now completely disappeared from the opposite normal kidney, while on the side containing the calculus the renal shadow is much less dense but the calyces, renal pelvis and ureter are filled with urine containing opaque medium of moderate density.

Subsequent radiographs taken at intervals of 2, 3 or even up to 24 h may show that opaque medium remains, casting a moderately dense shadow of the kidney on the affected side, and the shadows of the pelvis, calyces and ureter may now be quite dense and may demonstrate a hydronephrosis and hydroureter (down to the level of the stone, which can then be identified on the radiograph).

The technique of the acute intravenous pyelogram finds its greatest use in a patient with ureteric colic, where the plain radiograph does not reveal a shadow which can be identified with certainty as a calculus, or at most reveals a tiny doubtful shadow (perhaps not very dense) in the line of the ureter, which may scarcely have been noted. The tell-tale column of radio-opaque urine within a dilated ureter on the intravenous pyelogram, ending abruptly at the very doubtful shadow and even obscuring it, provides convincing evidence of the presence of a very small calculus arrested in the ureter. Many small stones which were formerly missed can be diagnosed with virtual certainty by the use of this technique.

Stones in the Intramural Ureter. The diagnosis here is sometimes helped by a cystogram, which may delineate on the radiograph the trigone and the ureteric ridge, especially in males in whom they are well developed. This useful feature can be achieved if the central beam of the X-ray apparatus is so directed as to give a tangential view of the trigone and the base of the bladder [22].

With the patient in the supine position, the anteroposterior axis of the bladder is inclined several degrees in the caudo-cranial direction, when the interureteric ridge may be visualized as having a crescentic contour with the concavity looking cranially [20].

When a stone is impacted in the intramural ureter, there is often a great deal of periureteric oedema (which can be confirmed cystoscopically), which increases the normal distance (2–3 mm) between the lumen of the ureter and the interureteric ridge. Such a finding, along with the presence of a calcific shadow, may indicate the correct diagnosis of ureteric stone.

Large filling defects or radiolucent zones (cylindrical, tulip-shaped, oval or rounded) may be observed around the stone or the dilated ureter when there is extensive periureteric oedema, mimicking somewhat the radiographic appearance of a ureterocele. Sometimes irritation and oedema round the intramural ureter may even cause a strictly unilateral spastic contraction of the bladder for a short time after the stone has been voided.

Radiography Following Passage of an Opaque Catheter. Although the topography of the shadow of the probable ureteric calculus and the intravenous pyelogram together usually make the diagnosis of the ureteric calculus virtually certain, in a few patients the passage of an opaque ureteric catheter to the level of the stone or past it is needed to establish the diagnosis. Anteroposterior and oblique radiographs jointly demonstrating that the suspected shadow is in contact with that of the catheter, renders the diagnosis of ureteric stone quite certain.

Stereoscopic X-rays may also help at this stage. Thus in a dilated ureter, between the shadow of the supposed stone and that of the opaque ureteric catheter, there may be a clear space, which may be correctly interpreted by the help of stereoscopic X-rays. The injection of opaque medium (which may adhere to the calculus) along the ureteric catheter so as to give an additional shadow continuous with that of the catheter may give assistance if the catheter is arrested for some reason 1 or 2 cm below the shadow of the supposed stone. The shadow of the injected opaque medium must then be in continuity with that of the suspected stone, or the suspected shadow must be visible within the shadow of the dye or be completely obscured by it.

The use of the parallax method may help in the diagnosis of ureteric stone. After the opaque catheter has been passed, if possible beyond the stone, a film is exposed, following which manoeuvre the X-ray tube is moved transversely 6–10 cm and a second exposure of the X-ray is made on the same film. If the opacity believed to be that of a stone lies in the ureter, the same relationship of the shadow to that of the ureteric catheter is maintained in the two images. A ureteric calculus can often be visualized using image-intensifier control, especially if a ureteric catheter is passed and opaque medium injected along it; the image of the stone and the opacified ureter can be projected onto a television screen.

Radiolucent Ureteric Calculi. Calculi composed of uric acid or xanthine which come to rest in the ureter can be suspected on the radiograph by the presence of a rounded or ovoid filling defect or translucent zone in the ureterogram (for example, during intravenous pyelography), the ureter above the stone then being seen to be dilated or in a state of spasm, and the lacuna resulting from its presence being partly surrounded by opaque medium. A stone may be partly radio-opaque (usually at the centre) and partly radiolucent at the periphery. Care must be taken to exclude radiotranslucence resulting from the presence of air-bubbles introduced accidentally, for example, when injecting the contrast medium up the ureteric catheter. Filling defects in the ureteric shadow may also be present in the ureterogram of ureters containing tumours, the medium then surrounding them.

A double kidney should be recognized from the pyelogram and a calculus may obstruct the ureter from one half of such a kidney, the other half being of normal calibre. There may be delayed (or no) secretion from one half of an obstructed double kidney, with normal secretion from

the other half; the shadow of the supposed stone may then be thought to be outside the ureter and the existence of a double kidney may not be evident.

Benign Peripelvic and Periureteric Urinary Extravasation. During intravenous pyelography this anomaly has sometimes been observed and diagnosed during radiography for patients with ureteric calculi causing partial ureteric obstruction and also following the application of ureteric compression by an abdominal binder during intravenous pyelography. The condition may also (possibly quite commonly) occur in association with ureteric colic resulting from the lodgement of a stone in the ureter; the patient may experience pain. The extravasate tends to spread into the renal sinus possibly through a leak at the calyceal fornix (and not from a gross rupture of the renal pelvis), and thence by way of the renal hilus into the retroperitoneal space and downwards along the course of the ureter [25, 32, 45, 47]. The condition seems to resolve fairly readily and it does not lead to dire consequences.

4. Cystoscopic Examination

In most patients with an aseptic renal calculus in a calyx or the renal pelvis during the quiet phase, the cystoscopic appearances of the bladder mucosa and the corresponding ureteric orifice are usually normal. Occasionally there is slight oedema of the orifice, which may be dilated and injected if a calculus has been voided recently (following renal colic), smoky urine or actual blood being discharged from the ureter if the examination is conducted during an attack of haematuria.

After a calculus has entered the ureter, the corresponding ureteric orifice and mucosa over the adjacent intramural ureter may be seen to be oedematous, patulous and rigid, and to be beset with tiny red punctiform or stellate haemorrhagic zones with modified colour changes as the stone descends. Though the ureteric orifice may be seen to contract vigorously, there is either no efflux (urine being temporarily held up by the stone) or it is sluggish and intermittent (with incomplete obstruction) and possibly blood-stained. Such changes may be observed for a few days following the attack of colic and then slowly disappear.

If the urine is infected, a turbid, muddy or purulent efflux from an oedematous, swollen or pouting ureteric orifice is indicative of the presence of pyelonephritis; with a pyonephrosis, ribbon-like accretions of thick pus may be discharged intermittently (perhaps with a small efflux of urine).

When the stone lies in the ureter just outside the bladder wall, only slight ureteric changes (or sometimes none at all) may be recognizable cystoscopically, though sometimes the relatively immobile ureteric orifice may be gaping and fixed (and red and oedematous if the urinary tract is infected). When the stone lies in the intramural part of the ureter, typically there is well-marked oedema around the ureteric orifice, and, when the stone is firmly impacted there is a swollen or pouting collar of mucous membrane, sometimes beset with spawn-like bullae of varying size and radiating folds (sometimes mimicking a villous vesical tumour), which render the actual rigid and motionless ureteric orifice difficult to identify unless the dark-coloured stone is actually presenting at the orifice. If the stone lies 0.5 in. or so from the orifice, a local elongated swelling of the distended ureter extending upwards and outwards from the swollen orifice, indicates the position of the calculus in the ureter; the orifice may still be surrounded by the swollen mucosal collar just described.

If the stone has been extruded into the bladder shortly before cystoscopy it may be seen lying loose in the trigone, and (accord-

ing to the time that has elapsed) the ureteric changes will be judged to have receded. Rarely, a stone ulcerates through the intramural wall of the ureter (above the ureteric orifice) into the bladder leaving a ragged fistulous opening above and to the outer side of the true ureteric opening, which can be recognized separately from the fistula.

5. Isotope Renography

Isotope renography with the I^{131} Hippuran renogram yields useful information in the investigation of patients with ureteric calculous obstruction, though the necessary information can usually be obtained by radiography; it is useful in comparing the function of the two kidneys in diseased conditions. The normal renogram shows an initial vascular phase, followed by a secretory phase reaching a peak within 4 min, and an excretory phase which falls to half the peak count rate within 10 min. The tracing indicating the obstruction of the kidney shows a continuing rise in the secretory phase after 4 min, with a delayed excretory phase, representing the accumulation of I^{131} Hippuran within the obstructed collecting system. If an acute obstruction persists for longer than 72 h the trace flattens to show a pattern of non-function, which may be reversible on relief of the obstruction (Fig. 10.5, see p. 206).

VII. Urolithiasis in Children

The incidence of urinary calculi in children in the United States and Canada is less than that in England, according to Williams [57], who considered that the discrepancy could not be accounted for by dietetic differences [24].

In a series of 133 children under the age of 12 with urinary calculi (observed during a 12-year period) reported by Williams, 13

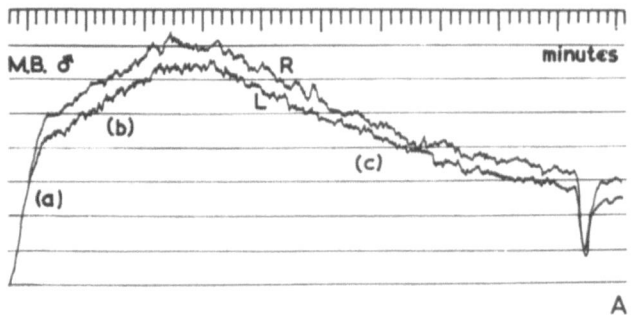

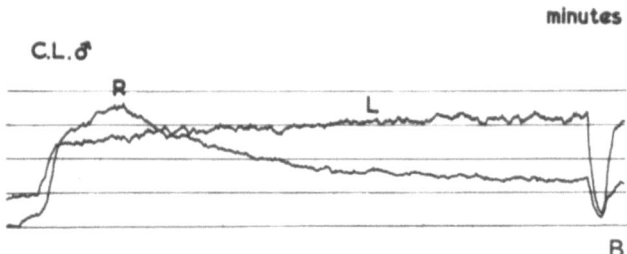

Fig. 10.5. Isotope renography:
A. The normal renogram.
B. Renogram showing left
ureteric obstruction due to a
stone. (By courtesy of Mr. P.
Smith, F.R.C.S.)

had a metabolic origin (cystinuria, hyperoxaluria, recumbency), in 34 the stones had
formed in dilated renal pelves or ureters,
and 75 were characterized as idiopathic.
Stones which had formed in non-infected
urine were found at any age within the
group and usually contained calcium
phosphate.

Williams [57] reported that infected renal
calculi (usually associated with *B. proteus*),
found usually during the first 3 years of life,
are the most common calculi seen in
children in Britain today, being mostly composed of ammonium magnesium phosphate with smaller amounts of other
substances and probably initiated by infection. They were thought possibly to belong
to the group of stones in which Murphy and
Pyrah [42] had believed that the colloid
element had been laid down first, crystallization in the matrix occurring later. These
calculi (usually multiple and sometimes
staghorn calculi) were found often bilaterally in the renal pelvis and the calyces
(and sometimes also in the bladder) and

were usually hard in consistency, though
sometimes soft and radiolucent.

Urinary calculi in children may complicate congenital anatomical defects in the
urinary tract (pelviureteric hydronephrosis,
horseshoe kidney, ureterocele, obstruction
of the bladder neck) or metabolic disorders
(primary hyperoxaluria, cystinuria, the uric
acid syndrome, the familial type of hyperparathyroidism [49]). In Winkel-Smith's
[59] series of 71 cases of urolithiasis in
children, anomalies of the urinary tract
were found in 58. In the series of 24 cases
reported by Daeschner [15] infection and
obstruction were the etiological factors in
14 and metabolic factors in 5. Bilateral
calculi are often found in children as in
adults [9, 34].

The symptoms resulting from the presence of renal stone in infants and young
children may be difficult to interpret
because they are unable to describe them
meaningfully. Some children with calculi
have had the appendix removed possibly
unnecessarily because of difficulty in diag-

nosis. The most common clinical symptoms are fever, abdominal pain, recognizable renal colic (though less common than in adults), haematuria and pyuria; painless haematuria has been reported [16].

On the negative side of diagnosis the palpable mass in the loin or elsewhere in the abdomen (an important clinical finding in some infants and young children who are too young to describe their symptoms) seems very rarely to have been the result of renal calculous disease (and indeed in none of the 615 infants and children with this syndrome reviewed by Melicow and Uson [40], the commonest diagnosis then being large hydronephrosis, Wilm's tumour of the kidney and renal cystic disease). Anuria was recorded (the stone presumably not having been previously recognized) in 12 cases in children reported by Campbell [13], in 3 resulting from bilateral calculous obstruction from among 75 cases of urinary lithiasis in children reported by Eckstein [19], and in single patients recorded by Gürsel [30] and by Bower and Fowler [8] in a single functioning kidney. In children as in adults calculi may be voided spontaneously, as in 26 of 71 cases reported by Winkel-Smith [59].

The composition of the stone in children has varied in different series; thus in Winkel-Smith's [59] series of 71 cases (the stone having been analysed in 33), in 31 it was composed of calcium oxalate with phosphate and urate, only 2 being infected stones. In Campbell's [13] series one-third of the cases were composed of uric acid, while in Myers' [43] series a high proportion were phosphatic.

Successful operations similar to those carried out in adults can usually be done in children if indicated; thus in Winkel-Smith's [59] series, of 63 operations performed on 53 patients nephrectomy was done in 7, simple removal of the stone in 36, and multiple operations in 9. Stones were successfully removed in three children by Delta and McKendry [16].

VIII. Renal and Ureteric Calculus in Pregnancy

Renal calculi observed during pregnancy, but which must have originated at an earlier date, have been reported in the literature largely because of the special problems they have created. The dilatation of the upper urinary passages during pregnancy may be expected to encourage the spontaneous voiding at least of small renal and ureteric calculi. The associated urinary infection which sometimes occurs during pregnancy may be expected to encourage stone formation, though in fact such infection rarely seems to do so; however, renal stone and infection sometimes are present in the same patient [26].

1. Clinical Picture

A renal stone may be completely symptomless during pregnancy. While symptoms when present may often be characteristic of stone, they are not always the expected ones, and hence may easily be overlooked. Examples of their recognition under unusual circumstances were seen in Walsh's [56] three cases. The first patient complained of pain in the fourteenth week and two stones were removed by nephrolithotomy. The second patient was thought to have had a toxic albuminuria with associated oedema, when a routine radiograph revealed a large, apparently symptomless, branched calculus, a functionless kidney being removed 3 months after an induced delivery. The third patient developed an extraperitoneal abscess which complicated a large stone in the right kidney.

Of 20 patients with renal or ureteric calculi reported by Arnell and Getzoff [4], 9 had surgical procedures, 6 during pregnancy. In McVann's [38] 12 patients with calculi (one in the renal pelvis and 11 in the ureter) 8 had been recognized during the second and 3 in the third trimester.

Of 35 cases of patients with renal calculi seen during pregnancy, reported by Harris and Dunnihoe [31] those seen in the early months presented usually with renal colic while in those seen after the fourth month of gestation an associated renal infection was a more common indication of their presence. In 10 the stone was voided spontaneously and 5 needed operative treatment.

2. Treatment

While the management of urinary calculi in pregnant women should be as conservative as possible for fear of precipitating an abortion, it is relatively safe to remove stones from the kidney or from the upper part of the ureter by open operation during the first 3 months and even during the second 3 months of pregnancy if symptoms seem to indicate this. A small stone in the ureter should, if possible, be dealt with by perureteral instrumentation in preference to operation. Operative removal of a stone from the lower end of the ureter must be physically almost impossible during the last 3 months of pregnancy and is contraindicated. It is generally agreed that termination of the pregnancy is not indicated simply because of the presence of a stone.

References

1. Abeshouse,B.S.: Rupture of the renal pelvis. Surg. Gynecol. Obstet. 60, 710 (1935)
2. Abeshouse,B.S.: Renal and ureteral fistula of visceral and cutaneous types; report of four cases. Urol. Cutan. Rev. 53, 641 (1949)
3. Ambos,M.K., Bosmiak,M.A.: Tomography of the kidney bed as an aid in differentiating renal pelvic tumour and stone. Am. J. Roentgenol. 125, 331 (1975)
4. Arnell,R.E., Getzoff,P.L.: Renal and ureteral calculi in pregnancy. Am. J. Obstet. Gynecol. 44, 34 (1942)
5. Baker,R., Connelly,J.P.: Bilateral and recurrent renal calculi: evidence indicating renal collagen abnormality and results of salicylate therapy. J. Am. Med. Assoc. 160, 1106 (1956)
6. Bell,E.T.: Study of approximately 25,000 autopsies for reported incidence of urolithiasis. In: Renal diseases. Philadelphia: Lea and Febiger 1946
7. Bollack,C. et al.: Spontaneous rupture of the upper urinary apparatus (4 cases). J. Urol. Nephrol. (Paris) 77, 850 (1971)
8. Bower,D.B., Fowler,D.B.: A case of anuria due to ureteric stone in a child. Br. J. Urol. 31, 164 (1959)
9. Bruezière,J. et al.: Idiopathic renal lithiasis in infants. Report of 40 cases. J. Urol. Nephrol. (Paris), 80, 589 (1974)
10. Bülow,H. et al.: Spontaneous kidney perforation, at present a rare complication of kidney calculi. Med. Welt, 27, 87 (1976)
11. Burch,P.R.J., Burwell,R.G.: Self and nonself. A clonal induction approach to immunity. Q. Rev. Biol. 40, 352 (1965)
12. Burch,P.R.J., Dawson,J.B.: A biological implication of the sex and age distribution of renal lithiasis. In: Renal Stone Research Symposium. Hodgkinson,A., Nordin, B.E.C. (eds.). London: Churchill 1969
13. Campbell,M.F.: Clinical pediatric urology. Philadelphia: Saunders 1951
14. Cibert,J. et al.: Painful symptomatology of caliceal calculi. J. Urol. Nephrol. (Paris) 78, 197 (1972)
15. Daeschner,C.W., Singleton,E.B., Curtis, J.C.: Urinary tract calculi and nephrocalcinosis in infants and children. J. Pediat. 57, 721 (1960)
16. Delta,B.G., McKendry,J.B.: Urolithiasis in children; report of three cases and review of the literature. Can. Med. Assoc. 82, 353 (1960)
17. Dempsey,E.F.: Urinary oxalate excretion in relation to renal stone formation. J. Clin. Invest. 36, 882 (1957)
18. Dempsey,E.F., Forbes,A.O., Melick,R.A., Henneman,P.H.: Urinary oxalate excretion. Metabolism 9, 52 (1960)
19. Eckstein,H.B.: Calculous anuria in children. Br. J. Urol. 32, 269 (1960)
20. Edling,N.P.G.: Further studies of the interureteric ridge of the bladder. Acta Radiol. 30, 69 (1948)
21. Edwards,N.A., Hodgkinson,A.: Phosphate metabolism in patients with renal calculi. Clin. Sci. 29, 93 (1965)
22. Emmett,J.L.: Clinical radiography: an atlas and textbook of roentgenologic diagnosis. 2nd ed. Vol. I. Philadelphia and London: Saunders 1964

23. Garvey,F.K., Boyce,W.H.: Diagnostic and therapeutic problems incidental to surgical management of 'malignant' renal calculous disease. J. Int. Coll. Surg. *25*, 318 (1956)
24. Ghazalis,S., Barratt,T.M., Williams,D.I.: Childhood urolithiasis in Britain. Arch. Dis. Child. *48*, 291 (1973)
25. Ginsberg,S.A.: Spontaneous urinary extravasation in association with renal colic and ureteric calculus. J. Urol. *94*, 192 (1965)
26. Gödde,S.: Urinary calculi and pregnancy. Dtsch. Med. J. *21*, 536 (1970)
27. Goldblatt,H., Lynch,J., Hanzal,R.F., Summerville,W.W.: Studies on experimental hypertension. J. Exp. Med. *59*, 347 (1934)
28. Goldstein,A.E.: Familial urological diseases. Am. J. Surg. *17*, 221 (1951)
29. Gram,H.C.: Heredity of oxalic urinary calculi. Acta Med. Scand. *78*, 268 (1932)
30. Gürsel,A.E.: Sur un cas d'anurie chez un enfant de 8 ans. J. Urol. Med. Chir. *58*, 1212 (1952)
31. Harris,R.E., Dunnihoe,D.R.: Incidence and significance of urinary calculi in pregnancy. Am. J. Obstet. Gynecol. *99*, 237 (1967)
32. Hinman,F.: Peripelvic extravasation during intravenous urography, evidence for an additional route for backflow after ureteral obstruction. J. Urol. *85*, 385 (1961)
33. Ljunghall,S., Hedstrand,H.: Epidemiology of renal stone in a middle-aged population. Acta Med. Scand. *197*, 439 (1975)
34. Malek,R.S., Celalis,P.P.: Pediatric nephrolithiasis. J. Urol. *113*, 545 (1975)
35. Marshall,V., White,R.H., De Saintonge, M.C., Tresidder,G.C., Blandy,J.P.: The natural history of renal and ureteric calculi. Br. J. Urol. *47*, 117 (1975)
36. McGeown,M.G.: Heredity in renal stone disease. Clin. Sci. *19*, 465 (1960)
37. McIntosh,J.F., Read,M.K.: Oxalic acid excretion in oxalate lithiasis. J. Urol. *80*, 272 (1958)
38. McVann,R.M.: Urinary calculi associated with pregnancy. Am. J. Obstet. Gynecol. *89*, 314 (1964)
39. Melick,R.A., Henneman,P.H.: Clinical and laboratory studies of 207 consecutive patients in a kidney stone clinic. N. Engl. J. Med. *259*, 307 (1958)
40. Melicow,M.N., Uson,A.C.: Palpable abdominal masses in infants and children: a report based on a review of 653 cases. J. Urol. *81*, 705 (1959)
41. Murphy,B.T., Purton,M.J.: Personal communication: unpublished results (1968)
42. Murphy,B.T., Pyrah,L.N.: The composition, structure, and mechanisms of the formation of urinary calculi. Br. J. Urol. *34*, 129 (1962)
43. Myers,N.A.: Urolithiasis in childhood. Arch. Dis. Child. *32*, 48 (1957)
44. Mylvagnan,H.B.: An unusually large renal calculus. Lancet *II*, 898 (1920)
45. Narath,P.A.: Extrarenal extravasation observed in the course of intravenous urography. J. Urol. *39*, 65 (1938)
46. Narath,P.A.: Renal Pelvis and Ureter. New York: Grune & Stratton 1951
47. Olsson,O.: Studies on back-flow in excretion urography. Acta. Radiol. *24*, 411 (1948)
48. Pridgen,D.B., Resnick,M., Goodman,H.D., Boyce,W.H.: Inheritance of calcium renal stones. Lancet, *I*, 537 (1968)
49. Pyrah,L.N., Hodgkinson,A., Anderson, C.K.: Primary hyperparathyroidism. A critical review. Br. J. Surg. *53*, 245 (1966)
50. Richaud,C. et al.: Spontaneous urinary extravasation associated with nephritic colic (à propos of 4 cases). J. Urol. Nephrol. (Paris) *78*, 148 (1972)
51. Schumann,H.J. et al.: Nephrolithiasis, unilateral pyelonephritic kidney, cirrhosis and hypertension (a statistical autopsy study). Zentralbl. Allg. Pathol. *113*, 229 (1970)
52. Silver,T.M., Koff,S.A., Thornbury,J.: An unusual pathway of urine extravasation associated with renal colic. Radiology, *109*, 537 (1973)
53. Smith,R.M. et al.: Tomography for evaluation of renal lithiasis. J. State Med. Soc. *128*, 144 (1976)
54. Sutherland,J.W.: Recurrence following operation for upper urinary tract stone. Br. J. Urol. *26*, 22 (1954)
55. Thomas,J., Berge,D., Brunschwig,J.F., Abouker,P.: Caractères sexuals et facteurs génétiques des trois grandes variétés chroniques de lithiases renales: urique, oxalique phosphatiques. Rein Foie *8*, 147 (1966)
56. Walsh,C.H.: Renal calculus in pregnancy. Br. Med. J. *I*, 814 (1936)
57. Williams,D.I.: Urinary calculi in England. Urologists' Correspondence Club 11/2/72 p. 10, 1972
58. Williams,R.E.: Long-term survey of 538 patients with upper urinary tract stone. Br. J. Urol. *35*, 416 (1963)
59. Winkel-Smith,C.C.: On urinary lithiasis in childhood. Clinical study of 71 cases of urinary calculi in children. Acta Chir. Scand. *90*, 179 (1944)

Chapter 11

Some General Considerations in the Surgical Treatment of Renal and Ureteric Stone

Before considering the techniques of the various operations in use for the treatment of renal stone, it is appropriate to consider some of the factors relevant to the operations for the removal of renal calculi taken as a whole. Some limitations to operative procedure are imposed by the anatomy of the renal vasculature. The extent to which incisions can be made in the renal parenchyma without too much resultant damage, the amount of the total renal tissue in the body which can be removed without jeopardizing the health of the patient, and the extent to which a completely obstructed kidney can recover after removal of the obstruction, have considerable relevance to the surgery of renal stone.

In a kidney which is the seat of what may be called the surgical diseases (stone, infection and obstruction) renal function is never a static attribute. The kidney possesses a surprising degree of functional dynamism which varies with the pathology. If one kidney is removed the opposite kidney can undergo functional hyperplasia, thereby providing more than enough renal tissue to sustain life.

I. Blood Supply of the Kidney

A massive array of data concerning the blood supply of the kidney [8, 10, 23] has revealed the fact that the ordinary text-book description applies (in full detail) to only about one-third of the population [32]. In the kidney (and also in the liver and the suprarenals) the anatomical arrangement of the blood supply varies greatly in different individuals. Renal angiography has enabled a further contribution to be made to its study.

Hyrtl [23] showed that the renal artery divides into branches which supply the dorsal and ventral parts of the kidney respectively, making a natural division between the two arterial trees. The zone between these two vascular systems, which lies 0.5 in. dorsal to the convex border, is the so-called exsanguinated renal zone of Hyrtl or the non-vascular zone.

Brödel [8], using corrosion casts of the kidney, confirmed this contention and maintained that the anterior division of the renal artery supplies three-quarters of the kidney, while the posterior division supplies one-quarter. In order to select a relatively avascular area and avoid the division of the collecting tubules of the posterior pyramids, he suggested that the incision into a kidney for the removal of a calculus should be made just posterior to the convex border along a line which came to be called the 'bloodless line of Brödel'. Anatomical studies of the arteries of the kidney demonstrate, in fact, how impossible it is to select a strictly 'bloodless' incision in any part of the kidney. The chief importance, however, of Brödel's incision is that it probably avoids the principal arterial trunks and divides only smaller arterioles; since the renal arteries are usually said to be end-arteries it perhaps reduces the extent of the necrosis of renal tissue to a minimum.

Recent studies of the renal vasculature have been made by Graves [11, 12, 14]. The renal arteries of more than 30 human kidneys removed at autopsy were injected with liquid polyester resin, which was allowed to set, after which the renal parenchyma was removed by corrosion in concentrated hydrochloric acid, enabling casts of the renal vessels to be prepared. Angiograms were also prepared by injecting 50% and 70% diodone into the renal artery and vein. He found that the kidney was divisible into several segments (apical, upper anterior, middle anterior, lower and posterior), each of which was supplied by its own artery. The main stem of the renal artery divides at a variable point between the aorta and the hilum of the kidney into two branches or divisions: the anterior division, which gives rise to the upper, middle and lower segmental arteries and usually the apical segmental artery; and the posterior division, which continues into the kidney to supply only the posterior segment, though it may also give rise to the apical segmental artery. The apical segment of the kidney is a cap of tissue on the medial side (and mostly on the anterior surface) of the upper pole of the kidney.

The main arteries subdivide into smaller branches after entering the renal substance. The posterior segmental artery, which is a continuation of the posterior division of the renal artery, enters the posterior aspect of the hilum running from front to back across the upper border of the renal pelvis, after which it passes behind and in close association with the junction of the upper calyx and the pelvis (a constant landmark), and then divides into three groups of branches supplying the posterior surface of the calyces and renal parenchyma.

No evidence was found of a collateral blood supply between the segments, when, for example, the segmental arteries were injected separately with the resin. If a segmental artery was ligated before resin was injected into the main stem, a 'bare area' was subsequently found in the cast corresponding to the segment excluded by the ligated artery. The course of the renal vein and its tributaries was found to be similar to that of the arteries but a free venous

anastomosis within the kidney was shown to exist.

A practical application of the study is that the ligature of a segmental artery will produce a bloodless field of operation if the segment is subsequently exactly resected. Moreover, the segmental arteries can often easily be seen in the hilum and sometimes at points nearer the aorta. Temporary compression of a division of the main renal artery results in a purplish discoloration of the area supplied, and its recognition assists in determining the amount of tissue which should ideally be resected. Examination of the renal casts confirmed that the so-called bloodless line of Brödel [8] is by no means bloodless. The segmental arterial pattern of the kidney in patients with renal calculous disease was not found to be materially different from that seen in a normal kidney. Other studies on the renal blood supply were made by Renon et al. [42], Smithius [46], and Syme [51].

Many of the so-called aberrant or accessory renal arteries are really normal segmental vessels with a precocious origin, and the presence of additional vessels at the hilum is due to an early division of the main renal artery [10].

The lower segmental artery, which can usefully be ligated before the performance of a lower polar partial nephrectomy, may have its origin from the aorta or from the trunk of the main renal artery close to its origin in the aorta; sometimes the main artery does not divide until it reaches the hilum.

Merklin and Michels [32], who examined dissections of the blood supply of 185 kidneys, found that the renal artery was one single vessel in 72%, was double in 10% of the cases examined, and that (rarely) triple or even quadruple renal arteries occur. Superior polar arteries arise from the aorta in 7% and from the renal artery in 12% of cases; aortic inferior polar arteries occur in 5.5% and renal inferior polar arteries in 1.4%. These workers confirmed the **work of**

Graves [11, 12] concerning the segmental distribution of the branches of the renal artery.

II. Amount of Renal Tissue Needed to Sustain Life

Clinical observations on the ability of an individual to survive, when both kidneys are known to be badly diseased from any cause, are commonplace. Many patients with bilateral chronic glomerulonephritis or bilateral staghorn calculi (both kidneys being infected) with considerable impairment of renal function, may live for several years and many can even work with little apparent embarrassment. In a different context the whole of one kidney and a considerable part of the remaining kidney have not infrequently been removed surgically for malignant tumour and for various other conditions; the quality of life under such circumstances may be finely balanced.

A similar problem arises in relation to the performance of operations for calculous disease as to how much of the total renal tissue in the body can safely be removed surgically without impairing health. The amount of normal renal tissue needed to maintain life varies within a certain range in different species of animals. Dogs and cats need 25% of their total renal tissues; rats can exist with only one-sixth of theirs, rabbits with 40% and goats with 10%–15% [1].

In man it is possible to live when one kidney and at least one-third and probably even one-half of the other kidney has been removed, provided the remaining portion of the second kidney is healthy. Probably at least 300,000 nephrons are removed during the standard operation of partial nephrectomy. It follows that approximately one-fourth of the total renal substance in the body (or one-half of one kidney) is necessary to sustain life.

It is known that after the removal of one diseased kidney the other kidney undergoes functional hyperplasia (or hypertrophy). But after partial nephrectomy of the solitary kidney Bitker and Bitker [5] found that the creatinine clearance averaged about 30% and the PAH clearance 62% of the values prior to the operation. These parameters of function stabilized eventually at about 55% and 53% respectively of their preoperative values. Osmolar clearances were lower than the control value. These workers found, therefore, no compensatory increase in function in the remaining renal tissue after excision of about one-third of the solitary hypertrophied kidney; this finding is referred to in the following section.

The removal of one kidney and of one-third of the other kidney by partial nephrectomy was successfully accomplished in 10 of 296 patients submitted to partial nephrectomy collected from the literature by Abeshouse and Lerman [1]. In the author's department a similar combination of operative procedures has been carried out successfully on at least four occasions for renal calculous disease. In carrying out such a bilateral operative programme for the treatment of advanced calculous disease, when the total renal tissue is to be reduced to near the limits of safety, the procedure should be done in stages. Probably an interval of at least 2–3 weeks is desirable following the removal of the first diseased kidney, before partial nephrectomy is carried out on the second kidney. Similarly the operation of bilateral partial nephrectomy should be timed so as to allow a suitable interval between the two operations.

III. Compensatory Hypertrophy of the Kidney Following Nephrectomy

When one kidney has been removed in man, the remaining kidney undergoes considerable enlargement. There is no increase in the number of nephrons (that is, there is no growth by hyperplasia). The total blood supply to the remaining kidney gradually increases, the individual nephrons and renal cells enlarge and there is an increase in its functional capacity (that is, there is growth by hypertrophy). It has been suggested that the hypertrophy is under the control of a renotropic hormone. Work in the experimental animal has thrown light upon the structural and physiological changes of compensatory hypertrophy.

1. In the Experimental Animal

Allen [2] resected one kidney and a part of the remaining kidney in dogs, the largest fraction of total renal tissue to have been removed being not less than three-fourths. It was found that as little as one-fourth of the renal substance left behind was capable of maintaining a normal concentration of the blood urea. The larger the proportion of total renal substance resected (but not in excess of 70%) the greater was the relative hypertrophy (glomeruli and tubules) which occurred. In rats and rabbits fed with a protein-rich diet or one which contained 30% urea, much larger kidneys developed following the removal of one kidney than in the control animals on a standard diet. In animals fed on a diet containing 15% concentration of sodium chloride, the kidneys secreted a much larger amount of urine but did not grow larger than in the control animals. It was suggested that compensatory hypertrophy is a physiological reaction.

Levy and Blalock [25] showed that after the removal of one kidney the amount of blood which flowed through the remaining kidney slowly increased, and that in 3 months it had reached approximately that which normally passed through the normal kidneys. Oliver [35] showed that the removal of one and one-half kidneys resul-

ted in a fivefold increase in the size of the proximal tubule but in only a twofold increase of the residual total renal mass.

Using rats, Platt et al. [37] removed the upper and lower poles of one kidney, and after 10–14 days the whole of the opposite kidney. A variable degree of hypertrophy of the surviving renal remnant took place which in four cases exceeded 100%, affecting mainly the middle and terminal portions of the proximal convoluted tubules and the loops of Henle. Block at al. [6] found that following the removal of one kidney in the rat, the remaining kidney increased by 20%–88% in weight, and that there was a rapid increase in its functional capacity.

In the dog, Rous and Wakin [44] found that the functional capacity of the remaining kidney started to increase as early as 24 h after operation and that later there was a decline in functional activity for a few weeks, following which it increased to the levels which were obtained just after operation. They found, however, that no compensatory increase in function occurred in the remaining renal tissue after excision of about a third of a solitary hypertrophied kidney.

The production of the compensatory hypertrophy of the opposite kidney following unilateral nephrectomy is thought to be influenced by many factors such as the added solute excretory load placed on the remaining kidney [34], by anabolic hormones and dietary proteins, and by the action of the anterior lobe of the pituitary.

Specific Renotropic Factors. The possibility that a specific renotropic factor found in the body following unilateral nephrectomy, stimulates hypertrophy of the remaining kidney, has received attention in recent years. In the search for a possible kidney-specific, mitosis-stimulating humoral factor in the serum of the experimental animal following unilateral nephrectomy, Ogawa and Nowinski [34], using renal tissue culture techniques, concluded that 42 h after nephrectomy the serum of rats contained such a factor.

Lowenstein and Stern [28] found that the effect of the renotropic substance formed in the rat after unilateral nephrectomy was abolished by heating the serum at 50°C for 30 min, or by freezing it for more than 72 h [27]. From their own experimental evidence and that of others, Silk et al. [45], using isotope techniques, considered that in the serum of unilateral nephrectomized rats and puppies there is a specific renotropic factor which is non-dialysable and non-species-specific, and which brings about an increasing rate of cellular division in the kidneys of intact mice exposed to the action of the serum.

Lytton et al. [29] investigated the problem of compensatory hyperplasia in the kidney in parabiotic rats by determining the uptake of tritiated thymidine into DNA in the kidneys of the intact parabionts, 48 h after unilateral nephrectomy on the partner. Bilateral nephrectomy was also done on one of the parabionts in each of five pairs. They found a mean increase of 71% in the mitotic activity in the kidneys of the intact animals following unilateral nephrectomy in the partners, as compared with that in sham operation controls. Following bilateral nephrectomy or partial hepatectomies there was no increase in mitotic activity in the kidneys of the intact partner. It was believed, therefore, that after the removal of one kidney, a tissue-specific serum factor was elaborated by, or in the presence of, the remaining renal tissue, which stimulates compensatory cellular hyperplasia in the remaining kidney. The presence of the second kidney, however, appeared to be necessary for the elaboration of this factor.

2. In Man

In cases of unilateral renal disease in man the healthy kidney undergoes hypertrophy and may well compare with that found in

the experimental animal. Functional studies after nephrectomy have shown that the renal blood flow and the glomerular filtration rate of the healthy remaining kidney may increase to reach about 80% of that of the two normal organs [22]. In subjects under the age of 30 hypertrophy of the solitary kidney after nephrectomy is complete in a few months. In subjects between the ages of 30 and 50 the process may last up to 20 years and in subjects over the age of 50 the compensatory hypertrophy is probably never completed [5]. The rate of hypertrophy in the remaining kidney is affected by various collateral circumstances, being retarded by constriction of the renal artery and by starvation.

IV. Recovery of Function After Ureteric Obstruction

It is of importance for the urologist to know for how long a ureter can be obstructed completely or partially (for example, by stone) and yet recover its function in whole or in part; the time interval is almost certainly longer than has been generally believed. Does the presence or absence of a normally functioning kidney on the unobstructed side influence favourably or not at all the potential for recovery of the obstructed kidney?

Such knowledge determines the timing of operative interference upon the ureter. Surgeons have tended, for reasons partly based on experience and partly from precepts handed down, but not necessarily completely verified, to accept certain indications, in particular a moderate degree of ureteric obstruction, as an indication for removing the offending ureteric calculus for fear of permanent damage to the kidney.

1. In the Experimental Animal

Beer [4] tied the lower end of the ureter in the dog and 7 days later implanted the upper divided end into the bladder. The opposite kidney was removed after the animal had recovered from the operation and the dog lived for 3 months with no sign of renal insufficiency. In the experimental animal Hinman and Morison [21] found that if the ureter was obstructed for 3 weeks, the corresponding kidney underwent atrophy unless the opposite kidney was removed. The theory here was that the unobstructed kidney underwent hypertrophy when the obstruction in the other kidney had persisted for 3 weeks and that there was then no stimulus for the obstructed kidney to recover its function. When the unobstructed kidney was removed, however, there was a stimulus for the obstructed kidney to resume its function.

The effects of complete ureteric obstruction for periods of 7, 14, 21 and 28 days in the dog and the rate of recovery of function following the release of obstruction, were examined by Kerr [24], renal clearance methods being used to assess renal function. In dogs in which the ureter had been obstructed for 2 weeks the glomerular filtration rate (GFR) and the renal plasma flow (RPF) were significantly less, 1 h after release of the obstruction, than when the ureter had been obstructed for 1 week. Dogs in which the ureter had been obstructed for only 1 week showed much greater improvement in the GFR and the RPF after the release of the obstruction than dogs which had been similarly obstructed for 4 weeks. When the opposite normal kidney (used as a control) was removed 2 days after the release of the obstruction from the operated kidney, there was a prompt increase in the rate of urine formation by the previously obstructed kidney in all groups. The ability of the previously obstructed kidney in all the groups to concentrate urine was impaired, but the ability to dilute the urine or to produce an alkaline or acid urine was not impaired. In three dogs in which the contralateral kidney had been removed some days after apparently

maximum recovery had been achieved in the kidney operated upon, in each case renal clearances increased still further. Hence, even after long periods of stabilization (amounting to approximately 2 years in one animal), these kidneys could still be stimulated to increase the GFR and the RPF.

2. In Man

In the human, the maximum duration of ureteric obstruction compatible with subsequent total or partial recovery of function is still not universally agreed. The extent to which the normal unobstructed kidney can influence the quality of recovery of the obstructed kidney after the obstruction has been removed is also still not fully known [39]. The degree (partial or complete) of ureteric obstruction, the level in the ureter at which obstruction occurs, the presence of urinary infection (probably because associated oedema physically increases the degree of obstruction) are important features in the assessment of a given case. If the ureter can be shown to be completely obstructed by a medium-sized stone, 3 weeks is believed to be as long as it is safe to defer operation for its relief.

If the ureter is only partially obstructed by stone so that urine can seep past it into the bladder, operation is less urgent. Calculi are known to have remained in the ureter for many months without giving rise to any permanent harm; indeed, complete recovery of function has been known to occur following their removal. Obstruction in a single kidney (or a single functioning kidney) constitutes an emergency. The appearance of the nephrogram effect (Chap. 10) on an intravenous pyelogram is evidence of a considerable, though not necessarily complete obstruction; but the picture may change from day to day. A further intravenous urogram taken only a few days later may reveal a near-normal urogram. If, on cystoscopy, no methylene blue is excreted from a ureter following its intravenous injection, and none is voided into the urine for some hours, it is certain that the obstruction is at that moment complete, though the finding may be reversed after a few days.

In a more empirical vein, if proved ureteric near-total obstruction resulting from a stone seems to be unlikely to be relieved by its spontaneous voiding or migration, or if the obstruction results from external pressure on the ureter, early removal of the obstruction should, generally speaking, be undertaken. In the female patient, aged 42, reported by Lewis and Pierce [26] the right ureter had been ligated during an emergency hysterectomy done for severe haemorrhage. A complete obstruction of the ureter was demonstrated at operation 69 days later, when the ureter was divided above the point of the obstruction and reimplanted into the bladder. An excretory urogram 2.5 months postoperatively showed normal function of the affected kidney with no hydronephrosis, and a radioactive Hippuran renogram 19 months postoperatively showed a normal curve.

Badenoch [3] illustrated the varied problems and the difficulties of assessment in a report of seven cases of ureteric obstruction, two apparently complete and five apparently incomplete. The first patient had a ureteric stone giving rise to incomplete obstruction, which during 2 years and 11 months had slowly descended from the kidney, down the ureter and ultimately into the penis, where it was found in the fossa navicularis. Another patient (a man of 54) had had stones in a partially (but nowhere near completely) obstructed left ureter with few symptoms in 11 years, during which period the stones had gradually moved down the ureter, the pelvis and ureter showing very little dilatation above the stones. In another patient the ureters had been damaged during a Wertheim's hys-

terectomy for cancer of the uterus, one ureter having been completely obstructed for 9 weeks and 4 days (having been occluded by a silk ligature which had been tied completely round it). Normal function was restored to that kidney following a successful operation. In a further case a stone had been present for 101 days before it was removed, after which renal function was reasonably good and equal to that of the normal opposite side. These varied experiences show the difficulty of predicting in advance what would be likely to happen in any given case. Recovery of function can be demonstrated by the use of the radioisotope renogram [43].

V. Prevention of Infection

In aseptic cases, the surgeon has to decide whether to carry out the operation to remove the stone (for example, partial nephrectomy) under the cover of antibiotics commencing, say, 36 or 48 h before the operation and continued for 4 days after operation, in order to prevent postoperative infection in the wound and within the urinary tract; or whether to reserve the use of antibiotics for the treatment of cases in which active postoperative infection has actually occurred. If the former method is practised, protection can be expected only against organisms which are sensitive to the given antibiotic though the use of broad spectrum antibiotics could be protective. Infection by non-sensitive organisms would not be prevented. If the latter method is adopted, infection may occur which could have been prevented and which has then to be cured.

The question as to whether the use of antibiotics can encourage a persistent wound infection by antibiotic-resistant organisms, is part of a wider problem which affects every surgical operation, and a full discussion is beyond the scope of this book.

The prevention of postoperative infection following operations for renal stone, in which the kidney is uninfected before operation, involves the application of many basic principles:

1. Meticulous aseptic technique in the operating theatre;
2. The protection of the skin edges of the wound by suitable cloths applied after the incision has been made;
3. Meticulous haemostasis at all stages of the operation;
4. Gentle handling of tissues and of the kidney itself;
5. The avoidance of unnecessary dissection of tissues;
6. The careful suturing of the urinary passages (renal pelvis, calyces, ureter) which it had been necessary to open during the operation, in order to avoid altogether or to minimize the postoperative escape of urine;
7. The removal of rubber drains inserted into the wound as soon after operation as possible;
8. The reduction to a minimum of postoperative dressing of the wound except, for example, for the removal of the drainage tube, or for the patient's comfort.

One suspects that an over-reliance upon antibiotics has resulted in many of these desiderata, so strongly advocated by surgeons in the pre-sulphonamide and pre-antibiotic era, being applied less meticulously and rigidly than they might be. Recent enquiries in various hospitals into the incidence of wound infection after operation in 'clean' surgical cases, even when the patient has had the benefit of antibiotic cover, have come as an unpleasant surprise and have led to a re-advocacy of the principles of aseptic operative surgery just referred to.

The author has usually taken the view that in addition to making every effort to minimize postoperative infection, there is more to be gained than lost by using during the period of an operation ampicillin, for 6 days, beginning 36 h before operation and continuing for 5 days after. (Formerly, penicillin 500,000 units with streptomycin 0.5 gm, morning and night, was used.)

If, however, it is known that there is or has been an infection in the urinary tract before operation, the appropriate antibiotic to which the micro-organism is sensitive should be given for some days before and after operation. The danger of antibiotic-resistant organisms being in a wound (say, during convalescence), possibly following the use of antibiotics, has to be recognized and if such a view is strongly held, some may feel that operations for the removal of renal calculi should be done without any antibiotic cover in non-infected cases. The urologist must choose between these two alternatives.

VI. Temporary Control of Bleeding

Mechanical methods of temporary control of the renal pedicle during the operations of nephrolithotomy and partial nephrectomy are available which enable the operation to be done in a field relatively or absolutely free from blood. Complete permanent arrest of bleeding can be done at the conclusion of the operation. A sufficient length of the renal artery and vein must be dissected out.

Pressure on the pedicle may be maintained for as long as 20 min without damage to the kidney. The objective can be achieved by manual compression by the fingers of the assistant, placed one on either side of the pedicle, though the procedure can be fatiguing. Prather [38] used a semi-flexible Doyen's curved 9-in. intestinal clamp covered by 'soft rubber boots' to clamp the vascular pedicle, releasing it at the end of 8–10 min for 20–40 s, after which it is reapplied. A simple angled clamp, the blades of which are covered with soft rubber tubing [47] can be applied to the pedicle.

The author has used two rubber-covered bulldog clamps applied close to each other on the renal pedicle. The pressure of one of these may not be sufficient to arrest the bleeding but two clamps placed one above the other have proved satisfactory [40]. The spring of the clamps must be just sufficient to occlude the vessels but not tense enough to risk causing damage to the intima of the artery and veins.

A distensible tourniquet clamp devised by Stewart [48] consists of two curved pieces of metal hinged at one end and joined at the other by a ratchet. When closed the clamp is oval in shape. Each blade is covered by an inflatable cuff of poly-ethylene, which is attached to a long rubber tube fitted with a pressure gauge, the degree of pressure in the rubber tourniquet being regulated by the anaesthetist. With rapid inflation of the bag there is little risk of venous congestion. The clamp, which is made in three sizes, should not be left in position for more than 15–20 min. The author has used this clamp on many occasions with satisfactory results.

White and Spence [53] described a tourniquet suitable for compression of the renal pedicle. Marshall et al. [31] used a tourniquet composed of a soft rubber catheter passed through the holes of a Lane's orthopaedic plate.

VII. Cooling Techniques

In order to allow for the prolongation of a period of renal ischaemia without any consequent harm to the body, techniques have been devised which will enable the kidney to be cooled down to, say, 2.0°C for the duration of a longish operation for the removal of calculi, so that the rate of meta-bolism and the consumption of oxygen by the renal parenchyma can be reduced; such a procedure might be expected to ensure the survival and return to normal function of the kidney in a healthy condition.

1. The Experimental Animal

The principles of earlier background studies relating to the effect on the kidney of the experimental animal of temporary circulatory arrest have been summarized by Wickham et al. [54]. Histological studies by various workers have shown that during a period of circulatory arrest in the healthy mammalian kidney, the proximal renal tubular epithelium suffers histologically demonstrable damage if the duration of the ischaemia has exceeded 35 min, while the glomeruli and the intrarenal vascular tree seem to be relatively free from damage; and also that the residual renal function (result-ing from renal tubular damage) diminishes in proportion to the duration of the period of arterial occlusion. Animals which have been subjected to occlusion of the renal artery for a period in excess of 3 h have shown gross deterioration of renal function. With occlusion for a period of 4–6 h, the amount of resulting renal damage deter-mined a fatal uraemia.

In the dog the optimum renal tem-perature consistent with minimal functional and structural changes was found by Stueber and his associates to be between 0° and 5°C [49, 50]. Wickham et al. [54] con-cluded from their review of the available data and their own experimental evidence that in the human kidney, if it is desired to arrest the blood supply, in order to avoid any permanent cellular damage, the warm ischaemia time should not exceed 30 min; and to avoid even the minimum depression of function, the warm ischaemia time should not exceed 10 min.

In the experimental field many ingenious methods of cooling the kidney have been tried [54]: perfusing the renal artery with a hypothermic fluid; surrounding the kidney by a device to cool the renal parenchyma directly; reduction of the temperature of the entire body.

2. In Man

In the clinical application of cooling techniques to the human kidney for the removal of renal calculi by the operation of nephrolithotomy (especially, for example, in the solitary kidney), various methods have been used.

Stewart [48] cooled the kidney by the use of closed polyethylene bags (the outside temperature being 40°F or 4.5°C) containing cooled isotonic saline, sealed at each end, and placed beneath each side of, and around the kidney and the renal pedicle, replacing them from time to time. He reported satisfactory results in partial nephrectomy operations. The aim was to cool the outside of the kidney to 21°C in 10 min. For the rapid estimation of temperature, the sensitive probe of one thermistor was placed on the surface of the kidney through the capsule at the pole which was to be removed, and that of the other was inserted into the pole for a distance of about 1 cm; a difference of about 10°F between the two readings was necessary if cooling to the required temperature of 70°F was to be achieved in 10 min.

Other methods have included a metallic heat exchanger through which a coolant mixture could be circulated [9], sterile iced water in a plastic bag surrounding the kidney [13], and sterile crushed ice packed against the renal substances.

Wickham et al. [54], for the operation of nephrolithotomy for staghorn calculi, used a continuous length of coiled silastic rubber tubing arranged in the form of twin biconcave discs, which could be sterilized by boiling and through which the coolant liquid (which was alcohol cooled by dry ice) could be pumped. The kidney was exposed in the ordinary way and the renal artery was occluded with a bulldog arterial clamp

and the cooling capsule was applied to the kidney. An average period of 8.5 min was needed to achieve a temperature in the coil of 7° to 8°C, as monitored by two thermistor probe electrodes introduced respectively into the renal cortex and medulla, the temperature of which fell to 20°C. If the temperature fell below this level there was apt to be freezing and adhesions between the renal capsule and the coil. The coils were then removed and a bulldog clamp placed on the upper end of the ureter to prevent the downward migration of stones, and nephrolithotomy was carried out in a relatively dry field, the complete removal of the calculi being checked by the use of a contact radiograph incorporating a local grid [16]. Haemostasis by the ligature of individual vessels, was secured after the stones had been removed, the renal collecting system being then closed with a 000 chromic catgut suture [15, 17, 18]. Cases operated upon using this technique are referred to in Chapter 13.

VIII. Radiography of the Exposed Kidney

From the time of the first introduction of radiodiagnosis attempts have been made, attended by ever-increasing success, to obtain satisfactory pictures of the stone-containing kidney when exposed at operation. Fenwick, as long ago as 1897, used the X-rays which had been discovered by Roentgen only 2 years before, together with a photographic film placed behind an exposed calculus-containing kidney to make a picture.

Braasch and Carman [7] were among the pioneers of renal fluoroscopy on the operating table, used in recent years by others [33]. Small cassettes made of aluminium to hold the photographic plate, were placed in the wound in the loin behind the kidney by Quinby [41]. Willan [55] used small films in sterile cotton containers. Olsson [36] used easily sterilizable flexible cassettes containing an intensifying screen, which were placed in a flat rubber bag. Radiography of the exposed kidney during removal of the stone with television guidance has been successfully used by Hellstrom and Franksson [19]. Untermeyer et al. [52] suggested the use of the radioisotope thulium 170 as an alternative source of energy to make the pictures.

Unless the surgeon has decided before operation to perform nephrectomy, a radiograph of the kidney when exposed and mobilized on the operating table should always be made before proceeding to remove the stones, as a necessary part of the operation, in order to determine the extent of the calculous disease.

A good modern portable X-ray unit (of which several models are available), is powerful enough to produce an accurate photograph of the calculi known to be present as well as of tiny calcific particles in the renal parenchyma and calyces, which may not have been visualized on the plain radiograph.

The technique used by the author has been employed with modifications and improvements in his hospital since 1933 [40]. The kidney with its vascular pedicle, as well as the upper part of the ureter, is mobilized and placed in a cotton sling, traction upon which enables the assistant to draw it as far as possible out of the wound. A metal clip or a wire suture is placed through the renal capsule at the upper pole for the purpose of its identification on the film. A small flexible X-ray film in a thin flexible plastic cassette wrapped in a sterile container of thin cotton, is placed in the wound, closely applied to the side of the exposed kidney remote from the X-ray tube. Attached to the X-ray tube is a detachable cone or cylinder of metal or glass, which is sterilized before it is mounted, and introduced in a sloping position into the wound. The distal end of the cone is sufficiently large to allow of the exposed

kidney being gently placed within it when the portable X-ray unit has been moved into position. Pressure on the cassette by the assistant helps to retain the kidney in position if necessary.

One radiograph is taken before, and one or more during or after the operation, to ensure that the removal of the calculi has been as complete as possible. If thought necessary after an inspection of the first radiograph, it is possible to locate with considerable accuracy the position of the stone in a calyx by passing a straight needle through the renal substance to the depth and the position where the stone is believed to be. A radiograph (in two planes if possible) is then taken to enable the surgeon to gauge the distance of the stone from the needle. A metal grid consisting of thin interlacing wires in the form of squares, with an attached sling to hold the kidney, placed in contact with the kidney before the radiograph is taken, helps in the localization of calculi [16, 30, 55].

In the author's cases of radiographs taken of the exposed kidney in the operating theatre, amounting to some hundreds, there have been examples in which an intended pyelolithotomy was changed to partial nephrectomy, since the former operation would have resulted in paracalyceal calcific particles being left behind which had not been visible on the preoperative radiograph. Two calculi instead of the one assumed to be present from the preoperative radiograph have several times been observed on the radiograph taken at operation, especially when one renal stone (or stones) lies posterior to a second calculus.

Unsuspected cases of localized medullary sponge kidneys can be detected. In badly infected stone-bearing kidneys, the radiograph sometimes demonstrates the presence of a surprising accumulation of fine, gritty, calcific particles in or around all the dilated calyces, so numerous and so widely spread that they cannot possibly be removed at operation, a finding which will incline the urologist towards nephrectomy rather than the simple removal of the stones.

By injecting opaque medium along the exposed ureter, having clamped it below the point of injection, a pyelogram can be obtained which may be useful in the localization of some calculi.

MacKelvie and McKelvie [30] found that their provisional preoperative choice of operation in 17 of 75 patients was changed as a result of the radiograph of the exposed kidney. Partial nephrectomy was preferred to pyelolithotomy in 9; in 2 in whom a partial nephrectomy had been contemplated because of the presence of calyceal calculi as well as a pelvic stone, it had been possible to demonstrate on the radiograph that all the calyceal material had been removed during the pyelolithotomy procedure.

IX. Closure of the Wound

When the definitive operative procedure on the kidney has been concluded, the fascia of Gerota is drawn together by a few interrupted sutures. The muscles are sutured in two layers. Deep catgut stitches are placed about 1 in. apart through the muscle, care being taken to include the internal oblique muscle, which tends to retract upwards and downwards beneath the more superficial layers of muscle. A second row of interrupted stitches is inserted through the superficial layer of the muscles, a rubber drainage tube is placed down to the kidney through the fascia of Gerota and is removed as early as possible.

The excellent muscular mass with a good blood supply, beneath this incision, makes for sound healing, but a hernia may result from inadequate suturing of the wound as well as from infection. In the repair of wounds in patients who have had an earlier renal operation, it may be found that the parietal muscles are thin, possibly because

of earlier wound infection; the different layers must be identified as clearly as possible before suture in an effort to prevent postoperative hernia.

References

1. Abeshouse,B.S., Lerman,S.: Partial nephrectomy versus pyelolithotomy and nephrolithotomy in the treatment of localized calculous disease of the kidney, with a report of 17 partial nephrectomies. In: International Abstracts of Surgery. Surg. Gynecol. Obstet. *91*, 209 (1950)
2. Allen,R.B: Experiments on the physiology and cause of compensatory renal hyperplasia. Proc. Mayo Clin. *9*, 333 (1934)
3. Badenoch,A.W.: Observations on the management of the obstructed ureter. Br. J. Urol. *35*, 386 (1963)
4. Beer,E.: Experimental study of the effects of ureteral obstruction on kidney function and structure. Am. J. Urol. *8*, 171 (1912)
5. Bitker,M.P., Bitker,B.: Compensatory hypertrophy and functional adaption of the remaining kidney after unilateral nephrectomy. J. Chir. (Paris) *97*, 95 (1969)
6. Block,M.A., Wakim,K.G., Mann,F.D.: Appraisal of certain factors influencing compensatory renal hypertrophy. Am. J. Physiol. *172*, 60 (1953)
7. Braasch,W.F., Carman,R.D.: Renal fluoroscopy at the operating table. J. Am. Med. Assoc. *73*, 1751 (1919)
8. Brödel,M.: The intrinsic blood vessels of the kidney and their significance in nephrotomy. Bull. Johns Hopkins Hosp. *12*, 10 (1901)
9. Cockett,A.T.K.: The kidney and regional hypothermia. Surgery. *50*, 905 (1961)
10. Gerard,G.: Les artères rénales (Note statistique d'après l'étude de 150 paires de reins). J. Anat. Physiol. *47*, 531 (1911)
11. Graves,F.T.: The anatomy of the intrarenal arteries and its application to segmental resection of the kidney. Br. J. Surg. *24*, 132 (1954)
12. Graves,F.T.: Anatomy of the intrarenal arteries in health and disease. Br. J. Surg. *43*, 605 (1956)
13. Graves,F.T.: Renal hypothermia: an aid to partial nephrectomy. Br. J. Surg. *50*, 562 (1963)
14. Graves,F.T.: The Arterial Anatomy of the Kidney. Bristol: J. Wright and Sons 1971

15. Gregoir,W.J.: Surgery of renal calculi using refrigeration. Urol. Nephrol. (Paris) 79, 533 (1973)

16. Hanley,H.G.: Flexible renal grid-sling for localizing stones during lithotomy. Lancet I, 661 (1967)

17. Hanley,H.G.: The removal of a staghorn calculi under local renal hypothermia. Br. J. Urol. 44, 731 (1972)

18. Hanley,H.G., Joekes,A.M., Wickham, J.E.A.: Renal hypothermia in complicated nephrolithotomy. J. Urol. 79, 517 (1968)

19. Hellstrom,J., Franksson,C.: Operative urology I. In: Encyclopaedia of urology. Dix,V.W., Weyrauch,H.M., Wildbolz,E. (eds.), Vol. 13. Berlin, Heidelberg, New York: Springer 1961

20. Hinman,F.jr.: The pathophysiology of urinary obstruction. In: Urology I. Campbell,M.F. (ed.), Ch. 8. Philadelphia: Saunders 1963

21. Hinman,F., Morison,D.M.: An experimental study of the circulatory changes in hydronephrosis. Trans. Am. Assoc. G-U Surg. 16, 7 (1923)

22. Hogeman,O.: Clearance tests in renal disorders and hypertension. Acta Med. Scand. (Suppl. 216a) (1948)

23. Hyrtl,J.: Handbuch der topographischer Anatomie I, p. 834. Vienna: Branmeller 1882

24. Kerr,W.F.Jr.: Effects of complete ureteral obstruction in dogs on kidney function. Am. J. Physiol. 184, 521 (1956)

25. Levy,S.E., Blalock,A.: The effects of unilateral nephrectomy on the renal blood flow and oxygen consumption of unanaesthetized dogs. Am. J. Physiol. 122, 609 (1938)

26. Lewis, H.Y., Pierce,J.M.: Return of function after relief of complete ureteric obstruction of 69 days duration. J. Urol. 88, 377 (1962)

27. Lowenstein,L.M., Lozner,E.C.: Demonstration and partial characterization of a humoral renal growth factor. Clin. Res. 14, 383 (1966)

28. Lowenstein,L.M., Stern,A.: Serum factor in renal compensatory hyperplasia. Science 142, 1479 (1963)

29. Lytton,B., Schiff,M.jr., Bloom,T.N.: Compensatory renal growth; evidence for tissue specific factor of renal origin. J. Urol. 101, 648 (1969)

30. MacKelvie,A.A., McKelvie,G.B.: Operative radiography in the surgery of renal stone. Lancet II, 15 (1963)

31. Marshall,V.F., Lavengood,R.W., Kelly,D.: Complete longitudinal nephrolithotomy and the Shorr regime in the management of staghorn calculi. Ann. Surg. 162, 366 (1965)

32. Merklin,R.J., Michels,N.A.: The variant renal and suprarenal blood supply with data on the inferior phrenic, ureteral and gonadal arteries. J. Int. Coll. Surg. 29, 41 (1958)

33. Nicholson,N.J.: Radioscopy in nephrolithotomy. Br. J. Urol. 31, 249 (1949)

34. Ogawa,K., Nowinski,W.W.: Mitosis stimulating factor in serum of unilaterally nephrectomized rats. Proc. Soc. Exp. Biol. Med. 99, 350 (1958)

35. Oliver,J.: Renal Morphology. Harvey Lect. 40, 102 (1944–45)

36. Olsson,O.: X-ray examination of exposed kidneys. J. Urol. 61, 1032 (1949)

37. Platt,R., Roscoe,M.H., Smith,F.W.: Experimental renal failure. Clin. Sci. 11, 3 (1952)

38. Prather,G.C.: A method of haemostasis during nephrostomy for large kidney calculi. J. Urol. 32, 578 (1939)

39. Pridgen,W.R., Woodhead,D.M., Younger,R.K.: Alteration in renal function by ureteral obstruction. J. Am. Med. Assoc. 178, 563 (1961)

40. Pyrah,L.N.: Personal communication (1960)

41. Quinby,W.C.: Note on localization of renal calculi by aid of X-ray film made during operations. J. Urol. 13, 59 (1925)

42. Renon,C.M., Illes,J., Gouaze,A.: Segmental systematization of the vessels of the kidney: its application to regulated partial nephrectomy. J. Urol. (Paris) 60, 208 (1954)

43. Ross,J.C., Edwards,E.C., Kulke,W., Haggart,B.G.: Recovery of renal function as demonstrated by the radioisotope renogram. Br. J. Urol. 35, 394 (1963)

44. Rous,S.N., Wakin,K.G.: Renal function before, during and after compensatory hypertrophy. J. Urol. 98, 30 (1967)

45. Silk,M.R., Homsy,G.E., Merz,T.: Compensatory renal hyperplasia. J. Urol. 98, 36 (1967)

46. Smithius,T.: The problem of renal segmentation in connection with the modes of ramification of the renal artery and renal vein. Arch. Chir. Neerl. 8, 3 (1956)

47. Stewart,H.H.: In: British surgical practice. Carling, Ross (eds.). London: Butterworth 1953

48. Stewart,H.H.: The surgery of the kidney in the treatment of renal stone. Br. J. Urol. *32*, 392 (1960)

49. Stueber,P.J.,   Kovacs,S.,   Koletsky,S., Persky,L.: Regional hypothermia in acute renal ischaemia. J. Urol. *79*, 793 (1958)

50. Stueber,P.J.,   Mahoney,S.,   Kolestsky,S., Persky,L.: Late effects of regional renal hypothermia. J. Urol. *92*, 87 (1964)

51. Syme,R.A.: The blood supply of the kidney in relation to the surgery of stone. Br. J. Urol. *44*, 730 (1972)

52. Untermeyer,S.,   Spedding,F.H.,   Daane, A.H.,   Powell,J.E.,   Hasterlik,R.:   Portable thulium-X-ray unit. Nucleoics *12*, 35 (1954)

53. White,E.jr.,   Spence,H.M.:   Use   of   the Rumel tourniquet for intermittent renal vascular occlusion. J. Urol. *86*, 373 (1961)

54. Wickham,J.E.A.,   Hanley,H.G.,   Joekes, A.M.: Regional renal hypothermia. Br. J. Urol. *39*, 727 (1967)

55. Willan,R.J.: Radiography during operation for renal calculus. Br. Med. J. *II*, 552 (1930)

Chapter 12

The Conservative Treatment of Renal and Ureteric Calculi

I. Conservative Treatment

The management of the treatment of patients with renal calculi calls for a consideration of various possibilities. A few examples of the spontaneous disappearance of renal calculi have been reported but such an unusual event only exceptionally concerns the urologist in determining the treatment for a given patient. Many small renal (calyceal and pelvic) calculi are voided spontaneously after negotiating the ureter, and such a possibility is always relevant. When a stone moves from the kidney into the ureter the problem then becomes one of aiding its removal. Various alternative forms of treatment are open to the urologist. Ureteric calculi may be voided spontaneously or they may require instrumental or operative intervention.

1. Spontaneous Disappearance of Some Renal Calculi

Renal calculi occasionally undergo what is sometimes referred to as spontaneous disappearance or dissolution, as distinct from being voided spontaneously. Such an event may result from an almost complete reversal of the biochemical, physical or hormonal conditions which have been responsible for their formation and which it should usually be possible to trace.

The large, soft, putty-like renal calculi composed mainly of apatite, which occasionally complicate the advanced skeletal type of hyperparathyroidism, may disappear spontaneously a few weeks after parathyroid adenomectomy. The disappearance of such calculi is dependent upon the return to normal of the high preoperative serum calcium level and the consequent considerable reduction in the high level of the urinary calcium, enabling the urine to take up the calcium phosphate in the calculi into solution (especially if it is kept acid in reaction). Soft phosphatic renal calculi, which have formed as a complication of prolonged recumbency for the treatment of spinal or other injuries or of poliomyelitis, provided the urine is free from infection and acidified, may disappear when the mobility of the patient has been restored to normal. Elliott [35] collected 13 cases from the literature (mostly recumbency calculi) and added four examples of his own of spontaneous disappearance of renal calculi; some others are included in Table 12.1.

2. Spontaneous Voiding of Some Renal and Ureteric Calculi

Renal Calculi. Some small calyceal or pelvic renal stones are voided spontaneously. The assessment as to whether a calculus may possibly be voided spontaneously after migrating into the ureter depends upon its size and its topographical character, including the presence or absence of spiculation. The statistical probability that such an event will occur has a bearing. Stones of a size smaller than 0.5–0.75 cm which are not causing obstruction (provided the urine is sterile) may be treated conservatively in the hope that they will be voided spontaneously, probably following an attack of colic. If a patient is known to have voided small calculi previously, it is possible that he will pass further small stones spontaneously. Stones which are

Table 12.1. Cases of spontaneous disappearance of renal calculi (complete or partial) (taken mostly from paper by J.S. Elliott, 1954)

Author	Year	Status of stones	Age and sex	Time after disappearance	Factors contributing to stone formation or associated disease	Treatment
Scheele	1924	4 renal calculi	F 34	4 years (reduction in size)		
Hellstrom	1925	(1) Large recurrent stone, left (2) Renal stone (3) Bilateral calculi	F 24 F 26 M 45	5 years (disappearance)		
Hasselstrom	1926	Large left renal calculi	F 40	1 month	Recumbency for fractured femur Chronic gastric ulcer	
Barney	1929	Bilateral renal calculi	M 22	3 months	Recumbency for fractured femur	
Kearns	1935	Large renal calculi	F 42	Several months		Drank beer
Sisk, Bunts	1935	Bilateral renal calculi	F 13		Recumbency for coxitis	
Gibson	1938	Bilateral renal calculi	M 48	4 years	Big stone removed right kidney; staghorn disappeared from left kidney; infection of urine	Nil
Nadeau	1939	Several stones left solitary kidney	F	6 months		Drank 1 gallon distilled water daily
Lassen	1939	Bilateral renal calculi	F 17	1 year	Recumbency for hip disease	
Walker, Thompson	1942	Bilateral renal calculi				
Wesson	1950	Bilateral renal calculi	M 21	6 weeks	Recumbency for fractured femur	Ammonium chloride with acid-ash diet
McCrae, Van Buskirk	1951	Bilateral renal calculi			Recumbency for fractured femur	
Elliott	1954	(1) Large left renal calculus	M 75	4 months	Carcinoma prostate	Stilboestrol; no other treatment
		(2) Left renal calculus	F 23	1 month		No treatment
		(3) Bilateral renal calculi	F 39	8 months (great reduction in size)	Urinary infection	Low-phosphorus diet; fluids; Amphogel
		(4) Large staghorn calculus		Great reduction in size		
Pyrah, Hodgkinson, Anderson	1966	Bilateral renal calculi	F 18	8 weeks	Primary hyperparathyroidism	Parathyroidectomy
Pyrah, Fowweather	1937	Bilateral renal calculi	F 16	12 weeks	Spinal tuberculosis	Mobility; ammonium chloride

larger than those which were first passed can often be voided down the ureter, possibly because its lumen has undergone some degree of permanent dilatation following the passage of one stone. If it is decided not to operate on a patient with a small renal stone, 6-monthly plain radiographs would demonstrate any increase in the size of the stone.

Ureteric Calculi. Many small calculi are voided after an attack of colic, often without the patient being aware of it, and probably most ureteric stones pass spontaneously. The question of the conservative treatment of ureteric calculi has a somewhat different relevance from that of renal calculi, since such stones have already descended from the kidney.

The percentage of ureteric calculi voided spontaneously in different series has been between 30% and 76%. The general configuration (ellipsoidal or barrel-shaped) and the character of the surface of the stone (spiculated or nodular) as well as the size have a bearing upon the likelihood of spontaneous voiding. It is not usually stated whether patients with renal colic in whom radiography has been negative are included in the published series, and probably usually they are not, but many such patients have probably voided small calculi.

In our own series one-third were passed between 1 month and 1 year after the onset of symptoms, and a further 18.6% after the passage of a ureteric catheter, though it is impossible to determine whether this simple procedure influenced their passage.

Size of Stone. In our series, in all but 5 cases the ureteric stone which passed spontaneously (89 of 292 (30.5%)) had a diameter smaller than one-third of a centimetre. Ninety-one percent of calculi with a narrowest diameter of 0.5 cm or less, passed spontaneously or with the assistance of endoscopic procedures. No stone was passed which had a diameter greater than 0.5 cm [40].

Wax and Frank [101] found that 83% of stones of 4 mm or less in diameter and 36% of stones between 5 mm and 1 cm in diameter were voided spontaneously; of 18 stones which were 1 cm in diameter only 2 were passed spontaneously.

A careful study of the size of stones which would pass spontaneously down the ureter was made by Sandegard [85, 86] in a series of 541 patients with ureteric calculi assessed during the period 1951–1954. If there was no indication for early intervention, most cases were treated expectantly and the descent of the stones noted in relation to their size and position when first diagnosed, the stones being divided into three groups according to their transverse diameter as measured on the plain radiograph. He found that small stones (less than 4 mm) in the lower half of the ureter passed spontaneously in 93% of the cases; medium stones (4–6 mm) in 53%; large stones (more than 6 mm) only rarely passed spontaneously (1 in 24). Approximately half of the medium-sized stones in the upper half of the ureter migrated to the lower half but large stones rarely did so.

Position of Stone. Many stones which come to rest in the upper third of the ureter are too big to pass spontaneously and if larger than 0.5 cm in diameter should usually be removed by operation; this seems to be a consensus view among urologists.

In our series of 292 cases [40] of ureteric stone, none with a diameter exceeding 0.5 cm and being located in the upper part of the ureter were voided spontaneously in the time allowed, though some might have done so had we waited longer. Obstructive symptoms (hydroureter and hydronephrosis) were present more frequently and to a greater degree with stone in the upper part of the ureter than with stones lower down, symptoms which favour early operation. For smaller calculi which had been watched for a time and had failed to descend, operative removal was usually done; 28% of the cases when first seen were in the upper ureter. A factor favouring early operative removal of stones in the upper and middle thirds of the ureter is the comparative ease of the operation itself, and the absence of complications. The same arguments apply to stones in the middle third of the ureter. Small calculi (less than 0.5 cm) may be voided spontaneously.

It may be thought that a stone which has descended to the lowest third of the ureter will probably be voided spontaneously though possibly after a considerable interval. Dix [24] favoured leaving small stones in the lower third to be voided, and Davidson [22] believed that one could leave a small stone in the pelvic ureter for months. Winsbury-White [103] stated 'that if a stone has reached the pelvic floor, months can be allowed to elapse without the likelihood of renal damage and with good prospects that the stone will ultimately pass'.

The author agrees with these views concerning small stones subject to the patient having a periodic radiograph. It is, however, the general view that stones more than 0.5 cm in diameter should have active interference of some kind especially if there is early dilatation of the ureter. Endoscopic removal has been reported in varied proportions of patients in different published series for calculi in the lower third. Some urologists have preferred such methods because of the supposed difficulty of the operative removal of calculi especially in the lowest 2 in. of the ureter, a procedure which, however, in the author's opinion is a satisfactory surgical procedure.

Effect on Renal Function of a Stone Remaining for a Long Time in the Ureter.
Many stones which have lodged in the ureter for long periods of time have not resulted in serious damage to the kidney.

The degree of obstruction is of greater importance than the length of time alone.

Sandegard [85] found that the quality of the excretion and the density of the contrast medium in the urogram were normal, and that there was no dilatation of the renal pelvis or ureter in 86 patients with ureteric stone who had been treated conservatively, when urography was done 5–8 years after the passage of the stone. By contrast he found in 26 patients who had been treated by active intervention (for large stones) that renal function was normal and that there had been no dilatation of the renal pelvis in all except two cases, where renal function was impaired or lost (one of these had a subsequent nephrectomy). He concluded that many stones may remain in the ureter for a long period without there being any subsequent renal damage and that the presence of a (small) stone, therefore, is not necessarily an indication for early active intervention but can be treated expectantly.

In our own series of 292 cases, 46 follow-up urograms in patients who had voided the stone spontaneously showed mild hydronephrosis in only one patient who had passed a stone only 2 weeks previously and who also had a stone in one of the lower renal calyces. No relation was found between the degree of initial dilatation of the upper urinary tract, the duration of time before the stone passed and the return of the renal collecting system to normal, provided the stone passed spontaneously [40] (Table 12.2, see p. 228).

3. Expectant Treatment

If it is considered that active interference of any kind should be deferred for a time for renal or ureteric calculi, suitable measures may assist the passage of a small stone.

Little is known with real accuracy of the precise effect of a high fluid intake, on the urinary output of the affected side (though that of the healthy kidney must be

Table 12.2. The spontaneous passage of ureteric calculi

Author	Year	Total	Passed spontaneously
Chwalla	1929	91	36% of 91 cases
Hellstrom	1935		Between 24% and 36%
Arneson	1940	113	66
Boeminghaus	1940		+50%
Busch	1943		+50%
Dix	1951	225	100 (operations done on 115 cases)
Prentiss et al.	1952	423	53.7%
Sandegard	1956⎫ 1958⎭	518	76.0%
Dodson et al.	1957	1732 (from 6 reports)	12.9%
	1957	651 (from their own hospital)	90 (In this period 89 had renal colic with negative X-ray, but probably they had stones)
Prince and Scardino	1960	922	260 (27%)
Higgins and Straffon	1963		17.1%
Fetter et al.	1963		Between 24% and 36%
Fox et al.	1965	292	89 (30.5%)
Wax and Frank	1965	220	124 (56%)

increased), but if ureteric obstruction is incomplete, peristaltic contractions of the ureter are probably stimulated. Fluids should therefore be generously taken. Vigorous exercise, which has been suggested as an aid to the passage of a stone, could result in much loss of fluid from the skin and the lungs, thereby reducing urinary output and also the peristaltic activity of the ureter. Patients in hot countries in whom the urinary output is often small and ureteric activity consequently reduced not only form renal calculi but often expel them down the ureter [24].

It is doubtful (and is probably impossible to prove) whether the administration of diuretics is any more effective than a simple increased intake of fluids. Commonly recommended have been potassium citrate and diuretin. Antispasmodics, such as belladonna, atropine, are sometimes prescribed in the hope that ureteric spasm may be reduced.

Lapides [65] stated that change in the urine volume induces changes in the peristaltic activity of the urine, and that stretching of the ureteric muscle by the urine is the normal stimulant to its activity. He found that rhythmic contractions and tone of the intact human ureter were not directly affected by the administration of prostigmine, atropine, trasentin, papaverine, pitressin, benadryl, ephedrine or morphia.

Renal Colic. The severe pain of acute renal colic calls for urgent relief by the injection of 100 mg pethidine, or of one-third of a grain of omnopon (repeated after 1–2 h) or of one-quarter of a grain of morphia (repeated if necessary). If relief is not obtained in this way, the passage of a catheter along the ureter beyond the stone (which may not be possible) should provide drainage of urine (which may be bloodstained) from the distended upper tract and usually gives prompt relief. For the relief of renal colic McLean et al. [71] used a thoraco-lumbar sympathetic block in 13 patients (injecting 2% procaine through a long needle) and claimed relief of pain within a few minutes. The injection facilitated the spontaneous passage of the stone which, in fact, happened in eight cases.

II. Attempted Dissolution of Renal Calculi

1. General Considerations

Attempts have been made to cause calculi in the renal pelvis to go into solution by the use of various solvents introduced by way of a ureteric catheter. Similar attempts have also been made to dissolve vesical calculi by irrigation of the bladder with solvents, sometimes successfully.

Among early efforts to cause renal calculi to go into solution by irrigating the renal pelvis with supposed solvent solutions were those of Keyser [54–56], who used dilute aqua regis, phosphoric acid and some organic acids. In 1932 he accomplished what was probably the first almost complete disintegration of a calcium phosphate stone in the kidney by the irrigation through a large ureteric catheter left in situ, with a solution of dilute aqua regis aided by the administration of an acidogenic diet to render the urine acid in reaction. In partially successful experiments using various reagents he found that the superficial portions of most phosphate stones could be dissolved, but that the stone then became covered with a mucoid organic substance which hindered further action by the solvent and which he tried to dissolve by introducing various enzymes into the irrigating medium (urease, pepsin, diastase, trypsin) with partial success. He stated that he had caused nine stones in the renal pelvis to go into dissolution partially or completely.

2. Irrigation Through an Indwelling Catheter

The ideal irrigating fluid for attempts to cause the stone to go into solution should act within a relatively short period of time. It should be non-irritating to the epithelium of the urinary passages. It should be non-toxic, since some of the components of the fluid are almost certain to be absorbed. It should be easy to prepare and store and be reasonably inexpensive. Such combinations are not easy to achieve.

A large-size ureteric catheter (No. 10F) is passed along the ureter through a cystoscope to the renal pelvis, its final position being confirmed by radiography or by television amplifier [98]. The end of the catheter (and its eyes) should be lodged as close as possible to the stone in the renal pelvis. When it has been established that free drainage of urine is taking place by way of the catheter, irrigation is commenced with the selected fluid, either intermittently or by slow continuous drip from a reservoir placed at a suitable height above the patient.

A double (biluminar) ureteric catheter (9–12 F), one being for the introduction of the irrigating fluid, the other for its voiding, may be used, the pressure within the renal pelvis being recorded by means of a U-tube and manometer attached to one of the catheters. The irrigation may be continued for several days.

Some urologists have left the catheter in situ for a few weeks, in attempts to dissolve large staghorn calculi [18], the patient himself being taught the routine of controlling the supply of the irrigating fluid.

Dormia et al. [29] devised an apparatus which allows the automatic perfusion of renal cavities (for days or even weeks), which is suitable for irrigation of the renal pelvis containing stones composed of ammonium magnesium phosphate, calcium phosphate and/or calcium oxalate. The apparatus allows of the rhythmic filling and emptying of the renal cavities by the solvent solution kept at a constant temperature. The patient himself can interrupt the injection if he experiences pain.

The chief danger is the introduction of infection of the upper urinary tract, which when established may be difficult to eradicate, but which may be countered by the use of urinary antiseptics or antibiotics by mouth, or in small concentrations in the irrigating fluid. If the infecting micro-organism is the *B. proteus* or the *Ps. pyocyaneus*, further stone formation may be encouraged rather than prevented, especially if the urine is allowed to become alkaline.

Temporary obstruction in the lumen of the catheter by muddy debris, derived either from the disintegrating calculus (especially one composed of ammonium magnesium phosphate) or from plugs of fibrin or pus resulting from infection of the urinary passages, can lead to retention of urine in the renal pelvis, pain and fever. Such an event would have to be countered by gentle irrigation through the catheter with sterile saline to remove the obstruction, or failing relief, the catheter may have to be withdrawn and replaced later. Using various irrigants, observers have reported occasional cases of complete or partial dissolution of stones. Most dissolution techniques have, however, been disappointing; some calcareous debris usually remains, in which case recurrence is likely.

For patients who have had most but not all of the calculi removed surgically (for example, by nephrolithotomy), continuous or rapidly repeated irrigations of the stone-bearing (and frequently infected) kidney through a nephrostomy tube with or without the use of associated ureteric catheters, tidal irrigators and hand syringes, has been frequently tried. Sooner or later, however, such irrigation has often led to local discomfort in the renal area and sometimes to fever and added infection. Since some calcific foci may lie almost buried in the renal tissues or tightly surrounded by dilated renal calyces, it could be almost impossible for the irrigating fluid to reach the site of such stones or even the closely knit clefts of a branching staghorn calculus. The final test of success is the achievement of a negative radiograph indicating that the residual calculi have disappeared. In the

author's department the results of such treatment have been disappointing.

3. Sodium Citrate–Citric Acid Solution: Solution G

A major effort to find solutions which would dissolve urinary calculi when used as irrigating fluids was made by Albright, Suby and their co-workers [3, 4, 93–95]. It was shown that solutions of sodium citrate and citric acid could dissolve calcium phosphate calculi in vitro [3]. Solutions of many different organic acids were examined under various conditions to see which combination was most appropriate. They considered that weakly dissociated acids buffering between pH 4.0 and 4.8 were the most effective, and the following organic acids were listed in the order of their efficiency: citric, phthalic, succinic, laevu-linic, β-hydroxybutyric, acetic, malonic, propionic, gluconic, lactic and pyruvic. Further details were given in their papers.

In 1939, Albright et al. [4] successfully dissolved vesical calculi in a patient with a 'cord' bladder by using an isotonic citrate solution at pH 4.0. The irritability of the bladder to various possible irrigating fluids (in the dog and the rabbit) was studied by cystoscopic methods.

After examining solutions of many substances, solution G, usually known as Suby's solution, was found to be most effective in respect of the ability to dissolve calcium phosphate and the lack of irritability to the bladder. Its composition is: citric acid monohydrate, 32.4 g; magnesium oxide (anhydrous), 3.8 g; sodium carbonate (anhydrous), 4.4 g; in distilled water, 1000 ml at pH 4. Solution M (which was less acid in reaction and not quite as irritating as solution G), was also developed, the formula for which being: citric acid monohydrate, 32.5 g; magnesium oxide anhydrous, 3.84 g; sodium carbonate anhydrous, 8.84 g; distilled water,

1000 cc. They reported the use of the solutions on about 20 patients with partial or complete dissolution of their renal calculi (as shown radiographically) in 6, calculi composed mostly of calcium phosphate responding best. They gave sulphathiazole as a protective against infection.

In spite of the drawback of the method of irrigation and the risk of infection, solution G has been used with comparative success by many workers, irrigation treatment being tolerated by some patients for comparatively long periods [18]. Pelot et al. [77] used solution G with success by irrigation through a nephrostomy tube in a tetraplegic patient with calculi in the renal pelvis. Elliott et al. [36] reported the results of irrigation treatment in nine patients with renal phosphatic calculi (eight being young adults paralysed following poliomyelitis), in three of whom the stones were completely dissolved and in five, markedly reduced in size. Solution G is useful for irrigation of the bladder when an indwelling catheter has to be used for longish periods (as in patients with spinal injury) to prevent encrustation of the catheter with phosphatic debris.

4. EDTA (Versene)

EDTA or versene, which was first described in 1937 for use in the German dye industry [42] is the aqueous solution of the tetra-sodium salt of ethylene diamine tetra-acetic acid (EDTA; calsol). It is non-toxic, readily soluble in water, it is completely ionized in solution (since it is a salt of a strong base), it is easily crystallized from aqueous solution (as a hydrate of the bisodium salt) and it forms a crystalline precipitate on the addition of strong acids.

Abeshouse and Weinberg [1] found that a 10% solution is an effective solvent in vitro for calculi composed of calcium carbonate and mixed alkaline earth phosphate, and to a lesser degree for the dissolution of calcium oxalate calculi in pure

or combined forms. Gehres and Raymond [42], who independently suggested the use of EDTA as a solvent for calculi, used a 3% solution of the following composition, the pH being adjusted to between 7 and 8: calsol, 100 g; sodium hydroxide, 40 g: water to 1 litre. They reported moderately successful results in irrigation treatment mostly for some vesical calculi.

Brodzinski et al. [9, 10] successfully used continuous irrigation of the renal pelvis with a 2.5% solution of disodium ethylene diamine tetraacetate buffered at pH 8.6, with 3% triethanolamine, for the dissolution of calcium oxalate renal calculi, 150–200 ml of the irrigant being used hourly. Dormia and Zardina [28] used EDTA in combination with nitrilo-tetraacetic acid as an irrigant for the treatment of renal calculi with varied results.

Timmermann and Kallistratos [98, 99] reported the results of the treatment of 260 patients with renal calculi by irrigation of the stone with chemical solvents. The solutions which were used to give an alkaline pH (to aid the binding property of EDTA), were: solution A (0.05% pluronic F68 and 1.0% sodium polyphosphate) to help dissolve the organic matrix in the outer layers of the stone and to bind the calcium; and solution B (EDTA with polyvinyl-pyrrolidone, a buffer, and chloramphenicol as an antibiotic) to dissolve the mineral part of the stone. Of 125 patients treated between 1961 and 1963, total dissolution was achieved in 66% and partial dissolution in 34%. During the 5-year period 1961–1967, chemolysis used for recurrent stones judged to be not more than 6 months old resulted in 100% dissolution.

5. Renacidin

Renacidin was introduced into urological practice by Mulvaney [72–74] as an irrigation fluid specifically for the dissolution of renal and soft vesical calculi composed of calcium phosphate and magnesium ammonium phosphate, and of calcareous phosphatic deposits around indwelling urethral or suprapubic cathethers and in the urinary bladder. It is also used to dissolve particles left in the bladder following lithotrity, calcified debris in the prostatic cavity, and the calcific incrustations in alkaline phosphatic cystitis.

Renacidin is a composite substance, its principal components being citric acid, magnesium acid citrate, acid gluconate and glucocitrates, magnesium and calcium bicarbonate, d-gluconic acid and glucorolactone. It is a white powder which bubbles when added to water and is buffered close to a pH of 4.0 in a 10% concentration and seems to be able to generate acidic ions; it increases solubility of calcium salts through the formation of water-soluble complexes.

Mulvaney [73] reported his results in 45 patients with urolithiasis who had been treated by irrigation with Renacidin: of 13 patients with renal stones, good results were obtained in 9, the stones either disappearing completely or being shown to have been reduced in size on radiological examination. There were four failures; in one case the stone was reduced in size to one-half, leaving an insoluble calcium oxalate centre. Of 10 patients with vesical calculi, good results were obtained in 5, large vesical stones of mixed composition being softened and partly dimineralized by the irrigation. He found few irritating side-effects unless the catheter became blocked with sandy debris. Some paraplegic patients with vesical calculi were able to supervise their own irrigation treatment for some weeks with ultimate complete elimination of the stones.

Although successes were reported with the use of Renacidin, experiences published by Abeshouse et al. [2] included some indifferent results. Russell [84] reported the complete dissolution of bilateral infected staghorn renal calculi in 10–13 days in a woman with disseminated sclerosis who was relatively insensitive and who tolerated the treatment well, there being no recurrence of stone 18 months later.

With the increasing use of the remedy, some severe reactions began to be reported, and also cases of fatal pyelonephritis [82]. In Kohler's [58] patient sudden death occurred after treatment with Renacidin for about 12 h. Fostvedt and Barnes [39] reported four deaths from renal infection (two of their own cases and two from the practice of other surgeons) during a course of lavage therapy with Renacidin for the treatment of advanced renal calculous disease. Servadio and Caine [89] reported the use of irrigations of Renacidin through ureteric catheters in three patients with bilateral nephrolithiasis, some of whom encountered reactions, one patient dying in coma 10 days after the cessation of treatment.

It appears that Renacidin is an irritant to some calculous patients when used to irrigate the renal pelvis–calyx system. Moreover, it would appear that it may possibly give rise to toxic compounds during decomposition and that some patients may be allergic to it. Sludge may accumulate in the catheter leading to partial retention of the irrigating fluid (which has a low pH), and the procedure is then not free from danger. The cause of death in the fatal cases may have been an exacerbation of the existing renal infection.

The use of Renacidin is not recommended for the treatment of renal calculi, either by injection through ureteric catheters, or by way of a pyelostomy or a nephrostomy tube. When used to assist in keeping clean an indwelling urethral catheter, 1 oz. 10% solution three times daily, injected using a small syringe, will usually keep the catheter free from phosphatic deposits.

6. Irrigation or Operation?

The use of the various irrigating solutions in the attempt to dissolve phosphatic renal calculi in situ has shown that such a result is sometimes possible. Some good results have been achieved by the use of solution G, and by the use of other solutions by Dormia et al. [26–29] and by Timmermann et al. [98, 99]. A disadvantage of the method is that some part of the stone, especially that composed of calcium oxalate, may be left behind. The tedious nature of the treatment and the amount of personal attention and observation required, the length of time needed to achieve a result as well as the risks of infection and obstruction, combine to make the method a less satisfactory mode of treatment than operation for most patients.

For the treatment of patients with advanced bilateral infected staghorn calculi, in whom renal function is poor, some surgeons have chosen irrigation in preference to a sometimes hazardous operative treatment or to an attitude of complete inactivity.

The principle of the use of chelating agents for the purpose of dissolving or preventing calcification in the urinary tract is an attractive one. If a suitable agent in this group could be found which could be administered orally, is non-toxic, and the chelating properties of which were unmasked only during its excretion through the kidneys, a real advance would have been achieved. Calgon given in the drinking water, which was shown in the author's department to prevent the formation of calcification around foreign bodies introduced into the bladder of rats [16] comes most closely to this ideal; it is not suitable, however, for oral use in man.

7. Encrusted (Alkaline) Phosphatic Cystitis

Although a vesical condition, this may be referred to in a discussion concerning the dissolution of crystalline elements in the urinary tract. By alkaline phosphatic cystitis is meant the deposition upon the mucous membrane of the chronically inflamed bladder of massive deposits of calcium phosphate; in some cases, though not in all, the urine is infected. The condition is sometimes found in association with carcinoma of the bladder. Patients of both sexes are affected, usually during middle life.

The clinical importance of the condition lies in the distressing nature of its symptoms and in the probability, sooner or later, of the association of an ascending infection. There is severe pain in the urethra on micturition and, largely owing to the greatly reduced capacity of the bladder and the solid phosphatic debris within it, there is great diurnal and nocturnal frequency of micturition. The worst case in the author's series, a man of 50 years, was compelled to void urine almost hourly doubled up on hands and knees. The general health suffers on account of pain and loss of sleep. The capacity of the bladder may be reduced to 2 oz or less and only after prolonged washing out can a clear medium be obtained to allow of a cystoscopic examination.

In the fully developed case plaques of whitish phosphatic debris of various sizes are seen sometimes scattered in separate areas round the sides and vault, the base and the trigone and bladder neck. The mucosa between the encrusted areas, which is nowhere healthy, presents either a severe angry engorgement with here and there plaques of adherent lymph, or a red angry surface impaled by the phosphatic masses during micturition from which drops of blood ooze; it is often impossible to distinguish the position of the ureteric orifices. The upper urinary tract is radiologically normal.

Earlier treatment of this distressing condition by vesical irrigants such as dilute acetic acid solution and solution G used intermittently to 'dissolve' the calcium phosphate has been unsatisfactory, as seen in some patients who have been referred to the author. Indeed such occasional bathing of the masses of crystalline phosphatic material can hardly be expected to have been beneficial. The old treatment known as 'grand lavage' of the bladder carried out by the patient himself was also unsatisfactory.

The crystalline masses, however, can always be dispersed if the patient is given oral acid therapy for a continuous period of 4–6 weeks. It is necessary to be certain that renal function is normal so that the large doses of acid administered can be safely excreted in the urine, and also that the patient's stomach can tolerate it. The patient is given an acidogenic diet together with ammonium chloride (in capsules) in gradually increasing doses, which may reach as much as 30 grains 4-hourly. In the worst cases, in order to expedite the result of treatment, the author has given mandelic acid in addition. The effect of such treatment has been dramatic. The phosphatic masses have gradually passed into solution leaving the wall of the bladder still red, but free from debris. In at least three of the author's patients much of the debris was not voided per urethram but was clumped together to form one or more sizeable white phosphatic calculi, which were then crushed with a lithotrite and evacuated after 4 weeks of treatment. The capacity of the bladder gradually returned to normal and the patient became symptom free. In an occasional case it is necessary to continue the acid therapy in modified doses for a considerable time after the completion of the first phase of treatment to prevent recurrent symptoms. Antibiotics are needed in infected cases.

The treatment by acidifiers should not be abandoned because the bladder urine cannot at first be rendered acid to the litmus test, since that is to be expected; but with the recommended dose of acidifiers (given that the kidneys are healthy), the urine delivered into the bladder by way of the ureteric orifices must be acid in reaction, though on reaching the bladder it is at once neutralized by the presence of the phosphatic debris in the bladder, at least until the debris is much reduced in amount.

III. Perureteral Instrumental Methods for the Treatment of Ureteric Stone

1. General Considerations

The chances of the spontaneous passage of a ureteric calculus have been referred to. Some stones which are halted in their downward course (especially those in the lower third of the ureter) may be induced to descend to the bladder by suitable instrumentation, thereby avoiding an open operation. There is no general consensus of opinion regarding the precise indications for the use of manipulative and/or of operative treatment. Some urologists have acquired great expertise in the use of manipulative perureteral methods for the treatment of their patients (except those with very large calculi) while others have favoured operative treatment much more if spontaneous voiding has been seen to fail, yet there is much common ground of opinion. The simpler the technique, the wider its appeal and its usefulness.

The indications and contra-indications for manipulative treatment and also the proportion of cases treated by manipulation in various series are given below. Several variants of the instrumental or manipulative treatment of ureteric calculi include: instruments used to dilate the ureter and to cause it to contract in the hope that the stone will be voided; instruments used to extract the stone, including baskets and corkscrew-like appliances; special instruments and techniques for the treatment of stone in the intramural ureter and at the ureterovesical orifice, some of which are widely used.

The procedures to be described should usually be carried out in hospital under general anaesthetic, with the full ritual of a surgical procedure and with appropriate care and gentleness. Skilfully performed. perureteral instrumental treatment can be a great boon to the patient in appropriate cases. There is an incidence of injury to the ureter during these procedures, which is referred to below (Table 12.3, see p. 236).

Indications

1. Stones in the lower third of the ureter of between 0.5 and 1 cm in diameter which fail to pass spontaneously.

2. Small stones at the entrance to the bladder wall.

3. Stones in the intramural part of the ureter or at the ureteric orifice.

Contra-indications

1. Stones in the upper and middle third of the ureter.

2. Stones in the lower third of the ureter more than 1 cm in diameter.

3. When the affected kidney is moderately or markedly hydronephrotic and the ureter above the stone is greatly dilated, indicating firm impaction of the stone; a little dilatation of the ureter as shown in the intravenous pyelogram does not contra-indicate instrumentation.

4. Urinary infection and especially when the kidney is the seat of severe pyelonephritis or pyonephrosis.

5. A moderately or greatly dilated ureter (for example, congenital megaureter), where surgical treatment of the ureter as well as removal of the calculi may be necessary.

6. Congenital anomalies of the ureter.

7. An unyielding intramural ureter which resists dilatation.

8. Bad reaction (severe or recurrent colic, fever, undue pain, mental stress) to the first attempt at manipulation; or in any case when a number of earlier attempts at instrumental removal have not been successful.

9. When simple cystoscopy has been badly tolerated.

10. A spiculated stone (as determined radiographically), since it may be firmly anchored.

11. A stone present in the ureter for a long time with little downward movement; it is then probably firmly impacted.

12. Associated prostatic enlargement causing symptoms, since the ureter may be distorted at its lower end.

13. Recurrent attacks of colic following which the stone has not descended nor been expelled.

14. When the patient has previously voided ureteric calculi spontaneously.

15. Multiple calculi or long cylindrical calculi.

2. Passage of Ureteric Catheters and Dilators; Indwelling Catheters

The passage of a ureteric catheter to, or beyond, the calculus, may dislodge a small ureteric stone, change its axis, alter slightly the degree of its impaction and stimulate ureteric contraction so that it may be voided spontaneously a few hours or days later. To relieve spasm, 1 or 2 ml 2% novocaine may be injected around the stone, together with a small amount of sterile olive oil or liquid paraffin to act as a lubricant, the effect being uncertain. The catheter must be passed beyond the stone to achieve its maximal effect.

One or more ureteric catheters may be left in situ in the ureter beyond the stone for 12–48 h, and (if more than one) may be twisted on each other, a procedure sometimes attended by renal colic. Occasionally during the procedure a stone may be pushed upwards into the renal pelvis. If bleeding occurs the catheter must be withdrawn. If the catheter remains in position for 48 h or more, the subsequent descent of the stone may be painless, possibly because the ureter has become

Table 12.3. Proportion of cases treated by manipulation and by operation in various series

Surgeon	Year	Total cases	Successful manipulative treatment	Operative treatment	Spontaneous passage
Bugbee	1923	347	326		
Kretschmer	1923	140		28%	
Crowell	1924	98	88		
Bumpus and Thompson	1930	1001	348 successful (85%) 72 failed manipulation	529 (252 lower third of ureter) (228 in upper and middle third) 372 ureterolithotomy 51 nephroureterectomy 37 nephrectomy 3 ureterectomy 66 combined operation	
Squires	1930	606	87.15%		
Alyea	1938	377	72%		
Thompson and Kibler	1941		361 ('An almost equal number of 361 were treated expectantly because of the small size of the stone, or the absence of symptoms')	392 (in 25 manipulation failed)	
Councill (extractions mainly)	1945	504	374		
Dourmashkin	1945	1550	93.3%		
Dix	1951	225 (During a 27-month period at Urological Centre M.E.F. during the war; in same period 112 patients who had had renal colic were also seen; although they had negative radiographs, probably small calculi had been passed).		115	100
Winsbury-White	1954	230		23%	
Dodson et al.	1957	561 (large stones; 15 mm or more in diameter)	85.9%		
Dodson et al.		689 (small stones; 5 mm or less)	99.7%		
Dodson et al.		283 (patients with normal ureter)	37.5%		8.4%
Dodson et al.		102 (patients with a dilated ureter)	14.0%		3.3%
Dodson et al.		413 (in a 5-year period)	244 (stone passed spontaneously or removed by manipulation)	169	
Dodson et al.		4947 (collected series)	68.2%		
Prince and Scardino	1960	861	31% attempted (successful in 65.4% of these)	227	260 (27%)
Fetter et al.	1963		48.1%		
Fox et al.	1965	292		109	

dilated. The catheter first passed may be replaced by a slightly larger one after a day or two. Antibiotics should usually be given when indwelling ureteric catheters are used. Conical-ended or olivary-tipped ureteric dilators passed to, and if possible beyond the stone may be used instead of a ureteric catheter to try to dislodge the stone. A successful result could depend upon the degree of dilatation of the ureter produced; an estimate of their value compared with that of ureteric catheters is difficult.

Dourmashkin [30–32] published a series of papers recording a large and successful experience of the use of instrumental methods for the treatment of ureteric calculi. Using tunnelled and tapering metallic radio-opaque bougies (12–22 F) measuring 2 cm in length, screwed to the end of a ureteric catheter lined with a fine flexible silver tube, and introduced through the middle compartment of a Brown–Buerger operating cystoscope or through a McCarthy panendoscope, he contrived to push the stone upwards into the dilated segment of the ureter above the point where it was impacted and then, if possible, to pass the bougie a further distance of at least 2 cm beyond the stone. Oil for lubrication was injected through the bougie and urine could drain downwards through the tunnel. Treatment with the bougie was repeated after an interval if necessary and was most effective for the release of calculi in the lower third of the ureter.

In 1926 he modified and extended this method; a rubber bag 3 cm in length was fitted over the tunnelled bougie (which was screwed onto the end of the catheter) and tied to it by silk. The tunnelled bougie with the rubber bag attached, was introduced through the operating cystoscope into the bladder. The rubber bag was then distended by injecting either air or water through a syringe attached to the proximal end of the catheter, and introduced along the ureter. A number of cases were successfully treated by the method, the stone

dropping out within 2 or 3 days of the treatment.

In 1945 he described the further development of his rubber bag technique for the treatment of stones in the upper 20 cm of the ureter and even for stones in the renal pelvis which it was thought were of a size which could be made to descend the ureter. The ureter was first dilated with an inflatable rubber bag (distended with not more than 12 minims of liquid) attached as before to an olive-tipped catheter and passed through an operating cystoscope. Ideally the stone is now pushed upwards for a few centimetres, and dilatation of the ureter with the distended rubber bag then begun at the segment of the ureter which had contained the stone, following which dilatation was proceeded with centimetre by centimetre, throughout the entire length of the ureter below the stone; it was hoped that the stone would then be voided.

A remarkable degree of success was achieved by his methods, sometimes stones of considerable size being extracted. In his series of 1253 patients treated with his metallic bougies and rubber bag catheter, 1171 (93.5%) were successful, and in no patient was there a rupture of the ureter. In the hands of other workers, however, ruptured ureter was encountered occasionally. Many of the large calculi treated by Dourmashkin in the way described would now preferably be removed by open operation.

Injection of Air Along the Ureter. Flesch [38] recommended the attempted disimpaction of ureteric calculi by the injection of air along a ureteric catheter passed to the level of the stone; if drainage of urine could not be established because the catheter could not be passed beyond the stone, 4 cc air were slowly injected along it; following a momentary increase of pain, there was normally a gush of urine through and around the catheter. If the air failed to pass beyond the stone, it bubbled back into the bladder and no pain was experienced. A larger catheter was then used so as to occlude the ureteric orifice and the procedure repeated.

3. Instruments for Extracting Ureteric Calculi

The extraction of calculi from the ureter with different instruments has been in use for a long time. Various devices including loops attached to bougies have been used by earlier urologists to try to extract ureteric calculi.

Basket Extractors. Different workers have devised various forms of wire or nylon baskets, some of which are currently in use [87].

Councill [19, 20] devised an expandable wire basket or cage consisting of six flexible wires about 7 cm in length, arranged side by side in the form of a spindle, the proximal end of which is attached to a flexible metal shaft and the distal end to a short filiform bougie. In order to bend the wires and open the spindle a central wire is added (which passes from the distal end of the spindle through the shaft to a handle at the proximal end of the instrument), traction upon which causes the ends of the spindle to be approximated to one another, thus opening the wires of the spindle. The stone may then be caught in the basket, which is withdrawn; the ureter is dilated before the instrument is introduced, which must be passed beyond the stone. The results of treatment in a series of 504 cases of ureteric stone (57 in the upper third, 86 in the middle third and 361 in the lower third) included the successful removal of 364 stones (26 from the upper, 67 from the middle and 271 from the lower third). Councill was unable to pass the extractor beyond the stone in 12.9% but in the cases in which this was possible, 84.8% were removed.

Howard [49] developed an extractor consisting of a spiral or corkscrew wire with an olivary point, which was introduced into the ureter and moved upward with a screw-like movement, the hope being that the stone would engage in the coils and that gentle traction on the instrument would cause it to descend. This instrument is best used for calculi low down the lower third of the ureter.

Johnson's extractor [52], a modification of Councill's basket [19], consists of four thin, flexible wires arranged in the form of a spindle and attached proximally to an insulated flexible wire shaft and distally to a fine bougie. The spindle, which is the effective part of the instrument, varies from 2.5 to 3.0 cm in length and its greatest diameter when expanded is a little less than 1 cm.

Dormia's Spiral Basket. Dormia [27, 28] constructed a spiral basket for the extraction of stones in the ureter which has won wide acceptance and has been used in the author's department with considerable success. The apparatus consists of a Neoplex ureteral catheter (No. 5 Char.), which is traversed by a flexible metal rod carrying at its proximal end a screw mounting, by which its position is controlled. The distal end carries the basket, consisting of three or four stainless steel wires twisted to form a helical bobbin spindle, which is surmounted by a small cylindrical cap of the same small calibre as the catheter. When the rod is pulled down the wires of the basket are approximated and become lodged entirely within the catheter, the terminal cap alone remaining visible without any outward projection. When the rod is pushed upwards the wires emerge and because of their elastic construction they emerge as the spiral basket. The same principles of inserting the basket, engaging the stone, and use of radiography apply as with the Councill and Johnson baskets.

Thread Extractors. McKay [70] passed up the ureter a filiform whalebone bougie to which four long silk threads were attached; by pushing forward the bougie and pulling the threads downwards and twisting them, the bougie was bowed, and it was then hoped that the stone would be enmeshed and then extracted. Zeiss [104] employed a ureteric catheter to the distal end of which was attached a long piece of silkworm gut, the end of which was made to enter the lumen of the catheter some centimetres below its tip and to emerge from the proximal end. The loop, which was intended to enmesh the stone, was formed by traction upon the thread.

Ellik's Looped Catheter. Ellik [33] devised a looped catheter (using a No. 5 whistle-tip) at the distal end of which (6 cm from the tip) a hole is made by a hot hypodermic needle. A long piece of surgical steel suture wire (gauge No. 32 and 35) is threaded through the distal end of the catheter until it comes out at the base where it is anchored, the other end of the filament (the 'pull' filament) being threaded downwards through the newly created hole until it also appears at the base; a loop is then formed at the distal end, which can be used for traction. The instrument is passed down the cystoscope and the pull filament drawn on to enable the catheter to be pushed up, usually to the renal pelvis when it has passed the stone. The loop, which is more easily formed within the pelvis than within the ureter (its size being determined by radiography), is withdrawn slowly (1 cm every 10 s), some resistance being encountered when it engages the stone. The instrument is secured by tape to the abdomen, when traction is not being applied; most stones come away within 24 h. Ellik extracted 131 stones of various sizes and in different positions during a period of 34 months.

4. Stones in the Intramural Part of the Ureter and at the Ureterovesical Orifice

Stones may remain in the intramural part of the ureter for a considerable time but if their spontaneous passage is unduly delayed they should be encouraged to descend into the bladder by an intravesical manipulative procedure. The intramural part of the ureter is somewhat rigid and resists dilatation. Perurethral treatment is usually successful in enabling a stone to fall into the bladder either at the time of treatment or within a few days. The methods of treatment used are: simple diathermy of the orifice; incision of the orifice by the use of meatotomy, diathermy, Collings knife or Buerger's cystoscopic scissors; extraction of the stone by Howard's stone extractor.

Diathermy of the Ureterovesical Orifice. Furness [41] first used fulguration of the oedematous vesical opening of the ureter for the treatment of cases of stone at or near the orifice. In a group of 12 patients in whom the ureteric mound presented the appearance of a red oedematous swelling Dourmashkin [31] fulgurated the mass at random (the ureteric orifice being sometimes difficult to define) for a few seconds until the mucosa became white without resorting to any intraureteric dilatation, a procedure which was usually followed by prompt relief of pain, by the rapid disappearance of the 'tumour' (because of the release of fluid from the engorged area) and by the subsequent early voiding of the stone after a few days.

Dix [24] used electro-coagulation of the whole of the oedematous area around the ureteric orifice with a diathermy electrode introduced through an operating cystoscope. The procedure was followed by fibrosis of the peri-ureteric tissues and an actual enlargement of the ureteric orifice, the stone being usually extruded into the bladder after a few days; in 27 of 37 patients treated, the stone was voided after an average time of 11.3 days; in 17 in whom the exact time of the voiding of the stone was known, the average was 7.8 days.

Various Techniques for Stone at the Ureterovesical Orifice. A stone, the tip of which is seen on cystoscopy to be presenting at the ureteric orifice, or which is shown by the passage of a ureteric catheter and the appearance of the orifice to be just within it, may be dealt with by the use of Lane's meatotome The instrument, which is the size of a No. 5 ureteric catheter, is passed into the bladder through a catheterizing cystoscope, and the end of the instrument is moved to the proximity of the ureteric orifice. The central wire electrode of the meatotome is then caused to project from its sheath for 1 cm by pressure on the button at its proximal end and is introduced into the ureteric orifice just above the stone; depression of the proximal end of the cystoscope produces a little upward pressure by the wire electrode onto the upper lip of the ureteric orifice; when the cutting current is turned on for a few seconds a small neat linear cut is made which enlarges the orifice, when the stone may fall out into the bladder immediately or during the next 24 h, when it may be voided spontaneously.

Linear diathermy to divide the lip of the ureteric orifice in an upward and outward direction for 1 cm starting at the ureteric orifice may be used for the treatment of stones at or just within the ureteric orifice. The Collings knife is a small knife (which may be used as an electrode) introduced through a cystoscope or a panendoscope for the purpose of incising the lower end of the ureteric orifice where the impacted stone is situated. The incision begins at the meatus (or at the swelling caused by the stone) and is carried upwards over the swelling.

Howard's [49] spiral stone extractor, previously referred to, may be used for the extraction of a stone just visible within or at the ureteric orifice, the olive tip of the instrument being passed between the calculus and the wall of the ureter to engage the stone within the curve of the spiral, and then to withdraw it.

Cystoscopic scissors, introduced by Buerger [12] have been used to cut one lip of the ureteric orifice in order to liberate a stone which is retained there. The scissors, which are mounted on a long flexible stem, which can be passed into the bladder through an operating cystoscope, have one sharp-pointed blade, the other being probe-pointed for passage into the ureteric orifice for 0.5 cm. The opening and closing of the instrument are controlled by two handles at the proximal end of the instrument; a sharply executed cut divides the orifice. The instrument has been largely replaced by the meatotome.

The Bransford Lewis dilator [67, 68], which consists of two moveable expanding terminal blades mounted on a long, flexible stem working on the principle of a Kollman dilator and controlled by a handle at the proximal end of the instrument, may be used to dilate the lowest 2 cm of the ureter. The instrument is introduced into the ureter through an operating cystoscope, the blades being closed. By pressure on the handles the blades are cautiously opened to stretch (but not to tear) the wall of the ureter, the procedure being repeated after rotating the instrument through 90°. It can be effective if used with care.

Transurethral Endovesical Ureterolithotomy. Davis et al. [23] used the loop of a resectoscope to slice off the bulge at the lower end of the ureter, resulting from an intramural stone, which was then disclosed to view and dislodged, bleeding from the edge of the incision being controlled by the coagulating current. If the stone is very low in the ureter the resected tissue may include the ureteric orifice, with possible subsequent undesirable reflux; they reported 20 cases relieved by this method without serious complication.

Ureteric Reflux. Division of the ureteric orifice by scissors, knife, diathermy or resection may lead to ureteric reflux of urine by damaging the normal valve-like action, with the subsequent development of hydroureter, hydronephrosis and possibly infection. The oblique course of the intramural portion of the ureter through the bladder wall produces a valve-like action allowing urine to be normally voided into the bladder but preventing an upward reflux. When the procedures just referred to are carried out at the ureteric orifice, the size of the slit produced by meatotomy should be such as to allow the stone to be voided and no more. Multiple divisions of the orifice are undesirable and may be followed by a large ureteric opening and reflux.

Bruber (quoted by Macalpine [11]) found that after the ureteric orifice had been excised completely, reflux up the ureter was invariable and hydroureter followed. Jacobsson et al. [51] reviewed 20 patients who had had division of the ureteric orifice by various methods for the relief of stones which had varied in size from 3 to 13 mm in diameter, and which lay either within the orifice itself or in the ureter just outside the bladder wall. Four patients were subsequently found to have reflux when investigated 14 days to 2.5 years later.

5. Injuries of the Ureter Following Instrumentation

A little blood may be discharged from the ureter even after a perfectly smooth catheter has been passed along it for diagnostic purposes and later withdrawn, the mucous membrane having suffered slight trauma. Such bleeding is more likely if the tip of the catheter becomes looped within the lumen, or if larger or multiple catheters are introduced. The ureter is a long muscular tube disposed in a series of gentle curves which can safely be stretched longitudinally by instruments passed along it only within certain limits.

Instruments designed to be passed along the ureter must be perfectly smooth and be rigid enough not to buckle but to ride easily along its curved course. Local segments of the wall of the ureter may be weakened by infection associated with the stone and may therefore be vulnerable to instrumentation.

When any instrument (catheter, bougie, looped catheter) is to be passed along the ureter, it must be examined to see that it is mechanically sound and that the filiform end of a wire basket (for example) is screwed home. The instrument itself must be introduced with the greatest gentleness. Since a wire basket may traumatize the ureteric mucous membrane it probably should not be used unless at least a ureteric catheter can be negotiated past the stone. When traction is exerted upon, say, a wire basket containing a spiculated stone, some trauma to the wall of the ureter can scarcely be completely avoided; but the consequences may be minimized if an indwelling catheter is retained for a few hours after the procedure has been completed and antibiotics given before and after the procedure.

One type of injury causing limited damage to the wall of the ureter results in temporary obstruction or retention of urine within the renal pelvis. Another more serious injury is the removal of a long strip of ureteric mucous membrane when the extracting instrument (especially a basket) is withdrawn with or without the calculus inside it. Such an injury may lead to stenosis of the ureter, hydronephrosis and even to serious ascending renal infection and to nephrectomy. The next grade of injury in order of severity is a perforation or tear of the wall of the ureter leading to extravasation of urine, which may be limited and perhaps not of any great consequence, or gross, leading to the formation of a periureteric abscess requiring drainage.

Any of the injuries referred to may be associated with retention of part of the catheter or basket, which may have broken off and which may lodge partly within and partly outside the lumen of the ureter. Some such injuries may be evident at once from

Table 12.4. Injuries of the ureter following instrumentation

Author	Year	Type of injury	Note
Klika	1931	Ureteric catheter tied into knot	Operation needed
Ruschė and Bacon	1940	1. Perforation of ureter; extravasation of urine usually with retroperitoneal abscess; 13 cases 2. Ureter split by buckled catheter leading to extravasation (1 case) 3. Pieces of broken catheter or instrument left in ureter (2 cases)	From summary of 16 cases of ureteric injury; nephrectomy in 3; 2 died
Councill	1945	Ruptured ureter; 3 cases	From series of 504 cases
Ellik and Newton	1951	Ruptured ureter with Ellik loop (4 cases)	From series of 104 cases; nephrectomy in 1 case
Taylor	1953	Following use of Dourmashkin bag (4 cases): 1. Rigor and pain after failed extraction 2. Periureteric abscess; infected hydro-nephrosis in 15 years 3. Ruptured ureter with extravasation 4. Long period of treatment; badly functioning kidney	Nephrectomy 18 months later Drainage operation Drainage operation Nephrectomy needed
Iwano and Bunts	1953	Injury to ureter in 9 cases: 1. Parts or whole of Johnson basket broken off; 2 cases 2. Injury resulted in non-functioning kidney 3. Injury following use of Ellik looped catheter and/or Johnson basket 4. Ureteric mucosa stripped following tension on looped catheter 5. Ruptured ureter with Dourmashkin bag (2 cases)	Operation needed Nephrectomy needed One needed nephrectomy
Sandegard	1956	1. Zeiss catheter broken in ureter 2. Zeiss catheter with stone impacted in the ureter 3. Mucosa stripped from ureter on withdrawal of instrument	Operation needed Operation needed for removal
Prince and Scardino	1960	1. Ruptured ureter, 4 cases 2. Basket wedged in ureter, 1 case 3. Broken basket 4. Rupture of ureter; pyonephrosis	Drainage operation Basket and stone removed Basket and stone removed Nephrectomy needed
Grasset	1968	Injury with Dormia basket	Boari bladder flap operation to repair gap in ureter

inspection of the apparatus after its withdrawal, and by the early pain and rise of temperature experienced by the patient. Sometimes the instrument and the stone have become so firmly engaged in the ureter that they cannot be withdrawn and an open operation has to be performed for their removal.

Rarely, a patient develops symptoms and signs of the injury to the ureter only after he has left hospital, when he may return with an abscess in the loin requiring drainage or occasionally nephrectomy.

Injuries to the ureter reported by various urologists are summarized in Table 12.4. Dodson et al. [25] stated that between 1940 and 1957, 12 authors had reported 67 instances of ureteral injury; 6 required drainage operations; nephrectomy was necessary in 7 patients and 4 died; at least 9 of these injuries had resulted from the use of the looped catheter.

6. Ultrasonic Fragmentation of Calculi

Ultrasonic lithotresis is a technique introduced by Lamport and his co-workers and designed to effect the fragmentation of ureteric calculi by a process of drilling the stone [60–64]. Low-frequency ultrasonic vibrations, about 20,000/s are transmitted mechanically through a metal wire from outside the body through a catheter passed along the ureter to a tiny drill-tip in contact with the calculus. The technique is unsuitable for the treatment of calyceal or pelvic stones. It was thought that if by instrumental means a ureteric stone could be broken into fragments with little associated trauma, it would void spontaneously. Tiny particles may linger in the ureter after instrumentation and be a disadvantage. Ouchi and Takahashi [76] reported some good results in the disintegration of small ureteric calculi by means of ultrasonic vibration, using an apparatus of their own design. The stone was first caught in a basket in the ureter and then given 3 s ultrasonic vibration with an ultrasonic wire drill introduced up the ureter.

7. Summary of Results of Instrumental Methods

Alyea [5] in a series of 236 patients reported that in 72% the stones were removed by cystoscopic manipulation while 18% had operations. Thompson and Kibler [97] reported a series of 361 cases of ureteric stones of varying sizes (mostly in the lower third), treated by the various transurethral methods referred to earlier: in

28% the stones measured 5 mm or less in their greatest diameter, in 19% between 5 and 10 mm, in 46% from 1 to 2 cm and in 2% slightly above 2 cm. The stone was completely withdrawn in 246; in 103 the stone was not extracted at the time of manipulation but in 35 of these it was voided within a few days and in 28 more within a few weeks. In 27 (7.5%) the stone was removed later by operation. The removal of calculi by means of intraureteric instrumentation has been facilitated in recent years by direct visual guidance of the instrument under fluoroscopic control [92].

Unsuccessful Manipulation of Ureteric Calculi. Manipulation may have failed because the stone was too large or spiculated. It may not have been possible to pass a ureteric catheter (nor of course the extractor) beyond a tightly impacted stone. The basket may fail to engage the stone, even when it has been passed beyond it.

The curved lower end of the ureter in patients with prostatic hyperplasia may not allow the instrument to be passed up the ureter. Occasionally the extractor may displace the stone upwards even to the kidney, when a further manipulative attempt will be useless. A friable stone may be fragmented during extraction, the main part of the stone being withdrawn, and the fragments descending to the bladder later; radiography is then necessary to ensure that removal has been complete.

After failed manipulation another attempt may be made a few days later, but the surgeon (and the patient) may feel that ureterolithotomy is then indicated. Unsuccessful manipulation may be followed by pain (requiring morphia), occasionally by renal infection (which could have unpleasant or even dangerous results) and still later by temporary hydronephrosis. Following the successful removal of a stone, a ureteric catheter may be left in the ureter for 24 h (though this is not always necessary) depending upon the amount of trauma which the ureter is judged to have suffered.

References

1. Abeshouse,B.S., Weinberg,T.: Experimental study of solvent action of versene on urinary calculi. J. Urol. *65*, 316 (1951)
2. Abeshouse,G.A., Abeshouse,B.S., Doroshow,L.W.: Use of renacidin as a solvent for vesical calculi. J. Urol. *8*, 69 (1961)
3. Albright,F., Sulkowitch,H.: Further studies in the in vitro and in vivo dissolution of calcium phosphate urinary calculi. J. Clin. Invest. *19*, 786 (1940)
4. Albright,F., Sulkowitch,H.W., Chute,R.: Non-surgical aspects of the kidney stone problem. J. Am. Med. Assoc. *113*, 2049 (1939)
5. Alyea,E.A.: Cystoscopic removal of ureteral calculi. J. Urol. *30*, 83 (1938)
6. Arneson,A.: Der akute Nierensteinanfall. Z. Urol. Klin. *45*, 94 (1940)
7. Barney,J.D.: Spontaneous dissolution of renal calculi. Trans. Am. Assoc. G-U Surg. *22*, 55 (1929)
8. Boeminghaus,H.: Konservative und Chirurgische Behandlung des Harnleitersteins. Leipzig: Thieme 1940
9. Brozinski,M., Sengbusch,R.von, Timmerman,A.: Renal calculi dissolution in man by the formation of complexes. Urol. Int. *10*, 307 (1960)
10. Brozinski,M., Knothe,W., Sengbusch, R.von, Timmerman,A.: A chemical solvent for oxalate stones in the human kidney. Germ. Med. Monthly *6*, 105 (1961)
11. Bruber,: Quoted by Macalpine,J.B. Urography and cystoscopy. London: Wright 1949
12. Buerger,L.: A new method of facilitating the passage of descending ureteral calculi (and of dilating the ureter). Am. J. Surg. *27*, 151 (1913)
13. Bugbee,H.G.: Intraureteral manipulation of ureteral calculi. Trans. Am. Assoc. G-U Surg. *16*, 183 (1923)
14. Bumpus,K.C., Thompson,G.J.: Stones in the ureter. Surg. Gynecol. Obstet. *50*, 106 (1930)
15. Busch,F.: Bericht uber einem Fall von singularer, angeborener ureterstenose und deren operation. Z. Urol. *36*, 172 (1943)
16. Care,A.D., Wilson,G.: The prevention of vesical calculi in rats by the oral administration of polysodium metaphosphate. Clin. Sci. *15*, 183 (1956)
17. Chwalla,R.: Das Spatschicksaal unserer Nieren und Uretersteinfälle. Z. Urol. Chir. *26*, 157 (1929)
18. Colby,F.: Personal communication (1947)
19. Councill,W.A.: New ureteral stone extractor and dilator. J. Am. Med. Assoc. *86*, 1907 (1925)
20. Councill,W.A.: The treatment of ureteral calculi; report of 504 cases in which Councill stone-extractor and dilator was used. J. Urol. *53*, 534 (1945)
21. Crowell,A.J.: Discussion on renal calculi. J. Urol. *12*, 425 (1924)
22. Davidson,G.R.: Treatment of ureteric calculi. Med. J. Austr. *1*, 840 (1952)
23. Davis,E., Lee,L.W., Davis,E.jr.: Transurethral endovesical ureterolithotomy with resectoscope. J. Urol. *67*, 634 (1952)
24. Dix,V.W.: Discussion on stones in lower third of the ureter. Proc. R. Soc. Med. *44*, 933 (1951)
25. Dodson,A.I., Sipe,W.R., Lord,K.H.: The treatment of patients with ureteral calculi. J. Urol. *78*, 575 (1957)
26. Dormia,E.: Considerazioni su 93 casi di calcolosi urinaria cureti con litolisis. Arch. Ital. Urol. Nephrol. *41*, 85 (1968)
27. Dormia,E., Bassi,R.: Radiological collaboration in the endoscopic removal of ureteric stone with the Dormia extractor. Urologia, *28*, 355 (1961)
28. Dormia,E., Zardini,C.: Experienze di Laboratorie su une nuova soluzione litica par i calcoli delle vie urinaire (Soluzione DZ). Arch. Ital. Urol. *36*, 167 (1963)
29. Dormia.E., Cantanzari,F., Tomboline,P.: Resultati della litolisis con perfusove automatici. Atti Soc. Ital. Urol. 42nd Congress (1969)
30. Dourmashkin,R.L.: Concerning the use of tunnelled bougies and the hook-catheter in the treatment of ureteral calculi. J. Urol. *13*, 85 (1925)
31. Dourmashkin,R.L.: Dilatation of ureter with rubber bags in treatment of ureteral calculi; presentation of a modified operative cystoscope; a preliminary report. J. Urol. *15*, 449 (1926)
32. Dourmashkin,R.L.: Cystoscopic treatment of stone in the ureter. J. Urol. *54*, 245 (1945)
33. Ellik,M.J.: Looped catheter ureteral stone-extractors: perplexities in its construction and use. J. Urol. *61*, 351 (1949)

34. Ellik,M.J., Newton,L.A.: Ureteral calculi: experiences in looped catheter management. J. Urol. *65*, 532 (1951)
35. Elliott,J.A.: Spontaneous dissolution of renal calculi. J. Urol. *72*, 331 (1954)
36. Elliott,J.A., Adamson,J.P., Lewis,L.: Dissolution of phosphate calculi by retrograde irrigation. J. Urol. *81*, 56 (1959)
37. Fetter,T.R., Zimskind,D.P., Graham, R.H., Brodie,D.E.: Statistical analysis of patients with ureteral calculi. J. Am. Med. Assoc. *186*, 21 (1963)
38. Flesch,W.L.: Air disimpaction of ureteral calculi. J. Urol. *81*, 96 (1959)
39. Fostvedt,G.A., Barnes,R.W.: Complications during lavage therapy for renal calculi. J. Urol. *89*, 329 (1963)
40. Fox,M., Pyrah,L.N., Raper,F.P.: Management of ureteric stone: review of 292 cases. Br. J. Urol. *37*, 660 (1965)
41. Furness,H.B.: Renal and ureteral calculi. J. Am. Med. Assoc. *61*, 1322 (1913)
42. Gehres,R.F., Raymond,S.: Dissolution of urinary calculi. J. Urol. *65*, 474 (1951)
43. Gibson,T.E.: Problems in the surgical treatment of renal calculi. Arch. Surg. *37*, 211 (1938)
44. Grasset,D.: An injury with the Dormia basket necessitating Boari flap replacement. J. Urol. Nephrol. *74*, 851 (1968)
45. Hasselstrom,E.: Ein Fall von spontaner Verkleinerung eines Nierensteines. Ups. Lakforen Land. *31*, 703 (1926)
46. Hellstrom,J.: Einige Erfahrungen über Entstehung Wachstum und spontanen Abgang von Nierensteinen. Z. Urol. Chir. *18*, 248 (1925)
47. Hellstrom,J.: Njur-och uretarsten. Nord Kirug. For Fordandl. Kopenhafen 1935
48. Higgins,C.C., Straffon,R.A.: In: Urology. Campbell,M.F. (ed.). Philadelphia: Saunders 1963
49. Howard,F.S.: Stone extractor. J. Urol. *56*, 319 (1928)
50. Iwano,J.H., Bunts,R.C.: Complications arising from transureteral manipulation of ureteral catheters. J. Urol. *70*, 708 (1953)
51. Jacobsson,B., Sundin,T.: Vesico-ureteral reflux following slitting of ureteral orifice. Acta Chir. Scand. *125*, 261 (1963)
52. Johnson,F.P.: New method of removing ureteral calculi. J. Urol. *37*, 84 (1937)
53. Kearns,W.M.: The complete dissolution of a large renal calculus. Wis. Med. J. *34*, 179 (1935)
54. Keyser,L.D.: Urinary lithiasis; its cause and prevention: dissolution and disintegration of a renal calcium phosphate calculus by irrigation of the kidney with dilute aqua regis and by acidifying the patient's urine with acid diet and dilute aqua regis by mouth. South Med. J. *25*, 1031 (1932)
55. Keyser,L.D.: Studies in urinary calculosis. J. Urol. *54*, 194 (1945)
56. Keyser,L.G., Scherer,P.C., Claffey,L.W.: Studies in the dissolution of urinary calculi: experimental and clinical aspects. J. Urol. *59*, 826 (1948)
57. Klika,M.: Kompaktinsel oder ein Nierenstein und eine spontane Kröpfung des Uretercatheters im Ureter. Z. Urol. *25*, 590 (1931)
58. Kohler,F.P.: Renacidin and tissue reaction. J. Urol. *87*, 102 (1962)
59. Kretschmer,HL.: Stone in the ureter. J. Am. Med. Assoc. *80*, 1425 (1923)
60. Lamport,H.: Average distribution of light flux by a narrow slit vibrating in amplitude-modulated harmonic motion. J. Opt. Soc. Am. *48*, 760 (1958)
61. Lamport,H.: Ultrasonic fragmentation of calculi: final progress report 1960–64. Department of Physiology New Haven, Connecticut (1964)
62. Lamport,H., Newman,H.F.: Ultrasonic lithotresis in the ureter. J. Urol. *76*, 520 (1955)
63. Lamport,H., Zinsser,H.H.: Strain gauge measurement of output of magnetostrictive ultrasonic transducer—pitfalls of optical measurement. J. Acoust. Soc. Am. *31*, 435 (1959)
64. Lamport,H., Newman,H.F., Eichhorn, R.D.: Fragmentation of biliary calculi by ultrasound. Fed. Proc. *9*, 50 (1950)
65. Lapides,J.: Physiology of the intact human ureter. J. Urol. *59*, 501 (1948)
66. Lassen,H.K.: Spontan opløsuing af myreton. Nord. Med. *2*, 1569 (1939)
67. Lewis,Bransford: The removal of ureteral stone by cystoscopic methods. Trans. Am. Urol. Assoc. *6*, 169 (1912)
68. Lewis,Bransford: Ureteric stones; the techniques of their removal by cystoscopic methods. Surg. Gynecol. Obstet. *20*, 462 (1915)
69. McCrae,L.E., van Buskirk,K.E.: Spontaneous disintegration of staghorn calculus due to recumbency. J. Urol. *66*, 640 (1951)
70. McKay,R.W.: Stone dislodger. J. Am. Med. Assoc. *95*, 794 (1930)
71. McLean,J.J., Carroll,J.J., Greaves,H.B.: Treatment of ureteral colic and ureteral calculus by thoraco-lumbar sympathetic

block: preliminary report. J. Urol. *61*, 204 (1949)

72. Mulvaney,W.P.: A new solvent for certain urinary calcifications. J. Urol. *82*, 546 (1959)

73. Mulvaney,W.P.: Clinical use of renacidin in urinary calcifications. J. Urol. *84*, 206 (1960)

74. Mulvaney,W.P.: The hydrodynamics of renal irrigation with reference to calculus solvents. J. Urol. *89*, 765 (1963)

75. Nadeau,: Quoted by Elliott,J.S. (1954). Spontaneous dissolution of renal calculi. J. Urol. *72*, 331 (1939)

76. Ouchi,T., Takahashi,H.: Disintegration of urinary calculi by means of ultrasonic vibration. Kongr. Int. Ges. Urol. München, July 1967 (1967)

77. Pelot,G., Voetlin,R., Masson,B.: Dissolution des calculs uretèreux et pyeliques par la solution G. J. Urol. *65*, 585 (1959)

78. Prentiss,R.J., Mullenix,R.B., Whisenaud, J.M.: Management of ureteral stone; guide for physicians in general practice. Calif. Med. *77*, 7 (1952)

79. Prince,C.L., Scardino,P.L.: A statistical analysis of ureteral calculi. J. Urol. *83*, 561 (1960)

80. Pyrah,L.N., Fowweather,F.S.: Urinary calculi developing in recumbent patients. Br. J. Surg. *26*, 98 (1937)

81. Pyrah,L.N., Hodgkinson,A., Anderson, C.K.: Primary hyperparathyroidism: a critical review. Br. J. Surg. *53*, 245 (1966)

82. Ries,S.W., Malament,M.: Renacidin: a urinary calculus solvent. J. Urol. *87*, 657 (1962)

83. Rusché,C.F., Bacon,S.K.: Injury of the ureter due to cystoscopic intraureteral instrumentation: report of 18 cases. J. Urol. *44*, 777 (1940)

84. Russell,M.: Dissolution of bilateral renal staghorn calculi with renacidin. J. Urol. *88*, 141 (1962)

85. Sandegard,E.: Prognosis of stone in the ureter. Acta Chir. Scand. (Suppl. 219) (1956)

86. Sandegard,E.: The results of expectant treatment of urolithiasis: follow-up study of kidney function and recurrence. Acta Chir. Scand. *116*, 44 (1958)

87. Scardino,P.L.: Editorial: Stone basketry. Urology *1*, 379 (1973)

88. Scheele,K.: Über spontane Verkleinerung von Nierensteinen. Z. Urol. *18*, 528 (1924)

89. Servadio,M.D., Caine,M.: Some hazards of renacidin therapy of renal calculi. Isr. Med. J. *22*, 28 (1963)

90. Sisk,I.R., Bunts,R.C.: Spontaneous dissolution of renal calculi. Trans. Am. Assoc. G-U Surg. *28*, 149 (1935)

91. Squires,C.B.: Disposition of ureteral calculi at Crowell Clinic from 1915 to 1930. J. Urol. *24*, 461 (1930)

92. Stevenson,J.J., Fergusson,J.D.: The use of television in X-ray diagnosis. Lancet *I*, 713 (1961)

93. Suby,H.I.: Quoted by Keyser,L.D., Scherer,P.C., Claffey,L.W. (1948). J. Urol. *59*, 826 (1948)

94. Suby,H.I., Albright,F.: Dissolution of phosphatic urinary calculi by the retrograde introduction of a citrate solution containing magnesium. N. Engl. J. Med. *228*, 81 (1943)

95. Suby,H.I., Suby,R.M., Albright,F.: Properties of organic acid solutions which determine their irritability to the bladder mucous membrane and the effect of the magnesium ions in overcoming this irritability. J. Urol. *48*, 549 (1942)

96. Taylor,W.N.: Lumbar ureterolithotomy. J. Urol. *69*, 77 (1953)

97. Thompson,G.J., Kibler,J.M.: Treatment of ureteric calculi with particular reference to transurethral manipulation. J. Am. Med. Assoc. *114*, 6 (1941)

98. Timmermann,A., Kallistratos,G.: Modern aspects of chemical dissolution of human renal calculi by irrigation. J. Urol. *95*, 469 (1966)

99. Timmermann,A., Kallistratos,G., Fenner, O., Sommer,E.: In: Renal Stone Research Symposium. Hodgkinson,A., Nordin, B.E.C. (eds.). London: Churchill 1969

100. Walker,R.M., Thompson,J.W.: Disappearance of phosphate deposits from the urinary tract. Br. J. Surg. *29*, 336 (1942)

101. Wax,S.H., Frank,I.N.: A retrospective study of upper urinary tract calculi. J. Urol. *94*, 28 (1965)

102. Wesson,M.B.: Spontaneous dissolution of bilateral renal calculi. Urologists Correspondence Club 31st May (1950)

103. Winsbury-White,H.P.: Stone in the urinary tract, 2nd ed. London: Butterworth 1954

104. Zeiss,L.: New sling catheter for conservative therapy of ureteral calculi. Z. Chir. Urol. *31*, 681 (1937)

Chapter 13

Operative Treatment of Renal and Ureteric Calculi

Before deciding the question of operation for the removal of a renal calculus in any given patient, the possibility of spontaneous voiding of the stone will have been considered. In a very few cases some urologists will have considered the possibility of treatment by irrigation of the renal pelvis. The choice of operation depends upon the position of the calculi (calyces, renal pelvis, intracystic), upon their number and extent and upon the presence of any associated infection or other concomitant disease.

The indications for the operative removal of renal calculi are the following; the special indications for ureterolithotomy and for nephrectomy and nephroureterectomy are referred to later in the chapter:

1. A stone a centimetre or more in diameter causing symptoms.

2. Frequently recurring severe attacks of renal colic.

3. Evidence of increasing obstruction, causing hydrocalycosis and/or hydronephrosis.

4. Persistent urinary infection associated with the calculus, because of danger to the kidney.

5. Persistent or recurrent attacks of haematuria.

6. Rapid increase in the size of the stone.

7. Calculi in a solitary kidney larger than the size referred to above.

8. Associated ureteric calculus.

9. A stone associated with other renal pathological conditions (tuberculosis or neoplasm).

10. A stone associated with a cyst or a cystic condition of the kidney may call for operation.

11. In a patient who is moving to a place remote from surgical assistance.

I. Simple Pyelolithotomy and Its Variants

In the operation of pyelolithotomy the renal pelvis is opened by a simple incision for the removal of one or more stones of medium size. Various extensions and modifications of the operation have been introduced over the years for the removal of stones which are too large to be extracted through the usual incision or which lie in an intrarenal pelvis. A small non-adherent calyceal stone may sometimes be removed through a pyelolithotomy incision, for example, by syringing the calyx with saline or by the use of appropriate forceps. A stone lodged within and adherent to the wall of a minor calyx cannot usually be removed across the renal pelvis. Although the proximal part of the renal pelvis lies hidden in the renal sinus, in which a large part of the calculus may sometimes lie, and which may therefore be relatively inaccessible, in most patients there is a biggish extrarenal pelvic segment containing the major part of the stone. The major calyces and their infundibula, if considerably dilated from the presence of calculi, are sometimes accessible for the removal of calculi across the renal pelvis. The operation of pyelolithotomy may be used not only in combination with nephrolithotomy but also with partial nephrectomy in order to remove calyceal and pelvic stones at a single operative procedure.

The kidney and the renal pedicle with the upper end of the ureter are mobilized through an incision in the loin to the extent which will allow a radiograph of the exposed kidney to be obtained, in order to exclude the presence, for example, of tiny hitherto unsuspected calculi. Mobilization also enables the various forms of extended pyelolithotomy to be done without difficulty.

1. For a Calculus in a Mainly Extrarenal Pelvis

The presence of the stone in the pelvis and its exact position will have been confirmed by palpation when the kidney is held forward or partly lifted out of the wound during exposure. It is usually easily possible to strip away from the posterior aspect of the renal pelvis the soft peripelvic fat (or even a firm oedematous pad of fat which is sometimes present), by dissection with scissors or gauze. Sometimes such a pad may need to be deliberately incised with a scalpel in a longitudinal direction from just below the renal sinus to a point close to the pelviureteric junction, until the bluish wall of the renal pelvis appears, when the pad can be dissected away. The pelviureteric junction is freed and inspected for the presence of narrowing or of adventitious fibrous bands or aberrant vessels giving rise to a hydronephrosis, which would need to be corrected later in the operation.

A cotton sling is now placed around the kidney and a radiograph of the exposed kidney is taken to give a picture of any unsuspected additional calculi. If the stone is large in relation to the size of the renal pelvis, it may be difficult to extract it from the pelvis through a simple incision without tearing the renal pelvis. In such a case one of the extensions of the incision referred to below may be needed. If the renal pelvis is wholly or almost entirely intrarenal, palpation of the entire stone may be difficult or impossible though its apical part may be felt above the pelviureteric junction. Assuming

that a medium-sized stone is lying in a fairly normal extrarenal pelvis, the surgeon proceeds to remove it, the assistant holding the kidney out of the wound by drawing on the cotton sling. Gauze swabs having been laid in front of and behind the kidney to absorb any urine which may escape, a vertical incision is made into the posterior wall of the pelvis directly onto the stone starting a few millimetres below the renal sinus and ending just above the pelviureteric junction, the incision being large enough to allow the stone to be extracted without further tearing of the pelvic wall. A grating sensation is noted when the knife comes into contact with the stone, which is then extracted with suitable straight or curved stone forceps or scoop, or it may be squeezed out by pressure from the surgeon's thumb.

A search is made for possible additional calculi and the number of stones removed should correspond with those seen on the radiograph taken in the operating theatre. If one or more small stones are difficult to find they may be discovered by repeated search with curved stone forceps or a scoop; or irrigation with a stream of sterile saline may cause them to be voided onto the gauze. Gentleness is needed during these manipulations if fragmentation and the dispersal of crystals from the surface of the stone are to be avoided.

A transverse incision across the renal pelvis, a few millimetres below and parallel to the renal sinus, is sometimes appropriate for the removal of a stone of large transverse diameter. For the removal of a large pyramidal calculus lying in the renal pelvis, a suitable additional exposure of the portion of the renal pelvis which lies beneath the lip of renal parenchyma within the renal sinus can be obtained by the use of adequate retraction of the overhanging lip of renal tissue, thus allowing an extension of the incision. In some cases a curved transverse incision high up in the posterior wall of the widest part of the pelvis is appropriate, the overhanging lip of parenchymal tissue having been retracted; when the lower flap of the divided renal pelvis is turned downwards a slightly larger curved retractor can be inserted beneath the upper flap of the pelvis, when the ostium leading to the infundibulum of a calyx together with the extension of a biggish stone inside it, may then come into view; the calculus can be drawn down by forceps introduced between the stone and the calyceal wall.

2. In Situ

The technique of pyelolithotomy just described implies the fairly complete mobilization of the kidney together with the renal pedicle and the renal pelvis. It is possible, however (and sometimes quite easy), to remove medium-sized calculi from the renal pelvis without complete mobilization of the kidney. Some surgeons have considered that extensive mobilization of the kidney is undesirable and that only its posterior aspect with the renal pelvis should be fully exposed for the removal of calculi. Hellstrom [49] and also Hellstrom and Franksson [50] considered that extensive mobilization of the kidney encourages the formation of postoperative adhesions, and that the free mobilization of the kidney may lead to the displacement or even to the fracture of the renal calculi and may marginally increase the chance of postoperative recurrence of stone. They therefore advocated minimal mobilization of the kidney, and designated their technique 'pyelolithotomy in situ'. With the limited exposure referred to the kidney is mobilized only to an extent which will allow access to the dorsal aspect of the hilum and the posterior surface of the pelvis. The lip of renal parenchymatous tissue at the margin of the renal sinus is retracted by the use of one or more spatulae so as to render visible as much of the renal pelvis as is necessary,

following which an adequate incision is made into it for the extraction of the stone.

3. Transparenchymal Extension

More room for the extraction of a large, partly intrarenal stone from the renal pelvis, and sometimes even from a major calyx or its infundibulum, can be obtained by extending the vertical incision in the renal pelvis through the adjacent parenchyma; two such techniques have been used. In the operation of *pyélotomie élargie* [72], the renal pelvis is exposed and a vertical incision is made through the middle of its posterior wall from just above the pelviureteric junction to the overhanging lip of renal tissue. The incision is continued in the same line through the renal parenchyma in a curved direction so as to extend the pelvic opening even into a stone-bearing calyx if thought desirable to enable the stone to be extracted. It is necessary to secure the retropelvic artery either before or after making the incision through the renal parenchyma by underrunning it with a catgut suture.

In the operation of inferior pyelonephrolithotomy [86, 120], the incision into the pelvis (for the removal of a large pelvic stone extending into the lowest calyx) is made at its lower border rather than on its posterior surface and is then carried through the inner convex border of the lower pole of the renal parenchyma, and gradually deepened (using a guide if necessary) until the entire lowest calyx is opened up in continuity with the renal pelvis. Haemostasis of the divided parenchyma is achieved by underrunning it with fine sutures. The procedure has the disadvantage that some local necrosis of the kidney in the neighbourhood of the incision inevitably follows and indeed secondary haemorrhage is a possible late complication in infected cases. The large stone is extracted from the renal pelvis and its extension into the calyx is removed. The divided renal tissue and the renal pelvis are closed by simple sutures.

Alternatively a side-to-side anastomosis of the opened calyx to the lowest part of the opened pelvis or even to the upper end of the ureter may be done, if the lowest calyx is dilated and the renal parenchyma overlying it is not too thick (ureterocalycostomy). If the renal tissue overlying the dilated calyx is thin, the renal capsule can be reflected and a limited partial nephrectomy then done, covering the resected renal surface with the reflected renal capsule without attempting any reconstruction of the renal parenchyma over the calyceal closure [114].

4. Subcapsular Pyelolithotomy

In order to obtain more room and better access for the removal of large stones in the renal pelvis, Handley [45] introduced what he described as subcapsular pyelotomy, reporting nine unilateral and two bilateral cases (Fig. 13.1). After the kidney has been exposed, a curved incision 3 in. in length was made through the renal capsule along the long axis of the posterior surface of the kidney and mid-way between the convex border and the renal sinus. The capsular flap thus defined was stripped down to the hilum of the kidney (to a position beneath the overhanging lip) where it becomes fused with the posterior surface of the renal pelvis. By continued dissection the pocket thus formed was gradually deepened until the line of entrance of the renal pelvis into the renal parenchyma was reached. The posterior surface of the pelvis was then incised transversely at the bottom of this capsular pocket so that a pair of forceps, or the surgeon's finger if necessary, could be introduced to locate and remove the stone. The incision into the renal pelvis was left unsutured. The risk of injury to the retropelvic artery from this procedure is small;

the approach can be used for the removal of an associated biggish calyceal stone which cannot easily be removed across the pelvis. With one finger inside the pelvis thus opened up and one on the outside of the kidney, it should be possible to locate precisely the position of such a stone and remove it by nephrolithotomy. Similar procedures were used by Aboulker [2], Rovinescu et al. [103], and Resnick et al. [99].

5. Extracapsular Extended Pyelolithotomy

Gil-Vernet [38, 39] suggested that more room to visualize and then to incise a considerable length of the posterior wall of the renal pelvis (and especially an intrarenal pelvis) together with its attached major calyces could be obtained by dissecting in the plane of cleavage between the peripelvic fat and capsule, and the muscular coat of the renal pelvis. A considerable space within the hilum of the kidney can be opened up. The fibrous capsule of the kidney hives off some fibres, which become attached to the entire circumference of the renal pelvis forming a kind of capsular diaphragm. This shuts off the entrance to the renal sinus [82] and can be separated or avulsed from the renal pelvis by blunt dissection with scissors, enabling the entire intrarenal pelvis to be demonstrated, without injury to the retropelvic vessels. The adventitious tissue surrounding the renal pelvis can be separated from the peripelvic adipose cellular tissue, exposure being helped by the insertion of a curved retractor under the lip of the renal parenchyma, which is not then injured during the dissection. The retropelvic artery remains intact. A thin strip of wet gauze, which is first introduced into the renal sinus outside the pelvis as the dissection progresses, to assist the separation of tissues, is then withdrawn to allow another longer-bladed retractor to be introduced, after which gauze can be reinserted. The infundibulum of the calyces can be gradually brought into view, allowing of the extraction of biggish calyceal stones and prolongation into a calyx of mushroom-shaped pelvic calculi. A longitudinal incision along the calyceal infundibulum facilitates a direct approach to the stone, which can be (if necessary) fractured first at its narrow neck with appropriate forceps. A large calyceal stone may be removed by making an incision through the (often thinned) renal cortex, which is then sutured. When the transverse pelvic incision is sutured the renal parenchyma falls into position over it and makes any leakage of urine less likely.

He reported the use of the extracapsular extended pyelolithotomy method in a large series. Calculi were removed from the renal pelvis in 237 cases; staghorn calculi were removed from 19 patients with no subsequent recurrence. In 27 patients multiple pyelocalyceal calculi were removed; in 41, calyceal calculi were removed, 36 of which were dealt with by incisions through the infundibulum of the stone-containing calyx (calicolithotomy), while in five (which were examples of large stones occupying the entire calyceal system and were associated with a thin renal cortical parenchyma) the stones were removed by nephrolithotomy.

Blandy and Tresidder [9], who used the procedure for the removal of staghorn calculi from 30 kidneys in 28 patients, found that the definition of the plane of cleavage was sometimes difficult when there had been an earlier operation on the kidney [108]. Others have reported good results [15, 71].

6. Conclusion of Operation

After the stone has been removed by any of the above methods, a ureteric catheter is passed into the renal pelvis and down the ureter to the bladder to ensure patency of the ureter and to exclude the presence there

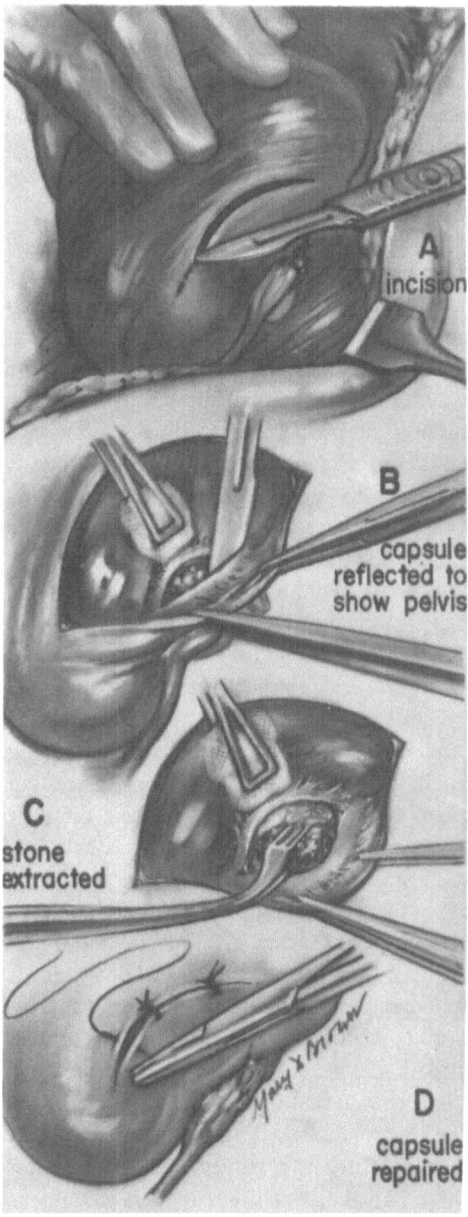

Fig. 13.1. Removal of medium-sized stone lying mainly in an intrarenal pelvis (Sampson Handley's method). **A.** The renal pelvis has been exposed; a curved incision 1 in. above the hilar lip of the renal parenchyma is made through the renal capsule. **B.** The renal capsule is reflected and the renal parenchyma retracted as described in the text, thus exposing the intrarenal pelvis overlying the stone. **C.** The pelvis is incised transversely and the stone removed. **D.** The renal capsule is sutured

of associated calculi or pieces of grit in the ureter (which, if found, should be removed). The pelvis and calyces are finally irrigated with a stream of sterile saline in order to wash away gritty particles, fragments of stone accidentally detached, or pieces of fibrin or of clot.

The incision in the pelvis is sutured with fine interrupted non-chromic 0000 sutures mounted on a tiny atraumatic curved needle, inserted fairly close together, avoiding as far as possible any penetration of the mucous membrane by the sutures. Such a suture-line properly introduced is water-tight, and is to be preferred to a continuous suture with its slight risk of rendering avascular parts of the edges of the pelvic incision and therefore of delayed healing. Finally the flaps of the peripelvic fat which had been made before opening the renal pelvis are brought together by interrupted stitches over the suture line in the pelvis.

Some surgeons do not always close the renal pelvis by sutures, preferring to leave it open, or they merely approximate the cut edges of the renal pelvis with one or more sutures. The chance of temporary but undesirable external drainage of urine and even the accumulation of small loculated collections of urine around the kidney is reduced by accurate suturing. The kidney is replaced in its bed and the perirenal fat disposed round it. The parietal wound is closed, leaving a thin rubber drain through the perirenal fat down to the renal pelvis but not in contact with the suture line. The drainage tube is removed after 48 h unless there is leakage of urine (which is rare), in which case it may be retained for a longer period.

7. Associated Calyceal Calculi

Generally speaking, the operation of pyelolithotomy can be used only for the removal of calculi in the renal pelvis and not for the removal of small or medium-sized associated calyceal calculi, since these cannot be extracted across the narrow calyceal neck, which is usually too narrow to allow of the introduction of either a finger or a stone forceps to remove the stone. Moreover, a calyceal stone may be spiculated and firmly attached to the renal papilla within the calyx. Occasionally, a calyceal stone has migrated from a calyx into the infundibulum, and its tip can be felt by a finger introduced into the opened pelvis to be presenting into its proximal part; and when the renal pelvis is opened it may be possible to displace such a stone by the finger, or even to grasp it and withdraw it by forceps introduced into the pelvis. The position of such calculi can sometimes be recognized on the radiograph of the exposed kidney, since they are seen to lie appreciably nearer to the renal sinus than to the convex border usually definable on the radiograph. Alternatively, having located the calyceal stone in the manner described it may be removed by an incision directly over it through the renal parenchyma (nephrolithotomy). Partial nephrectomy for calyceal stone may also be combined with pyelolithotomy.

8. Anterior Pyelolithotomy

Although an approach to the renal pelvis by exposing the posterior wall seems to be most sound anatomically, with a small risk of injury to the renal vessels, some surgeons have used an anterior approach, the pelvis being incised either below the renal vessels or even between them; it has been said that there is less risk of postoperative leakage of urine following such an incision. In doing a pyelolithotomy for a calculus in a horseshoe kidney or an ectopic kidney, an anterior pyelolithotomy may be appropriate. The fat in front of the lower pole of the kidney is displaced revealing the ureter, which is then followed upwards to the renal pelvis; the renal vein may have to be retracted before the pelvis is incised to remove the stone [89].

9. Transperitoneal Pyelolithotomy

Since the renal pelvis lies behind the renal vessels an approach to it from across the peritoneal cavity (which is also an anterior approach) seems to be less logical anatomically than a lumbar approach. Gridner [43] reported the removal of two calculi by this route and claimed that the advantage of the route was that it avoided mobilization of the kidney. Poutasse [89] found the transperitoneal route satisfactory for the removal of recurrent calculi in some patients.

10. Coagulum Pyelolithotomy

In order to assist in the removal of gritty particles and small concretions from the renal pelvis and calyces, Dees and Fox [27] attempted to find a coagulable non-toxic substance the components of which were fluid, and which could therefore be injected separately into the renal pelvis in order to fill it completely, and which would then coagulate uniformly within a period of time long enough to ensure that the gritty particles were enmeshed in the clot. It was essential that the coagulum when formed had sufficient tensile strength to enable it to be removed intact when it had done its work, and that it would dissolve or disintegrate within a few days if portions were left behind in the renal pelvis.

Solutions of human and also of bovine fibrinogen coagulated by the addition of clotting globulin (a fraction of rabbit plasma globulin prepared by Lederle) were found to fulfil most nearly the theoretical criteria. The upper part of the ureter is temporarily occluded with a small clamp; through a small incision in the renal pelvis, a round-headed mushroom catheter (14 or 16 F) is introduced, the pyelotomy opening

then being closed round the catheter with fine catgut. All urine is first aspirated from the renal pelvis, the capacity of which is estimated by injecting saline through the catheter until it is distended; the amount of fluid injected is then withdrawn and measured.

Fibrinogen equal in amount to 90% of the estimated capacity of the pelvis is injected along the catheter, while simultaneously, through a syringe (the needle being introduced through the wall of the catheter), an assistant injects the thrombin solution (30 units/ml) equal in amount to 10% of the capacity of the pelvis. The two solutions intermix and form the coagulum, and 5 min later the pyelotomy incision is opened sufficiently to remove with ring forceps the resultant clot containing the enmeshed tiny calculi. The existence of a small intrarenal pelvis would contraindicate the method because of the difficulty in extracting the clot, as would also biggish calyceal stones. In 35 of 73 cases so treated, all the calculi shown to be present had been removed; there were seven technical failures and in the other cases only some of the stones were removed [21–27, 83]. Successful results using the treatment were reported by Harrison and Trichel [48], by Hoffman [53] who extracted some 40 tiny concretions, and by Moore and Sweetsen [79], who claimed to have made a tougher coagulum [85, 96]. The method may have a limited application for the removal of gritty debris from the renal pelvis.

11. Complications

Laceration of the Wall of the Renal Pelvis may follow an attempt to extract a large stone through an opening in the renal pelvis which is too small for the purpose; if the tear is located near to the renal sinus, subsequent suturing may be somewhat difficult. An incision into a largely intrarenal pelvis which has not been extended by one of the manoeuvres previously described, in order to achieve easy access to the stone, may be complicated by a tear, which may not be easy to repair by simple sutures. A flap of the renal capsule, rotated downwards, may be useful as a graft to repair the rent. Trouble rarely arises from this complication.

Injury to the Pelviureteric Junction may occur if the incision made for the operation of pyelolithotomy is carried too close to the junction. The subsequent repair by sutures could result in slight narrowing and to a consequent hydronephrosis.

Postoperative Pyelitis or Pyelonephritis may follow operation on an infected kidney and may need antibiotics. Ferrier and Bliss [35] recorded a case of infection by gas-producing organisms (*B. welchi*) following a pyelolithotomy operation; recovery followed multiple incisions, irrigation and antitoxin.

Fistula. Prolonged drainage of urine from the wound or even fistula may occur if suturing of the renal pelvis has been inadequately carried out, or if no sutures were used, or if a small stone or some gritty debris or blood clot has been left behind in the upper part of the ureter, or if there is a co-existent refluxing lower ureteric orifice (which would then call for correction). Drainage of urine following pyelolithotomy is usually either completely absent or is limited to a few days, lasting for no more than 2 weeks. If it persists for such a time, the passage of a ureteric catheter to the renal pelvis and its retention for 2 or 3 days to allow the downward drainage of urine is usually curative.

Renal Function following a successful pyelolithotomy in the absence of infection and complications, seems unlikely to be affected. If the retropelvic artery (a branch of the renal artery) which lies in the renal sinus close to the overhanging hilar lip of renal tissue, is injured (for example, during the procedure of *pyélotomie élargie* or one of its modifications), a limited amount of the renal tissue supplied by this artery must be rendered functionless, but total renal function is scarcely affected.

Pararenal Pseudohydronephrosis. This condition occasionally complicates the operation of pyelolithotomy, though it is non-specific in the sense that it may occasionally complicate the traumatic rupture of a normal kidney (for example, following a road accident) or the spontaneous rupture of a diseased kidney.

The conditions usually necessary for such a lesion to be produced are: (1) There must be a tear in the renal pelvis or at the pelviureteric junction, resulting from operative trauma, external injury or renal disease. (2) In cases of renal trauma there is a tear in the renal cortex extending from the outer surface of the kidney into a calyx or into the renal pelvis. The complete division of the renal cortex into two separate fragments following an injury has occasionally fulfilled this requirement. Or the renal pelvis must fail to heal, or alternatively it must not be sealed off with blood clot before leakage of urine in any quantity has taken place. Such a failure to heal may be the consequence of a wide separation of the fragments of the torn renal pelvis or of the ruptured kidney. (3) There must be an obstruction of the ureter, which may result from fibrosis and scarring resulting from the injury, or from a previous pathological condition or from external pressure by blood clot.

Some degree of hydronephrosis of the kidney is usual in the fully developed syndrome unless retention of urine within the renal pelvis is impossible because of the size of the tear in the renal parenchyma or in the renal pelvis. A perforation of the renal pelvis alone may be sufficient, providing the third condition just referred to coexists.

In cases seen as a complication of the operation of pyelolithotomy, the symptoms, which may come on gradually, consist of discomfort in the loin, with the subsequent development of a palpable swelling. In those which follow rupture of the kidney, there may have been initial shock and possibly haematuria, but symptoms may subside after a few days and if a swelling has not appeared in the loin the patient may soon be well enough to leave hospital. At some time later pain or discomfort in the loin appear gradually or suddenly. A swelling may then be discovered in the region of the kidney which may lead to the diagnosis. In the case reported by Johnson and Smith [56] the cystic swelling was discovered accidentally 37 years after the injury. The swelling is usually tender and fluctuant, it does not move on respiration, it may be localized to the perinephric region or it may extend from the diaphragm to the pelvis and across the middle line of the abdomen. The condition has to be differentiated from a cyst which has originated from a large haematoma following a ruptured kidney, from the various pararenal cysts and from cysts resulting from calyceal diverticula; in such cases there is no history of injury.

The wall of the pseudocyst, which surrounds the kidney almost entirely, is composed of dense fibrous tissue and the lining is shiny though not covered by epithelium. Fatty, fibrous or oily debris, altered blood clot, crystalline urinary salts or even altered fragments of renal tissue have been found in the cavity. The wall of the cyst in course of time may undergo localized or generalized calcification. The cyst is intimately connected with the surrounding parietal muscles, fascia, ribs and great vessels. The kidney or the renal pelvis is actually in the wall of the cyst.

Crabtree [19] collected 20 cases of this condition from the literature between 1834 and 1935 and added 3 cases of his own, the youngest being 3 years and the oldest 70 years. Of the 2 cases reported by the author [94] the first was a young man who had had a run-over accident many years before and who presented with a soft cystic swelling in the loin giving rise to aching discomfort. The second case developed within a few weeks of operation of pyelolithotomy for the removal of a stone from an intrarenal pelvis during which the pelviureteric junction had been divided and subsequently repaired; leakage of urine during the postoperative period had gradually led to the formation of the cyst. Sauls and Nesbit [105] reported four cases of pararenal pseudocyst, one of which complicated a pyelolithotomy operation after 2 years; another had complicated a ureterolithotomy operation.

Operative treatment, which is usually necessary, involves a careful dissection and removal of the cyst from the kidney and vessels to which it is adherent, and also removal of the damaged kidney.

II. Nephrolithotomy

The term nephrolithotomy is used to describe the removal of calyceal calculi through one or more incisions across the renal parenchyma. Until comparatively recently it was the operation of choice for the necessary removal of small or medium-sized calyceal calculi, but because of the subsequent high rate of recurrence of stone, the operation of partial nephrectomy has largely replaced it.

The operation is still used by some surgeons for the removal of calyceal stones in a non-infected kidney, and in a mildly infected kidney in which partial nephrectomy may be thought to carry a somewhat greater risk of postoperative trouble. The operation is also used for the removal of multiple biggish calyceal calculi (which cannot normally be removed across the renal pelvis), which are too widespread to be treated by partial nephrectomy, and for which nephrectomy is not indicated. It is also used for the removal of one medium-sized or large calyceal stone which is causing pain, from a kidney in which there are tiny multiple calcific foci in or around other calyces which it is impossible to remove, but for which the surgeon does not wish to do a nephrectomy, perhaps, for example, in a solitary kidney.

When very large staghorn calculi are present in both kidneys (or when they occur in a solitary kidney), and when the association of chronic infection and impairment of function is causing deterioration of the general health, the choice has to be made between complete inactivity (except for the medicinal treatment of the infection which is then only of limited value), and the removal of the calculi first from one kidney and later from the other. Until comparatively recently it was the common practice among urologists not to remove multiple large bilateral staghorn calculi from badly infected and damaged kidneys through long incisions across the renal parenchyma. It was argued that in such cases the renal infection (commonly by urea-splitting organisms) could not be eradicated, that the risk from primary haemorrhage of operation and of secondary haemorrhage after operation was consequently considerable, and that early recurrence of the calculi was very likely to take place. The use of extensive incisions across functioning and highly vascular renal parenchyma must lead to some permanent destruction of renal tissue with still further resulting loss of renal function as a direct consequence of the operation itself. In recent years the gradual improvement in the treatment of renal infection by the use of suitable antibiotics, with the possible reduction of the incidence of secondary haemorrhage, and the employment of cooling techniques at operation allowing of a longer period of renal ischaemia to enable the removal of stones to be done carefully and thoroughly, have

enabled a more aggressive approach to be adopted towards the removal of such staghorn calculi. Surgical opinion has thus moved in favour of the principle of removing at least some of the larger staghorn (pelvic and calyceal) stones.

1. For Calyceal Calculi

The patient is placed in the lateral position as described for the operation of pyelolithotomy, the kidney and the renal pedicle are mobilized, and inspection of a radiograph of the exposed kidney will allow the precise details of the operation to be decided. While a small calyceal stone is impalpable from without if the renal parenchyma is of normal thickness, a medium-sized stone in a dilated calyx covered by partially atrophied renal tissue can often be recognized as a firm intrarenal mass.

The mobilized kidney is held by the assistant in a cotton sling so disposed as to leave uncovered the part of the kidney to be incised, and the selected method of controlling bleeding by temporary occlusion of the renal pedicle is then applied; cooling techniques may be used with advantage. The incision through the renal parenchyma should be made as nearly as possible over the stone, and long enough to enable it to be extracted without undue laceration of the tissue around the incision. The position of the so-called bloodless line of Brödel can be noted as a guide. Although a longitudinal incision through the renal parenchyma has become conventional, a transverse incision is sometimes appropriate. Multiple small incisions through the renal parenchyma for the removal of several calculi are, if practicable, to be preferred to one long longitudinal incision.

2. For a Small Solitary Calyceal Stone

An incision through the renal cortex (1 in. in length at first, but enlarged as required) is made over the stone-containing calyx usually along a straight line a short distance behind and parallel to the convex border of the kidney. A long straight needle or probe passed into the renal parenchyma to impinge if possible on the stone, sometimes helps to localize it precisely. Using a narrow-bladed knife passed alongside the probe or needle the incision is gradually deepened until the stone is reached when it is extracted with forceps together with any associated gritty particles. The resulting cavity is irrigated with a stream of lotion to remove other tiny concretions if present. It is not necessary or even practicable to suture the wall of the stone-bearing calyx after a stone has been extracted. Two or three interrupted sutures of No. 1 non-chromic catgut introduced 1 cm or less from the edge of the incision deeply into the renal parenchyma, but not so as to penetrate the wall of the calyx, serve to draw the renal tissue into sufficiently close apposition to achieve haemostasis leaving no dead space. Mattress sutures should not be used; the clamp on the renal pedicle is relaxed and one or more further stitches may be inserted if there is bleeding. The insertion of muscle or fat grafts into the renal incision to arrest bleeding before suturing is neither desirable nor necessary. Broad catgut bands tied round the kidney have been used by Lowsley and Bishop [67] to reinforce the sutures in the arrest of bleeding. No drainage tube should be inserted into the renal substance.

3. For a Medium-sized Stone in a Dilated Calyx

With such a stone the altered consistency of the kidney resulting from the underlying stone and the slightly thinned or even partially atrophied overlying cortical tissue may be apparent to the examining finger. A short incision parallel or at right angles to the convex border through the renal paren-

chyma will enable the stone to be reached without difficulty and often with little bleeding.

4. For Multiple Small or Medium-sized Calyceal Stones

Multiple short longitudinal or transverse incisions through the renal cortex may be appropriate for the removal of calculi from more than one calyx (for example, a middle and a lower calyx) separated from each other by a few centimetres. The trauma to the kidney is less than if one longer incision had been made.

5. The Bivalve Procedure

Multiple massive stones may be removed across the renal parenchyma by the so-called bivalve procedure; alternatively, a combination of the operation of extended pyelolithotomy with nephrolithotomy (for the less accessible stones) is good practice. A judicious combination of nephrolithotomy with a limited partial nephrectomy of a group of calyces badly damaged and perhaps partly atrophied from infection and obstruction, may sometimes be preferred to a complete longitudinal nephrolithotomy [8, 75, 76, 97, 102, 119].

The bivalve procedure carries a risk of secondary haemorrhage and temporary fistula formation, which has to be set against the chances of long-term improvement and success. The conditions needed for its successful performance are: adequate temporary control of the renal pedicle to prevent loss of blood, preferably with cooling of the kidney to enable the period of renal ischaemia to be prolonged as long as is deemed necessary; good visualization of the operative field by adequate opening of the renal cavities; and one or more radiographs of the exposed kidney, before, during and at the end of the operation, as the only final check that all the smallest concretions have been removed.

A long incision extending from pole to pole of the mobilized kidney, 1 in. behind and parallel to the convex border may be needed in the worst cases of massive stone formation occupying the renal pelvis and all the calyces; multiple shorter incisions are sometimes adequate. The incision is carried through the renal parenchyma to the calyces, pus and gritty debris being removed or sucked away. Individual stone-containing calyces are opened and then slit up on their longitudinal axes with scissors, and finally the renal pelvis (which is usually large and contains a big calculus) is opened widely. Since bleeding is controlled by the pedicle clamp, attention can be given to the deliberate removal of the fibrino-purulent debris, grit and calculi which are usually composed mainly of magnesium ammonium phosphate, many of which are soft and crumbly. Forceps, scoops, the fingers and a stream of sterile saline and suction are the necessary tools for the removal of the calculi and debris.

When it is thought that all the calculous material has been removed, a radiograph of the exposed kidney at a certain stage may reveal still more hidden particles or small calculi in minor calyces. The search must go on until a negative radiograph has been obtained; the divided vessels (which are usually visible) are now grasped by mosquito forceps and ligated, or underrun with fine sutures and tied, a procedure which is the best safeguard against reactionary and secondary haemorrhage. The pedicle clamp may be released for a few seconds and then reapplied, in order to help to locate unligatured vessels. The openings into the divided calyces and the renal pelvis are accurately closed by a continuous suture of 0000 fine non-chromic catgut, after blood clot and debris have been sucked out, care being taken not to narrow the calyx lest a later stricture should develop. Deeply placed interrupted non-chromic catgut sutures are

then inserted to draw the divided surfaces of the kidney together, obliterating dead space; mattress sutures should never be used.

Marshall et al. [73] recommended the use of three encircling straps of plain ribbon gut inserted under slots in the renal capsule as an aid to haemostasis. Drainage tubes passed through the renal parenchyma into the renal pelvis are best avoided. The divided renal capsule is approximated by fine stitches, though some room may be left for blood and serum to seep out of the repaired kidney.

Brady [14] reported 19 nephrolithotomy operations for staghorn calculi (2 being in a solitary kidney); 7 of 9 cases followed up had recurrent stones, 2 of them needing nephrectomy. Petrovic and Ostojic [88] did 51 kidney-splitting operations for staghorn calculi in 50 patients (23 male, 27 female), 45 of whom had badly infected urine. Relatively recently, Hanley, Wickham and their co-workers [46, 118] have done nephrolithotomy on 22 patients with massive renal calculi, some of the stones being almost a cast of the kidney. The use of the cooling technique allowed an average time of occlusion of the renal vessels to be 50.6 min (with a range of 25–84 min in the series). They achieved a relatively dry operation field with relatively little loss of blood. In one-third of the cases, following the operation, there was a mild depression of renal function, which invariably returned to normal within 10 days. Subsequent radiographs showed that the calculous material had been removed in 19 of the 20 cases; in 12 of 13 patients in whom the urine was infected preoperatively it was rendered sterile within 3 weeks of operation. They have not been able to demonstrate any permanent postoperative renal damage as assessed by subsequent renal function tests and by isotope renography. Indeed renal function improved following the complete removal of multiple infected renal calculi in most of the cases.

6. Lateral Resection of Renal Tissue

This method (first used experimentally in the pig) has been used by Maddern [69] in nine patients with large branched calculi not suitable for removal by less extensive operations such as pyelolithotomy alone or combined with partial nephrectomy. A series of shavings of renal tissue was cut from the lateral surface of the kidney, using an amputation knife, until the most lateral calyces containing calculi had been opened. Thereafter the other stone-bearing calyces and the renal pelvis were opened and calculi removed. For details of the operation, which therefore has many features in common with the guillotine method of partial nephrectomy, the original paper should be consulted. This ingenious procedure would appear to have too many built-in risks of persistent urinary fistula to be generally acceptable.

7. Complications

Reactionary Haemorrhage. This may occasionally be considerable if suturing and haemostasis of the incised kidney have been inadequate; it may occur during the first 24 h after operation, and is manifested as external bleeding through the wound or as severe haematuria. Persistent bleeding may necessitate a re-opening of the wound and the insertion of sutures into the renal parenchyma.

Secondary Haemorrhage. This used to be a complication greatly feared as a consequence of infection; its prevention required as complete a control as possible of any renal infection known to be present before the operation, and continued treatment during the postoperative period. The cause of secondary bleeding is to some extent inherent in the operation itself, and follows the local ischaemia, the subsequent infarction and necrosis of the incised renal tissue

and its subsequent separation from living parenchyma with the consequent opening of blood vessels.

Secondary haemorrhage usually occurs between 7 and 12 days after operation but can be as late as 3 weeks. There is a heavy discoloration of the urine with blood, and clots may be voided leading to temporary urinary retention. Alternatively there may be bleeding from the external wound in the loin or a tender lump may be observed in the region of the kidney. The degree of pain and shock will depend upon the severity of the bleeding, which may threaten life and require blood transfusion or even the removal of the kidney. The bleeding may cease spontaneously (permanently or temporarily) to be followed after an interval by further bleeding, which may call for a secondary nephrectomy. The frequency of secondary haemorrhage following nephrolithotomy is illustrated by reported cases from the literature (Table 13.1).

Secondary haemorrhage even in recent years is still a problem and points to the selection of one of the extended forms of pyelolithotomy (with only limited nephrolithotomy) as being the most suitable procedure for the removal of large calculi. Hypoprothrombinaemia was thought to be a contributory cause of the bleeding in a case of secondary haemorrhage following nephrolithotomy reported by Jordan and Tomskey [58]. The patient had received terramycin for some days before and after operation, and it was believed that the formation of vitamin K had been inhibited because of the sterilization of the lower bowel, the bleeding ceasing as soon as the antibiotic was discontinued and vitamin K prescribed.

Urinary Fistula. This may complicate the operation on an infected kidney. It may also be the result of an uncorrected obstruction (by grit, a small concretion or infected debris) in a calyx, at the pelviureteric junction or in the ureter itself. Prolonged

Table 13.1. Secondary haemorrhage following nephrolithotomy

Author	Year	Cases operated on	No. with haemorrhage	Notes
Rehn	1921		10%–12%	
Braasch and Foulds	1923	150	8	Secondary nephrectomy in 3
Israel	1923	204	23 (11.5%)	17 fatal cases
Cifuentes	1923	626	85 (13.6%)	Secondary nephrectomy in 36
Mikkelsen	1935	204	23	Secondary nephrectomy in 1
Joly	1929	67	2 (6%)	Secondary nephrectomy in 1
Hellstrom (for Hedenberg)	1949	63	9	
Abeshouse and Lerman	1950	1482	156 (10.5%)	From series of eight different surgeons between 1922 and 1929; secondary nephrectomy in 67
Jordan and Tomskey	1957	75	7 (9%)	Secondary nephrectomy in 5
Petrovic and Ostojic	1965	51 (kidney-splitting operation)	9 severe haemorrhage 15 moderate bleeding	One patient died from haemorrhage
Marshall et al.	1965	50 (kidney-splitting operation)	8	Secondary nephrectomy in 2
Maddern	1967	30		Secondary nephrectomy in 3

retention of a nephrostomy tube (if one has been used) may contribute to fistula formation. Even a temporary leakage of urine from the wound in the loin during the first few days after operation is undesirable since infecting organisms may gain entry; such a leakage may be one of the causes of recurrent calculus or of a persistent infection of the kidney. Fistulous drainage of urine in small amounts usually clears up spontaneously after a few days, as soon as drainage down the ureter has become normal. The treatment has been referred to in Section I of this chapter. The rare persistent fistula may be an indication for nephrectomy provided the opposite kidney is healthy. The difficulties and risks in the pre-sulphonamide days are shown in the 1247 cases of nephrolithotomy collected by Abeshouse and Lerman [1] from series of cases by eight different surgeons between 1894 and 1930 in which there were 156 cases (12.5%) of persistent urinary fistula. The incidence differed widely in different series, from 3.65% in the 82 cases reported by Brongersma [16] to 21.1% in 288 operations recorded by Tardo [113]. Persistent fistula occurred in 6 of 75 cases following nephrolithotomy reported by Jordan and Tomskey [58], in all of which there had been severe renal infection, the kidney having been drained by nephrostomy.

Wound Infection. This may complicate the postoperative period in patients whose kidney is known to have been infected, though its incidence is nowadays much reduced. Perinephric abscess may follow operations on an infected kidney.

Impairment of Renal Function. In a kidney already badly damaged by multiple (stag-horn) calculi and infection and submitted to an extensive nephrolithotomy procedure (and especially the bivalve operation) there may be subsequent impairment of function. Much will depend on how much or how little injury has been done to the blood supply during the operation. In 15 of 17 patients submitted to a kidney-splitting operation for the removal of large calculi during a 10-year period, Helsby [51] found that the kidneys later functioned satis-factorily as determined by intravenous pyelography; rapidly growing recurrent calculi were found in two cases, in both of which the urine had been infected with *B. proteus*. Improvement in renal function following operation was reported by Baker et al. [4], by Petrovic and Ostojic [88] and by Marshall et al. [74]. The functional results reported by Wickham et al. [118] have already been referred to. Occasionally the combined damage to the kidney result-ing from disease and the operative trauma may determine in the end a functionless kidney, a risk which is intensified in patients who have a secondary haemorrhage. In two of 75 cases of nephrolithotomy reported by Jordan and Tomskey [58] and in three patients reported by Petrovic and Ostojic [88] the kidneys became functionless after operation.

Renal Arteriovenous Fistula. This has been reported as a complication of nephrolitho-tomy [59, 117]. In the case reported by Kelly [59] recurrent calculi were observed 1 year after nephrolithotomy. A palpable mass was then observed in the loin and a bruit was heard over the left renal area. The clinical diagnosis of renal arteriovenous fistula was confirmed after a successful nephrectomy.

8. Mortality

The operation of nephrolithotomy has in the past been associated with the highest mortality of the conservative operations for the treatment of renal stone. Thus in the series of 1767 patients submitted to nephro-lithotomy collected by Roseno [10] be-tween 1910 and 1925 the surgical mortality was 5.8%. Mimpriss [78] reported 17 cases without mortality though there was haema-turia in 3. Even in the series collected by Abeshouse and Lerman [1] of patients operated on between 1926 and 1949, totalling 378 cases from various published cases, the mortality was 27 or 7.1%, and in some individual series quoted by these authors it exceeded 11%. Death apparently from renal failure resulted from 4 of 51 (8%) bivalve operations reported by Baker et al. [4]. There were three deaths in 16 patients submitted to nephrolithotomy reported by Papathanassiadis and Swinney [84], and a further case in the group needed secondary nephrectomy. With the passage of time the mortality of the operation has been reduced.

III. Partial Nephrectomy

Partial nephrectomy implies the removal of a part (usually but not necessarily one pole) of the kidney for the purpose of extirpating disease in a localized part of the kidney (Fig. 13.2). The operation has a wide appli-cation in the treatment of a variety of renal abnormalities including renal calculi. It has been used for the treatment of localized renal tuberculosis, cysts, simple and malig-nant tumours of the kidney, and for certain cases of trauma and hypertension. The term heminephrectomy refers to the removal of one-half of a horseshoe or sigmoid kidney, or the diseased segment of a duplex kidney associated with double ureters with or without ureteral ectopia.

1. For Renal Calculous Disease

The usual indication for partial nephrectomy for calculous disease (now accepted by most urologists) is the presence of one or more calculi in a calyx. The operation is now done in preference to nephrolithotomy for the treatment of such cases. The aim of the operation is to remove not only the stone but also the calyx in which it has formed or matured (which may have been damaged by the stone), together with its narrow neck, with the object of preventing subsequent recurrences. Partial nephrectomy is especially appropriate for the treatment of a stone lying in a calyx shown radiologically to be dilated, or to have a narrowed neck in which additional gritty calcific particles are also present. While the operation is done most commonly for lower calyceal stone (the commonest site of the calcium oxalate calculus) it is often performed for upper calyceal stone and less frequently for stones in a middle calyx.

The operation can safely be done in selected cases of solitary stone-containing kidneys [11, 18, 29, 37, 70, 74, 87, 93, 110, 111]. Gross infection of the kidney usually contraindicates partial nephrectomy because of the risk of secondary haemorrhage. In less severe grades of renal infection associated with stone, preliminary treatment by antibiotics may render the operation safe. Infection with urea-splitting organisms is usually a contra-indication. The operation is usually unsuitable for the treatment of calculi in several calyces of one kidney. However, lower- and upper-polar partial nephrectomy for calculi in these situations is not infrequently done in óne operative procedure.

Fixity of the kidney in its bed following earlier operations or as a consequence of infection, may render its mobilization difficult, and the satisfactory performance of the operation technically difficult or impossible. Partial nephrectomy as a second or third operation on one kidney may be difficult and even inadvisable. In some congenitally abnormal kidneys the unusual blood supply may render the kidney unsuitable for the operation. Partial nephrectomy would not usually be indicated in a kidney in which unrelated diseases (tubercle, malignant disease or polycystic kidney) were found in association with calculus. The aims of the operation are to remove the appropriate amount of renal tissue necessary to extirpate the disease including the stone-containing calyx, to control the bleeding during and at the end of the operation and to close the urinary passages.

Three different principles or techniques are in use: In the wedge-shaped method of resection the stone-bearing calyces are removed by deliberate incisions along with a considerable surrounding cuff of renal tissue as described below. In the guillotine method of resection a simple transverse resection of renal tissue in the lower or upper pole of the kidney is made followed by haemostasis. Partial resection of the kidney by blunt dissection was used by Semb [106, 107] as a method for the partial resection of the tuberculous kidney. In removing the diseased tissue by transverse section through healthy tissue, the renal parenchyma was divided by dissection with a blunt instrument, such as the handle of the scalpel.

An early variant of partial nephrectomy for the treatment of calculous disease was simple calycectomy, whereby a relatively small amount of renal parenchymal tissue containing the stone and the calyx which contained it, were removed. Twinem [115, 116] reported 10 such cases, later radiography showing no recurrence in 9. In 41 cases in the series reported by Culp and Hendricks [20], simple calycectomy was performed while in 42 others all or most of one pole of the kidney was excised.

2. Exposure and Control of Bleeding

The kidney is exposed through an incision across the bed of the resected twelfth rib and is fully mobilized together with the renal pelvis, the pelviureteric junction and the vascular pedicle. It is suspended in a cotton sling and a radiograph of it is taken to establish finally the position and number of the calculi.

Temporary control of bleeding by the use of clamps must be provided or permanent control established by the ligature of appropriate vessels in continuity. For permanent haemostasis the vessels on the cut surface of the kidney must be identified and ligated, infarcted renal tissue thereby being reduced to a minimum.

Ligature in continuity of the branch of the renal artery (lying in the renal sinus) which supplies all or most of the portion of the kidney to be resected, as an alternative to, or complementary to the ligature of their divided ends at the beginning of or during the operation, is a relevant and satisfactory procedure. It has the disadvantage that it is not possible to make the ultimate line of section of the kidney correspond exactly with that part of the renal tissue supplied exclusively by the artery which is ligated. Either a small part of the renal parenchyma left behind has been infarcted, or alternatively the ligature does not completely arrest bleeding when the kidney is sectioned. In practice the second alternative usually applies, a point which removes some of the objections which have been made to the method, some vessels in the divided surface of the kidney then subsequently needing to be ligated. On balance, the author believes that this is a good method to achieve secure haemostasis and has usually used it.

In applying the method of ligature in continuity, if it has been decided to do a lower polar partial nephrectomy, the branches of the renal artery within the renal sinus are exposed. Dissection with fine forceps and scissors usually reveals a branch of the artery (together with a tributary of the renal vein) leaving the main trunks at a variable distance from the kidney, within the renal sinus, and of a size which the surgeon judges would supply blood to approximately the lower third of the kidney. Digital compression of such an artery usually causes some discoloration and demonstrates the part of the kidney supplied by the vessel. If an artery and vein of the size which seems to be appropriate to the segment of the kidney to be removed have been found, they are ligatured in continuity. If there is any question as to the exact zone of the kidney served by the vessel in question, indigo-carmine may be injected into it before ligature, after which the involved portion of the kidney becomes softer and darker than normal [89].

Puigvert and Gittes [92] prefer the individual ligature of arterial branches as they enter the affected pole, with guidance from an arteriogram. Bleeding can be finally controlled by the individual ligature of divided vessels on the cut surface of the kidney after the resected part has been removed.

3. Wedge-Shaped Resection

The object is to remove a wedge of renal tissue containing the stone with the calyx in which it lies up to its junction with the renal pelvis, together with any adjacent minor calyces which drain upwards into the renal pelvis and which could, if left behind, prevent dependent drainage of urine into the renal pelvis after the operation has been concluded. The wedge of renal tissue which is removed should not be such as to leave long thin tapering flaps of renal tissue but broad flaps with an adequate blood supply. The procedure was strongly advocated by Stewart [110, 111]. The use of the wedge-shaped method of resection has not been without critics. Power [90] claimed that the apposition of flaps of renal tissue by sutures does not add to the security of the operation, since they are of uncertain viability especially towards their margins and apices, and that the renal tissue in them has virtually no excretory function, having been largely destroyed. Whatever the theoretical objections, the method seems to work well in practice.

In the case of a lower-polar partial nephrectomy an incision is first made through the renal capsule along the convex border of the lower third of the kidney and is continued over the lower pole and the inner border of the kidney towards the hilum. The cut edges of the capsule are picked up with fine forceps and reflected by the use of the flat handle of a scalpel. A thin capsule may be torn if it dips into furrows or scars on the surface of the kidney which have resulted from past attacks of inflammation. The separation of the capsule is carried out to a level in the kidney somewhat higher than the proposed line of section. The kidney is then sectioned with a knife in two places so as to excise a large wedge of tissue, the two incisions meeting each other deep in the renal substance at the lower border of the renal pelvis. As the incision is deepened, the neck of the major calyx containing the stone comes into view close to its junction with the renal pelvis, and is cut across either with the knife or with the scissors. The entire lower major calyx must be removed along with the sector of renal tissue. If a truncated stump of the major calyx (or minor calyces which empty into it) have been incompletely excised, they have in some instances acted as diverticula (or a sump) for the stagnation of urine, and have been the seat of subsequent stone formation (Fig. 13.2).

When the wedge of renal tissue has been resected, the number of stones removed must be seen to compare numerically with those shown on the radiograph. Syringing the renal pelvis at the end of the operation assists in the removal of all calcific particles of macroscopic size, as well as pieces of blood clot. A radiograph of the kidney on the operating table is desirable to demonstrate the complete removal of all calculi. The cut surface of the kidney is now inspected for the divided openings of arteries and veins, which are picked up with mosquito forceps and ligated, or underrun by fine catgut sutures and ligatured. Temporary relaxation of the haemostatic clamp on the pedicle helps to identify bleeding vessels.

The divided major calyx at its junction with the renal pelvis is closed accurately with a continuous suture of fine 0000 non-chromic catgut to prevent any late accumulation of blood clot from entering the renal pelvis. The repaired pelvis must be quite smooth. The cut surfaces of the kidney are then brought into apposition by interrupted sutures of 00 non-chromic catgut, not tightly drawn together and placed fairly close together, the sutures passing through the renal tissue inwards to the depths of the divided parenchyma and picking up the cut border of the turned-in capsule. Some urologists have interposed grafts of fat or muscle, oxycel packs or fibrin foam; foreign bodies such as these carry some disadvantages. Nephrostomy tubes to drain the renal pelvis and splinting catheters are no longer considered to be necessary.

4. Guillotine Method

In this method the stone-containing segment is removed by a simple transverse section of the kidney followed by arrest of the bleeding and closure of the urinary tract. Partial control of bleeding by ligating the vessel to the segment to be resected can be done as in the wedge-shaped method. The renal capsule is stripped from the part of the kidney to be resected after making a circumferential incision distal to the line of section; the kidney is then divided transversely at a level to include the stone-con-

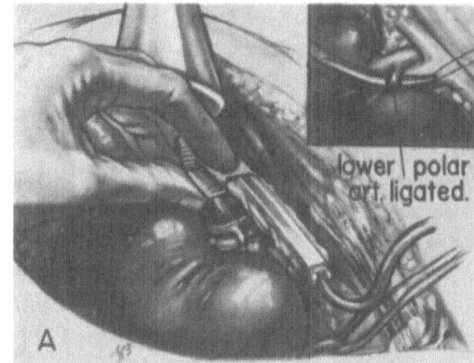

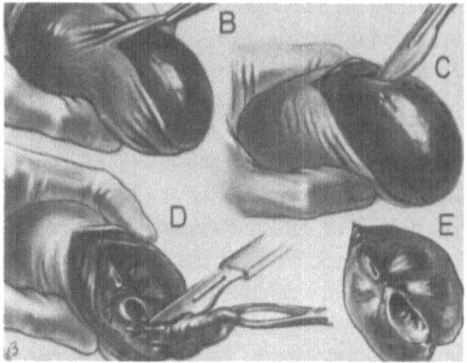

Fig. 13.2. Lower-polar partial nephrectomy.
A. The kidney and the renal vascular pedicle are mobilized; the artery to the lower pole of the kidney is defined and ligated in continuity; a Stewart's haemostatic clamp has been applied to the renal vascular pedicle (*see text*). **B.** The renal capsule overlying the lower pole is incised and retracted beyond the line of incision through the kidney. **C.** The line of the first incision through the renal parenchyma. **D.** Wedge-shaped resection of the lower third of the kidney, including the lowest stone-containing calyx. **E.** Resection completed, the lowest calyx remaining open at its junction with the renal pelvis. **F.** The opening into the pelvis is repaired by a fine continuous catgut stitch. **G.** The renal capsule is folded inwards over the cut surface of the renal parenchyma. **H.** The renal tissue is repaired by interrupted stitches. **I.** The suture of the kidney is completed

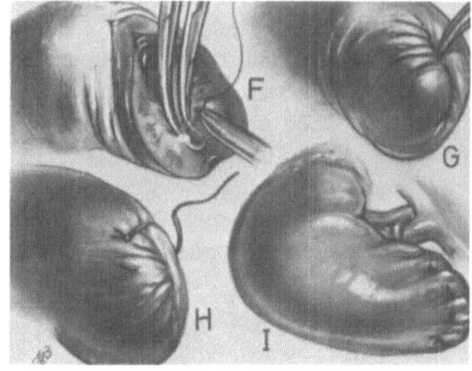

taining calyx in the resected part. The larger divided vessels are picked up with mosquito forceps and ligated, or underrun individually, and the opened major calyx or renal pelvis is closed with plain catgut sutures. Both the vessels and calyceal openings are readily accessible on the surface of the kidney instead of being in the deeper parts of a wedge-shaped cavity. The reflected renal capsule, or alternatively a flap of fatty or muscle tissue is sutured to the raw surface of the kidney with catgut sutures; alternatively a piece of Gelfoam may be used.

5. Blunt Dissection

In this method as much renal tissue as necessary is removed by a blunt instrument, such as the handle of a scalpel; the vessels, being more resistant than the soft renal parenchyma, stand out as the dissection proceeds and can be identified, clamped and ligated [18, 63, 89, 106, 107]. The opened major calyx or renal pelvis is then closed with plain catgut sutures. The author has used the method of resection by blunt dissection for a few cases of tuberculous kidney and found it to be satisfactory. For the operation of partial nephrectomy, Poutasse [89], who has mostly used the anterior approach to the kidney (using a subcostal or paramedian incision), used a combination of blunt and sharp dissection to excise the selected portion of the kidney. He identified and ligated the branches of the renal artery in the renal pedicle and sinus which supplied the part of the kidney to be resected. The reflected capsule was used to cover the bare area of the kidney without any attempt to reconstruct the kidney.

After the completion of the operation of partial nephrectomy, the kidney is secured in its normal position in the renal fossa by the use of a few stitches passed through the renal capsule and into the parietal muscles, in order to provide natural downward drainage of urine and to avoid kinking of the ureter. The fatty coverings below the kidney are brought together by sutures so as to form a sling or shelf to prevent late undue mobility of the kidney, which is now reduced in size.

6. Type of Operation

Lower-polar partial nephrectomy is the procedure most commonly used. Upper-polar partial nephrectomy is performed occasionally for a calculus in an upper calyx. An incision through the bed of the resected eleventh rib gives a perfect exposure for the operation, in which removal of the stone-bearing calyx alone (simple calycectomy) may be sufficient to give a good result, the other upper minor calyces (which will have

free dependent drainage of urine into the renal pelvis) being left behind. There is then less sacrifice of renal tissue than with a lower-polar partial nephrectomy. Partial nephrectomy of a middle calyx containing multiple calculi and which is itself the seat of a hydrocalycosis (congenital or acquired) with the excision of a cuff of renal parenchyma, is a satisfactory operation. Simple calycectomy may be preferred and may be adequate for the treatment of a solitary biggish dilated stone-containing calyx. The incision through the renal capsule (which is then reflected) is made transversely across the central part of the kidney from the region of the renal sinus in front to a corresponding place behind. The wedge of renal tissue removed is also disposed transversely and must include the stone-bearing calyx and extend to the renal pelvis, which is closed by a continuous suture at the conclusion of the operation. The steps for the control of bleeding and repair of the kidney are the same as for lower-polar partial nephrectomy.

Abeshouse and Lerman [1] reviewed 193 cases of partial nephrectomy for calculous disease from the literature and added 17 of their own. Stewart [110, 111] reported 152 partial nephrectomies performed on 144 patients for calyceal calculi of which 29 were for upper-polar calculi, 5 for upper- and lower-polar calculi and 6 for calculi in the lower pole and middle calyx. Hamm and Finkelstein [44] reported 46 cases, 39 of which were performed for calculous disease alone or in association with ureteropelvic obstruction and 6 for a duplex kidney, in 2 of which calculi were present. Poutasse [89] reported 51 cases, mostly for stone. Puigvert and Gittes [92] reported 208 cases for calculus, including a proportion with mixed staghorn phosphatic calculi. The author has done about 100 cases of partial nephrectomy for stone with overall satisfactory results. In Kilpatrick's [60] cases of partial nephrectomy for calculous disease 57 were for lower-polar calculi, 6 for upper-polar calculi and 3 for the removal of a hydrocalyx; the operation was combined with pyelolithotomy in 7 cases.

7. Combined Procedures

Patients who have a stone in the renal pelvis and one in the lower calyx should usually be treated by a combined operation of pyelolithotomy and partial nephrectomy (assuming that a biggish calyceal stone cannot be removed across the pelvis).

In patients who have had pyelolithotomy or ureterolithotomy for calculi in the renal pelvis or the upper part of the ureter, if the radiograph taken of the kidney exposed during the operation showed pathological changes or particles of grit in a lower calyx, suggesting that the ureteric calculus had matured in that calyx and that a subsequent recurrence could be expected, Stewart [111] recommended that partial nephrectomy should be done in sequence to the primary operation, and did it in 23 cases. It cannot always be easy to decide whether such an addition to the operation of pyelolithotomy or ureterolithotomy is really justified, since it adds materially to the total surgical trauma; there is always the possibility that such particles could be voided spontaneously in course of time.

8. Complications

The operation of partial nephrectomy carried out in carefully selected cases and with painstaking technique is an operation with few complications and which has established itself as the most important procedure for the treatment of calyceal stone.

Reactionary Haemorrhage may occasionally follow a repair of the kidney which has been less than perfect; if bleeding does not cease spontaneously and is severe, the wound should be reopened and further sutures placed in the kidney.

Secondary Haemorrhage may be a more serious complication occurring 8–12 days after the operation. It may be manifested by gross haematuria occurring after the initial postoperative discoloration of the urine has disappeared, by external bleeding from the wound, or by the development of a mass in the renal region. It may complicate an operation which has been done on an infected kidney. The bleeding may cease spontaneously (assisted possibly by blood transfusion); alternatively recurrent (and sometimes severe) haemorrhages may occur and secondary nephrectomy may be necessary if the bleeding is uncontrollable. Secondary haemorrhage following partial nephrectomy for calculous disease was recorded in 3.1% of 193 cases collected by Abeshouse and Lerman [1], and in 3.4% of a collected series of 819 cases of the operation done for various conditions by Murphy and Best [81], nephrectomy being necessary in 2.5% of them.

Drainage of Urine and Urinary Fistula. Following the operation, urine may occasionally drain from the wound in the kidney to the exterior or to the perinephric region. External drainage of urine may result from the incomplete or inadequate suturing of the calyceal system especially if the kidney was infected before operation. The sequence of events, the causes and the treatment are similar to those already referred to in the earlier section dealing with nephrolithotomy. In a series collected by Goldstein and Abeshouse [41] of 296 patients who had had partial nephrectomy by various surgeons for many types of localized disease of the kidney (including 58 for calculous disease), there were 13 cases (4.3%) of urinary fistula, 2 being in the calculous cases. In a later report by Abeshouse and Lerman [1] of 193 collected cases of partial nephrectomy for localized calculous disease, there was 1 case of temporary and 2 of persistent fistula. In Murphy and Best's [81] larger collected series of 819 cases permanent urinary fistula was reported in 3.9%. Fistula was reported by Hamm and Finkelstein [44] in 3 of 46 cases.

Provided there is no ureteric obstruction a urinary fistula usually closes spontaneously, occasionally after a period of drainage. If the fistula is associated with an infected kidney, some damage to renal function is almost certain to follow and the affected kidney may even undergo total destruction or require secondary nephrectomy. It may sometimes be possible to ascertain the extent of the fistula and any infected pockets derived from it, by a combination of intravenous urography and injection of opaque medium along the fistulous track. Drainage of infected pockets deep to the wound and even a resection of the fistulous track down to the kidney may sometimes be possible. A badly damaged fistulous kidney, however, should in general be removed.

Wound Infection. As with any renal operation, wound infection may be an occasional sequel if the kidney was infected prior to operation. Organisms may gain entry to the wound by way of the drainage tube especially if retained too long. Escape into the perinephric tissue of urine which does not drain into the dressing may be followed by perinephric abscess [60].

Renal Function seems to be but little impaired following the operation in aseptic cases. Intravenous pyelograms a few months later show a good concentration of medium and a satisfactory outline of the remaining calyces and the renal pelvis with, of course, the absence of the excised major calyx. There must, however, be some loss of renal function following the loss of more than one-third of the kidney. Thus, Herbst and Polkey [52] in their experiments on dogs showed that when part of the kidney

was resected, there was a decrease in renal function which was approximately proportional to the loss of excised secreting renal tissue, though there was some gradual return of function between the third and the fifth weeks, but never to normal.

Arteriovenous Fistula. This complication, which is discussed in Section V of this chapter [12, 42], has occasionally complicated partial nephrectomy. Kuhle and Schenker [62] reported a case in which an aneurysm which had developed following partial nephrectomy (and which may have been associated with the repair) was later responsible for a severe fatal haemorrhage. A case was reported by Houtappel et al. [54].

Snodgrass and Robinson [109], reported a female patient, aged 37, who had had a partial nephrectomy for lower polar calyceal calculi. Radiography 6 years later showed the presence in the lower pole of the kidney of a calcified ring shadow, which lay between the pelviureteric junction and the lowest remaining calyx, and in the neighbourhood of the earlier partial nephrectomy operation. The excised kidney showed a calcified aneurysmal sac, the lumen of which was continuous with the branch of the renal artery (which supplied the lower pole of the kidney) and from which a dilated major tributary of the renal vein emerged.

IV. Ureterolithotomy

An operation for the removal of a ureteric calculus will have been decided upon after consideration of the possibility of spontaneous voiding of the stone and sometimes after perurethral instrumentation to induce the stone to pass into the bladder. A ureteric calculus may change its position within a short period of time. The everpresent possibility of complete ureteric obstruction calls for careful watch. A small silent stone may be allowed to remain in the ureter for a time though in practice usually not longer than 6 months. A functionless hydronephrotic kidney may gradually develop in the presence of a stone supposedly under observation.

For the surgical removal of ureteric stones, an extraperitoneal operation is preferred and is virtually routine. The skin incision is made as far as possible directly over the stone. Transperitoneal operation may have a place for the occasional removal of recurrent stones and of bilateral stones in the lower third of the ureter. For the operative approach to the lowest 2 in. of the ureter, at various times the vaginal, the perineal and even the parasacral routes have had their advocates; the last two approaches are not easy and have now been discarded, but vaginal ureterolithotomy, which is also extraperitoneal, is still used occasionally.

The operation should be done under antibiotic cover in infected cases. Because of the mobility of some ureteric calculi, it is necessary to confirm radiologically the precise position of the stone immediately before operation. If this procedure is not carried out, occasionally it is found that during the exposure of the ureter (which in such cases is dilated) the stone has moved a few inches up the ureter, and occasionally into the renal pelvis. In some patients the mobility of two or more calculi in a dilated ureter can be demonstrated before operation on successive radiographs, one taken with the patient flat, and the second with the table tilted into a moderate Trendelenburg position. The surgeon then knows that he may have trouble and should ensure that both stones have descended to their lowest possible point in the ureter before commencing the operation, which must then be done with the patient in a reverse Trendelenburg position. In most instances a mobile stone only moves upwards for a short distance and, when found, can be milked down to the site of the first stone at operation. Once the stone has been located after exposure of the ureter, it must be held between the fingers, until tapes have been passed round the ureter at levels above and below the stone.

1. Indications for the Operative Removal of Ureteric Calculi

1. Frequently recurring severe attacks of renal colic, especially if they do not hasten the descent of the stone down the ureter.

2. Increasing evidence of obstruction as shown by increasing hydroureter and hydronephrosis.

3. Associated urinary infection, because of the danger to the kidney.

4. Rapid increase in the size of the calculus.

5. Persistent or recurrent attacks of haematuria.

6. Calculus in the ureter of a solitary kidney.

7. Bilateral ureteric calculi.

8. Calculi in the upper and middle third of the ureter, which are unlikely to be voided spontaneously or to descend into the pelvic ureter.

9. Calculi in the lower third of the ureter of more than 0.6 cm diameter for many surgeons; for some the indication is 1 cm in diameter.

10. Associated renal calculi, especially where renal function is already impaired.

11. Failed endoscopic manipulation.

12. In a patient who is to move to a place remote from urgent surgical assistance.

2. Upper Third of the Ureter

For the removal of a stone at or just below the pelviureteric junction the patient is placed in the lateral position as already described for an operation on the kidney. If the stone is situated some distance below, a semi-lateral position is appropriate, a small cushion being placed suitably behind the back. The incision used for exposing the kidney (extended downwards a little if necessary) is suitable for exposing the ureter from the level of the pelviureteric junction to that of the lower border of the fourth lumbar vertebra. Unless it is intended to remove an associated stone in the renal calyx at the same time as that in the ureter, it is not necessary to mobilize the whole kidney, though for a stone at or just below the pelviureteric junction the lower pole of the kidney will have to be partly freed in order to gain access to the ureter.

The fascia of Gerota is defined and incised in the upper part of the wound, and the fat covering the lower pole of the kidney (when indicated) and that lying in front of the ureter, is displaced forward by stripping it, along with the peritoneum, from the posterior abdominal wall towards the middle line. The ureter is lifted forward with the peritoneum and can be demonstrated with the help of a right-angled retractor. It is more easily recognized if it is dilated and it vermiculates if stroked with an artery forceps. Crossing the ureter from within outwards at the level of the third lumbar transverse process are the spermatic or ovarian vessels. At this stage the stone may easily be felt lying in ureter, which may be moderately or considerably dilated just above the stone. The areolar sheath of the ureter (often oedematous) is divided longitudinally before it can be mobilized at the site of the stone. If the stone has been impacted for a considerable time, fat of a firm texture surrounds the ureter at the site of the stone. The ureter for an inch or more above and below the stone is freed from its coverings by blunt dissection. For the removal of the stone, a small pair of scissors with sharply pointed blades, ureteric stone forceps, a ureteric catheter and a fine non-chromic catgut stitch in a fine atraumatic half-curved needle mounted on a needle holder, are made immediately accessible for the surgeon. A gauze pack is placed beneath the mobilized ureter to absorb the urinous discharge when it is opened.

If the ureter is not dilated a small longitudinal incision is made directly onto the stone, which is recognized by the grating sensation when it is touched with the scalpel. If the ureter is dilated above an impacted stone, and if it has been possible to milk the stone upwards, the incision is made into the dilated segment of the ureter over the stone. The incision may be extended upwards or downwards, to an appropriate size (using the fine-pointed scissors) which will allow of extraction of the stone. Urine (clear or turbid depending on the presence or absence of infection) may escape, when the stone may be coaxed out of the ureter or removed with forceps. In the case of a long or ellipsoidal stone, it is often unnecessary to incise the ureter for the full length of the stone unless it is very spiculated, since it can be made to present at a small opening and then be extracted by forceps. The ureter is palpated below the stone, to make sure that particles of grit or even a second small stone is not left behind, and a ureteric catheter is passed down the ureter to the bladder to ensure its patency. The incision in the ureter is now sutured accurately, with interrupted sutures of No. 0000 non-chromic catgut mounted on a very small half-curved atraumatic needle, penetration of the mucous membrane by the needle being avoided especially in infected cases. The periureteric fascia or fat is then drawn together over the ureteric incision by a few interrupted stitches. As with the renal pelvis, some surgeons do not advise suture of the incision in the ureter, believing that the urine will find its own way down the ureter to the bladder and that the wound will heal spontaneously, which it eventually does. There may then be free drainage of urine from the wound, perhaps for a few days after the operation, moreover an undesirable pocket of urine may collect retroperitoneally. The wound in the loin is closed, leaving a thin rubber drain down to the ureter near to the part which has been incised.

In Foley's [36] incision for the exposure of the upper ureter, an attempt is made to avoid cutting muscles by using a muscle-displacing incision, and secondly the fascia of Gerota is not incised, the ureter being approached after displacing it forwards. For the further details of this much-used incision, the original paper should be consulted.

Transverse Incision

A transverse incision in front of the abdomen extending from the outer border of the rectus abdominis in an outward direction for 10–12 cm has been used for the removal of stones in the upper third of the ureter. The external oblique aponeurosis and then the internal oblique with the transversalis muscles are divided in the direction of their fibres; the peritoneum is displaced inwards, retractors are introduced and the ureter is found attached to the peritoneum. The advantages claimed for this incision are that muscle is not cut, that bleeding is minimal and that no major nerves are divided.

3. Middle Third of the Ureter

In this group are included calculi situated from the level of the transverse process of the third lumbar vertebra to that of the brim of the true pelvis. For the removal of stones from the upper part of this segment of the ureter the patient is placed in the semi-lateral position, suitably supported by a small cushion. For the removal of stones located at or slightly above or below the bifurcation of the common iliac artery, the patient is placed flat on his back. The middle third of the ureter is approached through an oblique incision which is continued downwards in the same line and direction (but at a lower level) as that for

the removal of calculi in the upper third of the ureter. After incising the deep fascia the anterior part of the external oblique muscle (and its aponeurosis) is split in the direction of its fibres, and the fibres of the internal oblique and transversalis muscles are incised in the direction of the incision to the outer border of the rectus sheath, so as to demonstrate the transversalis fascia, which is then divided in the line of the incision. The peritoneum is reflected from the loin and from the iliac fossa towards the middle line, until first the external iliac artery and then the point of division of the common iliac artery comes into view. The ureter, which can then be seen, is drawn forwards with the peritoneum from which it is separated by blunt dissection, and freed upwards and downwards until the stone is located. The stone is then removed in the manner described for calculi in the upper third of the ureter. Calculi from a few inches above the brim of the pelvis to a level even 2 in. below it can be removed through this incision by a suitable selection of its level, though some of such calculi are strictly in the lower third of the ureter.

a) McBurney's Incision

For the exposure of a limited segment of the ureter at the level of the pelvic brim, where a stone occasionally becomes arrested, a simple McBurney's incision may be used, but if the stone is not found at the expected spot, the incision would need to be extended by division of muscular fibres. The patient is placed flat on his back; the skin incision, 4 in. long, crosses at right angles the line from the umbilicus to the anterior superior iliac spine at the junction of its upper and middle thirds. After division of the external oblique as described above, the fibres of the internal oblique and transversalis muscle, which lie roughly parallel to each other, are separated in the line of the incision, the two portions being then retracted. The operation then proceeds as described above.

b) Oblique Lateral Incision

This was described by Joly [57] and can be used for a stone at the brim of the pelvis. The patient is placed flat on his back. The incision begins about 1 in. in front of and above the anterior superior iliac spine and passes obliquely downwards to a point 1–1.5 in. above the pubis; it is, therefore, for the most part parallel to Poupart's ligament. The operation proceeds as when McBurney's incision is used, though it is usually necessary to ligate and divide the deep epigastric artery and vein.

4. Lower Third of the Ureter

The bladder is emptied by catheter. The patient is placed first on his back at the beginning of the operation but in the Trendelenburg position when the lower ureter has been exposed and a piece of tape has been passed round it above the stone to prevent it from then moving upwards towards the kidney if the ureter is dilated.

A vertical mid-line incision is made from the umbilicus to the symphysis pubis, the rectus sheath is incised in or near to the middle line and the rectus muscles are separated. The perivesical space is opened up with the finger below the semilunar fold of Douglas by separating the pelvic areolar tissue, while higher up the peritoneum is separated from the lateral wall of the pelvis and from the iliac vessels, when the empty bladder with its fatty coverings can be seen. The semilunar fold of Douglas marks the curved lower extremity of the posterior rectus sheath and it is usually desirable for better access to divide this for some distance in a vertical direction, by gentle touches with the scalpel; too vigorous cutting will carry the blade through the peritoneum. This manoeuvre allows the peritoneum to be stripped more readily from the iliac fossa and from the upper part of the iliac vessels. The deep epigastric artery

and vein, which will be seen coursing upwards and outwards underneath the rectus muscle, should not be injured during the dissection, though sometimes small branches passing to the peritoneum have to be sealed by diathermy coagulation. With a suitable retraction of the wound, designed to draw the peritoneum towards the middle line, the ureter comes into view, lifted upwards with the peritoneum, to which it remains attached. It is usually first recognized as a whitish muscular tube (especially if dilated) as it crosses the point of division of the common iliac into the external and internal iliac arteries.

If the ureter is moderately dilated above an impacted stone it should be more easy to define the stone by palpation, the ureter being freed from surrounding areolar tissue. This part of the operation can be easy or difficult depending upon the degree of periureteric fibrosis associated with the stone, its precise level (especially its proximity to the bladder) and the obesity of the patient. In some cases, by traction on the tape (passed behind the ureter), and with the finger behind the ureter, the stone can sometimes be reached without much difficulty. There are differences, however.

Since the ureter in its descent to its vesical termination, passes *behind* a part of the bladder before it enters the bladder wall to become the intramural part of the ureter, the presence of periureteric fibrosis secondary to the impacted stone may render difficult the surgical approach to the lowest 2 in. of the ureter, including the intramural part. The surgeon may have dissected the ureter downwards to a point where he thinks he should be able to palpate the stone, but instead of locating it, he finds a fibrofatty mass of tissue (often containing blood vessels) of varying size and toughness, almost surrounding the lower part of the ureter, closely involving the adjoining part of the bladder and lying in relation to the inner wall of the pelvis. If an attempt is made to cut through such a mass of tissue hoping to demonstrate first the ureter and then the stone, troublesome bleeding may ensue. A guide to the lowest part of the ureter at this point is, in the male, the vas deferens, which can be seen crossing the pelvis and which, if recognized and dissected, can be followed downwards to the lower end of the ureter, to which it is intimately related. In the female, the uterine artery crosses the ureter from without inwards in its lowest part (Fig. 13.3).

The most appropriate technique to mobilize the lowest 1.5 in. of the ureter in a difficult case is as follows: The lateral part of the bladder wall must be mobilized (by the surgeon's finger) fairly freely from the pelvic wall, to which it is only attached by areolar tissue. This step properly carried out renders relatively easy the approach to this segment of the ureter. Dissection with curved scissors through the periureteric and perivesical fibro-fatty tissue in front of the ureter (sealing a few small vessels by long diathermy forceps before they are divided) is then proceeded with under direct vision. Traction upon the tape already passed behind the ureter towards the middle line gradually enables the posterior wall of the bladder to which the ureter is attached, to be lifted up at least for 1 in., and its lateral border to be slightly rotated towards the middle line so as to make it present to the surgeon.

In the male the vesiculo-deferential artery (sometimes of considerable size), which is a branch either of the anterior division of the internal iliac artery or of the inferior vesical artery, and which if it cannot be easily displaced downwards during the dissection hinders the approach to the ureter prior to extracting the stone, will then have to be divided between ligatures; as the ends of the divided vessel separate, a little more of the ureter is freed.

In the female, the uterine artery can usually be demonstrated and dissected free from the ureter, enabling its lower end to be drawn upwards by gentle traction on the tapes, making subsequent removal of the stone easy in the manner previously described.

If the stone is impacted in the intramural ureter, not only perivesical fibro-fatty tissue but also some red muscular fibres of the bladder wall have to be divided before this segment can be adequately exposed. In teasing away the muscle fibres of the bladder wall, the blue vesical mucosa may be slightly tented upwards, and care must be taken not to cut it, otherwise there is an escape of urine as the bladder is opened.

If the steps in the technique described above are carried out in the wrong order and particularly if the side of the bladder is not mobilized, the surgeon may encounter troublesome bleeding, which may obscure his view, and he may then be tempted to open the bladder and remove the stone by incising the ureteric opening. In the author's experience this is never necessary and it is undesirable because it entails the subsequent repair of the bladder and the use of an indwelling catheter for a period.

The surgeon should never be tempted to open the ureter some distance above the level of the stone (because of the supposed difficulty of the dissection to reach the level of the stone), and insert ureteric stone forceps in the hope of grasping the stone and removing it. Except in the case of a greatly dilated ureter such a manoeuvre cannot succeed, since the blades of the forceps cannot be opened to a distance greater than the diameter of the impacted stone, which would be necessary if it has to be grasped. In such a situation (to deal with a stone very low down in the ureter) Dodson [31] recommended that an incision be made in the ureter above the stone through which a Howard spiral stone extractor be inserted to engage the stone and draw it upwards. The technique for the removal of the stone when the stone-containing segment of the ureter has been mobilized follows that described in earlier sections.

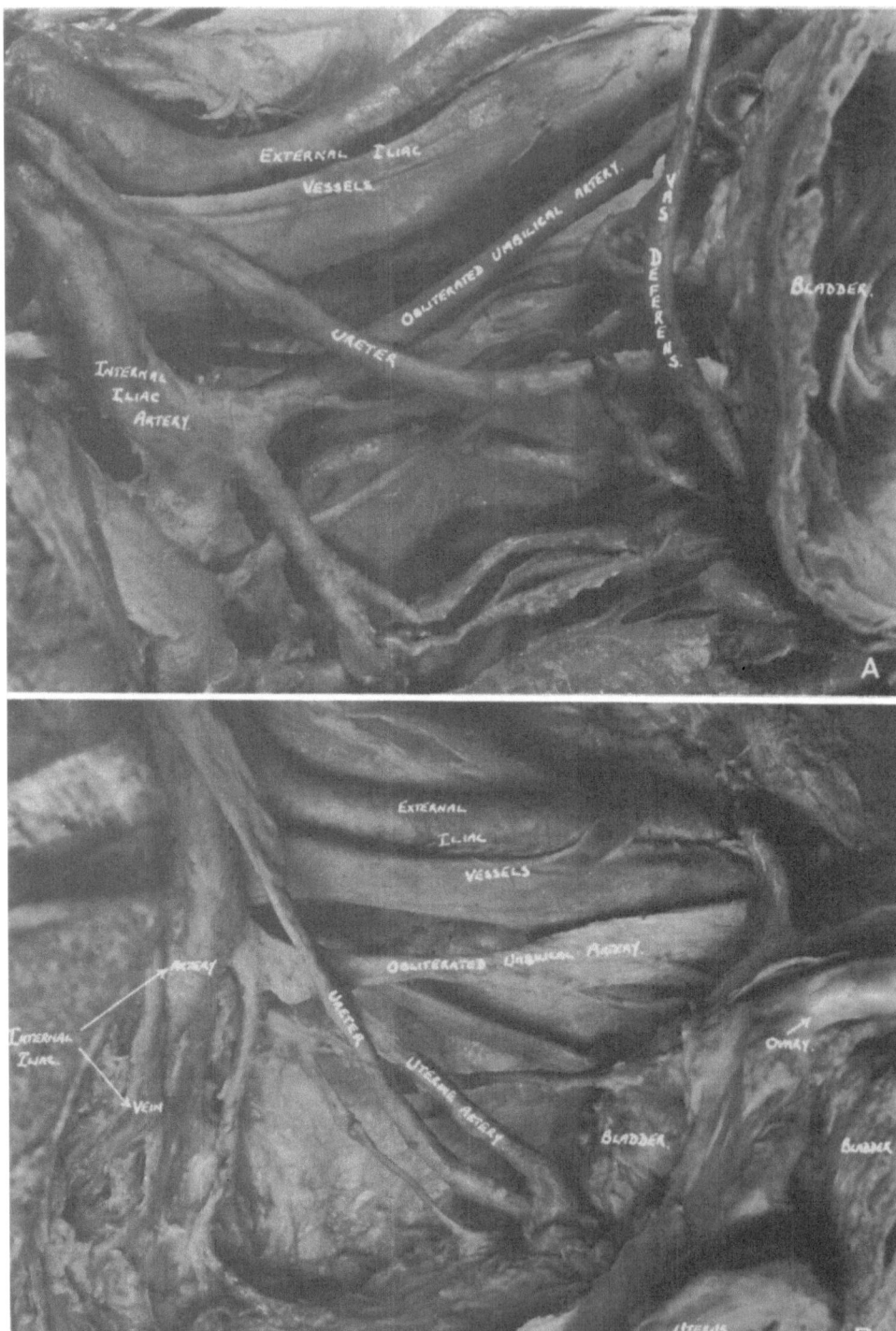

Fig. 13.3

A pararectal incision has been used for the removal of calculi in the lower third of the ureter especially in obese patients as an alternative to the more usual mid-line incision, to which in general it is inferior. The incision extends from just above the spino-umbilical line, a little distance internal to the outer border of the rectus muscle, and is carried downwards, internal and parallel to the outer border of the rectus muscle, to a point just above the inguinal ligament. The rectus sheath is incised in the line of the wound, enabling the rectus muscle to be displaced inwards towards the middle line. The subsequent course of the operation follows that described for a mid-line exposure.

a) Transvesical Ureterolithotomy

The operation of transvesical ureterolithotomy for the removal of stones impacted in the lowest inch of the ureter is rarely needed. Many calculi in that position descend into the bladder spontaneously or following instrumentation. Such an operation endangers the integrity of the sphincter mechanism at the ureterovesical junction, risking the development of ureteric reflux. It has already been stated that it is always possible to remove a stone in the lowest part (and even the intramural part) of the ureter by an extravesical operation from above, in spite of occasional difficulties. The procedure, however, is still practised by some surgeons and will therefore be briefly described.

Seven or eight ounces of sterile saline are run into the bladder through a urethral catheter, which is left in position. The patient is placed in the Trendelenburg position. The bladder is exposed either through a vertical or a transverse extra-peritoneal incision, is mobilized and freely opened longitudinally, and an illuminated bladder retractor is placed in position. The ureteric orifice of the affected side is identified and, with a stone of medium size its position can be seen by a bulge of the vesical mucous membrane at or just above the ureteric orifice. The ureteric orifice is divided using curved pointed scissors (or a diathermy electrode) upwards and outwards as far as the stone, which is then removed with long, fine, curved stone forceps, bleeding in the rather deep cavity being dealt with by diathermy. A suture, picking up the edges of the incision, may also be used to arrest haemorrhage, and helps to preserve the sphincter mechanism of the orifice. If a widely gaping orifice is left, subsequent postoperative reflux is probable. Some surgeons have raised a small semicircular flap of the whole thickness of the bladder wall above and to the outer side of, and about 0.75 in. from the ureteric orifice. When dissected back, this exposes the lowest inch of the ureter, which can then be incised to enable the stone to be removed. The ureter and the flap are repaired by interrupted sutures.

b) Transperitoneal Ureterolithotomy

The transperitoneal approach to the ureter was occasionally used by older surgeons for the removal of ureteric calculi, but it gradually fell into disuse as the extraperitoneal approaches were perfected. The chief disadvantage was the possible leakage of urine (especially if infected) into the peritoneal cavity with possible unpleasant sequelae. With the better control of infection now available urologists have been less reluctant than formerly to open various parts of the urinary tract across the

Fig. 13.3. **A.** Dissection of the lower third of the ureter in a *male* subject showing the relationship of the ureter to the vas deferens and the vesiculo-deferential artery. **B.** Dissection of the lower third of the ureter in a *female* subject showing its relation to the bladder, the uterine artery and the obliterated umbilical artery. (By courtesy of Mr. G. Wilson, F.R.C.S. by whom the dissections were done)

peritoneal cavity. The transperitoneal exposure of the middle segment of the ureter (which is closely related to the peritoneum) to a level well below the pelvic brim is an anatomically easy approach for the removal of stones. After opening the abdomen through a lower median, paramedian or muscle-cutting incision, the intestine including the caecum is packed off and the ureter located by direct vision or by demonstrating vermiculation by stroking it with a clip. It is usually easy to palpate the stone through the overlying peritoneum which is then incised, the ureter is dissected free for a limited extent and opened. The stone is extracted and the ureter sutured after passing a ureter catheter downwards to the bladder. The parietal peritoneum overlying the ureter may be sutured and an extraperitoneal drain inserted; alternatively the peritoneal cavity is drained for 2 days. Quist et al. [95] described 22 patients with stones in the middle part of the ureter treated in this way as an elective procedure, in 7 of whom the stone was impacted in the pelvic ureter above the level of the ischial spine; in one case there was drainage of urine for 10 days. Transperitoneal ureterolithotomy is often suitable for the removal of recurrent ureteric calculi (see later).

c) Vaginal Ureterolithotomy

The operation has been done for the removal of stones in the lowest segment of the ureter and especially for those close to the ureterovesical junction. De la Pena [28] who summarized the early literature and the surgical anatomy, reported 13 cases and considered that calculi located even 6–8 cm up the ureter could be removed by this route without difficulty.

The lowest part of the ureter lies from one-third to half-an-inch above and to the outer side of the lateral vaginal fornix, coming forward beneath the broad ligament and the uterine artery, lateral to the neck of

the uterus, from which it is separated by loose connective tissue. In a stout multipara in whom the vaginal tissues and the perineal muscles are relatively lax and in whom the calculus is palpable, the vaginal route has an advantage over the abdominal, in that the approach is direct and simple and the operation is accompanied by a minimal amount of shock and little pain. The dependent drainage after operation is an advantage. The possibility of an external incisional hernia is avoided.

The patient is placed in an exaggerated lithotomy position so as to render the plane of the perineum parallel with that of the operating table. The position of the stone is confirmed by palpation through the lateral fornix and if its recognition is difficult a catheter inserted in the ureter as a guide may help. Retractors are placed in the vagina, the cervix is grasped with tenaculum forceps and drawn downwards and towards the side opposite to the stone. An anterolateral incision 4 cm long is made over the stone in front of and lateral to the cervix through the whole thickness of the lateral vaginal mucous membrane, and is deepened until the stone can be palpated. A blunt hook placed round the ureter above the stone to prevent it from moving upwards is used to exert traction on the ureter which can be mobilized and drawn almost through the vaginal incision. The ureter is incised over the stone, which is then removed and the incision is repaired. The vaginal incision is left unsutured for drainage (which is dependent).

Fistula is rarely a problem. Injury to the bladder and to the peritoneum has been reported. The uterine artery, which lies above and medial to the ureter, could be injured if the dissection is carried upwards too vigorously, though its position is at a higher level in the pelvis than that of the lowest 2 in. of ureter. The operation has a place for the urologist and has been used by the author on a few occasions.

d) Perineal Ureterolithotomy

Lowsley and Kirwin [68] showed that a calculus impacted in the vesical end of the ureter may be removed through the perineum as an alternative to the abdominal route, though not in obese patients. The patient is placed in the exaggerated lithotomy position, a sound being passed along the urethra. A horseshoe-shaped incision is made in the perineum above the urethral bulb, the central tendon of the perineum is divided and the wound is deepened as far as the apex of the prostate. The recto-urethralis muscle is divided and the levator ani muscle separated from the prostate to expose its posterior surface. Traction upon a blunt-toothed retractor fixed at the base of the prostate enables the seminal vesicles to be drawn forward.

The operating table should now be elevated considerably, since the ureter is on the roof of the deep wound. The intervesicular fascia is then incised and drawn laterally to expose the ampulla of the vas and the seminal vesicle on the affected side, the rectum is retracted and the dissection is carried deeper until the ureter is exposed and isolated where it emerges above the tip of the seminal vesicle. Traction upon a tape passed round the ureter beyond the site of the stone enables the ureter to be lifted into the wound, when it can be incised and the stone extracted and the ureter repaired.

e) Parasacral Ureterolithotomy

The parasacral approach to the ureter was occasionally used by the older surgeons. The patient was placed in position on the operating table lying on his chest with the thighs dropping downwards at a right angle over the end of the table. An incision was made from the middle of the lateral border of the sacrum, deviating a little laterally, to just above the anal orifice. The skin flap was dissected towards the middle line, the coccyx resected, the pelvic fascia and also the levator ani on the side of the incision were divided enabling the rectum to be displaced to the opposite side of the wound. After defining the seminal vesicle the ureter was ultimately reached in the depths of the wound [10].

f) Combined Procedures

If the patient has a stone in the kidney, one in the ureter, and one in the bladder, the latter may be removed first by crushing, and the other stones dealt with later. If there are multiple infected stones in a disorganized kidney as well as one in the ureter, nephroureterectomy may be indicated.

If there is an uninfected, reasonably healthy kidney containing stones (and also a ureteric stone), a combined operation to remove the renal stone, for example, partial nephrectomy, with ureterolithotomy, may be done at the same time in a fit patient. If the patient is not fit the stone in the ureter should be removed first (or dealt with by cystoscopic manipulative treatment) and the renal stone dealt with appropriately after an interval. The renal stone should not be removed first, since a renal urinary fistula would probably result. Conversely, if the ureteric stone is removed first, a small stone from a renal calyx or the pelvis may migrate down the ureter if too long an interval is left between the two operations.

If there are simultaneously stones in both ureters, the patient is at risk to develop calculous anuria, so that early surgical removal of both stones is indicated. If anuria has not yet developed, both stones may be removed at the same operation and the advantages of such a course probably outweigh the risks. If one or both stones are in the upper third of the ureter, the appropriate incisions should be made in the loin or loins, while if both stones are in the lower half of the ureters, a transperitoneal approach is suitable.

5. Complications

The surgical removal of a stone in the ureter is nearly always easy and there should be no difficulty in locating either the ureter or the stone. The procedure can usually be carried out without incident except occasionally in the case of stone lying just outside the bladder when the procedure may sometimes be difficult. For these reasons it often takes priority in the practice of many urologists over the perurethral instrumental methods of treatment.

Haemorrhage. Reactionary haemorrhage following operation must be virtually unknown, while secondary haemorrhage possibly resulting from the injudicious placement of a drainage tube close to the wall of a medium-sized artery is excessively rare.

Infection. Postoperative infection, retroperitoneal cellulitis and severe ileus should usually be preventable by appropriate anticipatory treatment. Preoperative urinary infection (if present) should disappear after removal of the stone with appropriate treatment before and after operation, providing the appropriate operation has been done. If a nephroureterectomy rather than a ureterolithotomy should have been done, the renal infection may persist, and may need further treatment later; it is possible to be too conservative in dealing with some cases of infected ureteric calculi.

Fistula. The complication of urinary fistula following the other renal operations, and its causes and treatment has already been referred to. Dix [30] summarized cases of temporary leakage of urine from the wound in his series of 177 cases of ureterolithotomy. There were 12 temporary fistulae of an average duration of 10.4 days in 68 operations for stone above the pelvic brim; and 11 of average duration of 10.7 days in 109 operations for stone below the pelvic brim. The shortest period of drainage was 3 days and the longest 30 days. The appropri-

ate treatment has been referred to in an earlier section. In 1 case the fistula persisted for 65 days, nephrectomy then being done.

Injury to Adjacent Organs (colon, duodenum) or blood vessels (iliac vessels) during the course of operation should be avoidable, though the larger pelvic vessels are vulnerable during operations on the lower third of the ureter. Permanent injury to the ureter itself during operation may be important and may be followed by ureteric stricture or fistula in the shorter term, or by renal infection and ultimate deterioration in the longer term. Postoperative ureteric stricture is rare, the ureter apparently possessing a remarkable degree of recovery following the temporary impaction of a stone, so that presumably complete epithelialization leads to healing of the ureter without residual ulceration and fibrous contraction. Such is usually the case even following temporary fistulous drainage of urine. Occasionally, a slight dilatation of the ureter at the site of impaction can be demonstrated by a ureterogram taken a year or so following the voiding or removal of the stone. Sandegard [104] reported postoperative stricture in 3 of 62 cases of ureteric stone.

Renal Function. An impacted ureteric stone causes at least a temporary depression in renal function, which is recovered from in whole or in part, probably depending upon how long the stone has been impacted. Even a considerable hydronephrosis resulting from a stone may recover completely following ureterolithotomy though sometimes recovery is incomplete.

V. Nephrectomy and Nephroureterectomy

While the aim of treatment of renal calculous disease is primarily to remove the calculi, as much renal tissue as possible must be conserved. Yet a grossly, progressively infected and badly functioning kidney sometimes becomes a continuing menace to health and has to be removed. A decision to remove one kidney, however, can only be taken when it has been established that the opposite kidney is either healthy or that it can at least function sufficiently well to sustain life. In the present context the term nephrectomy implies the removal of the diseased kidney to a point a short distance below the pelviureteric junction. The term nephroureterectomy implies removal of the kidney together with either the entire ureter down to the bladder, or a considerable part of it down to a level below a firmly impacted stone; in such cases the ureter is involved in the total pathological process. The indications for these operations are the following:

1. Indications for Nephrectomy

1. Severe calculous hydronephrosis with advanced renal atrophy.

2. Severe calculous pyonephrosis.

3. Multiple unilateral staghorn calculi with advanced pyelonephritis.

4. Occasional cases of unilateral multiple calyceal calculi in kidneys which are either not infected or only slightly infected, are giving rise to recurrent pain, and have not responded to treatment by conservative operations.

5. Renal fibrolipomatosis with calculi and almost complete renal atrophy.

6. Renal calculi in association with some malignant tumours of the kidney and renal pelvis.

7. Renal calculi with pyonephrosis in association with a duodenal or a colonic fistula.

2. Indications for Nephroureterectomy

1. Calculous pyonephrosis, pyelonephritis or hydronephrotic atrophy of a degree of severity calling for nephrectomy, when found in association with one or more impacted calculi in the ureter.

2. Renal calculi associated with simple or malignant papillary tumour of the kidney; such tumours may metastasize in any part of the ureter.

3. Renal calculi and renal tuberculosis in the same kidney, the ureter being usually involved in the disease.

4. Calculous pyonephrosis needing nephrectomy in association with ureteric reflux from the bladder.

5. Some cases of renal and ureteric calculi in an infected kidney associated with ureterocele.

In severely infected calculous kidneys an examination of the kidney when it has been exposed at operation usually confirms that the decision tentatively made before operation has been appropriate, the scarred renal surface presenting soft zones of thin and atrophied renal cortical tissue overlying distended calyces obviously full of pus or purulent urine. If it was felt that a conservative procedure (such as bivalve nephrolithotomy) to remove the calculi would be followed by an early recurrence of stone, and that it is unlikely that the infection can be eradicated by the use of antibiotics (because of the presence of urea-splitting organisms resistant to antibiotics), and that the destruction of renal tissue which has already taken place will proceed further if conservative treatment is adopted, nephrectomy will usually be decided upon.

If there is a functionless pyonephrotic calculous kidney on one side, with one or more calculi in the opposite kidney, nephrectomy on the bad side may still be desirable and reasonable, the stones from the better side being removed at a separate operation. Some surgeons would then prefer to remove the calculi from the better side first, in order to prevent further deterioration of that kidney if, for any reason, operation on that kidney has to be deferred. There is much to be said, however, for removing a functionless, toxin-producing pyonephrotic kidney first, thereby probably relieving the patient of pain or discomfort and improving the general health.

Small pyonephrotic calculus-containing kidneys, and kidneys that are the seat of advanced renal lipomatosis (in which there are stones, but often minimal remaining renal tissue) should be treated by nephrectomy, if there are clinical symptoms; and there is usually no difficulty in reaching a decision. In a patient with severe calculous disease in both kidneys, the problem is that of the treatment of bilateral calculous disease.

3. Extracapsular Nephrectomy

This is the procedure which is most often appropriate and it applies to most of the conditions listed in the indications for nephrectomy. Anatomically, it is indicated when the renal capsule can be fairly easily separated from the surrounding tissues. In secondary operations for infective calculous disease, when the kidney is perhaps beset with formidable adhesions, a subcapsular nephrectomy may be preferred. The operation is usually done extraperitoneally through a lumbar incision in the loin. Very rarely, as in some patients with calculi associated with a duodenal fistula, a transperitoneal nephrectomy is appropriate.

The aim of the operation is to remove the calculous kidney complete in its capsule without soiling the wound with pus and urine. The kidney, which is exposed as previously described, can usually be mobilized without undue difficulty, though in infected cases the perirenal fat may be oedematous, sodden and fibrous. Fibrofatty adhesions when encountered, should usually be divided with scissors after defining the renal capsule instead of attempting to break them down, a procedure which may result in tearing the renal parenchyma. The renal pelvis and the upper part of the ureter,

which may be surrounded by a dense cuff of oedematous fat, are defined and dissected free, after which the renal vessels are freed from the renal pelvis to the level of the inferior vena cava. On the right side the duodenum is separated. The ureter is ligated some distance below the pelviureteric junction (and below any associated ureteric stone if one be present) at two points 0.5 in. apart and divided by diathermy.

An aberrant or accessory renal artery, which occasionally enters the upper part of the renal sinus from the aorta, must be ligated and divided if present. The renal artery and vein are defined separately by careful dissection, and ligatures are passed around each of them in turn and tied as deeply as convenient in the wound prior to dividing them between pedicle clamps, and applying a second ligature to the entire pedicle. It is never desirable to tie the renal vascular pedicle by one stout ligature applied round a large clamp holding the divided renal artery and vein with the surrounding fat. However slowly and cautiously the clamp is released by the assistant, there is a danger that the ligature may break, or that the pedicle may slip away from the grip of the ligature as it is drawn tight. Seizure of such a slipped pedicle with ring (sponge) forceps may be the most effective method of checking temporarily the flow of blood. It may be desirable, however, to pack gauze swabs into the wound, pressing the renal vessels against the vertebral column, a procedure which will check the bleeding and provide opportunity for mopping away the blood and clots before the bleeding can be definitively dealt with.

4. Subcapsular Nephrectomy

Joly [57] gave a clear description of the procedure, which was first described by Albarran [3]. In many calculous patients with an associated pyonephrosis, the author has found that this operation often has the advantage over the operation of extra-capsular nephrectomy, in that it is easier to perform and is especially suitable for the bad risk patient. Kittredge and Fridge [61] reached a similar conclusion after comparing 53 cases in which subcapsular nephrectomy had been performed at the Ochsner Clinic with 285 'classic' extra-capsular nephrectomies. The procedure is often the operation of choice for the removal of the kidney for calculous pyonephrosis if there has been an earlier operation for drainage of a pyonephrotic kidney or for the removal of calculi, when the tissue planes between the renal capsule and the surrounding structures may as a consequence have become so obscured from dense adhesions that definition of the true plane of cleavage between them may be difficult. The perirenal fibrosis is usually densest along the convex border of the kidney, where an earlier operation has most obviously left its mark, and this must now be the starting point for the proposed new operation. The operation, which may be difficult, must be referred to in some detail (Fig. 13.4, see p. 282).

It is appropriate to decide to do a sub-capsular nephrectomy quite early in the operation, the surgeon basing his decision upon the difficulty of the initial approach to the kidney. An incision from pole to pole of the kidney is made through the renal capsule, which is then separated from the parenchyma over the anterior and posterior surfaces by blunt dissection until the renal sinus is reached. The separation (which is usually easily accomplished except at furrows on the surface of the kidney resulting from past infection) is continued until a point is reached when no further progress can be made, since the line of junction or fusion between the capsule and the renal pelvis has been reached.

The bulky renal pedicle has then to be dealt with. It is usually impossible (and it is certainly undesirable) to ligate en masse the entire renal pedicle at that point without further dissection, since it is not only oede-matous as a result of obstruction and infection but also extremely thick, containing as it does the renal vessels, the peripelvic fat and the renal pelvis, which may contain calculi as well as pus. The method of dealing with the pedicle at this stage involves going through the renal capsule along the line where it has become fused with the renal pelvis.

The kidney is lifted by the surgeon or his assistant as far out of the wound as possible in order to put the pedicle on the stretch. The reflected renal capsule is then incised deliberately on its inner surface in a vertical direction from within outwards, using the point of the scalpel or scissors, at its line of juncture or fusion with the renal pelvis. The cut edges of the divided capsule (which may be quite thick) tend to separate from each other, revealing the fat around the pelvis and the upper end of the ureter (which gradually comes into view), which may be dense and fibrous, oedematous and easy to separate.

The dissection of the pedicle (now outside the renal capsule) is continued until the renal artery and vein are defined. In the anterior part of the pedicle it is continued completely round the renal sinus to free them completely on their posterior aspect. The kidney, now greatly freed, can be lifted somewhat further out of the wound so that a more complete exposure of the entire pedicle, including a reasonable length of the renal artery and vein becomes visible and easier to define; care must be taken not to injure the inferior vena cava at this stage.

The renal pelvis is lifted up to enable the pelviureteric junction and the upper part of the ureter to be defined. The ureter, followed by the renal artery and vein, are then separated from each other and divided individually between ligatures. When the kidney is finally lifted out, the residual renal capsule, which is left behind, can be seen encircling the cavity, and the line of its

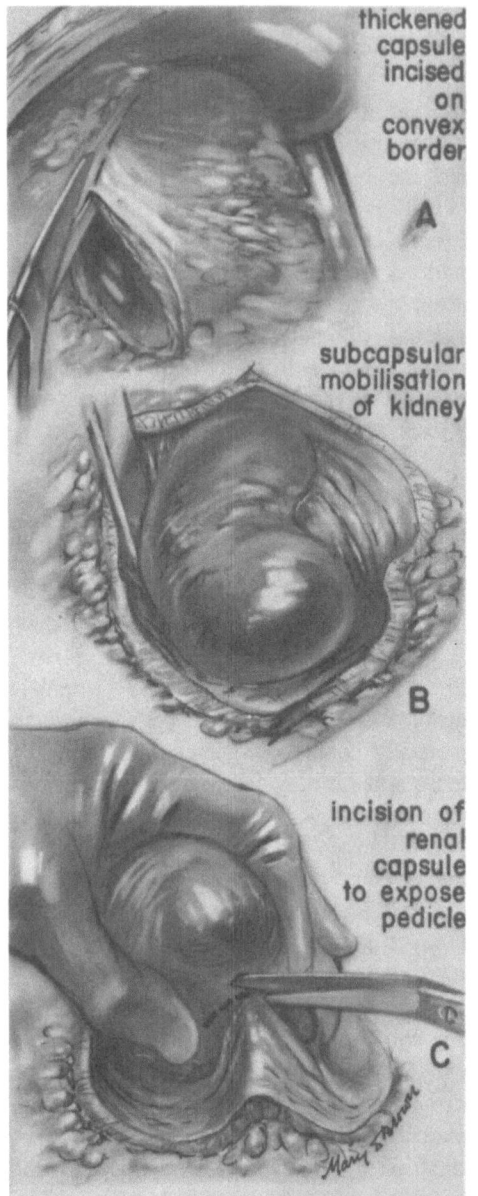
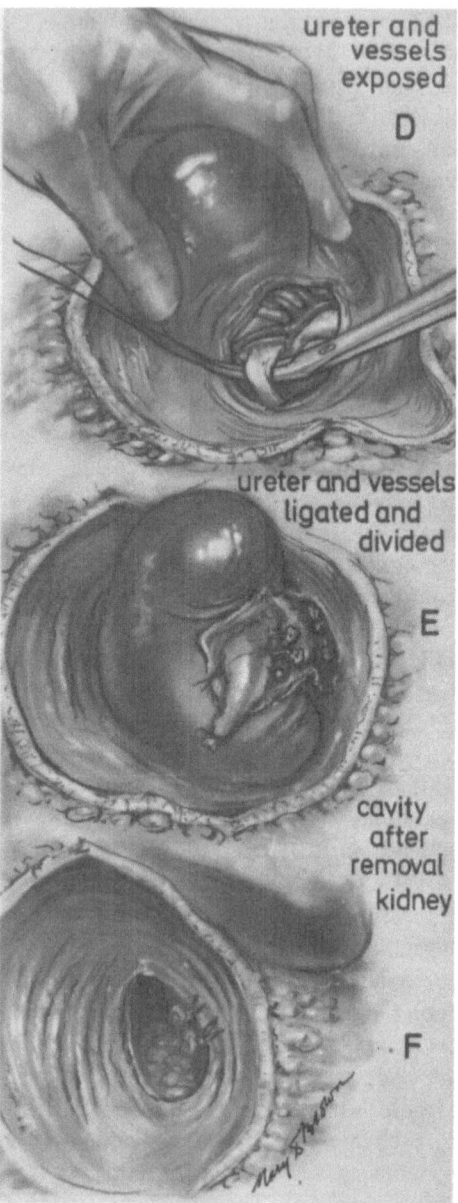

Fig. 13.4. Operation of subcapsular nephrectomy. **A.** The capsule of the badly infected kidney is exposed in the operation wound; a longitudinal incision through the thickened capsule is made on the convex border of the kidney to expose the subjacent renal parenchyma. **B.** The entire kidney is mobilized by blunt dissection with the finger beneath the renal capsule down to the hilum at the pelviparenchymal junction. **C.** The reflected renal capsule is incised at the hilum of the kidney with scissors or scalpel from within outwards to expose the structures in the renal pedicle lying in the peripedicular fat. **D.** The renal pelvis, the upper part of the ureter and the renal artery and vein are exposed and dissected prior to ligature and division; a good wide opening gives an adequate exposure. **E.** The ureter and vessels are ligated and divided, enabling the kidney to be removed. **F.** The cavity after removal of the kidney shows the inside of the thickened renal capsule and also the fatty tissue around the divided pedicle

division from the renal pelvis can be recognized in the depths. The wound is closed with drainage.

5. Transperitoneal Nephrectomy for Stone

The author has always managed to do even a difficult nephrectomy for calculous pyonephrosis (except in a few patients with severe scoliosis) through an incision in the loin. The transperitoneal route for the removal of an infected calculous kidney, so useful for the removal of some malignant renal neoplasms, has not found favour among most urologists because of the risk of peritoneal infection. However, the access to a difficult and adherent renal pedicle may not be easy through an upper abdominal transperitoneal incision.

The transperitoneal route may be used with advantage to do a nephrectomy for a largely disorganized kidney associated with a duodenal or colonic fistula. When the upper abdomen is opened through a paramedian incision, the colon overlying the kidney is displaced medially and a vertical incision is made through the retroperitoneum as it crosses the renal pedicle in order to expose the renal vessels, which are divided between ligatures. The ureter is similarly identified, ligated and divided. The kidney is then gradually freed starting with the posterior surface. The fistula is defined and the opening in the duodenum or colon closed. The peritoneum adherent to the anterior surface of the kidney may be removed with the renal mass.

In the rare circumstances in which a patient with severe kyphoscoliosis, needing a nephrectomy for calculous disease, has the ribs on the side to be operated on touching or even overlapping the iliac crest, there may not be sufficient room to provide the surgeon with access for the removal of the kidney through the loin. A transperitoneal operation using either a transverse incision across the upper abdomen and extending well back into the loin, or a paramedian incision may, when good retraction is applied, enable the kidney to be reached and removed. The author has removed three such kidneys transperitoneally through transverse incisions. In some such cases a combined thoraco-abdominal approach would be a suitable alternative.

6. Nephroureterectomy

If the decision to do a nephroureterectomy has been made before the operation is begun, and the ureteric calculi are in the upper two-thirds of the ureter (or even somewhat lower), a long single incision from the lumbar region to the level of the stone may enable the kidney, after ligature of its pedicle, together with the appropriate part of the ureter, to be removed in one piece, after dividing the ureter below the stone between ligatures.

If it is necessary to remove the kidney along with the entire ureter down to the bladder, because of an impacted stone in the lowest few inches or at the extreme lower end of the ureter, or because of associated ureteric tumours or serious ureteric reflux believed to be related to the presence of the renal calculi and infection, the operation should be done using two separate incisions rather than through one very long lumbo-ilio-inguinal incision, which was formerly used, dealing with the kidney first.

The operation proceeds as for simple nephrectomy and the renal artery and vein are ligatured and divided. The renal pelvis and the dilated ureter (which is often full of pus), are freed from the tissues of the posterior abdominal wall at least as far down as the brim of the pelvis. The kidney is delivered from the wound, attached only to the ureter and is allowed to hang down over the lower end of the wound, the incision being closed by layers of sutures, leaving a small gap in the muscle through which is inserted an untied suture (to be drawn together subsequently), around the emerging ureter. The patient is now turned on to his back in slight Trendelenburg position, the lower third of the ureter is exposed through a middle-line suprapubic incision and is mobilized to a point 1 in. or so below the stone or to the bladder as in the operation of ureterolithotomy, and divided between ligatures. If there are ureteric tumours it may be necessary to remove a small cuff of bladder wall. The kidney with the attached ureter is then drawn out through the upper part of the wound, which is closed with drainage.

Some surgeons prefer to expose and divide the pelvic ureter below the stone as the first step in the operation, the ureter then being freed to as high a level as convenient before the wound is closed, and pushed upward into the loin. The patient is then turned onto his side, the kidney being exposed and removed in the ordinary way.

It is, generally speaking, the sounder practice to remove the kidney and ureter from above downwards. If the patient is in poor condition and the removal of the kidney is difficult, the procedure can be terminated by removing the kidney and ligating the ureter as low down as possible in the kidney wound. The lower segment of the ureter with the stone can then be removed at a second operation 10 days later.

7. Complications

Reactionary and Secondary Haemorrhage. Bleeding from the stump of the renal vessels must be excessively rare if the renal artery and vein have been ligated separately and doubly ligated in the manner described. Reactionary bleeding could arise if the pedicle is ligatured en masse either because of a late break of the ligature, or because the mass of tissue in the renal pedicle escapes from the grasp of the ligature. Secondary haemorrhage from the renal vessels (which is always serious) may occur between the seventh and the twelfth day after operation in an infected case especially if the vascular pedicle was ligatured in an inappropriate way. A rapid opening of the wound with ligature of the bleeding vessels, together with the use of blood transfusion and other restoratives, is then probably the only way to save life.

Wound Infection may follow the removal of a badly infected calculus-containing kidney, the risk of which, however, is reduced by the appropriate use of antibiotics and by the insertion of a drainage tube.

Ureteric Sinus or Fistula. If the ureter below the kidney is normal when it is ligated and divided, no harm will follow from the stump of the ureter. If a simple nephrectomy has been done when a nephroureterectomy should have been preferred, early or late complications involving the residual ureter may follow. If the ureter below the point of ligature contains a calculus which should have been removed with the kidney at the earlier operation and is possibly therefore infected, or if it is dilated because of a hydroureter or pyoureter consequent upon a ureteric stricture (or spasmodic narrowing) near the bladder, or if there is ureteric reflux, a ureteric sinus or fistula may follow if the ligature on the ureter is shed or absorbed.

A ureteric fistula may appear as long as 23 years after the nephrectomy. The complication will be manifested by the appearance of a persistent discharge of pus (sinus) or even of urine (fistula) in a patient with ureteric reflux, from the lower part of the operation wound. Radiography, which should include a sinogram following the introduction of a catheter along the track, will usually reveal the extent of the trouble (including the presence of a ureteric stone if one has been overlooked) and also the calibre of the ureter. Assistance in diagnosis may be achieved by cystoscopy and an ascending ureterogram. A sinus may close spontaneously. When a urinary fistula is present the residual ureter down to the bladder should usually be excised.

Fall in Blood Pressure. Among 18 normotensive patients from a group of 30 who had undergone surgical treatment for unilateral calculous disease reported by Pryn [91] (nephrectomy 15; partial nephrectomy 3), 6 showed a rapid, significant and sustained fall in blood pressure after operation (5 after nephrectomy; 1 after partial nephrectomy). Calculous pyelonephritis was demonstrated histologically in the kidneys which had been removed. The length of the follow-up ranged from 7 months to 6.5 years. The reason for the fall in blood pressure was not clear, but they may have been early examples of unilateral renal hypertension.

Arteriovenous Fistula. Fistula between the renal artery and vein has been observed most often in the intact kidney, when it may have been congenital. It has been observed as an occasional complication of penetrating wounds involving the renal pedicle and of various renal surgical procedures including percutaneous renal biopsy [7, 12, 34]. Most reported cases have followed nephrectomy [32, 33] done for various conditions including pyonephrosis for renal calculous disease [40].

The steps in the operation of nephrectomy which, it has been thought, may lead to arteriovenous fistula, are mass ligation of the renal pedicle [59], transfixion of the renal pedicle as a preliminary to ligature (which in any case is dangerous), and the use of an aneurysm needle to carry the catgut used for the individual ligature of the renal artery and vein; the needle may then injure the wall of either the artery or the vein. When a fistula has developed after the renal artery and vein have been ligated separately, it has been suggested that the vessels may subsequently have become adherent to each other, that the intima may retract behind the ligature and that a low-grade infection at this site may allow the blood to track (after an interval of time) from the artery to the vein [40]. Symptoms of the aneurysm may occur as long as 5–35 years after nephrectomy [42]. In one case [80] the fistula was detected 29 years after the original nephrectomy; and in another following nephrectomy for renal calculous disease symptoms did not become prominent until 11 years after nephrectomy [40]. The patient may complain of local symptoms, including pain and discomfort, some time after such a renal operation, and the discovery of a thrill and a systolic bruit in the upper abdomen on the affected side, together with enlargement of the heart, leads to the diagnosis. A palpable swelling in the loin has occasionally been observed [59]. Hypertension following nephrectomy is a prominent and suggestive symptom and if untreated may be ultimately followed by cardiac decompensation, cerebrovascular lesions or renal failure [40, 47].

The treatment of arteriovenous fistula in the postnephrectomy cases consists of the exposure and dissection of the fistulous vessels through an incision in the loin, and their separate ligation above and below the fistula, with or without the removal of the associated aneurysmal dilatation; nephrectomy and occasionally partial nephrectomy have sometimes been done. In the case reported by Gokarn and Swinney [40] at operation a bilocular aneurysmal sac was found involving the renal artery and vein (both of which were twice the normal size) and the inferior vena cava and renal vein were found to be thick-walled and pulsating. The vessels were ligated individually and the aneurysmal sacs excised. A normal convalescence was subsequently followed by a considerable fall in blood pressure.

Residual Pyoureter. Unsound though the procedure is, probably in many patients for whom a simple nephrectomy has been performed, ureteric stones have been left behind at a level well below the ligature on the ureter. Such patients may experience no untoward symptoms whatever, provided the residual ureter can drain freely into the bladder. It has been shown above that if the lower ligature on the ureter sloughs away, a sinus or fistula is a likely sequel. However, the subsequent changes in a residual stone-containing ureter in which the ligature at its divided end remains in situ, but in which there is inadequate drainage, vary from an intermittent infection giving rise to relatively minor symptoms, to a pyoureter above the level of the stone associated with periureteritis or even a periureteric abscess. It has been suggested that stones may actually form in a residual ureter, though proof of this is lacking. Latchem [64] studied in the dog the fate of the ureter left behind after the kidney had been removed and showed that in the normal ureter after nephrectomy in the absence of obstruction, there was no atrophy of the mucous membrane nor any obliteration of its lumen; he showed that similar changes to those observed clinically in man occur in the dog, if there is obstruction and/or infection in the residual ureter.

The earliest consequences of a failure to remove a dilated pus-containing ureter to a level below that of the stone at the time that the kidney was removed, provided its upper end remains sealed off by the ligature, are intermittent vesical symptoms of greater or lesser severity. Often after months or even years, the patient may experience recurrent attacks of pain in the corresponding iliac fossa, sometimes associated with pain and frequency of micturition from the accompanying cystitis. Pus cells may be found in the urine even when symptoms are absent. In other cases there is severe and persistent pain, which may be associated with elevation of temperature (or even rigors), and of the pulse rate. In the worst cases there is chronic ill-health, persistent vague abdominal discomfort alternating with periodic exacerbations of pain, temperature, pyuria and anaemia. The condition has often posed difficult diagnostic problems.

On examination during the attacks of pain, there is tenderness in the abdomen in the line of the ureter especially above the level of the calculus. During the stage of purulent distension of the residual ureter, an acutely tender, palpable, sausage-shaped swelling or sometimes an indefinite mass may be detected in the iliac fossa; occasionally a tender swelling is palpable in a vaginal fornix. The plain radiograph will show the presence of one or more residual ureteric stones in the lower ureter and will provide the clue to the diagnosis, which may have been unsuspected, the case sometimes mimicking one of appendix abscess or diverticulitis of the colon. On cystoscopy during the active phase, the ureteric orifice is red and oedematous and there may be intermittent discharge of pus. In the quiet phase, the orifice may appear almost normal. Retrograde catheterization of the ureter and radiography will help to identify doubtful shadows as being those of calculi. The injection of opaque medium may demonstrate a grossly dilated ureter above the stone and even the existence of an abscess cavity continuous retroperitoneally with the upper end of the ureter. The time interval before the onset of clinical symptoms of sufficient severity to cause the urologist to remove the empyema of the ureteric stump has varied greatly. Best and Ormond [6] stated that it was usually from 1 to 4 years. Recorded intervals between the nephrectomy and the residual pyoureter have varied from 1 to 23 years.

The treatment used for some of the early recorded cases of residual pyoureter was conservative and has occasionally been successful. The measures included dilatation of the ureteric orifice by bougies, or a meatotomy through a cystoscope, followed by periodic irrigation of the dilated ureter with antiseptic solutions such as mercurochrome or 1% silver nitrate. Such treatment, however, had often to be carried out over several weeks, moreover the stone was left behind and gave further trouble later.

The stone has sometimes been removed from the pus-distended ureter as a definitive measure (possibly because of the operative difficulty of the removal of the pyoureter itself) in the hope that the distended ureteric stump would drain into the bladder and that the infection would disappear; though some successes have been reported, recurrence of symptoms would appear probable [65].

The rational and most successful treatment is the removal of the dilated residual ureter to a level below that of the impacted calculus or the stricture, a procedure which would not usually entail the removal of a cuff of the bladder wall, though this may be necessary occasionally. If there is an associated periureteric abscess or a fibrous periureteritis with dense adhesions, possibly in the neighbourhood of the iliac vessels, the procedure may be difficult and an abscess cavity if present should be evacuated and drained; the operation may ideally be carried out as an extraperitoneal procedure, but a transperitoneal operation may be appropriate in difficult cases under antibiotic cover.

Israel [55] reported that he had seen empyema of the ureteric stump in 4 of 900 cases of nephrectomy. Ljunggren [66] reported a case in which he had removed the stump of the ureter 18 years after nephrectomy for calculous pyonephrosis, during which time there had been intermittent troublesome symptoms. Stepita and Newman [112] collected reports of 11 patients in whom it had been necessary to remove a residual ureter a long time after nephrectomy; 4 of these had a residual pyoureter resulting from a stone in the lower part of the ureter, in 2 of whom the upper end of the divided ureter communicated with an abscess cavity. Rieser [100] found

that in the previous 25 years 37 cases of residual pyoureter had been reported by 18 observers; 17 were the result of residual calculi and 12 of ureteric stricture. The author has treated 3 cases of residual calculous pyoureter, 1 of which occurred 5 years after an earlier ureterolithotomy and was associated with an abscess.

VI. Nephrostomy and Pyelostomy for Calculous Pyonephrosis

It is sometimes necessary to drain as a matter of urgency (because of obstructive anuria) a pyonephrotic calculous kidney in a patient who is unfit for nephrectomy, or in whom the opposite kidney is relatively functionless although still present, or who has a pyonephrotic solitary kidney.

1. Nephrostomy

The object of the operation is to evacuate pus from the badly diseased kidney, to remove as far as possible any associated renal calculi which are easily accessible and to provide temporary continuous free drainage of urine in order to rescue the patient from uraemia.

With the patient in the lateral position, a short incision is made down to the kidney, which may be tense with a bulging capsule. Pus should first be aspirated through a thick-bore needle (or a trocar and cannula) before making the incision through the cortex, which must be long enough to allow two fingers to be introduced into the kidney to break down septa and loculi which may not communicate with the part of the swelling which has been first opened. Calyceal calculi which lie loose in the cavity are removed with forceps. The large obstructing calculus in the renal pelvis (which is usually present) is removed with the finger or with forceps. One or more large drainage tubes are placed in suitable loculi and possibly a de Pezzer catheter or a large tube in the renal pelvis. The incision through the cortex is loosely sutured around the tubes and the wound in the loin closed. Drainage through or around the tube must remain unimpeded for as long as necessary, and usually until the obstruction which the nephrostomy was designed to relieve has been corrected by removing all obstructing calculi.

A late complication of an indwelling nephrostomy tube is the incrustation with calcium phosphatic debris around the tube, which may interfere with drainage. In extreme cases this may prevent the easy periodic replacement of the tube, which is desirable. Such a complication is best prevented or minimized by giving fluids freely, and by keeping the urinary pH on the acid side of neutrality (if possible) by the administration of mandelamine and/or ammonium chloride, either of which can safely be given unless total renal function is grossly impaired.

2. Pyelostomy

In a patient who is gravely ill from obstructive anuria from any cause, including a stone in the ureter, if it is thought that the immediate removal of the stone would be difficult (as, for example, in the case of a recurrent stone in the pelvic ureter), a pyelostomy, or the insertion of a tube directly into the renal pelvis, to enable the drainage of urine to take place for some time, may be the easier procedure and may be life-saving.

References

1. Abeshouse,B.S., Lerman,S.: Partial nephrectomy versus pyelolithotomy and nephrolithotomy in the treatment of localized calculous disease of the kidney, with a report of 17 partial nephrectomies. International Abstracts of Surgery. Surg. Gynecol. Obstet. *91*, 209 (1950)
2. Aboulker,M.P.: Une nouvelle technique d'abord du bassinet intrarénal et des grands calices. J. Urol. Med. Chir. *66*, 407 (1961)
3. Albarran,J.: Medicine operatoire des voies urinaires, p. 255. Paris: Masson 1909
4. Baker,R., Maxted,W.C., Kelly,T., Laico, J., Longfellow,D.: Results of more than 10-year experiences with renal bivalve for calyceal compression defects and renal calculi. J. Urol. *92*, 589 (1964)
5. Begg,R.C.: Nephrectomy with partial resection of the other kidney. Br. Med. J. *I*, 385 (1945)
6. Best,J.W., Ormond,J.K.: Empyema of residual ureter. J. Urol. *61*, 904 (1949)
7. Blake,S., Hefferman,S., McCann,P.: Renal arteriovenous fistula after percutaneous renal biopsy. Br. Med. J. *I*, 1458 (1963)
8. Blandy,J.P., Singh,M.: The case for a more aggressive approach to staghorn stones. J. Urol. *115*, 505 (1976)
9. Blandy,J.P., Tresidder,G.C.: Extended pyelolithotomy for renal calculi. Br. J. Urol. *39*, 121 (1967)
10. Boeminghaus,H.: Konservative und chirurgische Behandlung des Harnleitersteine. Leipzig: 1940
11. Boeminghaus,F. et al.: Partial nephrectomy—experiences and result. Urologie (A) *11*, 121 (1972)
12. Boijsen,E., Kohler,R.: Renal arteriovenous fistulae. Acta Radiol. *57*, 444 (1962)
13. Braasch,W.F., Foulds, G.D.: Postoperative results in nephrolithiasis. Trans. Am. Assoc. G-U Surg. *16*, 155 (1923)
14. Brady,E.A.Jr.: Nephrolithotomy for staghorn calculi. Urol. Cutan. Rev. *55*, 724 (1951)
15. Brandstetter,L.H. et al.: Comparison of Gil-Vernet and classic flank approaches to pyelo- and ureterolithotomy. Urology *5*, 37 (1975)
16. Brongersma,H.: Report of Second Int. Soc. Urol. Conf. *1*, 351 (1924)
17. Cifuentes,P.: Postoperative results of nephrolithiasis. Trans. Am. Assoc. G-U Surg. *16*, 269 (1923)
18. Clark,F.B., Chute,R., Rudy,H.A.: Partial nephrectomy. J. Urol. *72*, 6 (1954)
19. Crabtree,E.G.: Pararenal pseudohydronephrosis with report of three cases.

Trans. Am. Assoc. G-U Surg. *28*, 9 (1935)

20. Culp,O.L., Hendricks,E.D.: Potentialities of partial nephrectomy. Surg. Clin. North Am. *38*, 887 (1959)

21. Dees,J.E.: Use of an intrapelvic coagulum in pyelolithotomy: a preliminary report. South Med. J. *36*, 167 (1943)

22. Dees,J.E.: Fibrinogen coagulum as aid in operative removal of renal calculi. J. Clin. Invest. *23*, 576 (1944)

23. Dees,J.E.: Fibrinogen coagulum in pyelolithotomy. J. Urol. *56*, 271 (1946a)

24. Dees,J.E.: Fibrinogen coagulum in pyelolithotomy. J. Am. Med. Assoc. *132*, 1039 (1946b)

25. Dees,J.E.: Coagulum pyelolithotomy. Am. J. Surg. *79*, 598 (1950)

26. Dees,J.E.: Coagulum pyelolithotomy. J. Urol. *73*, 445 (1955)

27. Dees,J.E., Fox,H.: Properties of human fibrinogen coagulum. J. Urol. *49*, 503 (1943)

28. De la Pena,A.: Transvaginal surgery of the pelvic ureter. Urol. Int. *1*, 267 (1955)

29. Dimopoulos,C. et al.: Role of partial nephrectomy in the treatment of renal lithiasis (apropos of 34 cases). J. Urol. Nephrol. (Paris) *78*, 159 (1972)

30. Dix,V.W.: Discussion on stones in the lower third of the ureter. Proc. R. Soc. Med. *44*, 933 (1951)

31. Dodson,A.K.: Urological Surgery. 2nd ed. London: Kimpton 1950

32. Dubost,C., Mathis,P.: Un cas d'aneurysme arterioveneux reno-renal après nephrectomie. Mem. Acad. Sci. *82*, 132 (1956)

33. Elliott,J.A.: Postnephrectomy arteriovenous fistula. Trans. West. Sec. Am. Urol. Assoc. *27*, 18 (1960)

34. Fernstrom,I., Lindblom,K.: Selective renal biopsy using roentgen television control. J. Urol. *88*, 709 (1962)

35. Ferrier,P.A., Bliss,W.P.: Pyelolithotomy complicated by gas bacillus infection originating in renal calculus. J. Urol. *20*, 471 (1928)

36. Foley,F.E.B.: Management of ureteral stone: operation versus expectancy and manipulation. J. Am. Med. Assoc. *104*, 1314 (1937)

37. Gellman,A.C. et al.: Partial nephrectomy in renal calculus disease. Urology *1*, 355 (1973)

38. Gil-Vernet,J.M.jr.: New surgery in renal calculus. 13th Congr. Int. Soc. Surg. London (1964)

39. Gil-Vernet,J.M.jr.: New surgical concepts in removing renal calculi. Urol. Int. *20*, 255 (1965)

40. Gokarn,A., Swinney,J.: Arteriovenous aneurysm of the renal artery after nephrectomy. Br. J. Urol. *34*, 15 (1962)

41. Goldstein,A.E., Abeshouse,B.S.: Partial resection of the kidney. J. Urol. *38*, 15 (1937)

42. Goldstein,A.G., Delaurens,D.A., Schwartz,E.J.: Post-nephrectomy arteriovenous fistula. J. Urol. *98*, 44 (1967)

43. Gridner,A.: Transperitoneal pyelolithotomy. Z. Urol. Chir. *39*, 165 (1934)

44. Hamm,F.C., Finkelstein,P.: Partial nephrectomy. J. Urol. *82*, 625 (1959)

45. Handley,W.S.: Subcapsular pyelotomy with remarks on the origin and treatment of renal calculi. Proc. R. Soc. Med. *16*, 21 (1923)

46. Hanley,H.G., Joekes,A.M., Wickham, J.E.: Renal hypothermia in complicated nephrolithotomy. Trans. Am. Assoc. G-U Surg. *59*, 25 (1968)

47. Harbison,S.P., Gregg,F.J., Gutierrez,I.Z.: Arteriovenous fistula following nephrectomy: report of a case complicated by severe azotaemia and congestive failure. Ann. Surg. *152*, 281 (1960)

48. Harrison,J.H., Trichel,B.E.: Experience with fibrin coagulum in pyelolithotomy. J. Urol. *62*, 1 (1949)

49. Hellstrom,J.: Some observations on the removal of kidney stones particularly by means of pyelolithotomy in situ. Acta Chir. Scand. *98*, 442 (1949)

50. Hellstrom,J., Franksson,K.: In: Encyclopedia of urology. Operative urology I. Alken,C., Dix,V.W., Weyrauch,H.M., Wildbolz,E. (eds.), Vol. 13, p. 147. Berlin, Heidelberg, New York: Springer 1961

51. Helsby,R.: The conservation of the severely damaged calculous kidney. Br. J. Urol. *34*, 493 (1962)

52. Herbst,R.H., Polkey,H.J.: Renal resection: an experimental study of postoperative function. Surg. Gynecol. Obstet. *51*, 213 (1930)

53. Hoffman,H.A.: Coagulum pyelolithotomy. Am.J. Surg. *79*, 598 (1950)

54. Houtappel,H.C., Reigns, G.A., De Wringer,T.P.: Intrahilararteriovenous fistula following lower pole resection of the kidney. A case report and a review of the literature. Arch. Chir. Neerl. *15*, 45 (1963)

55. Israel,J.W.: Postoperative results in neph-rolithiasis. Trans. Am. Assoc. G-U Surg. *16*, 321 (1923)

56. Johnson,C.M., Smith,D.R.: Calcified peri-renal pseudohydronephrosis; hydroneph-rosis with communicating perirenal cyst with calcification. J. Urol. *45*, 152 (1941)

57. Joly,J.A.: Stone and Calculous Disease of the Urinary Organs. London: Heinemann 1929

58. Jordan,W.R., Tomskey,G.C.: Compli-cations of nephrolithotomy with special reference to secondary haemorrhage. J. Urol. *77*, 19 (1957)

59. Kelly,D.G.: Renal arteriovenous fistula; a report of four cases and review of the literature. Br. J. Urol. *39*, 162 (1967)

60. Kilpatrick,F.R.: Partial nephrectomy for stones. S. Afr. Med. J. *37*, 767 (1963)

61. Kittredge,W.E., Fridge,J.C.: Subcapsular nephrectomy. J. Am. Med. Assoc. *168*, 758 (1958)

62. Kuhle,J., Schenker,J.R.: Aneurysm of renal artery following partial nephrec-tomy. J. Urol. *36*, 1 (1946)

63. Lattimer,J.K.: Partial nephrectomy for tuberculosis. Am. Rev. Tuberc. *66*, 744 (1952)

64. Latchem,R.L.: An experimental study of the ureter after nephrectomy: report of a clinical case of pyoureter. J. Urol. *8*, 257 (1922)

65. Livermore,G.R.: Stone in ureteral stump left when nephrectomy is done. J. Urol. *63*, 786 (1950)

66. Ljunggren,E.: Complications caused by stump of ureter after nephrectomy. J. Urol. *59*, 179 (1948)

67. Lowsley,O.S., Bishop,C.C.: New method of repairing kidney wounds. Surg. Gynecol. Obstet. *57*, 494 (1933)

68. Lowsley,O.S., Kirwin,T.L.: Clinical urol-ogy, 2nd ed. Baltimore: Williams and Wilkins (1944)

69. Maddern,J.P.: Surgery of the staghorn calculus. Br. J. Urol. *39*, 237 (1967)

70. Mahajan,V., Mahajan,K.C.: Partial neph-rectomy in a solitary kidney for calculi. Indian J. Surg. *26*, 585 (1964)

71. Mahmood,P., Morales,P.A.: Extended pyelolithotomy (Gil Vernet's pyelotomy). J. Urol. *109*, 772 (1973)

72. Marion,G.: Pyélotomie élargie. J. Urol. *13*, 1 (1922)

73. Marshall,V.F., Lavengood,R.W., Kelly, D.: Complete longitudinal nephrolitho-tomy and the Shorr regime in the manage-

74. Marshall,V.F., Singh,M., Tresidder,G.C., Blandy,J.P.: The place of partial nephrec-tomy in the management of renal calyceal calculi. Br. J. Urol. *47*, 759 (1975)

75. McDonald,D.F.: Surgical management of staghorn renal calculi. South Med. J. *67*, 1067 (1974)

76. Middleton,R.G., Marshall,V.F.: Complete longitudinal nephrolithotomy for staghorn calculi in children. J. Urol. *106*, 776 (1971)

77. Mikkelsen,O.: Haemorrhage after nephro-lithotomy. Br. Med. J. *II*, 962 (1935)

78. Mimpriss,T.W.: An investigation of the results of splitting the kidney. Lancet *II*, 921 (1934)

79. Moore,T.D., Sweetsen,T.H.Jr.: Coagulum pelvilithotomy. J. Urol. *67*, 579 (1952)

80. Muller,W.H., Goodwin,W.E.: Renal arteriovenous fistula following nephrec-tomy. Ann. Surg. *144*, 240 (1956)

81. Murphy,J.J., Best,R.: The healing of renal wounds. I. Partial nephrectomy. J. Urol. *78*, 504 (1957)

82. Narath,H.: Renal pelvis and ureter. New York: Grune & Stratton 1951

83. Narath,H., Dees,J.E., Fox,H.: Prepara-tion of human fibrinogen solutions: a pre-liminary report. J. Urol. *49*, 497 (1943)

84. Papathanassiadis,S., Swinney,J.: Results of partial nephrectomy compared with pyelolithotomy and nephrolithotomy. Br. J. Urol. *38*, 403 (1966)

85. Patel,V.O.: Coagulum-pyelolithotomy. Urologe *13*, 168 (1974)

86. Papin,E.: Chirurgie du rein, Vol. I, 1928

87. Pedersen,J.F.: Partial nephrectomy for nephrolithiasis. Scand. J. Urol. Nephrol. *5*, 171 (1971)

88. Petrovic,S., Ostojic,B.: Longitudinal nephrolithotomy in the treatment of stag-horn and multiple calculi. Urologia *32*, 554 (1965)

89. Poutasse,E.F.: Partial nephrectomy: new techniques, approach, operative in-dications and review of 51 cases. J. Urol. *88*, 153 (1962)

90. Power,S.: Note on the technique of partial nephrectomy. Lancet *II*, 1089 (1959)

91. Pryn,W.J.: Blood pressures after nephrec-tomy and partial nephrectomy for cal-culous disease. Lancet *I*, 675 (1960)

92. Puigvert,A., Gittes,R.F.: Partial nephrec-tomy in the solitary kidney. J. Urol. *100*, 238 (1968)

93. Pyrah,L.N.: Three personal cases of partial nephrectomy in solitary kidney. Unpublished observations (1974)

94. Pyrah,L.N., Smiddy,F.G.: Perirenal pseudohydronephrosis: a report of two cases. Br. J. Urol. *25*, 239 (1953)

95. Quist,G., Mahsen,J.J., Al-Waidh,M.: Transperitoneal ureterolithotomy. Br. J. Surg. *50*, 502 (1962)

96. Rathore,A., Harrison,J.H.: Coagulum pyelolithotomy using autogenous plasma and bovine thrombin. J. Urol. *116*, 8 (1976)

97. Redman,J.F., Bissada,N.K.: Extensive nephrolithotomy in previously operated solitary kidneys. J. Urol. *115*, 502 (1976)

98. Rehn,E.: Berl. Klin. Wochenschr. *58*, 1217 (1921)

99. Resnick,M.I. et al.: Symposium on renal lithiasis. Simple and extended pyelolithotomy. Urol. Clin. North Am. *1*, 319 (1974)

100. Rieser,C.: Consideration of ureteral stump subsequent to nephrectomy. J. Urol. *64*, 275 (1950)

101. Roseno,A.: Die Nephrotomie: Ihre Verhütung und ihre Gefahren. Z. Urol. Chir. *20*, 96 (1926)

102. Roth,R.A.: Current surgical management of branched renal calculi. Surg. Clin. North Am. *56*, 753 (1976)

103. Rovinescu,I., Belanger,P.M., Lapalme,R.: New technique for removal of staghorn calculi; the pyelorenal flap. Urol. Int. *231*, 326 (1968)

104. Sandegard,E.: Prognosis of stone in the ureter. Acta Chir. Scand. (Suppl. 219) (1956)

105. Sauls,C.L., Nesbit,R.M.: Pararenal pseudocysts: a report of four cases. J. Urol. *87*, 288 (1962)

106. Semb,C.: Renal tuberculosis and its treatment by partial resection of the kidney. Acta Chir. Scand. *98*, 457 (1949)

107. Semb,C.: Partial resection of the kidney; operative technique. Acta Chir. Scand. *110*, 132 (1955)

108. Stephenson,T.P., Bauer,S., Hargreave, T.B., Warwick,R.T.: The technique and results of pyelocalycotomy for staghorn calculi. Br. J. Urol. *47*, 751 (1975)

109. Snodgrass,W.T., Robinson,M.J.: Internal arteriovenous fistula: a complication of partial nephrectomy. J. Urol. *94*, 135 (1964)

110. Stewart,H.H.: Partial nephrectomy in the treatment of renal calculi. Ann. R. Coll. Surg. Engl. *11*, 32 (1952)

111. Stewart,H.H.: Partial nephrectomy. In: Modern trends in urology. Riches,E.W. (ed.), p. 80. London: Butterworth 1953

112. Stepita,C.T., Newman,H.R.: Empyema of ureteral stump with surgical excision; report of 15 cases. J. Urol. *63*, 500 (1950)

113. Tardo,G.V.: Report of Second and Third Congress of International Society of Urology. Cited by Joly,J.S. (1929). Stone and calculous diseases of the urinary organs. London: Heinemann 1924

114. Turner-Warwick,R.T.: Lower pole pyelocalycotomy, retrograde partial nephrectomy and ureterocalycostomy. Br. J. Urol. *37*, 676 (1965)

115. Twinem,F.P.: The relation of renal stone formation and recurrence to calyceal pathology. J. Urol. *44*, 596 (1940a)

116. Twinem,F.P.: Prevention of recurrent stone formation by calyceal resection. Surg. Clin. North Am. *20*, 299 (1940b)

117. Vest,S.A.: Renal arteriovenous fistula. Urologists' Correspondence Club Lett. 6th December (1954)

118. Wickham,J.E.A., Hanley,H.G., Joekes, A.M.: Regional renal hypothermia. Br. J. Urol. *39*, 727 (1967)

119. Wojewski,A. et al.: The treatment of bilateral staghorn calculi of the kidneys. Int. Urol. Nephrol. *5*, 249 (1974)

120. Zuckerkandl,O.: Ueber Nierenstein. Arch. Klin. Chir. *87*, 481 (1908)

Chapter 14

Special Groups of Cases of Stone and Their Treatment

I. Treatment of Bilateral Renal and Ureteric Calculi

1. Bilateral Renal Calculi

Calculi may occur in both kidneys and one or both ureters simultaneously, or in both kidneys in sequence and often at intervals of some years. If it is decided to remove bilateral renal calculi at two separate operations, the stone in the kidney adjudged to be better functionally should be removed first, the stone in the opposite kidney being removed after a suitable interval. Pain experienced in one kidney may influence the surgeon to operate on that side first. A tiny symptom-free calyceal stone on the contra-lateral (non-painful) side may be left to be voided spontaneously. The problem of operation for large bilateral calyceal and pelvic calculi of approximately equal size has already been touched on.

Medium-sized bilateral non-infected calculi in the renal pelvis (or in a renal pelvis and a contralateral calyx) in young fit adults, judged to need operative removal, can safely be removed at the same operation. Both kidneys are then restored to their normal function at the same time, with the need for only one course of antibiotics and one period of convalescence. If the surgeon is disinclined to do this for any reason (obesity of the patient; previous operation on one kidney; fear of chest complications) two separate operations at an interval of 10–14 days are appropriate. In fit patients with a calculous pyone-phrosis on one side for which nephrectomy is indicated, and an easily removable calculus on the other, both kidneys can still be operated on simultaneously [69, 70].

For the simultaneous operation the patient may be turned first on one side, then on the other and separate lumbar incisions made. Alternatively, he may be placed in the prone position on the operating table (which is broken as desired), the incision being made directly over each twelfth rib, which is resected. Hryntschak [35] reported 15 patients who had bilateral renal stone and were successfully operated on using simultaneous procedures, and he collected 19 other similar cases successfully operated on. Priestley and Schulte [54] reported 5 similar cases.

2. Bilateral Ureteric Calculi

If stones are present at the same time in both ureters, the patient is at risk to develop calculous anuria, so that early surgical removal of both stones is indicated, a procedure which may be done at one operation through appropriate incisions, depending on their positions. If both stones are in the lower third of the ureters, a trans-peritoneal approach or a suprapubic extra-peritoneal approach is suitable.

II. Treatment of Stone in a Solitary Kidney

Stone may present in a solitary kidney either because the contralateral kidney has been previously removed for calculous or other disease or for other reasons, or because there was congenital absence of one kidney, an abnormality which is said to vary from between 1 in 1500 [16] and 1 in 1000 subjects [9]. When one kidney is congenitally absent, the sole functioning kidney is appreciably larger than normal. When one kidney has been removed surgically the other undergoes compensatory hypertrophy. Patients who have had one kidney removed for calculous disease are at risk in respect of further stone formation. The removal of one kidney does not interfere with longevity in patients with renal calculous disease [26].

If a patient has only one remaining kidney and develops renal or ureteric stone, there should be no undue delay in his treatment (unless the stone is small enough for spontaneous voiding to be expected), and lithotomy or partial nephrectomy are well tolerated. The indications for surgical treatment of stone in a solitary kidney include recurrent and persistent pain, associated persistent infection, recurrent or persistent haematuria, which could be attributed to the stone, and calculous anuria from ureteric obstruction. A calculous pyonephrosis in such a kidney, possibly associated with an obstructing ureteric calculus, may have to be treated by simple drainage (nephrostomy) with removal of the ureteric calculus, the renal calculi being dealt with at a later date if the patient is acutely ill; the special difficulties are referred to later in this chapter.

In the series of 5323 patients with urolithiasis from the Massachusetts General Hospital collected by Suby [71], 2798 operations had been done, 343 (6.4%) having had nephrectomy; 8.4% of these required further surgical treatment for calculi in their residual solitary kidney; 55% of those who had had nephrectomy and who now had calculi in the remaining kidney, had had calculi in that kidney before the first kidney was removed, whereas 45% had formed stones in their solitary kidney after the other kidney had been removed.

Goldstein and Goldstein [27] collected a series of 717 patients with acquired and 30 with congenital solitary kidneys, in 92 of whom there was a pathological condition in the solitary kidney; the results of treatment showed that many such patients can survive for long periods. One patient had had his solitary kidney operated on four times. Of the 38 patients treated surgically for stone and other conditions 16 were alive from 1 to 19 years after operation, and 16 were known to have died between 1 and 17 years after operative treatment.

Dzhaudat [19] reported 62 patients seen between 1958 and 1968 with stone in a solitary kidney; of 46 for whom operative treatment was now needed, 38 had had the contralateral kidney removed, while 8 had had congenital absence of one kidney; recurrent stone had usually appeared in the contralateral kidney within 3 years of the nephrectomy.

III. Secondary Operations for Renal and Ureteric Calculi

1. Recurrent Renal Calculi

If it is necessary to remove renal calculi from patients who are known to have previously had one, two, three or more operations (pyelolithotomy, nephrolithotomy or partial nephrectomy) for renal stone, the difficulty of the procedure varies probably in direct proportion to the number of such earlier operations, and to the presence of earlier urinary infection.

Before embarking on the operation the surgeon must ascertain from the radiograph whether the twelfth rib had been removed in whole or in part at an earlier operation. Some of the parietal muscles beneath the earlier wound may have undergone a considerable degree of atrophy or have even been converted into a sheet of fibrofatty tissue, possibly associated with a slight bulge or even a hernia. The intravenous pyelogram may indicate that the kidney has taken up a slightly higher or lower, and a somewhat fixed position consequent upon earlier mobilization.

An incision, longer than that used for a primary operation for the removal of a stone, is usually necessary, the old scars being excised; the twelfth rib should be removed if this had not been done. It is easy for the knife to be carried through the parietes into the renal parenchyma (which is commonly adherent to the undersurface of the scar), unexpected bleeding announcing such an event. The peritoneum, which may have been drawn upwards and outwards in front of the kidney as a result of the earlier operation, may be easily divided. At the upper end of the incision the pleura may be injured more easily than at the primary operation.

The difficulties from then on vary with the nature of the primary operation. While in some cases mobilization is easy, in others it has to be dissected out literally inch by inch with a sharp scalpel or with scissors, by dividing fibrous tissue of varying degrees of toughness, attached especially to the convex border, the posterior surface and the upper and lower poles. Care is needed to avoid injury to the adrenal gland, the renal vessels, the pelvis and ureter and the duodenum.

Pyelolithotomy as a secondary procedure is not usually too difficult if care is taken to expose and mobilize the renal pelvis step by step. Hurried surgery can lead to its being torn. The extent of the adhesions may make the operation of pyelolithotomy in situ the procedure of choice, and a satisfactory radiograph of the exposed kidney may be difficult or impossible to obtain. If mobilization of the kidney and of the renal pedicle has been difficult, the performance of a satisfactory partial nephrectomy with temporary clamping of the renal pedicle may not be easy and may even be contraindicated. Subcapsular rather than extracapsular nephrectomy may be preferable if removal of the kidney is necessary.

2. Recurrent Ureteric Calculi

If a recurrent ureteric stone has become impacted at a point well above the site of the earlier operation, its removal usually presents no special problem. If it has come to rest at the site of the earlier operation on the ureter, removal may be difficult. Following the first ureterolithotomy, the ureter may have taken up a somewhat abnormal position, resulting in some kinking or angulation, which may have contributed to the arrest of the recurrent stone. Because of periureteritis, the ureter may have become adherent to the peritoneum.

If the recurrent stone is located in the upper half of the ureter (where the first stone also was), the usual extraperitoneal approach for its removal will entail a painstaking dissection through fibrous tissue. Exposure of the ureter for the removal of a stone at or just below the brim of the pelvis by the usual extraperitoneal route, because of the presence of fibrous tissue, will most likely result in the opening of the peritoneal cavity with possibly some prolapse of intestine and even the risk of injury to an iliac artery or vein. A transperitoneal operation for the removal of recurrent ureteric calculi at or below the iliac vessels could therefore be the method of choice, by way of a suprapubic mid-line incision extending to the umbilicus. The rectus sheath is divided and the rectus muscles separated.

The peritoneum will probably be found to be adherent to the underlying muscles. After packing off the intestine with swabs, an incision is made through the peritoneum on the posterior wall of the abdomen in the position where the ureter (and the stone) is expected to be, a procedure which may be easy if there is no retroperitoneal fat. Flaps of the peritoneum on either side of the incision are raised until the ureter comes into view, when it can be followed downwards in front of and below the iliac vessels to a level below that of the stone, which is then removed. The peritoneum is then repaired by a continuous suture. Ideally an extraperitoneal rubber drain should be provided, though if this is impossible because of adhesions, transperitoneal drainage should be provided.

IV. Recurrence of Calcium-Containing Stone in the Upper Urinary Tract After Operation

1. True and False Recurrence

'True recurrence' refers to a new stone in the kidney formed at a later date following operation, when it has been shown by radiography of the exposed kidney that all the original calculi have been removed during the operation. The promoting or associated causes of the stone formation (infection being important) still persist.

'False recurrence' refers to those calculi whose maturation has been dependent upon the presence in the kidney of small fragments of the original calculus removed at operation or of tiny concrements or small calculi which were present at the operation and which (for one reason or another) were not removed, and which with the passage of time have enlarged to form once again a definitive recognizable calculus. An example of the latter group would be the leaving behind of a tiny calyceal calculus during the operation of pyelolithotomy, for which many surgeons would have carried out a simultaneous partial nephrectomy. The term 'residual calculus' may be more appropriate to describe such calculi.

In the context of practical urology the operation for the removal of a stone (or its spontaneous voiding) may be regarded as a base-line for the study of the incidence of recurrent calculus in the affected kidney. Calculi very frequently appear (often at a later date) in the contralateral kidney. The rates of recurrence in series published before 1937 seem to show figures which are unrealistically low compared with those which would have emerged if a really long-term follow-up had been carried out.

There does not appear to be in the literature of renal calculous disease a complete documentation of the entire life history (including the operative treatment and other incidents) of a large group of calcium-stone-bearing patients. In reality the long-term incidence of recurrent stone formation is high, though many years may elapse before recurrence takes place.

2. Causes of Recurrence

False Recurrence (Pseudo-Recurrence). Calcific particles or actual concretions left behind at the operation.

True Recurrence. 1. Persistence of pre-operative urinary infection or the introduction of a new infection during the operation.

2. Failure to correct or neutralize a metabolic contributory cause after the stone has been removed:

Hypercalciuria
Hyperparathyroidism
Hyperoxaluria
Milk-alkali syndrome
Renal tubular acidosis
Cushing's syndrome
Recumbency
Environmental syndromes (phenacetin addiction; ingestion of silicate)
Prolonged dehydration

3. Failure to correct associated anatomical defects in the kidney or ureter, especially those which lead to obstruction and consequent stasis:

Calyceal stricture or hydrocalycosis
Pelviureteric hydronephrosis
Horseshoe kidney
Certain cysts and cystic conditions of the kidney

Retrocaval ureter
Stricture of the ureter
Ureterocele
Obstruction of the bladder neck

4. Imperfect operative technique.

5. Preference for conservative to 'radical' operative measures in the given case, leading sometimes to the inappropriate selection of the operative procedure.

6. Inadequate after-treatment following operation by such measures as are available.

Infection and Recurrence. In patients in whom calculi have been caused by, or are associated with or complicated by infection (especially by the urea-splitting organisms), or infection introduced into the kidney during operation or allowed to persist during the postoperative period, recurrence is likely to follow unless such infection can be permanently eradicated. The adverse effect of infection is exacerbated if anatomical defects in the kidney remain uncorrected. Chronic urinary infection was present in 49 of 212 (18%) cases in which stone recurred after operation in our departmental series. The incidence of stone in infected cases in some other series is given in Table 14.1.

Metabolic Abnormalities. Some abnormalities (hyperparathyroidism, Cushing's disease, idiopathic hypercalciuria etc.) may remain uncorrected after operative treatment of the stone by such methods as are available; even though they act very slowly or almost imperceptibly, they make the recurrence after surgical removal very likely.

Anatomical Abnormalities or Deformities. Such deformities of the kidney or ureter (or of the bladder neck) as interfere with the free normal downward drainage of urine from the pelvis-calyx system (if allowed to remain uncorrected) are contributory

Table 14.1. Incidence of recurrence of stone in relation to urinary infection

Author	Recurrence rate in patients with infected urine
Brongersma, 1924 / Oppenheimer, 1937	33%–35%
Hellstrom, 1949	46%
Sutherland, 1954	64%
Williams, 1963	31%

causes of recurrent stone formation. It follows that any operation for the removal of a renal stone is incomplete if such abnormalities remain uncorrected, or if any error of technique encourages ultimate stasis of urine (calyceal obstruction; permanently induced angulation of the pelviureteric junction after the kidney has been replaced in the loin after operation).

Surgical Technique. The various operations and their indications for the removal of renal calculi have been described earlier, but in the context of the question of recurrence of stone following operation, the need for careful technique, gentleness, precise attention to detail in the performance of the operation, and the choice of operation can be re-emphasized.

Recurrence of stone after operation takes place in some patients for whom no obvious cause can be determined and for whom therefore no remedial measures are as yet available. The incidence of recurrence of stone in kidneys submitted to various operative techniques for their removal, and also the incidence of 'recurrence' in the contralateral kidney can best be described by the experiences from the author's department.

3. Incidence of Recurrence in the Author's Series

An investigation was carried out in the author's department of 538 patients (male,

358; female, 180) who had had treatment for stone in the upper urinary tract between 1951 and 1961 and who were followed up for a minimum period of 10 years (and many for as long as 20 years), in order to ascertain the rate of recurrence of stone in the affected kidney after various operations, and also recurrence in the contralateral kidney, which had not been operated upon. The results were reported by Williams [78], whose paper gives more details than can be recorded here. When those who had voided the stone spontaneously and those who had had instrumental treatment were excluded, a total of 554 operations had been carried out during the period under review. Some patients had had more than one operation either on the same kidney or for the relief of recurrent stone in the opposite kidney.

Time of the First Recurrence. In 399 patients with recurrent calculi the time interval was known which had elapsed between the onset of clinical symptoms (or diagnosis) of the first stone and the onset of symptoms (or diagnosis) of the first recurrence (the stone being voided spontaneously, removed by a second operation or diagnosed radiologically), either ipsilateral or contralateral. Single-stone-formers (who did not have recurrent calculi) numbering 129 were excluded. The first recurrence of stone had occurred in less than 1 year in 54 patients (14%) of whom 37 had bilateral calculi on their first attendance.

It was between 1 and 4 years in 114 patients (28%), and in many patients up to and even beyond 20 years after the initial stone. The average time interval before recurrence was 9.5 years. In 42% recurrence occurred in less than 5 years, whereas in 20% the interval was 15 years or more. No significant difference was found in the time of recurrence between those patients in whom the first stone was passed spontaneously and those in whom it was removed by operation. The first recurrent stone was found on the same side of the

Table 14.2. The time interval between the initial stone and the first recurrence in 399 patients from the author's department

Time interval (years)	No. of patients
Less than 1	54
1–4	114
5–9	73
10–14	77
15–19	47
20–24	24
Over 25	10
Total	399

urinary tract as the initial calculus (ipsilateral) in 58%, and on the opposite side (contralateral) in 28%. Bilateral calculi were present when the patient was first seen in 12% (insufficient information being available in 8%), and if to this figure are added patients with a contralateral first recurrence (28%) at their first attendance it was found that 40% of patients then had stones on both sides of the urinary tract.

The time interval between operation and recurrence in a series reported by Braasch [6] was 2 years. In the series of staphylococcal calculi reported by Hellstrom [31] half the calculi had recurred within 1 year. In a series of 357 cases Baker and Connelly [3] found that the likelihood of recurrence following the spontaneous passage or removal of a stone was about 9%, that it usually occurred in 3–5 years and was infrequent after 8 years (Table 14.2).

Incidence of Postoperative Recurrence. Data recording the incidence of recurrence following conservative operations was available in 398 of 554 performed; 60% of the patients had developed a second stone, either ipsilateral or contralateral, which was voided spontaneously, removed surgically or demonstrated radiologically. A calculus present in the contralateral kidney or ureter at the time of the operation and subsequently voided spontaneously or removed

Table 14.3. The incidence of postoperative recurrence in the author's series

Operation	No. of patients	Average period of follow-up (years)	No. of patients with recurrence	Average period of time before recurrence observed (years)	No. of years before recurrence was observed		
					Less than 5 years Percentage	5–9 years	10 years or more
Nephrolithotomy	133	14.9	92 (69%)	7.1	54	28	28
Pyelolithotomy	117	11.8	66 (56%)	5.6	50	27	23
Ureterolithotomy	148	9.5	81 (55%)	5.9	63	17	18
Total	398						

Table 14.4. Previous investigations of postoperative recurrences

Author	Year	No. re-examined	Percentage recurrence following:			Average duration of follow-up (years)
			nephro-lithotomy	pyelo-lithotomy	uretero-lithotomy	
Cabot and Crabtree	1915	87	56	51	29	
Brongersma	1924	100	36	24		5 (minimum)
Twinem	1937	115	28 (ipsilateral)	21		
Oppenheimer	1937	141	59	24		4
Pyrah (various surgeons)	1954	156	60	35	21	5–20
Sutherland	1954	240	63	47	37	8.4

by operation was not counted as a recurrence. Fifty percent of patients who had nephrolithotomy, 30% who had pyelolithotomy and 20% of those who had ureterolithotomy were followed up for 15 years or more. It was only by following up patients for periods longer than 10 years that the true figure of recurrence was revealed (Table 14.3).

Other Series of Cases. The high recurrence rate reported in the present survey is comparable with that in long-term surveys reported by Oppenheimer [47] and by Sutherland [72], and in the earlier series collected by the author [55]. Other observers have reported lower figures for recurrence of stones probably with a shorter period of follow-up. Following a survey of urolithiasis by questionnaire in the United States, Burkland and Rosenburg [10] reported an average rate of recurrence of 14% (Table 14.4).

Immediate Results of Conservative Operations. The incidence of true ipsilateral recurrence following a given operation was calculated in the author's series after ascertaining the number of cases in which the ipsilateral upper urinary tract was proved by radiography to be free from calculi (that is to say, excluding residual calculi). It was shown that all ipsilateral calculi had been removed in 80%–84% of conservative operations. Residual calculi had usually been left by design rather than by accident; for example, following the operation of ureterolithotomy residual calculi were pre-

Table 14.5. True ipsilateral recurrence following conservative operation in the author's series

Operation	Total no. of patients	Immediate result after operation		Late results after operation	
		Ipsilateral kidney or ureter		True ipsilateral recurrence of cases known to be free from calculi after operation	Average interval of time before recurrence (years)
		Free from calculi	Residual calculi present		
Nephrolithotomy	121	97 (80%)	24 (20%)	49 (50%)	10.9
Pyelolithotomy	116	97 (84%)	19 (16%)	42 (43%)	7.7
Ureterolithotomy	133	110 (83%)	23 (17%)	37 (33%)	6.4
Partial nephrectomy	47			7 (15%)	3.1

Table 14.6. The late outcome of residual postoperative calculi

Operation	No.	Passed spontaneously	Operative removal	Position unchanged
Nephrolithotomy	24	7	13	4
Pyelolithotomy	19	7	5	7
Ureterolithotomy	23	4	13	6
Total	66	18 (27%)	31 (47%)	17 (26%)

sent in the corresponding kidney in 17% of cases not having been removed when the ureteric calculus was removed. The true ipsilateral recurrence rates were: 50% following nephrolithotomy; 43% following pyelolithotomy; 33% following ureterolithotomy; and 15% following partial nephrectomy (Table 14.5). The operation of partial nephrectomy is, of course, an attempt at a radical removal of the stone-bearing portion of the kidney; Stewart [68] reported a recurrence rate of 7.9% in a series of 139 cases of partial nephrectomy.

Residual Postoperative Calculi. Some calculi genuinely thought to be true recurrences in the ipsilateral urinary tract may really be false recurrences; such residual calculi are usually small and are situated at a place remote from the site of operation. The ultimate fate of these stones is of interest. Of 66 residual calculi in the series

investigated, which had not been removed by conservative surgery, 18 (27%) were voided spontaneously at a later date. The 49 calculi voided spontaneously or removed surgically represented an incidence of 13% false recurrences after 370 conservative operations; and if calculi demonstrated radiologically were included the incidence rose to 18% (Table 14.6).

In Oppenheimer's [47] series of 141 conservative operations 32 of 55 recurrences were due to residual calculi. In 51 kidney-splitting operations on 50 patients reported by Petrovic and Ostojic [51], of whom 38 were followed up, 3 had residual stones and 12 had recurrent stones. Recurrent stone was discussed by Wojewski [79] and by Shieber [63].

Contralateral Recurrence of Renal Stone. Following the operative removal of a renal stone (or when nephrectomy has been

Table 14.7. A. Contralateral recurrence following conservative and radical operations in a series of patients from the author's department

Original operation	Total no. of patients	True contralateral recurrence	Average interval before recurrence in years
Nephrolithotomy	121	39 (32%)	11.5
Pyelolithotomy	134	31 (23%)	8.8
Ureterolithotomy	116	32 (28%)	7.2
Partial nephrectomy	47	16 (34%)	3.1
Nephrectomy	101	34 (34%)	7.7
Total	519	152 (29.3%)	

B. Contralateral recurrence following nephrectomy in some reported series

Author	Year	Cases	Incidence (%)
Hellstrom	1933		11.0
Cahill	1935	128	34.0
		(These were cases of calculous anuria for which earlier nephrectomy in one kidney had been done)	
Oppenheimer	1937	169	15.0
Sutherland	1954	240	11.0
Civino and Gallivanone	1960	54	5.5

done), a calculus may appear in the opposite kidney (revealed by clinical symptoms, spontaneous voiding or radiography) a few months or many years later. Such a calculus is strictly a new clinical event rather than a complication of the first operation (though it emphasizes the general metabolic rather than the local character of so many cases of renal calculus). For the record it is convenient to designate such a stone in the opposite kidney as a true contralateral recurrence. The incidence is much higher than has been previously thought. In Table 14.7 the incidence of contralateral recurrence is shown; the presence of a calculus in the opposite kidney at the time of the first operation has been disregarded, only newly diagnosed contralateral calculi being included.

A true contralateral recurrence followed 152 (29.3%) of 519 operations. The time interval between the first operation and the observed contralateral recurrence was usually between 7 and 11.5 years. With a longer period of follow-up the percentage incidence of contralateral recurrence could well have been considerably higher. The incidence of contralateral recurrence after nephrectomy was 34%, which was almost the same as that following the operations of partial nephrectomy and nephrolithotomy.

The figures are of practical importance to the urologist, who often has to decide whether or not to remove the original stone-bearing kidney. The knowledge that the incidence of contralateral recurrence is high provides an argument for inclining towards conservative rather than radical surgery upon the first kidney if such a course is reasonable.

Recurrence of Ureteric Stone. Since ureteric stones originate in the kidney and not in the ureter, recurrence of ureteric stone depends usually upon the development and migration of a new stone in the kidney or upon the migration of renal stones known to exist. If a ureteric stone has been removed by operation, any associated renal stone should generally speaking also be removed, either at the same time or soon afterwards to prevent such a complication.

Unabsorbable sutures of silk or linen thread, which may easily penetrate the mucosa of the ureter, should not be used for its repair following ureterolithotomy, since they may eventually penetrate into the lumen of the ureter and form the nucleus of a further stone. The author has operated at least twice for recurrent ureteric caculi, the stones having come down from the kidney, and having lodged at the point of the earlier ureterolithotomy.

V. Serious Cases of Renal Calculous Disease

In the majority of cases, renal calculous disease pursues a relatively benign course through life; many patients void only one single stone, many are successfully operated on for the removal of calculi and even recurrent stones may be clinically benign. In a small number of patients whose calculi have not been successfully dealt with surgically, or who have themselves ignored the escalating clinical manifestations of advancing disease (or merely by chance) urgent symptoms ultimately appear either gradually or suddenly, constituting a threat to life from ultimate renal failure. These grave cases can be considered in two groups: those with advanced infective calculous disease either bilaterally or in a solitary kidney; and those associated with calculous anuria.

1. Renal Failure from Advanced Calculous Disease with Pyelonephritis

In this group some patients have often had more than one operation for the removal of calculi, both kidneys (or the solitary kid-

ney) having suffered some parenchymal damage with consequent impairment of renal function from large *B. proteus*-infected calcium-containing staghorn stones. Such patients may be approaching a critically low point of renal function.

Renal Function. The chief function of the kidney is the excretory function, whereby the excess of the waste products of metabolism (of which urea and creatinine are examples) is eliminated in order to maintain a relatively stable level of these substances in the blood. An elevated level of the blood urea or a depression of the urea clearance is indicative of some degree of renal excretory failure. The clinical expression of the failure of the excretory mechanism is uraemia.

The maintenance of homeostasis is the other chief function of the kidney, whereby the electrolyte balance of the blood is stabilized. The renal tubules absorb or excrete (at varying times) only as much of each of the electrolytes as is necessary to maintain the extra-cellular fluid in balance with respect to each important substance by modifying the fluid presented to them by way of the glomerular filtrate.

With a normal intake of food, a greater amount of fixed acid than of fixed base is produced by the metabolic processes of the body. In order to maintain the pH of the blood at about 7.4, the renal tubules by exchanging hydrogen ions for sodium ions, excrete an excess of anions over cations, thereby lowering the urinary pH; the renal tubules also form ammonia with which the anions can be excreted without accompanying fixed base (sodium and potassium), thereby conserving base.

The biochemical expression of the homeostatic renal failure is usually an acid-base imbalance (most typically an acidosis), a depletion of base (sodium, potassium or both), and, in the course of time, osteomalacia [5]. The clinical expression is renal failure, which is ultimately fatal. In some patients with severe bilateral renal calculous disease (and sometimes following the sudden relief of urinary obstruction) the kidneys may not be able to prevent very large amounts of electrolytes and water being poured out into the urine; serious clinical symptoms may then follow.

Among patients in this group with advanced calculous disease, some who would seem to be in a clinically hopeless condition live on even in the absence of treatment in a moderate grade of health, and many (after treatment) may even follow gainful employment for a long time, perhaps with periods of ill-health, always provided that a critical renal obstruction does not suddenly appear, so great, it would seem, is the potential functional reserve of renal tissue in the body.

Other patients, if untreated, move slowly and almost imperceptibly to a fatal renal failure gradually reaching a stage of poor health after many years with the characteristic clinical symptoms of renal failure (indifferent appetite, nausea, frontal headache, lassitude, some shortness of breath resulting from anaemia and an inability to do even light work). Even in such patients the quality of life may be improved and its duration prolonged for months or years by the use of conservative measures (adequate treatment of the urinary infection, correction of electrolyte imbalance and of the under-nutrition). An operation to remove obstructing calculi may be thought to be worthwhile and may be life-saving and life-prolonging.

Life may be terminated following a subacute renal episode or by an extrarenal disorder such as coronary thrombosis. Other patients, having been apparently well for a long time, move more or less suddenly to a potentially fatal crisis of unilateral ureteric obstruction (perhaps with calculous anuria), which may take the urologist unawares, because the patient has only a few days before been working and leading a relatively normal life.

Even if only one of the two badly functioning kidneys is blocked by a ureteric stone in such a patient and urine continues to be voided, not only will a calculous pyonephrosis probably develop in that kidney, but the slender margin of renal function needed to maintain life will have become still more eroded; the desirability of an urgent operation to remove the obstructing calculus has then to be considered.

Treatment. A patient presenting with such advanced bilateral renal calculous disease and with actual or impending grave renal failure must be urgently assessed, by examination of the urine (for the degree of infection), the blood urea, electrolytes, haemoglobin and by radiography.

The defects, some or all of which are present in such patients, and which must be recognized and corrected as far as possible if the patient is to survive, or even to be rendered moderately fit to withstand operative removal of his obstructing stones, are the following: (1) the urinary infection; (2) the grossly impaired renal excretory mechanism; (3) the electrolyte imbalance resulting from impaired renal homeostasis, including the possible presence of sodium-losing nephropathy; (4) anaemia; (5) under-nutrition resulting from prolonged failure of appetite. When these defects have been assessed and countered as far as possible there must also be considered: (6) the possible place of haemodialysis in his treatment; (7) the possibility of operative removal of calculi. Illustrative cases have been reported by the author [56], and by Pierce [52] and Camey [15] (Fig. 14.1).

Urinary Infection. The urinary infection in such patients is often resistant to medical treatment and is exacerbated by the obstructive element resulting from the presence of calculi. The amount of pus voided daily in the urine is a guide as to the gravity of the condition; the *B. proteus* and *Ps. pyocyaneus* and other urea-splitting

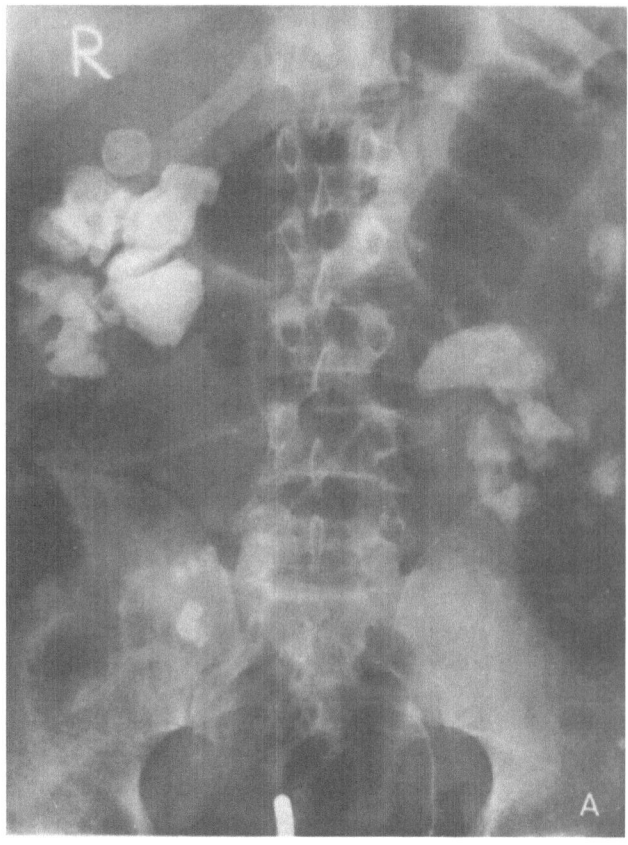

Fig. 14.1. Patient (G.H.W., male, aged 52). In 1953 he had huge bilateral renal calculi, the urine being infected with B. Proteus. An attack of left-sided renal colic, followed by persistent pain and elevated temperature (calculous pyonephrosis) was caused by a stone in the lower ureter (*A*). The ureteric stone was removed by operation and the pyonephrosis drained, as many stones as possible being removed. For 4 days postoperation his clinical condition was good. On 4th night he became mentally incoherent, his clinical condition deteriorated and he seemed likely to die from uraemia. Measures to correct the sodium deficit and the acidosis were taken (sodium lactate + sodium chloride + glucose i.v.). After 3 days his condition improved, he made a satisfactory recovery and was able to work for 4 years. The cause of the crisis on 4th day was postoperative diuresis following the sudden release of the ureteric obstruction which resulted in a net loss of body water, sodium and other electrolytes. **A.** Massive bilateral infective renal calculi in the pelvis and calyces of both kidneys, with a stone in the lower third of the left ureter (confirmed by passage of ureteric catheter), which was responsible for the crisis described above. **B.** Chart showing blood electrolyte levels and urine output commencing 5 days after the operation on the left kidney and ureter during and after the urgent crisis

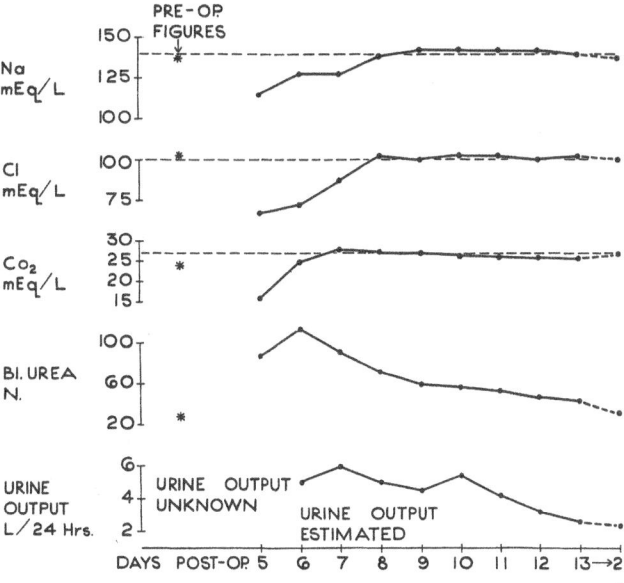

organisms (the most common ones to be encountered) should be treated by any antibiotic shown to be antagonistic to them (except streptomycin), though sulphonamides can hardly be used unless they can be adequately excreted through badly functioning kidneys. A developing pyonephrosis in such a patient increases the clinical severity of the illness and renders more urgent the need for a drainage operation to evacuate pus and calculi from the kidney.

Impairment of the Renal Excretory and Homeostatic Mechanism with Electrolyte Imbalance and Loss of Base. The blood urea level is usually gradually elevated, and during a crisis may be raised very much above normal. The protein dietary intake during the crisis period must be greatly reduced.

Electrolyte imbalance must be recognized and corrected. An acidosis (shown by the elevated serum chloride level and the reduced CO_2-combining power) should be treated by alkalis by mouth or in urgent cases by the intravenous infusion of sodium lactate together with sodium chloride in suitable proportions.

A severe sodium depletion resulting from a high urinary excretion of sodium in the urine is usually shown by a subnormal serum sodium level, and there is dehydration from heavy loss of water in the urine, the kidneys being unable to correct this by the normal reabsorption of water through the distal tubules. Clinically such a patient may have a dry, wrinkled skin with loss of its normal turgor, and sometimes impaired cerebration; sodium lactate should be given intravenously.

In a normal subject if the intake of sodium is high there will be a high sodium excretion, while if the intake of sodium is minimal or nil, he will excrete in the urine almost no sodium. If the oral intake of sodium falls below the quantity lost in the urine, sodium depletion follows: if the intake of sodium in the diet (equivalent to 10 mEq sodium/24 h) for 12 h prior to and during a 24-h collection of urine to measure the urinary sodium excretion, a base-line of sodium loss can be established.

If a timed collection of urine for several hours under conditions of sodium depletion and sodium restriction reveals a urinary excretion of over 100 mEq sodium (calculated on a 24-h basis) a severe sodium-losing state is present [52]. Examples of a severe sodium depletion have been reported in patients with renal tuberculosis [59], prostatic obstruction (Parsons, case 4 [48]), bilateral renal calculi and chronic pyelonephritis [52], chronic glomerulonephritis [40] and polycystic kidney.

Rapid loss of sodium may develop in a few days; there is a tendency to polyuria. If unrecognized the condition may lead to rapid sodium depletion, uraemia and death and in a patient who has to have (or has had) a severe operation, for example, for the removal of large staghorn calculi in patients with bilateral calculi, its presence untreated is almost a prescription for a fatality. In other patients in whom the syndrome of severe sodium depletion has been fully developed, clinical symptoms include loss of appetite followed by vomiting, which chiefly leads to further extrarenal depletion of salt and water thereby exacerbating the trouble still further. In a patient in whom severe loss of sodium has been detected the differential diagnosis of the cause lies between a sodium-losing nephropathy and an acute adrenal insufficiency [73].

The serum potassium level may be higher or lower than normal. If there is excessive urinary loss of potassium there may be weakness or paralysis of the muscles of the limbs, slurred speech, drowsiness and in the later stages paralytic ileus and heart failure. In some patients there is a dangerous retention of potassium manifested by elevation of the plasma potassium levels to 7.0 mEq/litre or higher, which may need to be corrected by the use of resins or in other ways.

Anaemia. Anaemia, which is common in patients with chronic renal failure including those with renal calculous disease, usually results from toxic action on the blood-forming centres in the bone marrow. It should be corrected as far as possible by intermittent blood transfusion (packed cells preferred) to render the patient fit for any operation thought to be necessary.

Undernutrition inevitably accompanies the period of grave illness when the patient will be unable to take solid food but may be able to accept fluids orally; in considering the diet it is necessary to suppress protein catabolism to the minimum and to reduce protein anabolism. Because of possible gastrointestinal upset following anaesthesia during the operative phase of treatment, the use of up to 2.5 litres of 20% or even 40% glucose solution (which helps to suppress protein catabolism) administered through a polythene tube inserted through the basilic vein and passed upwards into the great veins in the upper part of the chest, has been found useful, rapid dilution of the irritant glucose taking place. During convalescence protein can be gradually introduced into the diet during the period of recovery.

Haemodialysis and Peritoneal Dialysis. These measures have helped to provide a greater margin of safety before and/or after operation in some ill patients with advanced calculous disease, and in some cases have been life-saving. In the author's department valuable early experience in the use of haemodialysis was obtained in some patients with renal failure from long-standing prostatic obstruction and uraemia, and some of the beneficial results have been reported [21].

During a 10-year period (1957–1966) 83 patients with uraemia from severe obstruction of the upper urinary tract, in 10 of whom renal or ureteric calculus was the cause, were treated by haemodialysis [50]

or by peritoneal dialysis [21]. A second or third haemodialysis can be carried out during the early postoperative period if it seems to be indicated. A more rapid correction of the biochemical abnormalities is usually achieved by haemodialysis (which is especially appropriate for the severely infected cases) than by peritoneal dialysis; the table gives details of some patients with calculi in the author's department who have been treated by dialysis [49] (Table 14.8, see p. 306).

Removal of Calculi. Having achieved as great a degree of clinical improvement as possible in these serious cases the urologist has to consider whether an attempt to remove the calculi, first on one side, then on the other, is worthwhile. In considering whether to operate, the size and the number of the calculi and the practicability of their removal are relevant matters.

In many patients with large, bilateral staghorn stones in badly infected and damaged kidneys, or with massive stones in a solitary infected kidney, with grave impairment of renal function, the consensus of opinion in the past has often been against operation, not only because of the operative difficulties and risks but because early and rapid recurrence of the stones could be expected. The infection could probably not be finally brought under control and a possible further deterioration of renal function may result from the operative trauma.

In recent years, however, there has been a greater degree of success in operations upon these severe cases than in earlier years, though a return to completely normal risk-free health can hardly be expected. In a small group of patients with bilateral calculi, a crisis of considerable urgency may arise if a stone migrates into and becomes impacted in a ureter, leading to at least an obstruction of the kidney and at worst a resulting calculous oliguria or anuria, thereby posing the problem of urgent treatment. Such a patient will prob-

Table 14.8. Patients from the department with advanced renal calculous disease treated by dialysis before operation, (by courtesy of F. M. Parsons)

Case no.	Age	Sex	Blood urea on admission (mg/100 ml)	Dialysis Days after referral	H, haemodialysis P, peritoneal dialysis	Type of operation	Days after admission	Weeks in hospital	Blood urea on discharge (mg/100 ml)	Period of survival after operation
1	58	M	220	14 + 21	H	Nephrolithotomy	23	6.5	138	7 years
2	50	M	334	1	H	Nephrolithotomy and nephrostomy	3	6.5	73	
3	64	M	292	1	H	Nephrostomy	2	Died (pneumonia)		5 years
4	27	M	433	0 + 2	H	Pyelolithotomy	3	1		4 months
5	65	M	336	0.4 + 10	H	Pyelolithotomy and nephrostomy	1	Died (pneumonia)		13 months
6	55	F	279	0.2, 4, 11	H	Nephrolithotomy	6	Died		15 days
7	47	F	300	2	P	Ureterolithotomy	3	5	55	8 months
8	34	F	468	1	H	Ureterolithotomy	25	4	30	4.5 years
9	59	M	309	0	H			5.5	67	7 years
10	33	M	333	2, 4, 5	H	Exploration of ureter	6	6.5	37	5 years

ably have developed a pyonephrosis with pain, fever and an acute exacerbation of his illness, and an operation at least to remove the ureteric stone and to drain the kidney will probably be called for.

2. Calculous Anuria

A detailed consideration of the subject of anuria resulting from the many different pathological conditions which can give rise to it, is beyond the scope of this book but it is appropriate to enumerate briefly the broad division of its causes, since they come into the differential diagnosis of calculous anuria, one of the more serious complications of renal lithiasis.

Among a large series of patients with anuria referred to the author's department for haemodialysis we found that many who were believed to have anuria resulting from renal or even prerenal causes were in fact examples of undiagnosed obstructive (and sometimes of calculous) anuria.

Varieties of Anuria. Anuria or the total suppression of urine may be prerenal, renal or postrenal.

'Prerenal anuria' usually results from a fall in blood pressure following, for example, shock complicating trauma resulting either from multiple fractures or from a prolonged operation on the heart, lungs, major blood vessels or abdomen, involving considerable loss of blood. The renal glomerular pressure, as a consequence of which plasma filtrate passes through Bowman's capsule, is about 30–40 mm below the normal arterial pressure and is, therefore, about 90 mm Hg. Unless the glomerular vascular pressure exceeds that amount, filtration of plasma will not take place and anuria results.

'Renal anuria' may be the result of chronic glomerulonephritis. It may be a sequel to conditions such as poisoning by mercuric chloride (corrosive sublimate), which leads to such damage to the renal epithelium as will render it temporarily or sometimes permanently incapable of excreting urine.

'Postrenal anuria' is an obstructive condition usually resulting from pathological conditions within the renal passages and especially in the lumen of the ureter (stone; tumour; foreign body); or from conditions outside the ureter (pressure upon it resulting from malignant glands or growth such as advanced carcinoma of the uterine cervix); or from conditions involving the wall of the ureter (intrinsic ureteric growth or stricture; accidental ligature of the ureter at operation). In order that any of these conditions (including obstructive uropathies) may give rise to anuria, the suppression of urine must be bilateral, except in those patients who have only one kidney.

Calculous anuria may occur under the following conditions:

1. Obstruction of both kidneys or ureters by stone simultaneously (or in very close sequence).

2. Obstruction of a solitary functioning kidney by stone, the other kidney being congenitally absent, or having been previously removed.

3. Obstruction of one kidney or ureter by stone, the opposite kidney being the seat of advanced disease and its function being 'reflexly' suppressed.

The obstructing calculus in the ureter is usually fairly small. The commonest site of obstruction is in the upper third of the ureter though occasionally at the pelviureteric junction.

Apropos of reflex suppression of the function of the diseased kidney opposite to the one which is obstructed, Joly [36] referred to two cases (reported by Cabot and Ransahoff [13]) of calculous anuria in which a nephrostomy had been previously performed on one diseased kidney. When the opposite ureter became obstructed by a calculus, urine ceased to flow from the nephrostomy tube and only began to flow again after the obstructing stone had been removed. An alternative explanation for supposed reflex anuria could be a fall of the systemic blood pressure when the ureter of the better kidney is obstructed, resulting (as a consequence) in a prerenal anuria of the opposite badly functioning kidney. The kidney obstructed by a calculus so severely as to result in anuria becomes congested and somewhat enlarged. The renal pelvis may be distended with urine, though in some cases the urine within the renal pelvis does not seem to be under pressure, as if it had never been formed in the renal parenchyma under such circumstances. Thus Joly [36] found that when the obstructed kidney in a patient with calculous anuria was exposed at operation the renal pelvis sometimes contained little or no urine and was not distended.

Clinical Features. The patient who develops calculous anuria is usually known to have had recent clinical symptoms, previous operations for stone followed by recurrence, and perhaps long-standing precarious health because of advanced calculous disease. A patient with a solitary kidney, however, may develop obstructive anuria resulting from a renal stone which has recently migrated, and which had not given rise to earlier symptoms. A few patients have experienced discomfort over the affected kidney for some days before the crisis; a few have had polyuria for a short time [36].

The onset of the phase of anuria is usually sudden, and is ushered in by an attack of renal colic following which no urine is voided. Being unaware of the causes of the symptoms the patient may attempt to micturate but has neither the urge nor the capacity to do so. In some patients small amounts of blood-stained urine are voided for a short time after the attack of colic has subsided. In a few patients such oliguria is followed by short periods of relative polyuria, to be followed by absolute anuria. Occasionally the onset of the anuria is painless, the patient simply observing that he is voiding no urine; it is then difficult to decide which diseased kidney is responsible for the final blockage, and indeed both kidneys are then probably the seat of advanced disease.

For a variable number of days after the onset of the anuria there may be few further clinical symptoms of any kind. The patient does not feel ill though he is aware of the disability; during this period of tolerance, as it has been called, which usually lasts 5, 6 or 7 days and even up to 16 days, but sometimes for a much shorter time, the patient may be active and may continue to take food and liquids with an unimpaired appetite. There is no mental impairment.

The blood urea now rises rapidly to 250 mg in 3 or 4 days, in spite of the absence of clinical symptoms. Serious symptoms (being the non-specific symptoms of uraemia from any cause) now begin to appear during the period of intoxication, which gradually follows the period of tolerance. The mouth becomes dry, there is progressive thirst, the appetite disappears though there is a desire for water, hiccup is common; the bowels are constipated and the abdomen gradually becomes distended. Nausea followed by vomiting, which may be profuse, usually comes towards the end. Headache, lethargy, picking of the bed clothes, drowsiness, apathy, listlessness and inability to take food precede a gradual passage into a semicoma which may be preceded by a state of mental confusion. The breathing is slow and stertorous, and there may be terminal Cheyne–Stokes breathing; convulsions are rare. The pulse rate, which at first is slow or normal, becomes rapid towards the end. The blood urea by now may have risen to between 400 and 500 mg/100 ml or even higher.

Death follows within 2 or 3 days of the onset of the terminal stage. The majority of cases, if untreated, end fatally 10 days or so after the onset of anuria. In some cases the anuria passes off a few days after the attack of colic, presumably because urine has started to seep past the stone in the ureter, and the clinical symptoms subside as the flow of urine is re-established.

The existence of a state of anuria, presumed to exist from the history, must be confirmed by the passage of a catheter in order to exclude the more common condition of retention of urine, which is nearly always painful. When the catheter is passed either no urine at all, or only 1–2 oz blood-stained urine (which may contain pus cells) may be withdrawn. On abdominal palpation there is no distension of the bladder. The kidney on the affected side may be tender and slightly enlarged on palpation.

Diagnosis. The cause of the anuria has then to be determined and the diagnosis of calculous anuria (as well as the diagnosis of the side which is obstructed) has to be differentiated from the many other causes of obstructive anuria. Prerenal or renal anuria as the cause of the trouble can usually be excluded by a consideration of the patient's history. The extrarenal obstructive causes of urinary suppression include pressure on the ureter from masses of glands (simple or malignant) in the pelvis or abdomen, periureteric fibrosis, abdominal and especially uterine (cervical) cancer, and cancer of the bladder. The history will be helpful in the diagnosis of most of these conditions, though the diagnosis of periureteric fibrosis can only be made after investigation.

The commonest examples of calculous anuria in the author's experience are those in which one functioning kidney has become blocked by a calculus, the much reduced function of the opposite diseased kidney being reflexly suppressed. The obstructed side is that on which pain has first been experienced. Cases in which there is a simultaneous blockage of both ureters from calculi, both kidneys being functional, are rare.

In patients with calculous anuria the characteristic shadows of renal calculi and/or shadows in the line of the ureter, presumed to be ureteric calculi, will usually be demonstrable by radiography. In the case of uric acid calculi no shadows appear in the plain radiograph. A recent case in a gouty subject with only one kidney and a non-radio-opaque uric acid stone at the ureterovesical orifice has also been seen by the author. Intravenous pyelography cannot usually be attempted with much hope of success in patients with a rapidly rising blood urea, though in an early case of obstruction the intravenous urogram may demonstrate a dilated renal pelvis and ureter down to the level of the stone.

If a ureteric stone is present, cystoscopy may reveal redness, congestion, oedema and haemorrhages round the orifice of the ureter on the affected side. Usually there is no efflux though a small amount of blood-stained urine may be voided from it. Such a ureteric orifice is motionless though if there is a stone impacted a little distance above the surface, frequent contractions at the orifice may be observed. A ureteric calculus may occasionally be seen presenting at the orifice.

Usually it is necessary to pass a catheter up the ureter to determine the precise site of the obstruction and also in order to confirm by radiography the existence of a calculus. When this has been established, every effort should be made by using catheters of various sizes if necessary, to negotiate the tip of the catheter past the stone, when blood-stained urine escapes first in drops but gradually in a continuous stream (since it is usually under pressure) from the catheter. If radiography has shown the existence of a calculus in only one ureter, the surgeon must conclude either that the patient has only one solitary kidney or that the second kidney is so badly diseased that its function has been reflexly suppressed. It is usually desirable to try to assess the condition of the opposite kidney (if one be present) by passing a catheter up the opposite ureter and recovering urine if any be present. In the case of a congenitally absent opposite kidney, there may be no ureteric orifice and a badly developed trigone on that side.

A pelvic growth (the other common cause of extrarenal obstruction) usually arising in the cervix uteri and extending into the broad ligament and the pelvic cellular tissues, is the commonest cause of obstructive anuria from external pressure on the ureter and can be diagnosed on vaginal and pelvic examination. There has usually been a history of vaginal bleeding, or a previous hysterectomy or radiotherapy.

Carcinoma of the bladder in the terminal stages (a frequent cause of obstructive anuria) may obstruct both ureters, and can be diagnosed from the clinical history of recurrent haematuria, pain and frequency, from rectal and pelvic examination and from the early radiological and cystoscopic findings and history of earlier treatment. Compression of the ureter by bilateral periureteric fibrosis is usually diagnosed by showing the existence of obstruction of both ureters (usually in the middle third) by ureteric catheterization and pyelography. If a ureteric catheter can be passed beyond the obstruction on one or both sides the existence of a hydronephrosis and hydroureter can be demonstrated.

The diagnosis of the cause of the anuria may not be easy in those rare instances in which the onset has been painless or relatively so, but the principles of investigation outlined above apply here also.

Treatment. The role of the ureteric catheter in the diagnosis and treatment of calculous anuria has been referred to. If a catheter is negotiated past the obstruction (which may be sensed by the surgeon as he passes the catheter) it should be left in position for several hours or even 1–2 days; clinical improvement may be expected. If for any reason (such as blockage) the catheter has

to be withdrawn, urine may flow down the ureter and the acute incident may have passed. Probably the catheter should not be allowed to remain in situ in such patients for longer than 48–72 h before undertaking the definitive procedure to remove the obstruction. Occasionally the stone is voided after the catheter has been withdrawn, in which case operation may be deferred or may not be needed.

If a ureteric catheter cannot be passed to the renal pelvis, operation must be undertaken as an emergency, to relieve or remove the obstruction and to ensure free drainage of urine. If there is a staghorn calculus (and the patient is in poor condition) the meticulous removal of all the stones should be deferred and a simple drainage operation done, perhaps removing the most accessible calculi. There should be clear evidence at the operation from the presence of dilatation of the renal pelvis and/or the ureter on the operated side, that there has really been a calculous obstruction. If there is doubt (as there may be in the case of bilateral calculi), the opposite kidney should be explored and drained by nephrostomy or pyelostomy; the test of a successful operation is the abundant drainage of urine, followed by rapid improvement in the clinical condition and by a fall in the level of the blood urea.

If the patient is in good condition, for example, during the first 2 or 3 days of anuria, and the ureteric stone is easily accessible in a sparely built subject, the stone may be removed as a primary procedure. If there is any doubt concerning the presence of additional but inaccessible stones in the urinary tract, it may be desirable to drain the kidney also (nephrostomy). If the patient is in poor condition or if the cause of the obstruction is difficult to deal with surgically (because of obesity or because of earlier operations near the site of obstruction), a simple drainage of the kidney by a nephrostomy or pyelostomy may be done.

After operation the patient should be given intravenous 5% glucose and oral fluids as soon as possible, no protein food being given until the blood urea has been seen to be falling. While calculous anuria is essentially a surgical emergency all the available measures suitable for the management of serious cases (referred to earlier) to enable the patient to recover must be employed, including haemodialysis if thought necessary. When the patient has recovered from the emergency, the decision for the permanent relief of the calculous abnormality in the urinary tract must be made after due deliberation.

3. Symptomatic Relief for Patients with Rapidly Recurring Calculi

Replacement of the Ureter by Ileum. In some patients with bilateral staghorn calculi who also have multiple small calcium-containing or 'matrix' calculi in the dilated calyces of one hydronephrotic kidney, the function of the opposite kidney being either subnormal or totally absent, incidents of ureteric or pelviureteric obstruction resulting from the migration of calculi, grit or fibrinous debris (with or without temporary anuria) may provide a recurrently dangerous situation. Repeated direct surgical interference upon such a kidney may be badly tolerated.

In such patients reasonably satisfactory downward drainage of urine and also voiding of newly formed small calculi or grit, with a reduction in the severity of colicky pains, can be achieved by replacing the ureter with an isolated loop of ileum to link the renal pelvis or the lowest calyx to the bladder. Such isolated loops of ileum have been used in recent years to remodel the urinary tract in order to relieve a contracted bladder (ileocystoplasty) or to replace a part or a whole of the ureter (pyelonephrovesical anastomosis; ureteroileoneocystostomy), or as a conduit to drain urine to the surface following total cystectomy (ureteroileostomy).

The operation of ileal replacement in the present context is carried out through a long paramedian abdominal incision. An isolated loop of terminal ileum, sufficiently long to bridge the gap between the renal pelvis and the bladder without tension (the blood supply of the loop being carefully preserved), is prepared and continuity of the intestine is restored usually by an end-to-end anastomosis; the kidney and the renal pelvis are exposed in the loin and any calculi are removed before proceeding to make the anastomosis.

In some recorded cases, renal calculi may have been removed at an earlier operation, a permanent nephrostomy having been established, an inconvenience which itself would justify an attempt to obtain satisfactory closed urinary drainage by another method. Through the abdominal approach, mobilization of the renal pelvis or alternatively of an enlarged dilated lower renal calyx (perhaps after removing some of the overlying renal parenchyma) is then completed. The upper end of the loop of ileum is anastomosed by two rows of sutures to the renal pelvis (or calyx) and its lower end similarly to the postero-superior aspect of the bladder. The operation can be done so that the ileal loop lies within the peritoneal cavity, but it is best if possible to arrange that the two anastomoses lie extraperitoneally.

Replacement of part or the whole of a damaged or diseased ureter by an isolated segment of ileum has been carried out with good results by many surgeons for various diseases [2, 28, 29, 45]. In five patients with renal calculous disease Wells [77] successfully replaced the ureter with an isolated, isoperistaltic loop of ileum, following which stones were voided readily from the kidney to the bladder, whence they could be extracted if they did not pass spontaneously; symptoms were relieved and renal function seems to have been preserved.

VI. Treatment of Infection in the Calculous Urinary Tract

Treatment of urinary infection in patients with calculi in the upper urinary tract may be needed before operation (in order to minimize complications), and also during and after the period of operation. If the operative removal of the stone has been followed by infection such treatment, monitored by adequate follow-up, is necessary if recurrent stone formation is to be prevented. Patients for whom an indwelling temporary drainage tube has had to be placed in the kidney or the renal pelvis (nephrostomy or pyelostomy) carry the risk of having infection introduced; so do those patients who need an indwelling urethral catheter during the course of operative treatment upon the kidney (for unexpected acute urinary retention, or during the relief of unexpected postoperative haematuria). A closed urinary drainage system and suitable urinary antiseptics are essential for such patients.

Drugs which are used for the treatment of infections in the urinary tract should preferably be bactericidal and not merely bacteriostatic; they should have a low grade of toxicity especially if it is intended to use them for a long period of time and in patients with poor renal function. Following excretion by the kidney (the mode of which varies considerably among the different agents), their urinary concentration should be high enough to achieve the objective of destroying the micro-organisms.

Combinations of more than one urinary antiseptic, sulphonamide or antibiotic, acting perhaps synergistically if suitable combinations can be found, selected under the guidance of an interested bacteriologist, are more likely to assist in achieving a sterile urine than a more empirical approach.

Hexamine. This was first introduced into medicine, in 1900, by Nicolaier and Hagenburg [46] and was for many years the only drug capable of destroying bacteria in the urine [24] and it acts in virtue of the liberation by hydrolysis of formaldehyde (at appropriate strength) in acid urine of about pH 6. It is not effective for the treatment of urinary infection by the urea-splitting organisms, when the urine is alkaline; it still has a place in the treatment of organisms resistant to antibiotics.

Mandelic Acid. The use of mandelic acid followed the use of the ketogenic diet which was troublesome to organize and, to many patients, unpalatable. It is bactericidal, it passes into the urine through the kidney unchanged and it is rendered more efficacious in the presence of a low urinary pH, so that its value is enhanced when administered with ammonium chloride to achieve its maximal efficiency. Most organisms are susceptible to it except the urea-splitting organisms. Mandelic acid and hexamine are joined together as a chemical compound in mandelamine, which can render urine bactericidal and which also liberates formaldehyde.

Sulphonamides. The sulphonamides are usually able to deal effectively with infection due to *E. coli*. They are bacteriostatic and are excreted almost entirely by way of the kidney so that high urinary concentrations can be achieved. They are more active in an alkaline medium. The acetylated fraction, which varies with each drug, is inactive. Garrod and O'Grady [24] considered that there is little to choose between most of the sulphonamides as regards their antibacterial activity, an assessment which included sulphathiazole, sulphadimidine, sulphafurazole, sulphamethoxazole [41] and sulphamethizole [23].

Sulphonamides, which are rapidly excreted, produce the highest concentrations in the urine, while those which are more slowly excreted, including the long-acting sulphonamides such as sulphamethoxypyridazine, achieve levels of concentration which are higher in the tissues than in the urine, and may therefore be more suitable for the treatment of pyelonephritis than of infections in the lower urinary tract.

For the treatment of an acute urinary infection, the use of sulphadimidine or sulphafurazole (2 g initially, and 1 g 6-hourly), together with trimethoprim (100 g 6-hourly) for 7 days is appropriate [24]. When therapy fails it may be found that the original organism has become resistant to the therapeutic agent used, or that a species of organism has now appeared which is different from that which was originally isolated. Alternatively, the therapeutic agent may fail to reach the site of the infection, or the reaction of the organism in vivo to the agent may be different from that in vitro.

Nitrofurantoin (furadantin) is excreted in the urine and attains concentrations which render it bactericidal for most organisms, especially if the pH is on the acid side of neutrality; its beneficial effect is reduced at a urinary pH 8 or over. It has been found useful for coliform as well as *B. proteus* infection [67]; it is given in a total daily dose not exceeding 600 mg. There have been a few reports of anaphylaxis following its use.

Nalidixic Acid. This is used chiefly for the treatment of the gram-negative organisms, the gram-positive organisms being relatively resistant to it. The drug is easily absorbed from the gut and about 80% of the administered dose is rapidly excreted in the urine, partly unchanged and partly as derivatives, some of which are anti-bacterially active [24].

Antibiotics. Penicillin, streptomycin, poly-myxin, neomycin, kanamycin and ampi-cillin are bactericidal antibiotics. The pH of the medium in which they act is of importance. Thus, kanamycin, neomycin and streptomycin are respectively 16, 64 and 412-fold more active at pH 8.5 than 5.5 [24], so that alkalinization of the urine is necessary when they are administered.

Penicillin, which is excreted by the renal tubules, is indicated for the treatment of coccal infections; some strains of *E. coli* and *B. proteus* are sensitive to it though ampicillin has a greater degree of activity against the two latter organisms. Penicillin can, it seems, be administered orally for an indefinite period. Scowen et al. [62] reported the case of a boy who, after four operations for the removal of renal calculi, was finally cured of the infection which was responsible for the lithiasis by treatment with penicillin for many months. Streptomycin is excreted into the urine chiefly through the glomeruli [61]. Terramycin may be very valuable for urinary infections.

Other antibiotics which include the tetra-cyclines, chloramphenicol and cycloserine, are bacteriostatic rather than bactericidal but may be valuable in therapy. Chlortetracycline is more active in an acid medium. When chloramphenicol is given 90%–95% of it is excreted in conjugated and antibacterially active forms, so that its efficacy may not always be high; the cocci and *E. coli* are the most susceptible organisms. Cycloserine is excreted almost unchanged in the urine, its action is independent of the urinary pH [24] and it is especially useful for the treatment of acute urinary infections though toxic symptoms sometimes accompany its use.

Novobiocin is active against some strains of *B. proteus* as well as against the cocci but only about 2.5% of the administered dose appears in the urine. If treatment with one therapeutic agent (given as a short intensive course) has not produced a good response in 2 weeks, it is unlikely that the disease will yield to more prolonged such treatment. Some infections are caused by organisms which seem to be completely resistant to treatment by almost any drug or antibiotic.

VII. Medical Treatment of Calcium Phosphate-Containing Calculi

1. Aluminium Hydroxide

Calculi composed entirely or partly of calcium phosphate (providing the urinary tract is non-infected or relatively so), can sometimes be caused to go into solution wholly or partly or to disintegrate, by the use of orally administered aluminium hydroxide.

Shorr was the first to use the principle of the dietary restriction of phosphorus for the treatment of phosphatic renal calculi [64, 65]. He showed that the dietary phosphorus could be approximately balanced by giving orally an appropriate amount of aluminium gel, so that most of the phosphorus remained in an insoluble condition in the alimentary tract (forming insoluble aluminium phosphate), with a corresponding reduction in the urinary phosphorus.

A diet consisting of approximately 700 mg calcium and 1300 mg phosphorus daily was given, and 30–50 ml Basaljel (containing aluminium hydroxide) four times daily taken after meals. The urinary phosphorus level fell from an average of 1000 mg to less than 200 mg daily. In 19 patients with unilateral or bilateral renal stone treated on a phosphate-restricted diet and given the aluminium preparation, the calculi disappeared from two kidneys and became smaller in three [65]. The dietary regime is tedious and conducive to constipation, which may be countered by the daily administration of magnesia. It can be used with safety in patients with grossly impaired renal function, when it may bring about a reduction in the plasma phosphate level. It is not effective in patients with calculi composed predominantly of calcium oxalate, though partial success has been achieved in some patients with mixed calcium oxalate–calcium phosphate calculi; frequent radiological checks on the size of the calculi are desirable.

The treatment has to be used with care over a given period, since the failure to absorb sufficient phosphate from the gut for the needs of the body can have deleterious metabolic effects in the long term. Nutritional deficiencies in the rat resulting from a dietary deprivation of phosphorus had appeared earlier and in more severe form when aluminium was added to the diet [39]. Other workers [7, 18] showed that if aluminium, iron or beryllium were incorporated in the diet of rats in excess of its phosphorus content, the serum phosphorus level fell by 15%, the bone lost 30% of its ash and the animals developed rickets. Jones [37] showed that this kind of rickets resisted treatment with vitamin D and called the condition 'metal rickets'.

Freeman and Freeman [22] showed that when aluminium hydroxide was given orally (together with a low phosphorus diet) to children with chronic renal insufficiency there was a fall in the level of the urinary phosphate and in the level of the plasma phosphorus from 13.0 to 4.0 mg/100 ml. Vermeulen et al. [75, 76], using their experimental technique for the formation of vesical calculi round foreign bodies in rats, found that the use of Basaljel (aluminium hydroxide) reduced the incidence of calculus formation.

The value of the aluminium hydroxide therapy for the treatment of advanced renal phosphatic calculous disease was reported in a series of papers by Marshall and his coworkers from 1952 onwards. They showed the great value of the treatment if done with meticulous supervision in co-operative patients and their papers should be consulted for details [38, 42–44, 66]. In a group of 18 patients the aluminium treatment was instituted (to prevent recurrence) following extensive nephrolithotomies for staghorn phosphatic stones, a very exacting test of the aluminium treatment. In 14 patients who were followed up for periods of 1–7 years (average 3 years) no new stones had formed, nor were residual calculi shown to have increased in size (when checked by radiography), provided that the patient had adhered to the programme. The recurrence rate following such operations without the help of the aluminium treatment could be expected to have been between 30% and 70% [42, 43, 66].

In a review of 5842 of their departmental patients with urinary calculi of any type or at any site seen between 1940 and 1960, there were 725 patients whose calculi were shown on chemical examination to contain phosphate in more than trace amounts [38]. In 167 of 266 patients who had followed the dietary aluminium regimen strictly, there was a recurrent stone in only 8 (4%) reviewed for an average period of 3.5 years; in 99 who had adhered to the regimen only partially, stones had re-formed in 13 (13.1%) during a similar period of follow-up. Of 417 who had not adhered to the aluminium regime and who were followed up for an average period of 4 years, stones had reformed in 114 (27.3%). In 214 of the 70% of patients with infected urine, 272 in number (usually *B. proteus* and *E. coli*), who adhered to the regimen only 21 (7.8%) developed a recurrent stone having an average follow-up period of 4 years; while 82 (30.1%) of the 272 who did not accept the regimen developed a recurrence during a similar period. Satisfactory results from the use of aluminium compounds were reported by other observers [4, 20, 60].

In the author's department a series of 27 patients with renal calculi (6 having infected urine) were given carefully supervised treatment on the aluminium regime, mostly with Hyalgel for an 11-month period [58]. Before treatment was instituted these patients had had 61 operations for stone and 39 stones had been voided by them, 9 had had 3 or more operations and 1 had had 10. When treatment was begun 6 of the 27 patients, and 26 of their 50 kidneys, were free from stones; follow-up showed that the 26 kidneys which had been free from stone when treatment was begun were

still stone free, although 18 had either had stones previously removed by operation (15 cases) or stones had been voided spontaneously from them (3 cases). In 9 of these kidneys more than one operation for stone had been performed. Although a stone had increased in size in 1 patient, and in another a new stone had appeared, each of these incidents occurred during a period of inadequate control when it was known that the urinary phosphorus was at a high level. In 1 patient with multiple bilateral stones, the largest stone had diminished considerably in size though its neighbours had remained unaltered; in no case did an existing stone disappear completely (Fig. 14.2).

The available evidence supports the claims of Shorr [64, 65] as to the value of the aluminium treatment for the prevention of recurrence of phosphatic calculi. Treatment should be started immediately after the surgical removal of stones which have been shown to be composed mostly of calcium phosphate. The existence of hypercalciuria (which is more often associated with the calcium oxalate calculi than with those predominantly of phosphatic composition) may be one cause of failure. The use of antibiotics for intractable urinary infection, when given in association with the Shorr regime, may not always give the expected results: thus Albert and Reis [1] showed that chlortetracycline becomes firmly bound to the aluminium hydroxide in the gut if the two are given together by mouth, so that no effective antiseptic action can be expected from the use of that antibiotic under such circumstances.

2. Acidogenic Diet and Ammonium Chloride

Since calcium phosphate passes into solution in an acid medium, continuous acidification of the urine by the administration of ammonium chloride and/or an acid-ash

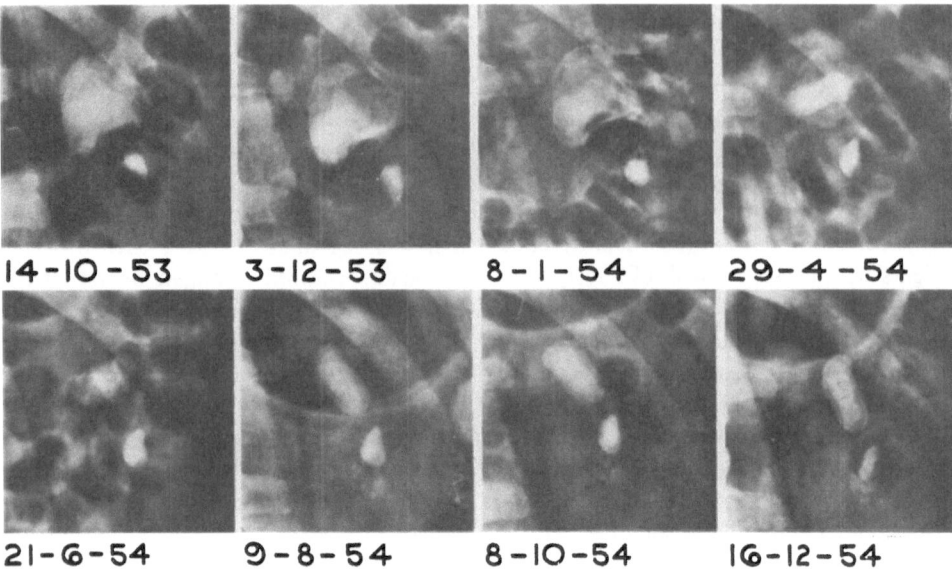

14-10-53   3-12-53   8-1-54   29-4-54

21-6-54   9-8-54   8-10-54   16-12-54

Fig. 14.2. A case of multiple calculi in the left kidney treated with a long course of aluminium hydroxide: the patient (J.O., female aged 37), who was referred on account of bilateral renal pain, was shown on radiography to have bilateral renal calculi, the urine being infected with *E. coli*. A stone impacted in the upper end of the right ureter (the kidney being hydronephrotic) was removed by pyelolithotomy in December 1953. For the treatment of the stones in the *left* kidney, which were laminated and therefore probably had a considerable content of phosphate, at least in the outer part of the stone, aluminium hydroxide was administered (Aludrox, 60 cc 4-hourly). Successive radiographs during a period of 12 months showed a diminution in size of the stones from that in January 1954, when treatment was started, until December 1954. The size of the large stone was reduced by about two-thirds of its content, but there was a cylindrical hard core which did not seem to change. A second stone became more compact and the peripheral part of the shadow became less dense. In May 1956, because of recurrent attacks of infection, a left lower-polar partial nephrectomy was done to remove the residual calculi. The stone after removal showed as expected a granular whewellite interior surrounded by a thin layer of apatite mixed with whewellite

diet has been used to cause phosphatic renal calculi (and also the calcific deposits found in phosphatic encrustation in the bladder) to disintegrate and to go into solution.

Higgins [33, 34] advocated the use of a planned acidogenic diet (with a high vitamin A content) designed to maintain the urinary pH between 5.2 and 5.4 in order to prevent the recurrence of phosphatic calculi (see Chap. 4); details of the diet are given in Higgins' papers. In patients with a urinary infection resulting from urea-splitting organisms (for example, *B. proteus*) attempts to acidify the urine by dietary or medicinal methods will probably fail to reduce the urinary pH to the desired level.

An acidogenic diet (with or without ammonium chloride) may be hazardous if renal function is markedly impaired, since its use may lead to an undesirable acidosis. The author [57] has used the method of induced acidification of the urine in appropriate patients to cause some calculi to go into solution (Chap. 4). When ammonium chloride is used to acidify the urine it should be given in doses of 30 grains, 4 or 6-hourly during the 24 h for periods of 3–6 weeks, though higher doses can be tolerated by some patients. The urine should be tested with litmus paper to ensure that acidification has been achieved.

VIII. Earlier Non-surgical Measures

Oestrogen, hyaluronidase and acetyl salycylic acid, which were in use a few years ago are probably no longer administered; for the details of these methods of treatment the original papers should be consulted [11, 53, 64].

References

1. Albert,A., Reis,C.: Incompatibility of aluminium hydroxide and certain antibiotics. Br. Med. J. *II*, 1028 (1955)
2. Askari,J.A., Moralles,P.A., Hotchkiss, R.S.: Replacement of ureter by ileal segment. J. Urol. *91*, 654 (1964)
3. Baker,R., Connelly,S.P.: Bilateral and recurrent renal calculi: evidence indicating renal collagen abnormality and results of salicylate therapy. J. Am. Med. Assoc. *160*, 1106 (1956)
4. Barrett,G.S.: Influence of aluminium gels on prevention of urinary calculi. J. Urol. *66*, 315 (1951)
5. Black,D.A.K.: Discussion on electrolyte imbalance in urology. Proc. R. Soc. Med. *47*, 582 (1954)
6. Braasch,W.F.: Clinical data on nephrolithiasis. Surg. Gynecol. Obstet. *24*, 8 (1917)
7. Brannion,H.D., Guyatt,B.L., Kay,H.D.: Beryllium rickets. J. Biol. Chem. *92*, 11 (1931)
8. Brongersma,H.: Rep. Sec. Int. Soc. Urol. Congr. *1*, 351 (1924). Quoted by Joly,J.S., 1929. Stone and calculous disease of the urinary organs. London: Heinemann
9. Burford,C.E., Burford,E.H.: Congenital solitary kidney. South Med. J. *48*, 934 (1955)
10. Burkland,C.E., Rosenburg,M.: Survey of urolithiasis in the United States. J. Urol. *73*, 198 (1955)
11. Butt,A.J.: The role of protective urinary colloids in prevention of renal lithiasis. J. Urol. *67*, 450 (1952)
12. Cabot,H., Crabtree,E.G: Frequency of recurrence of stone in the kidney after operation. Surg. Gynecol. Obstet. *21*, 223 (1915)
13. Cabot,Ransahoff: Quoted by Joly,J.S.

(1929). Stone and calculous disease of the urinary organs. London: Heinemann
14. Cahill,G.F.: Medical and surgical treatment of calculous anuria. J. Am. Med. Assoc. *104*, 1306 (1935)
15. Camey,M.: Chirurgie de la lithiase au cours de l'insuffisance renale chronique. Ann. Urol. *3*, 25 (1969)
16. Campbell,M.F.: Congenital unilateral absence of one kidney. Unilateral renal agenesis. Ann. Surg. *88*, 1039 (1928)
17. Civino,A., Gallivanone,A.: Recurrent renal stone on the non-operated side. Arch. Ital. Urol. *33*, 13 (1960)
18. Cox,G.J., Dodds,M.L., Wigman,R.B., Murphy,F.J.: Effects of high doses of aluminium and iron on phosphorus metabolism. J. Biol. Chem. *92*, 11 (1931)
19. Dzhaudat,R.: Stone formation in the solitary kidney: indications for surgical intervention and its results. Urol. Nephrol. *4*, 15 (1969)
20. Elliott,J.S.: Spontaneous dissolution of renal calculi. J. Urol. *72*, 331 (1954)
21. Fox,M., Parsons,F.M.: Value of dialysis in obstructive lesions of the upper urinary tract. Br. J. Urol. *41*, 197 (1964)
22. Freeman,S., Freeman,W.M.C.: Phosphorus retention in children with chronic renal insufficiency: the effect of diet and of the ingestion of aluminium hydroxide. Am. J. Dis. Child. *61*, 981 (1941)
23. Garrod,L.P.: R. Coll. Phys. Edinburgh. Publication No. 11 (1959)
24. Garrod,L.P., O'Grady,F.: Antibiotic and Chemotherapy, 2nd ed. Edinburgh and London: Livingstone 1968
25. Garvey,F.K., Boyce,W.H.: Diagnostic and therapeutic problems incident to surgical treatment of 'malignant' renal calculous disease. J. Int. Coll. Surg. *25*, 310 (1956)
26. Goldstein,A.E.: Longevity following nephrectomy. J. Urol. *76*, 31 (1956)
27. Goldstein,A.E., Goldstein,R.B.: Management of the diseased solitary kidney. J. Urol. *90*, 361 (1968)
28. Goodhard,T.E., Abbott,W.L., Abbott,A.C., MacDougall,J.T., Anderson,E.N.: The use of an isolated ileal loop for total replacement of the ureter. Can. J. Surg. *3*, 25 (1959)
29. Goodwin,W.E., Winter,C.C., Turner,R.D.: Replacement of ureter by small intestine: clinical application and results of ileal ureter. J. Urol. *81*, 406 (1959)
30. Hellstrom,J.: Recurrence of renal and

ureteral calculi after operation. Z. Urol. Chir. *37*, 83 (1933)

31. Hellstrom,J.: The significance of staphylococci in the development and treatment of renal and ureteral stones. Br. J. Urol. *10*, 348 (1938)

32. Hellstrom,J.: Origin, growth and spontaneous elimination of kidney calculi; etiological and therapeutic experiences concerning kidney and ureteric stones. Br. J. Urol. *21*, 9 (1949)

33. Higgins,C.C.: Present status of dietary regimes in the treatment of urinary calculi. Br. J. Urol. *9*, 36 (1937)

34. Higgins,C.C.: Renal lithiasis. Springfield, Ill.: C.C. Thomas 1943

35. Hryntschak,T.: Operative treatment of bilateral nephrolithiasis. Surg. Gynecol. Obstet. *58*, 103 (1934)

36. Joly,J.S.: Stone and calculous disease of the urinary organs. London: Heinemann 1929

37. Jones,J.H.: Metabolism of calcium and phosphorus as influenced by addition to diet of salts of metals which form insoluble phosphates. Am. J. Physiol. *124*, 230 (1938)

38. Lavengood,R.W., Marshall,V.F.: The prevention of urinary phosphatic calculi by the Shorr regimen. J. Urol. *108*, 368 (1971)

39. Leary,J.T., Sheib,S.H.: The effect of the ingestion of aluminium upon the growth of the young. J. Am. Chem. Soc. *39*, 1066 (1917)

40. Levere,A.H., Wesson,L.G.Jr.: Salt-losing nephritis: review and report of a case. N. Engl. J. Med. *255*, 373 (1956)

41. Linton,A.L., Chatfield,W.R.: A clinical trial of sulphamethoxazole on pyelonephritis with simplified methods of assessment. Br. J. Urol. *37*, 515 (1965)

42. Marshall,V.F.: The Shorr regimen for the prevention of urinary calculi of the phosphatic type. In: Treatment of urinary lithiasis. Butt,A.J. (ed.), p. 333. Springfield, Ill.: Thomas 1956

43. Marshall,V.F., Green,J.L.: Aluminium gels with constant phosphorus intake for the control of renal phosphatic calculi. J. Urol. *67*, 611 (1952)

44. Marshall,V.F., Lavengood,R.W., Kelly,D.: Complete longitudinal nephrolithotomy and the Shorr regime in the management of staghorn calculi. Ann. Surg. *162*, 366 (1965)

45. Morales,P.A., Askari,S., Hotchkiss,R.S.: Ileal replacement of the ureter. J. Urol. *82*, 304 (1959)

46. Nicolaier,A., Hagenburg,J.: Über Chinotropin (Chinasaures Urotropin), insbes. über den Einfluss desselben und ander. Hippusäurebildner auf die Harnsäureausscheidung. Zentralb. Stoffw. Verdaungskr. Göttingen *1*, 131 (1900)

47. Oppenheimer,G.D.: Nephrectomy versus conservative operation in unilateral calculous disease of the upper urinary tract. Surg. Gynecol. Obstet. *65*, 829 (1937)

48. Parsons,F.M.: Chemical imbalance in chronic prostatic obstruction: a preliminary survey. Br. J. Urol. *26*, 7 (1954)

49. Parsons,F.M.: Pers. comm. (1972)

50. Parsons,F.M., Hobson,S.M., Blagg,C.R., McCracken,B.H.: Optimum time for dialysis in acute renal failure: description and value of an improved dialysis with large surface area. Lancet *I*, 129 (1961)

51. Petrovic,S., Ostojic, G.: Longitudinal nephrolithotomy in the treatment of staghorn and multiple calculi. Urologia *32*, 554 (1965)

52. Pierce,J.M.: Sodium losing nephropathy in the urological patient: presentation of a case associated with renal calculus disease; differential diagnosis and therapy. J. Urol. *81*, 609 (1959)

53. Prien,E.L., Walker,B.S.: Studies in urolithiasis. IV. Urinary glucuronosides and calcium phosphate. J. Urol. *74*, 440 (1955)

54. Priestley,J.T., Schulte,T.L.: Simultaneous bilateral operation for renal and ureteric calculi. J. Urol. *47*, 255 (1942)

55. Pyrah,L.N.: Recurrent renal stone. Br. Med. J. *II*, 963 (1954a)

56. Pyrah,L.N.: Discussion on electrolyte imbalance in urology. Proc. R. Soc. Med. *47*, 586 (1954b)

57. Pyrah,L.N., Fowweather,F.S.: Urinary calculi developing in recumbent patients. Br. J. Surg. *26*, 101 (1938)

58. Pyrah,L.N., Raper,F.P., Smith,I.B.: The use of aluminium hydroxide to prevent recurrent renal calculi. Br. J. Urol. *28*, 231 (1956)

59. Rapoport,S., West,D.C., Brodsky,W.A.: Salt-losing condition: renal defect in tuberculous meningitis. J. Lab. Clin. Med. *37*, 552 (1951)

60. Satterthwaite,R.W.: In discussion on: Aluminium gels with constant phosphorus intake for control of renal phosphatic calculi. J. Urol. *67*, 611 (1952)

61. Satterthwaite,R.W., White,T.I.: Streptomycin in treatment of pyelonephritis, inter-

stitial cystitis, urethritis and tuberculosis of the genito-urinary tract. J. Urol. *60*, 678 (1948)

62. Scowen,E.F., Badenoch,A.W., Shooter, R.A.: Control of recurrent urinary calculus due to infection: report of case. Br. J. Urol. *29*, 140 (1957)

63. Shieber,W.: The need for adequate work-up in recurrent renal calculi. Surgery *78*, 126 (1975)

64. Shorr,E.: The possible usefulness of estrogens and aluminium hydroxide gels in the management of renal stone. J. Urol. *53*, 507 (1945)

65. Shorr,E., Carter,A.C.: Aluminium gels in the management of renal phosphatic calculi. J. Am. Med. Assoc. *144*, 1549 (1950)

66. Spellman,R.M., Marshall,V.P.: Aluminium gel dietary prophylaxis after extensive nephrolithotomy. J. Urol. *73*, 660 (1955)

67. Stewart,B.L., Rowe,H.J.: Nitrofurantoin (furadantin) in treatment of urinary tract infections. J. Am. Med. Assoc. *160*, 1221 (1936)

68. Stewart,H.H.: Calcification and calculus formation in the upper urinary tract. Br. J. Urol. *27*, 352 (1955)

69. Streenevasan,G.: The management of bilateral renal and ureteric calculi. Br. J. Urol. *42*, 736 (1970)

70. Streenevasan,G.: Bilateral renal calculi.

Ann. R. Coll. Surg. Engl. *55*, 13 (1974)

71. Suby,H.I.: Calculous disease in a single kidney. J. Urol. *81*, 369 (1959)

72. Sutherland,J.W.: Recurrence following operations for upper urinary tract stone. Br. J. Urol. *26*, 22 (1954)

73. Thorn,G.W., Koepf,G.F., Clinton,M.Jr.: Renal failure simulating adrenal cortical insufficiency. N. Eng. J. Med. *240*, 210 (1949)

74. Twinem,F.H.: Recurrence after operations for nephrolithiasis. J. Urol. *37*, 259 (1937)

75. Vermeulen,C.W., Grove,W.J., Goetz,R., Raggins,H.D., Correll,N.O.: Experimental lithiasis. I. Development of calculi upon foreign bodies introduced into bladders of rats. J. Urol. *64*, 541 (1950)

76. Vermeulen,C.W., Goetz,R., Ragins,E.D., Grove,W.J.: Experimental urolithiasis. IV. Prevention of magnesium ammonium phosphate calculi by reducing the magnesium intake or by feeding aluminium gel. J. Urol. *66*, 6 (1951)

77. Wells,C.: The use of the intestine in urology: omitting ureterocolic anastomosis. Br. J. Urol. *28*, 335 (1962)

78. Williams,R.E.: Long-term survey of 538 patients with upper urinary tract stone. Br. J. Urol. *35*, 416 (1963)

79. Wojewski,A.: On recurrences after surgical removal of renal calculi. Int. Urol. Nephrol. *6*, 53 (1974)

Chapter 15

Uric Acid Calculi

Uric acid is an end-product of purine metabolism. In most mammals the sparingly soluble uric acid is converted into the much more soluble compound allantoin by the action of the enzyme uricase. The first stage in purine biosynthesis is the formation of ribofuranosylamine-5-phosphate from 5 phosphoribosyl-1-pyrophosphate, a reaction which is catalyzed by the enzyme phosphoribosylamino-transferase [28]. This irreversible step possibly determines the site of action of a feed-back control mechanism which enables the end-products (adenine and guanine ribonucleotides) to regulate the rate of their own production. Possibly some cases of primary hyperuricaemia and gout may result from a defect in this self-regulating mechanism.

The first complete purine to be produced endogenously in the human body is inosinic acid; the basic precursors of the purine ring include glycine, formate, aspartic acid, glutamine and carbon dioxide. Purine bases are also supplied to the body exogenously, some of which are degraded to form part of the urinary uric acid [53, 58]. There is a direct route of conversion of inosinic acid to xanthine by way of xanthylic acid and xanthosine, or by way of guanylic acid and guanosine, or by way of hypoxanthine. These routes provide metabolic pathways by which any inosinic acid synthesized in excess of the body's requirements can be metabolized to xanthine and then to uric acid. The enzyme which catalyses the oxidation of hypoxanthine to xanthine and of xanthine to uric acid is xanthine oxidase, the chemical details of which are given by Watts [54].

Urine must be supersaturated with uric acid for uric acid calculi to form, and hyperuricosuria and a reduced urinary pH are the principal factors helping to create such a condition; hyperuricosuria, however, is not always found in patients with uric acid stone. In explanation of the low urinary pH, a reduction in the urinary excretion of ammonium has been suggested, though not all observers are agreed on this [25]. Gutman and Yü [36], using isotope techniques in gouty and normal patients, found evidence which suggested that in gouty patients there was a defect in the mechanism (possibly glutaminase) by which glutamine normally produces ammonia, which would reduce the urinary pH. This view has not, however, been accepted by other observers, some of whom have suggested decreased urinary excretion of ammonia to be normal in some elderly people.

The various enzyme reactions and abnormalities which can lead to the overproduction of uric acid in the body (and hence to hyperuricosuria) have been reviewed by Seegmiller [49] and by de Vries and Sperling [20]. Hyperuricaemia must result either from an increased rate of synthesis of uric acid or from a diminished rate of excretion (which could result from impairment of renal function).

An excessive synthesis of uric acid takes place in primary gout and in the myeloproliferative diseases, which can give rise to secondary gout. Since much of the daily production of uric acid is destroyed, the urinary uric acid does not represent quantitatively the extent of the purine synthesis. The endogenous urinary uric acid can be estimated by placing the patients on a purine-free diet, when the daily excretion of uric acid can be shown in approximately one-fifth of gouty subjects to be significantly greater than that in normal controls, thus providing evidence of the overproduction of uric acid in these patients. However, most gouty patients excrete an amount of urinary uric acid which is either comparable to or appreciably less than that excreted in normal subjects; some of the uric acid may have been disposed of into tophi.

Using isotopic methods it has been shown that the amount of uric acid which was excreted in 24-h urine ranged from 55% to 76% of the urate turnover, the deficit representing the loss of urate from the body pool by extrarenal pathways [8, 48]. The miscible pool of uric acid in the body is found by injecting isotopic uric acid intravenously, allowing it to mix with the uric acid in the body and doing urinary estimations of uric acid for several days. In a group of normal subjects the miscible pool averaged 1200 mg uric acid with a daily turnover of 695 mg; in gouty subjects the miscible pool reached 2000–4000 mg (or much larger amounts in severe tophaceous gout).

I. Pathology

1. Uric Acid Stone

Physical Characteristics. Uric acid stones voided spontaneously from the kidney are usually less than 1 cm in diameter, are multiple, rounded, ovoid and sometimes faceted, and the tiny ones are equal in size to grains of sand. A medium-sized pyramidal stone may occupy the renal pelvis or a calyx, and the staghorn stones may fill the renal pelvis and several calyces; those in the bladder are usually round or ovoid and often large. The stones usually have a smooth or finely granular surface but may have one or more round bosses. Most stones are hard though some are soft and friable. While the cut section of a small pure uric acid stone is usually homo-

geneous, that of a large stone may show concentric laminae of alternating light and dark colour, derived from the presence of extraneous pigment; alternatively the cut surface may reveal one or more yellowish nuclei composed of uric acid, sometimes surrounded by layers of calcium salts.

The stone may be composed of unoriented uric acid crystals aligned with the margins of the fibres of the matrix [46]. The fracture surface and thin sections of the calculi show radial striation and concentric banding (Fig. 15.1, see p. 322). Cavities may be found in the interior and tunnels occasionally penetrate the stone from end to end. A thin section of a uric acid stone shows the needle-shaped crystals oriented in an orderly radiating fashion.

'Urate' Constituents of Stone. What we call the 'uric acid stone' often contains not only uric acid but also urates and calcium salts. The stone is composed of matrix (about 2.2%–2.3% of the dry weight according to Boyce and King [12]) and crystalloid substances, the following substances being found: pure uric acid in either the anhydrous form or the dihydrate; uric acid with either calcium oxalate, calcium phosphate or magnesium ammonium phosphate or all together; uric acid with either ammonium hydrogen urate or sodium hydrogen urate monohydrate or both, and also with or without calcium salts.

Uric acid ($C_5H_4N_4O_3$) may be present in a calculus as the monoclinic, pseudo-orthorhombic crystals of the anhydrous acid, or as the orthorhombic crystals of uric acid dihydrate.

Ammonium hydrogen urate ($NH_4C_5H_3N_4O_3$) has been found only as an occasional constituent of renal uric acid calculi from western countries; in Lagergren's series [38] it was present in only one renal stone (as a thin layer on the surface of a uric acid calculus). In our own series of 500 cases of urinary calculi (mostly renal) submitted to crystal-

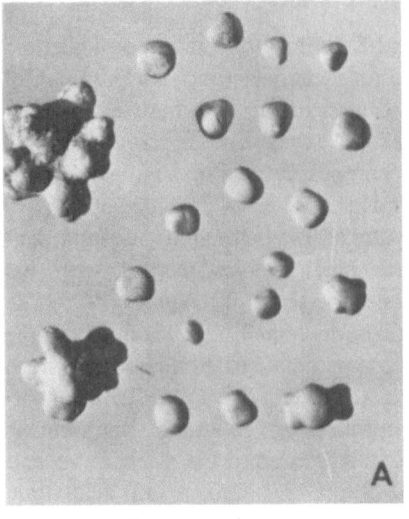

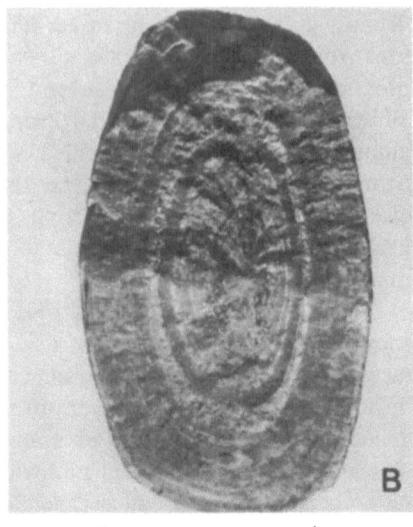

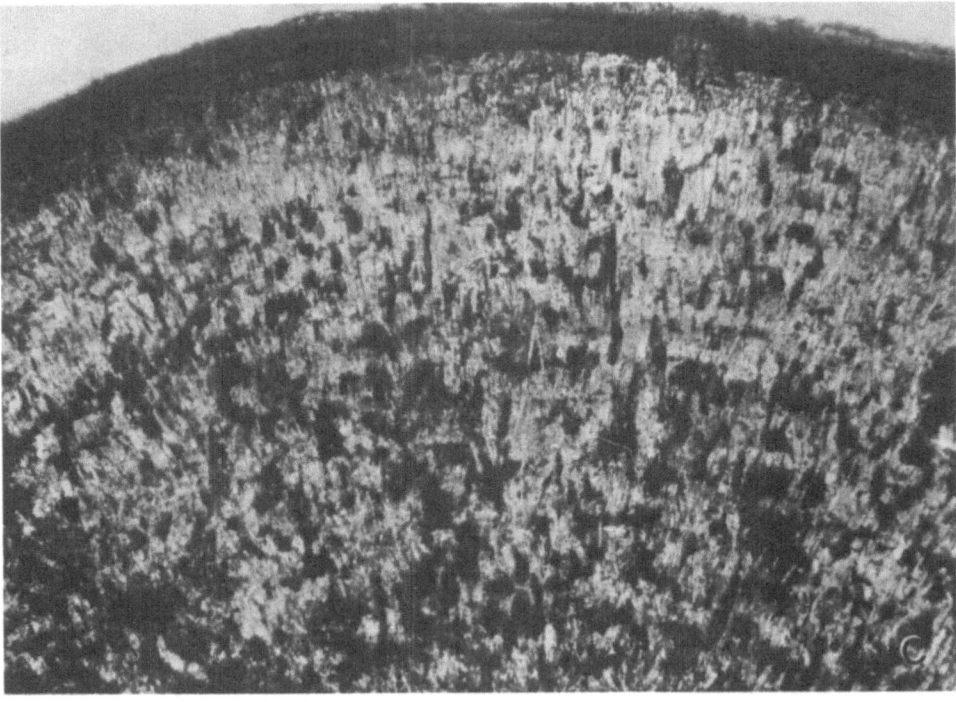

⊢ --- ⊣ = 1 cm

Fig. 15.1. **A.** Multiple uric acid vesical calculi with smooth white surfaces; some of the calculi have become loosely cemented together. **B.** Fracture surface of a uric acid calculus, showing prominent concentric layers of different shades of orange and brown and also radial striation of uric acid crystals; the layering and the striation is on a coarser scale than the pisolitic whewellite calculi. **C.** Photomicrograph of a uric acid calculus in ordinary light; the fracture surface of the calculus shows well-marked concentric laminations, although this does not show up well in the thin section; the radial orientation of the crystals can be seen.

lographic studies, ammonium hydrogen urate was found in 4 of 24 uric acid calculi, being in the nucleus in 2 [45]. In thin sections ammonium hydrogen urate, with a characteristic shade of brown, has the general appearance of uric acid, the crystals being radially oriented and slightly pleochroic. In some renal calculi (from one of our patients) composed of uric acid and ammonium hydrogen urate, there was a bright bluish-green layer about halfway between the centre and the periphery of the stone, which was shown by ultra-violet spectroscopy to be methylene blue, a substance known to form a complex with uric acid, and doubtless derived from a patent medicine taken by the patient.

Sodium hydrogen urate monohydrate $(NaC_5H_3N_4O_3 \cdot H_2O)$ was found in only one stone in their series of 1000 cases submitted to crystallographic examination by Prien and Frondel [46]. The salt formed a greyish-brown zone of needle-like crystals between a central nucleus of uric acid and an external zone of apatite. They found sodium urate in tiny plaques attached to the apices of renal papillae and also in the so-called uric acid infarcts of renal papillae. One renal calculus in our series of 500 cases of urinary stone [45] was composed of alternating layers of apatite, sodium hydrogen urate, ammonium hydrogen urate and whewellite, the thin layer of sodium urate consisting of an aggregate of needle-shaped crystals.

Mixed Stones. Uric acid with apatite and calcium oxalate stones are the most common. Uric acid may be found as the nucleus of stones composed of the other two substances, and calcium oxalate monohydrate has been found as the nucleus of a uric acid stone [46]. Apatite may be found in the interstices of coarsely porous uric acid calculi. In our series of 24 uric acid stones, calcium oxalate was present in 8 [45]. Of their 152 examples of uric acid calculi, Atsmon et al. [4] found that the stones were

composed of pure uric acid in 56%, the remainder being of mixed composition. The majority of the gouty patients had pure uric acid stones, whereas half of the idiopathic uric acid stones (which were medium-sized or large) were of mixed composition. A urinary infection was found in association with 34% of the pure uric acid calculi and with 57.9% of stones composed of uric acid and calcium salts (especially calcium phosphate), or of calcium salts alone.

The question arises as to how such different substances can form part of the same stone; it is possible that altered dietetic habits over a given period of time, or a temporary urinary infection (which may influence the urinary pH), or temporary hypercalciuria, coming together or separately could assume the promoting role in the final composition of the calculus.

Patients with uric acid lithiasis (or gout) sometimes have in addition calculi composed entirely of calcium salts. Kittredge and Downs [37] found 5 stones which did not contain uric acid among 14 stones from gouty patients. A patient with gout reported by Fineberg and Altschul [24] had a staghorn calculus composed entirely of calcium salts. Talbott and Terplan [52] stated that nearly 5% of gouty patients had calcium stones which contained no uric acid. The author had a hypertensive patient who had a pure calcium oxalate stone in one kidney and a pure uric acid stone in the other. In the large series of Atsmon et al. [4] 14.5% of their patients had voided or had had removed at least one stone composed of calcium salts only. Possibly such calcium-containing calculi might have had a uric acid nucleus if carefully looked for.

2. The Kidney

The microscopic renal changes seen in patients with idiopathic (non-gouty) uric acid lithiasis (as seen in subjects operated upon) may be minimal. In more advanced cases the kidney has cortical scarring similar to that associated with pyelonephritis from any cause. Still later, in association with staghorn stones and infection, or with a stone which has been impacted for a considerable time in the ureter, the kidney may show destructive changes; the small sclerosed kidney, contracted around the calculi within it, is the end-stage.

In the gouty subject renal changes may be marked and the associated uric acid calculi figure at first as an incidental finding. The earliest changes are tubular damage with a reaction in the renal interstitial tissues, glomerular sclerosis and fibrillar thickening of the basement membrane of the glomerular capillaries [31]; the loops of Henle may show dilatation, epithelial degeneration and pigmentation.

A distinguishing feature of the gouty kidney is the deposition of long slender crystals of sodium urate, arranged radially and disposed in sheaves, in the collecting tubules, which may suffer destruction of their tubular epithelium and become surrounded by foreign-body giant cells. Atrophy of the nephron and sclerosis of the renal pyramids follow [1]. Later there is cortical scarring resulting from the presence of dense wedges of pyelonephritic renal tissue with hypertrophy of nephrons between their zones. The epithelium of the convoluted tubules shows fine granular vacuolation in some places. There are sometimes cortical and medullary cysts and abscesses containing gritty masses [51]. The advanced nature of the histological renal lesions (vascular and pyelonephritic) usually seems to be correlated with the severity of clinical symptoms, though a few patients with tophaceous gout show only minimal clinical evidence of renal insufficiency. The vascular changes affecting the renal arterioles (and even the arteries) are comparable in some instances with those seen in patients with malignant hypertension [52].

Uric Acid Infarcts in Infants. This term is used to describe the yellow wedge-shaped deposits of uric acid crystals not uncommonly seen in the renal papillae in infants; in the newborn infant, in whom hyperuricaemia and hyperuricosuria are common, it has been suggested that there is a local deficiency of the enzyme urease, which may be responsible [1]. The spherical, well-defined, laminated crystals, individually of 10–20 μm in diameter, are found in the collecting tubules, where they form casts in association with granular protein and desquamated tubular epithelium; the tubule proximal to the casts may show no obvious dilatation and there is no evidence of interstitial inflammation.

II. Clinical Picture

Uric acid calculi, like calcium-containing calculi, are sometimes idiopathic, but are sometimes related to some extrarenal diseases or disorders, the chief of which are primary and secondary gout; the following groups of patients are referred to:

1. Uric acid calculi in association with primary gout.
2. Uric acid calculi in association with secondary gout.
3. Idiopathic uric acid calculi associated with a family history of stone.
4. Idiopathic uric acid calculi not having a history of gout nor a family history of stone.

1. Uric Acid Calculi and Primary Gout

Primary gout is a disorder of purine metabolism which is genetically determined and in which hyperuricaemia, attributable either to the overproduction or to an underexcretion of uric acid, is the cardinal

Table 15.1. A. The incidence of uric acid calculi in patients with gout

Observer	Country	Year	No. of patients with gout	No. or % with calculi
Brøckner-Mortensen (Reported by De Sèze and Ryckewaert)		1937	100	17%
Kittredge and Downs	U.S.A.	1952	324	14% (calculi actually re-covered, or shown on X ray; a further 3% had had renal colic; total 17%)
Gutman and Yü	U.S.A.	1957	300	9 (13.5%) 27 (11.5%)
Talbott	U.S.A.	1957		16%
De Sèze and Ryckewaert	France	1960		23%
Atsmon et al.	Israel (a stone clinic)	1963	67	50
Gutman and Yü	U.S.A.	1962	937 (primary gout) 44 (secondary gout)	189 (20%) 40%

B. The incidence of gout in patients with uric acid calculi

Observer	Country	Year	No. of patients with calculi	No. or % with gout
Armstrong and Greene	U.S.A.	1953		27.3%
Melick and Henneman	U.S.A.	1958		22.4%
Boyce (reported by Talbott, 1957)	U.S.A.	1957		10.0%
Badenoch	England	1960	21	2 patients
Atsmon et al.	Israel	1963	213	55 (25.8%) (23 had chronic gout with X-ray changes)

biochemical feature. Hyperuricaemia itself is initially asymptomatic, and was found in 25% of 136 asymptomatic blood relations of 27 gouty subjects by Talbott [50]. Wyngaarden [58] concluded that multiple metabolic aberrations may be responsible for hyperuricaemia, but that a single type of genetic defect is apt to characterize a given hyperuricaemic family. The incidence of uric acid calculi in gouty patients in reported series varies from 9% to 30% (Table 15.1).

2. Uric Acid Calculi and Secondary Gout

Secondary gout is an acquired form of the disease in which hyperuricaemia, arising as a consequence of another disease which is associated with an increased turnover of nucleoprotein, results in the development of arthritic and periarthritic changes similar to and indistinguishable from those of primary gout, and frequently renal insufficiency; it affects patients mostly in the fifth to the seventh decades.

Among the diseases or disorders which may lead to secondary gout are: polycythaemia vera, and occasionally the secondary polycythaemia which may accompany congenital heart disease; chronic myelogenous leukaemia; acute leukaemia; haemolytic anaemia; pernicious anaemia; and multiple myelomatosis. Attacks of gout in association with hyperuricaemia have also been reported as complications of the following: obesity, starvation, chronic glomerulonephritis, pyelonephritis and hypertensive cardiovascular disease, glycogen storage disease type I, miscellaneous conditions including sarcoidosis, psoriasis and hyperparathyroidism, choreoathetosis and mental retardation [58].

Secondary gout may also follow the treatment of polycythaemia vera and leukaemia by radiation or cytotoxic drugs, or by the administration of liver or vitamin B_{12} for pernicious anaemia; such forms of treatment increase the turnover of nucleoproteins and hence lead to the overproduction of uric acid [58]. Attacks of gout have also been reported as a result of hyperuricaemia following the administration of chlorothiazide, hydrochlorothiazide and pyrazinamide. Females are more frequently affected with secondary gout than with primary gout.

The incidence of renal uric acid calculi in patients who develop secondary gout is about 40% [26], though this figure does not of course represent the incidence of calculi in patients with the primary diseases which are complicated by secondary gout. Two cases of acute leukaemia (one myeloid, one lymphatic) in which, following radiotherapy, calculi obstructed the ureters, were reported by Bedrna and Polack [7]. Merrill and Jackson [43] found that nephrolithiasis was a frequent cause of renal failure in leukaemic patients. McCrea [41] reported an incidence of 4.67% of uric acid stones in leukaemic patients following treatment (for example, with nitrogen mustard), and that one mode of death may be urinary obstruction by uric acid crystals. The appearance of stone in several consecutive generations of these patients and the transmission of the tendency through father and mother, to children of both sexes indicated an autosomal dominant mode of inheritance with high penetrance.

3. Idiopathic Uric Acid Calculi Associated with a Family History of Stone

In a further group of patients with uric acid calculi not associated with gout, there is a family history of stone so that genetic factors have played an important role. Atsmon et al. [4] found that 45.5% of 187 patients with uric acid stones had relatives who had had renal calculi, compared with 38% of 150 with calcium salt urolithiasis and with only 13% in the group of normal subjects. They demonstrated a familial incidence of idiopathic uric acid lithiasis in 15 families in which at least two members had proven uric acid urolithiasis, and no hyperuricaemia either in the patients or in those members of their families who were available for examination.

In a detailed description of three of the families whose total members numbered 214, 60 or 28%, had idiopathic uric acid urolithiasis (33% males; 22% females). There was no instance of gout in any of the patients nor in any members of their families; the disease usually appeared in adult life (41% being above the age of 18) but at an earlier age in successive generations. The disease was clinically serious, sometimes proving fatal.

It was suggested that the condition here called idiopathic uric acid lithiasis is a genetically inherited disorder which is present in certain Jewish families, and probably in some families living in some Mediterranean countries (Italy, Turkey, France), thus explaining the relatively high incidence of uric acid urolithiasis in peoples of those countries.

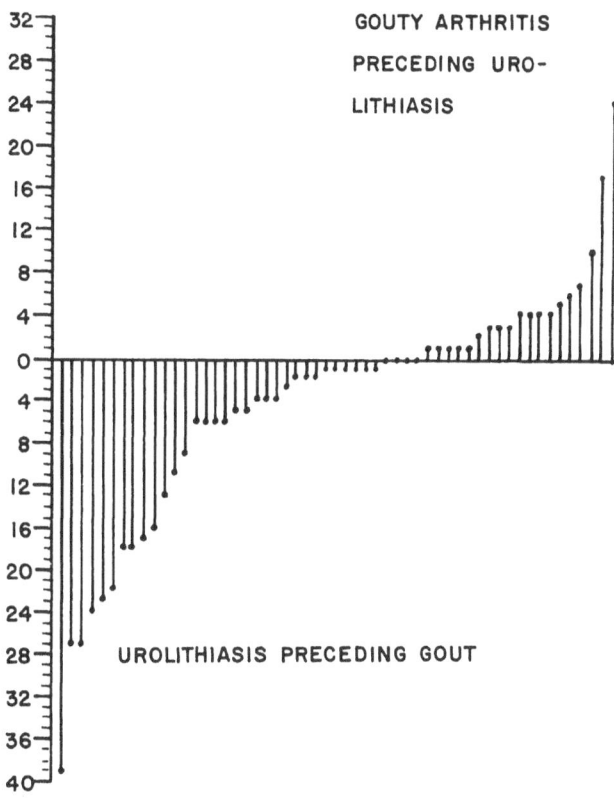

GOUTY ARTHRITIS
PRECEDING URO-
LITHIASIS

UROLITHIASIS PRECEDING GOUT

Fig. 15.2. Time relationship between the first manifestations of urolithiasis and of gouty arthritis in 55 patients with gout and uric acid lithiasis. The *vertical lines* represent individual patients; the *dots* on the zero line represent patients in whom both disorders were manifested at about the same time. (By courtesy of Drs. Atsmon, de Vries and Frank, 1963, and the Elsevier Publishing Company, London)

4. Uric Acid Calculi Without a History of Gout Nor a Family History of Stone

There exists a group of idiopathic uric acid calculi in the above sense; most of these patients do not have hyperuricaemia. The group, however, is not absolutely clear-cut, since some of these patients develop gout, but often not until many years after the development of the stone. It has been shown earlier that, conversely, many patients with gout develop uric acid calculi. In the large series of Atsmon et al. [4], the onset of the urolithiasis preceded that of the gout in 32 of the 55 patients, in 12 of whom the stone preceded the gout by more than 10 years, and in 1 by 39 years; while the gouty arthritis preceded the urolithiasis in 34.5% of the 55 patients by intervals often up to 4 years and exceptionally to 32 years.

Figure 15.2 shows the time interval between the first onset of urolithiasis and that of gouty arthritis (whichever started first), in 55 patients who all ultimately had both gout and uric acid lithiasis. In a patient with uric acid lithiasis, therefore, a negative history of gout having preceded the onset of the renal symptoms must be viewed with caution as regards the possible ultimate association of the two conditions.

5. Age and Sex Incidence

The maximum incidence of uric acid stone falls between the ages of 30 and 50, no age group being exempt; while in the gouty group males far exceed females, in the idiopathic group the ratio of males to females is approximately 3 : 2.

6. Symptoms

A patient who has had recurrent attacks of renal colic (either frequently or at long intervals) with spontaneous voiding of calculi and yet with negative urograms, and who has a family history of stone, may be suspected of having a uric acid calculus. Haematuria is said to occur less frequently in gouty patients than in those with idiopathic uric acid lithiasis. The passage of reddish gravel in the urine (consisting of tiny aggregates of crystals of uric acid or of urates) though found in many normal patients who have had neither renal colic nor uric acid calculi, may suggest the presence of a uric acid stone in patients with clinical symptoms.

Calculi may have been voided spontaneously and intermittently for years, sometimes unaccompanied by renal colic; such stones are usually small, round, yellow or reddish and occasionally they are voided in large numbers often from both kidneys. Badenoch [5] reported a patient who had passed some hundreds of uric acid calculi. Atsmon et al. [4] referred to a male patient who voided 300 stones within 2 months, and another aged 53 who for a time passed up to 50 stones daily. In spite of such a clinical picture renal function may remain good. Stones which remain in the kidney may increase in size to fill the renal pelvis and one or more calyces.

A variable number of patients with uric acid lithiasis in different series have had infected urine. In the small number of patients with uric acid calculi seen in the author's department, infection has been unusual and this has been the experience of some other observers.

There are the usual dangers of hypertension, gross renal impairment and uraemia. Calculous anuria has an incidence higher than that found in patients with calcium-containing stones and may result from the impaction of small stones simultaneously in both ureters or in a single ureter, if one kidney has been previously removed (Chap. 14). The author has seen at least three patients with calculous anuria from uric acid stones, in two of whom there were multiple massive, bilateral calculi, as well as smaller ureteric ones which were responsible for the anuria. Two cases of anuria were reported among Badenoch's [5] 21 patients with uric acid stones. Four of 16 patients with uric acid calculi, reported by Wrong [57], had had episodes of bilateral ureteric obstruction.

7. Associated Diseases

The association of primary hyperparathyroidism with gout and therefore with uric acid calculi has been referred to in Chapter 4, and the occasional association of cystine calculi and uric acid stones in the same patient in Chapter 16.

Ulcerative Colitis. Of Badenoch's [5] 21 patients with uric acid stones, 5 suffered from ulcerative colitis and 4 of these had had a partial or total colectomy and an ileostomy. All of the patients had a high serum uric acid level while 2 had a low serum calcium level. Ulcerative colitis is not one of the disorders usually said to be associated with hyperuricaemia, though starvation and possibly dehydration in such cases may be contributory factors. Several patients reported by Melick and Henneman [42] suffered from chronic diarrhoea. In an analysis of 583 patients with ulcerative colitis or regional ileitis from the Mount Sinai Hospital, New York, by Deren et al. [18] 28 patients had developed urinary calculi and of these nine were shown to be composed of uric acid and a further four were also believed to be composed of uric acid or urates. It was suggested that the potassium deficiency which is common in patients with ulcerative colitis may give rise to local renal tubular changes, which may have been partly responsible for the stone formation.

Maratka and Nedbal [40] referred to 512 patients with ulcerative colitis seen by them during a period of 30 years; urinary calculi had been observed in 10 patients, 9 being from the group of 74 patients who had had surgical treatment for their colitis (12%). Bennett and Jepson [9] reported an incidence of uric acid stones in 12.5% of patients in South Australia who had had ileostomies for ulcerative colitis, and there were similar reports from Gigax and Leach [27]. Of 465 patients with ulcerative colitis seen and followed up by Goligher [29] in Leeds between 1952 and 1963, 6 had developed urinary calculi, 3 being in the group of 297 patients treated along medical lines and 3 in the group of 168 patients treated surgically; there was no significant difference in the incidence of stone formation between patients treated medically and those treated surgically.

III. Investigation

1. Serum Uric Acid

The level of the serum uric acid varies within certain limits in respect of the age and sex of the subject, the diet (high protein, high or low purine) at the time that the estimation was made as well as the method of estimation used; probably the limits of normal vary between 6.4 and 7.5 in the male and 5.7–6.6/100 ml in the female. The level is raised if renal function is impaired, during prolonged starvation and in patients with pneumonia and a variety of other conditions. In their patients with gout and uric acid stones Atsmon et al. [4] found that the average serum uric acid levels were elevated, namely 7.5 mg/100 ml in 34 patients, and their average of the maximum and minimum was 9.0 and 6.0 mg/100 ml respectively. Some of these patients may have had impairment of renal function,

which would contribute to the elevation of the serum uric acid level. The average serum uric acid level in their patients with gout but without urolithiasis was almost identical; the average maximum and minimum levels being 8.8 and 6.1 mg/100 ml.

In patients with secondary gout and uric acid calculi the serum uric acid is usually raised, sometimes to a high level, an average figure being 12.0 mg/100 ml but much higher levels have been reported. In leukaemia levels as high as 68 mg/100 ml have been found.

In patients with idiopathic uric acid stones (without gout) most patients do not have hyperuricaemia, which was present in patients in various series as follows: Armstrong and Greene [3] 21%; Boyce (quoted by Talbott [11]) 20%; Melick and Henneman [42] 4 of 14 patients: Atsmon et al. [4] 16.5%.

2. Urinary Excretion of Uric Acid

Most normal adults excrete fairly constant amounts of uric acid when on a low-purine diet of between 300 and 600 mg daily [34]; while on a normal diet they excrete between 500 and 1000 mg daily, an amount which may be increased by purine-rich and protein-rich diets and decreased by a high-fat diet [17]. Uric acid filtered through the glomeruli is believed to be almost completely reabsorbed by the proximal renal tubules [59].

An abnormally elevated urinary uric acid excretion is found in about 25%–30% of patients with primary gout [32, 35], and in many patients with secondary gout. The mean daily urinary uric acid excretion in 27 cases of secondary gout recorded by Gutman and Yü [35] was 634 mg compared with 497 mg in 540 cases of primary gout. Gutman [33] stated that the incidence of uratic stone is higher in over-excretors of uric acid than in normo-excretors, and the greater the urinary uric acid excretion, the greater the incidence of stone, a condition which applies to secondary gout. Allen [2] considered that the hyperuricosuria is a prerequisite in patients with uric acid stone. But all patients with hyperuricosuria do not develop uric acid stones.

In 61 patients with primary gout (with or without uric acid stones) on a low-purine diet, Atsmon et al. [4] found that there was a broad distribution of daily urinary uric acid levels, 16 excreting uric acid in excess of 1000 mg/24 h (2700 mg/24 h in 1 patient). Of 96 of their patients with idiopathic uric acid stones, on a low-purine diet for 3 days, the average daily uric acid excretion was 400–700 mg in 44 patients, less than 400 mg in 16 and more than 700 in 36 (6 having a daily range of 1700–2200 mg). In 13 of 17 who excreted more than 1000 mg/day the serum uric acid level was normal, and it was considered that they had a uric acid clearance in excess of the normal values of 7–15 ml/min, and which may have so far prevented the development of clinical gout. It has been shown that hyperuricosuria is not necessarily present in patients with uric acid lithiasis, though it frequently is present.

In patients with idiopathic uric acid calculi (who had normo-uricaemia) Cottet reported normal urinary excretion of uric acid [15, 39]. When the uric acid urinary excretion is massive, as in some patients with secondary gout, following death from uraemia, there is commonly a blockage of both ureters by masses of uric acid crystals, but not of uric acid calculi. Similarly the so-called uric acid infarcts found sometimes in newly born infants result from a massive overloading of the kidneys by uric acid but uric acid calculi are not found. The same combination of circumstances may occur in some patients with primary gout.

The concentration of uric acid in the urine, though probably a promoting factor for calculus formation, even if it is much increased over the normal values is not necessarily the final determining factor. Thus Atsmon et al. [4] noted high concentrations of urinary uric acid during the daytime in some normal subjects (without calculi) in the hot southern part of Israel. Some additional factor must be present for uric acid calculi to be formed. The same reservation applies to patients with idiopathic hypercalciuria in respect of calcium—oxalate–containing renal stones, who seem to require also an abnormally high urinary oxalate excretion. Can the additional factor be a urinary mucoprotein?

Atsmon et al. [4] found that the urea clearance was impaired to a greater degree (below 50% of normal) in patients with idiopathic uric acid stones than in patients in a comparable series with calcium-containing renal stones (most of which were bilateral and/or recurrent), to an extent that was statistically significant. The combination of gout and uric acid stones had a more adverse effect upon renal function than had uric acid stones alone; the presence of gout also impairs the ability of the kidney to concentrate the urine. When the renal clearance of urate is considered it has been found that the mean C_{urate}/C_{inulin} ratios are slightly lower in gouty than in non-gouty patients and the disparity is more evident in normal excretor than in overexcretor groups; the clearance differences were accentuated in both non-gouty and gouty subjects when the serum uric acid was artificially increased [58].

Urinary pH. The pH of freshly voided urine in patients with uric acid urolithiasis and also in patients with gout, with or without calculi, is usually below 5.5 (and sometimes below pH 5.0) though it may be higher in patients with infected urine. The urinary pH in patients with calcium oxalate stone is usually between 5.6 and 6.6 and that in patients with phosphatic stone is above 6.6.

Uric Acid Crystalluria. Crystals of uric acid, which are commonly formed in urine of a pH of less than 5.8, are in the form of whetstones, rosettes, rectangles or quadrates, are usually tinted orange-yellow and are of variable size; crystals of sodium urate may be found in urine of pH 6.0 or higher but only rarely in association with crystals of uric acid. Crystals of calcium oxalate may be found along with those of uric acid. The absence of uric acid crystals in urine does not necessarily imply that the patient does not have a uric acid stone. A certain critical urinary concentration level of uric acid is necessary before crystals are deposited. Atsmon et al. [4] found urinary uric acid crystals in 89.7% of their patients with uric acid calculi in the early morning urine (which usually has a low pH). In patients with uric acid stone who had been given food with a high purine content (chocolate, liver) a heavy uric acid crystalluria has been found, but not in normal subjects, in whom, however, urinary uric acid crystals have been found following prolonged strenuous exercise, especially in a hot climate.

3. Radiodiagnosis

A pure uric acid stone, having a density equal to that of the soft tissues, is non-opaque to X-rays but if the stone has a small or moderate content of admixed calcium salts (sometimes as a complete encasement of the stone) an imperfect shadow of the stone may be cast on the radiograph. A ring type of shadow, or a non-homogeneous shadow of woolly appearance but with an attempt at a well-defined outline, or shadows showing concentric layers of differing density, may be that of a stone having a nucleus or alternating layers of uric acid. Air pyelography may enable small stones otherwise invisible to be recognized. Rarely the patient may have radio-opaque calcium-containing stones containing no uric acid, in

addition to radiolucent uric acid stones. A normal plain X-ray and urogram are not inconsistent with the presence of one or more small pelvic or calyceal uric acid stones.

Negative shadows or filling defects (rounded, ovoid or pyramidal) resulting from the presence of calculi, calyceal or pelvic, may be seen in the urogram. A small stone may not give rise to a recognizable filling defect on the radiograph, since there will usually be opaque medium in front and behind masking the stone, unless it happens to be in a minor calyx (Fig. 15.3, see p. 332). Sometimes there are darker and lighter zones in the translucent area, which may indicate the presence of annular deposits of calcium salts.

A combination of a large filling defect on contrast urography with a faint shadow on the plain film probably indicates the presence of a uric acid stone. A uric acid stone in a major calyx may obstruct some minor calyces, which are not then filled with opaque medium on pyelography; such an unfilled calyx was designated by Atsmon et al. [4] 'the sign of the invisible calyx'; the radiograph of the rare papillary tumour of one calyx may also give this sign. If a uric acid stone is causing partial obstruction, the urogram will show hydrocalycosis, hydronephrosis or hydroureter according to its position. In some cases of almost acute ureteric obstruction, there may be the nephrogram effect described for some calcium-containing calculi, a finding which is useful even though the stone itself is radiolucent; if the kidney has been destroyed by calculi there will be no pyelographic shadow.

A filling defect in the ureter caused by a uric acid stone usually has clear and regular margins, but may mimic that caused by a tumour of the ureter, the lower margins of which, however, may be indefinite and regular. Blood clot or papillary tumours of the renal pelvis, calyces or ureters give rise to filling defects on the urogram, and the

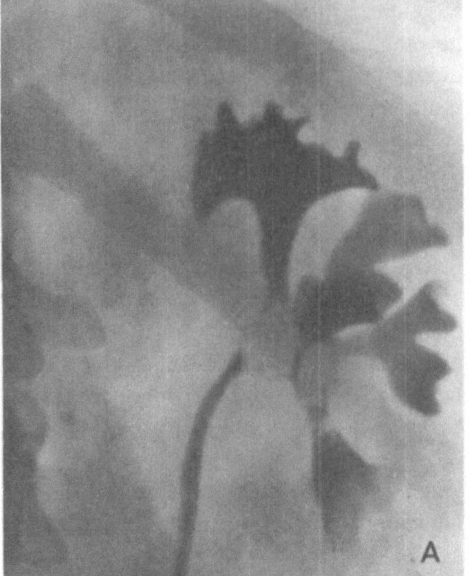

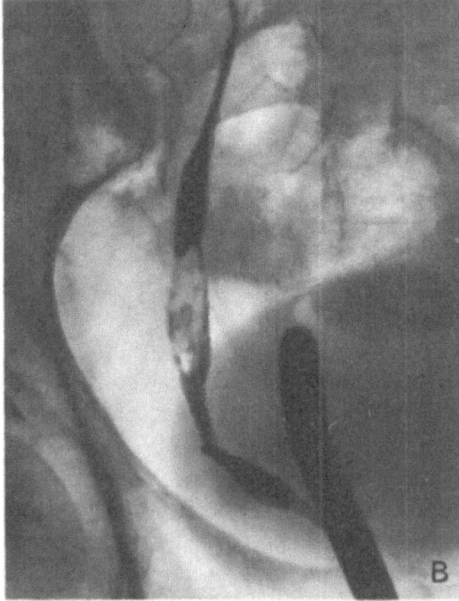

Fig. 15.3. **A.** Retrograde pyelogram (left kidney) of a European Portuguese National from Portuguese East Africa, showing uric acid calculi which are recognizable by filling defects on the radiograph; there is a stone (filling defect) in the pelvis and a second stone in the infundibulum leading to the lowest calyx and in the calyx itself. **B.** An ellipsoidal pure uric acid stone which had moved down from the right kidney to the pelvic ureter, identified by a filling defect on the radiograph. The stones were removed by Mr. R.M.Honey, F.R.C.S., Salisbury, Rhodesia

history of one or more attacks of haematuria or the detection of tumour cells in the urine are then of diagnostic importance. The very rare radiolucent xanthine stone gives rise to a filling defect on the urogram but the diagnosis is then made by the discovery of xanthinuria. Matrix calculi are radiolucent and can sometimes be diagnosed if the central soft mass of matrix is surrounded by a crust of radio-opaque calcium salts; the picture of the uric acid stone may mimic them very closely. An air bubble may lodge in the ureter or the renal pelvis and mimic a true filling defect, but a repeat pyelogram a day or two later should give a normal picture; moreover, an air bubble will not give rise to dilatation of the ureter, pelvis or calyces [23].

4. Diagnosis

The features which enable the urologist to make a tentative diagnosis of uric acid urolithiasis are:

1. The repeated voiding of small, reddish-yellow calculi.

2. Often a history of primary gout in the patient or in some of his relatives (some of whom may also have had urolithiasis) and the finding in some of them of evidence of gouty arthritis or tophi.

3. A history of secondary gout.

4. The presence of a negative plain radiograph (in the case of the radiolucent uric acid stone), or of one showing circular or irregular shadows alternating with translucent areas in one or both renal regions.

5. The presence of a negative urogram or one showing filling defects in the opaque medium in the renal pelvis, in one or more calyces or in one or other ureter.

6. The discovery of uric acid crystals in a urine with a pH less than 5.6.

7. The possible presence of hyperuricaemia or hyperuricosuria or both.

IV. Treatment

Uric acid calculi gradually increase in size and give rise to symptoms so that treatment, surgical or conservative, becomes necessary. Surgical diagnosis is hampered by the non-radiolucency of the stones. Conservative treatment on the other hand can achieve a great deal of permanent success in a co-operative patient.

1. Surgery

Probably more than half of uric acid stones are of such a size that surgical removal has to be considered, especially if they are bilateral and if calculous anuria is considered a hazard. A patient who has passed many small stones (with no suggestion of a large stone) is probably best treated by conservative measures. Preoperative infection should be treated as should residual postoperative infection to help to prevent recurrence. Large staghorn stones in a disorganized kidney (the other one being reasonably healthy) should usually be treated by nephrectomy.

Armstrong and Greene [3] reported surgical intervention in 60 of 117 (51.3%) patients with uric acid lithiasis. In Cottet's [16] series surgical removal of calculi was needed in 13% (one nephrectomy) while stones were voided spontaneously in 87%. In the series of 210 patients with uric acid lithiasis recorded by Atsmon et al. [4] surgical treatment was carried out in 54, with 73 operations in all (25.6%); operative treatment was needed more frequently in the patients with idiopathic (non-gouty) uric acid stones, often of mixed composition (38.2%), than in the gouty group, where the stones were more often of pure uric acid (13.9%). These observers also reported on the size of stones in the series of 183 patients with uric acid lithiasis: 61 had small stones only, 96 had small stones as well as medium-sized or large stones, 122

had medium-sized or large stones of which 23 (12.6%) were staghorn calculi.

These figures are of more practical importance in helping the surgeon to know what to expect at operation for radiolucent uric acid stones, than in the case of calcium-containing calculi, which can usually be counted on the preoperative radiograph before operative removal is undertaken.

2. Conservative Treatment

Conservative treatment is indicated for patients who have passed multiple small calculi frequently over a long period of time and who still have negative urograms. By strict adherence to the regime to be described, remaining existing calculi can usually be voided spontaneously and the formation of new stones prevented. A watch for calculous anuria must be kept in the early stages of treatment until residual stones have been voided. Sometimes it has been found possible by conservative measures to cause medium-sized uric acid stones to go into solution or to disintegrate. Medical treatment is indicated following the surgical removal of calculi to prevent recurrence.

Fluids. A high intake of fluids reduces the concentration of uric acid in the urine, and is complementary to treatment by alkalis. It has been shown that the amount of uric acid excreted in the urine increases to a urinary output of 2 ml/min as the urinary output rises, but remains constant at higher excretion rates, when its concentration in the urine gradually decreases, and the tendency for the precipitation of uric acid crystals is reduced [44]. A daily intake of fluid of between 2 and 3 litres should produce a urinary output of 2 ml/min and at least 2 litres daily. The regime should be supplemented by one to two glasses of water or other fluid before retiring and also between 2 and 3 a.m. to ensure adequate urinary excretion during the night.

An intake of fluids suitable for patients in temperate climates may be quite inadequate for the purpose in tropical and subtropical countries in which uric acid calculi are common; thus in some parts of Israel it is said that an agricultural worker must ingest 10–15 litres of fluid daily in order to void 1 litre of urine daily during a hot summer.

Alkalis. Uric acid is hardly soluble in urine below pH 5.6 but its solubility rises steeply above a pH of 6.5 to 6.8; a planned dose of alkalis should, therefore, be given to achieve a urinary pH of 6.0–6.5 or even to 7.0 at an approximately constant level throughout the 24 h [37]; no uric acid crystals are then present in the urine. If the pH is allowed to fall below 5.6 uric acid would be precipitated. A urinary pH of between 7.5 and 8.0 should never be aimed at, since large amounts of alkali carry the possible inconvenience of gastric upset, the possible danger of a metabolic alkalosis in patients with renal impairment and deleterious effects (from the ingestion of sodium) in patients with hypertension. Moreover, in patients with calculi and infected urine such high pH levels carry the probability of precipitation of calcium phosphate in the urine, which could result in an increase rather than a decrease in the size of the stone.

In patients with mixed calcium oxalate–phosphate–uric acid calculi, the above regime might be expected to cause the uric acid in the calculi to go into solution, but (theoretically) not the calcium salts, which might even increase in amount, thus causing the stone to increase in size. To render the urine alkaline a solution of potassium citrate and sodium bicarbonate can be used, and that recommended by Eisenberg et al. [21] (citric acid, 40 g; sodium citrate, 60 g; potassium citrate, 66 g; extractum aurantii, 6 g; with syrup to 600 ml; 15 ml or one

spoonful of the solution being taken three times daily), is appropriate; in hypertensive patients sodium citrate may be partly replaced by potassium citrate.

Diet. A diet low in proteins and in purines should reduce the urinary uric acid by up to 250 mg/24 h [15] and could be useful (though perhaps of limited real value) for gouty patients with uric acid calculi. A low-protein, low-purine diet is unappetizing and could be undesirable on general nutritional grounds. The ingestion of large amounts of fruit and vegetables is desirable and will tend to result in the production of an alkaline urine. Purine-rich foods (liver, sweetbreads, kidneys, brain, beefsteak, ham, beans, spinach) should be taken in moderation, and chocolate, sardines and anchovies should be avoided. Cereals, fruits and most vegetables, milk and eggs are almost purine-free.

Allopurinol should be given to reduce the hyperuricosuria by decreasing the total production of purines in the body including uric acid. It exerts an inhibitory action on the enzyme xanthine oxidase in the human jejunal mucosa so that oxidation of hypoxanthine and xanthine is inhibited. The oxidation of glyoxylate to oxalate, which is catalyzed by xanthine oxidase, is also inhibited [55, 56]. When given orally, allopurinol causes a prompt reduction in the levels of uric acid in the serum as well as in the urine in normal and hyperuricaemic subjects; it can be given along with uricosuric drugs if large gouty tophi have to be dispersed.

Allopurinol is usually given in doses of between 400 and 800 mg/24 h. Side-effects have been reported (gastrointestinal symptoms; acute gouty arthritis; and occasionally leucopenia, pruritus and fever). It has been found useful in the prevention of the acute uric acid nephropathy which occasionally complicates cases of acute leukaemia, in which there is a sudden increase in the rate of uric acid production from nucleoprotein, resulting in the blockage of the renal tubules with aggregates of uric acid crystals [56]. There is some danger of xanthine stone formation occurring when allopurinol is administered, since it induces a rise of urinary oxypurines, including xanthine, so that care should be exercised [30].

3. Results of Treatment

The results of the conservative treatment for largely pure uric acid stones using the fluid-alkali regime are in general very good provided the patient adheres closely to the instructions. In patients who have been passing small calculi composed of pure uric acid, sometimes for years, and often in considerable numbers, within 3 or 4 weeks of commencing treatment the attacks of colic usually cease and stone formation is reduced. Existing stones have to be voided and large stones in the renal pelvis may diminish in size gradually and ultimately disintegrate. This experience compares with the observations in vitro that small stones composed of pure uric acid may disintegrate within 1–2 weeks, when placed in an alkaline medium [13].

In patients with calcium oxalate–uric acid stones the results are not so dramatic in that a period (sometimes up to several months) must elapse before the patient ceases to void stones though it is probable that no new ones are formed. The calcium-containing fraction (often radiographically demonstrable) does not pass into solution but may later be voided as spherical shells of calcium-containing material, sometimes following attacks of renal colic.

Of 118 patients treated conservatively by Atsmon et al. [4], no new stones were formed in 96.6% of the patients during an average follow-up of 2.2 years. Of 30 patients who discontinued treatment, 86.7% had recurrent stone formation during an average follow-up period of 2.8 years.

Apart from the large calculi, previously mentioned, there were no significant differences in the results of treatment in the patients with pure uric acid stones from those with calcium oxalate–uric acid stones. Most patients with mixed calcium oxalate–uric acid stones who had successful treatment had observed the spontaneous voiding of small calculi, presumably containing the calcium element in the stone. The dissolution of pure uric acid stones took 1–6 months, while the time required for mixed stones was 6–18 months, after which time the calcific shadows had disappeared.

Stones in a non-functioning or very poorly functioning kidney cannot be dissolved especially if infected with urea-splitting organisms, since little or no urine is being excreted from that kidney. Operative removal of the stones with after-treatment by fluids and alkalis is the only hope for such patients. Renal function frequently improved especially in the non-gouty patients.

4. Drug Treatment for Gouty Patients

Colchicine and phenylbutazone (Butazolidine) are effective remedies for the treatment of the attacks of gout; the latter also has a uricosuric effect. The uricosuric drugs are believed to act by inhibiting the reabsorption of uric acid by the renal tubules and therefore increasing the urinary excretion and reducing the level of the plasma uric acid to the normal or near-normal range. They are effective in causing tophaceous deposits of sodium urate to go into solution and in the prevention of new tophi; they are useful in patients whose serum uric acid is consistently elevated and who have frequent attacks of gout in spite of adequate doses of colchicine. The aim is to reduce and maintain the serum uric acid level to below 6 mg/100 ml. Treatment should be begun during a quiescent phase of the disease because of the tendency of these drugs to initiate an attack of gout [47].

The uricosuric drugs have the potentiality of giving rise to uric acid calculi and should therefore be administered along with a high intake of fluids and alkalinization of the urine; small doses of the drug should be administered in the first 2 weeks of treatment and increased gradually. The uricosuric drugs include salicylates, sulphurpyrazone (Anturan) and zoxazolamine (Flexon), which sometimes have unpleasant side-effects.

Probenecid is a mild hyperuricosuric drug (given in doses of 0.5 g daily increasing to 1.5 g daily in divided doses) which causes an increased urinary excretion of uric acid in gouty subjects with a reduction of the serum uric acid level to below 7 mg/100 ml. In a patient of the author's, suffering from intermittent attacks of gout, treatment with probenecid gave rise to renal colic with the subsequent voiding of a uric acid stone. Bartels and Matossian [6], who recommended low doses of probenecid with a high daily intake of fluid at the beginning of treatment, reported that only 3 of 231 patients treated with probenecid over a 6-year period, developed uric acid calculi in spite of the fact that 10% of the patients had had a prior history of renal colic.

Allopurinol may have a place in the treatment of uric acid stones [10, 22].

References

1. Allen,A.C.: The kidney. New York: Grune & Stratton 1951
2. Allen,J.E.: Nonopaque ureteral calculus. Am. J. Surg. *101*, 258 (1961)
3. Armstrong,W.A., Greene,L.F.: Uric acid calculi with particular reference to determinations of uric acid content of blood. J. Urol. *70*, 545 (1953)
4. Atsmon,A., De Vries,A., Frank,M.: Uric acid lithiasis. Amsterdam, London, New York: Elsevier 1963
5. Badenoch,A.W.: Uric acid stone formation. Br.J. Urol. *32*, 374 (1960)
6. Bartels,E.C., Matossian,G.S.: Gout: six-year follow-up on probenecid (Benemid) therapy. Arthritis Rheum. *2*, 193 (1959)
7. Bedrna,J., Polack,J.: Akuter Harnleiterverschluss nach Bestrahlung chronischer Leukämien mit Röntgenstrahlen. Med. Clin. *25*, 1700 (1929)
8. Benedict,H.D., Forsham,P.H., Stetten De Witt,Jr.: The metabolism of uric acid in the normal and the gouty human studied with the aid of isotopic uric acid. J. Biol. Chem. *181*, 183 (1949)
9. Bennett,R.C., Jepson,R.P.: Uric acid stone formation following ileostomy. Aust. N.Z. J. Surg. *36*, 153 (1966)
10. Billings,A.A., Kandel,G.C., Shapiro,C.M.: Allopurinol therapy for renal uric acid calculi. J. Am. Med. Assoc. *210*, 2093 (1969)
11. Boyce,W.H.: Quoted by Talbot,J.H. (1957). Gout. New York, London: Grune & Stratton 1957
12. Boyce,W.H., King,J.S.: Effects of high calcium intakes on urine in human beings. Fed. Proc. *18*, 1102 (1959)
13. Boyce,W.H., Sulkin,N.W.: Biocolloids of urine in health and in calculous disease. III. The mucoprotein matrix of urinary calculi. J. Clin. Invest. *35*, 1067 (1956)
14. Brøckner-Mortensen,K.: Uric acid in blood and urine. Acta Med. Scand. (Suppl. 84) (1937)
15. Cottet,J.: Le syndrôme biochimique des lithiases urinaires. In: Handbuch der Urologie. X. Die Steinerkrankungen, p. 410. Berlin, Göttingen, Heidelberg: Springer 1961
16. Cottet,J., Weber A.: Intérêt pratique de l'analyse chimique des calculs urinaire. Pathol. Biol. *7*, 1975 (1959)
17. Dent,C.E., Philpot,G.R.: Xanthinuria. Lancet *I*, 182 (1954)
18. Deren,J.J., Poruch,J.G., Levitt,M.R., Knilnani,M.J.: Nephrolithiasis as a complication of ulcerative colitis and regional enteritis. Ann. Int. Med. *56*, 843 (1962)
19. De Sèze,S., Ryckewaert,A.: La goutte. Expansion Scientifique Française, Paris 1960
20. De Vries,A., Sperling,O.: Uric acid stone formation: basic concepts of aetiology and treatment. In: Scientific foundations of urology. Williams,D.I., Chisholm,G.D. (eds.), Vol. I, p. 297. London: Heinemann 1976

21. Eisenberg,H., Connor,T.B., Howard,J.E.: A useful agent for oral alkali therapy. J. Clin. Endocrinol. *15*, 503 (1955)

22. Elias,E., Lawrence,M.St.A. (for R. Hermon Dowling): Dissolution of renal uric acid stones complicating ileostomy. Proc. R. Soc. Med. *66*, 13 (1973)

23. Emmett,J.L.: Clinical radiography, 2nd ed., Vol. I, p. 452. Philadelphia, London: Saunders 1964

24. Fineberg,S.K., Altschul,A.: The nephropathy of gout. Ann. Int. Med. *44*, 1182 (1956)

25. Frank,M., De Vries,A., Atsmon,A., Kochwa,S.: Urinary pH, ammonia and calcium excretion in renal uric acid stone patients. Isr. Med. J. *12*, 299 (1960)

26. Gardner,F.H., Nathan,D.G.: Secondary gout. Med. Clin. N. Am. *45*, 1273 (1961)

27. Gigax,J.H., Leach,J.R.: Uric acid calculi associated with ileostomy for ulcerative colitis. J. Urol. *105*, 797 (1971)

28. Goldthwait,D.A., Greenberg,G.R., Peabody,R.A.: The involvement of 5-phosphorilboxyl-amide in the biosynthesis of glycinamide ribotide. Biochim. Biophys. Acta *18*, 148 (1955)

29. Goligher,J.C.: Personal communication (1972)

30. Greene,M.L., Fujimoto,W.Y., Seegmiller, J.E.: Urinary xanthine stones—a rare complication of allopurinol therapy. N. Engl. J. Med. *280*, 426 (1969)

31. Greenbaum,D., Ross,J.H., Steinberg,V.L.: Renal biopsy in gout. Br. Med. J. *I*, 1502 (1961)

32. Gutman,A.B.: Primary and secondary gout. Ann. Int. Med. *39*, 1062 (1953)

33. Gutman,A.B.: Urate urolithiasis in primary and secondary gout. Ann. Int. Med. *58*, 741 (1963)

34. Gutman,A.B., Yü,T.F.: Renal function in gout. Am. J. Med. *23*, 600 (1957)

35. Gutman,A.B., Yü,T.F.: Secondary gout. Ann. Int. Med. *56*, 675 (1962)

36. Gutman,A.B., Yü,T.F.: An abnormality of glutamine metabolism in gout. Am. J. Med. *35*, 820 (1963)

37. Kittredge,W.E., Downs,R.: The role of gout in the formation of urinary calculi. J. Urol. *67*, 841 (1952)

38. Lagergren,C.: Biophysical investigations of urinary calculi. Acta Radiol. (Stockh.) (Suppl. 133) (1956)

39. Loeper,M., Cottet,J.: Traitement de lithiases rénales. Paris: Doin et Cie 1955

40. Maratka,A., Nedbal,J.: Urolithiasis as a complication of the surgical treatment of ulcerative colitis. Gut *5*, 214 (1964)

41. McCrea,L.E.: Formation of uric acid calculi during chemotherapy for leukemia. J. Urol. *73*, 29 (1955)

42. Melick,R.A., Henneman,P.H.: Clinical and laboratory studies of 207 consecutuve patients in a kidney stone clinic. N. Engl. J. Med. *259*, 307 (1958)

43. Merrill,D., Jackson,H.Jr.: The renal complications of leukemia. N. Engl. J. Med. *288*, 271 (1943)

44. Mugler,A., Pernet,J.L., Pernet,A., Friedrich,S.: Le rôle du rein dans l'hyperuricémie d'après l'étude de 390 clearances de l'acide urique. Rev. Rhum. *22*, 320 (1955)

45. Murphy,B.T., Purton,M., Pyrah,L.N.: Personal communication (1962)

46. Prien,E.L., Frondel,C.: Studies in urolithiasis. I. The composition of urinary calculi. J. Urol. *57*, 949 (1947)

47. Seegmiller, J.E.: The present-day treatment of gout. Med. Clin. North Am. *45*, 1259 (1961)

48. Seegmiller,J.E.: Symposium on gout and other disorders of purine metabolism. Proc. R. Soc. Med. *59*, 287 (1966)

49. Seegmiller,J.E.: Symposium on clinical and biochemical features of X-linked uric aciduria. Arch. Int. Med. *130*, 181 (1972)

50. Talbott,J.H.: Serum urate in relatives of gouty patients. J. Clin. Invest. *27*, 749 (1940)

51. Talbott,J.H.: Gout. New York, London: Grune & Stratton 1957

52. Talbott,J.H., Terplan,K.L.: The kidney in gout. Medicine *39*, 405 (1960)

53. Watts,R.W.E.: Symposium on gout and other disorders of purine metabolism. Proc. R. Soc. Med. *59*, 287 (1966)

54. Watts,R.W.E.: Xanthinuria and xanthine stone formation. In: Scientific foundations of urology. Williams,D.I., Chisholm,G.D. (eds.), Vol. I, p. 310. London: Heinemann 1976

55. Watts,R.W.E., Gibbs,D.A.: Proceedings of Second Meeting of Federation of European Biochemical Societies. Abstract No. A278, p. 189. Vienna 1965

56. Watts,R.W.E., Watkins,P.J., Matthias,J.O., Gibbs,D.A.: Allopurinol and acute uric acid nephropathy. Br. Med. J. *I*, 205 (1966)

57. Wrong,O.M.: Symposium on gout and

other disorders of purine metabolism. Proc. R. Soc. Med. *59*, 287 (1966)

58. Wyngaarden,J.B.: Gout. In: The metabolic basis of inherited disease, 2nd ed. Stanbury, J.B., Wyngaarden,J.B., Fredrickson,D.S. (eds.). New York, London: McGraw-Hill 1966

59. Yü,T.F., Berger,L., Gutman,A.B.: Renal function in gout. Am. J. Med. *33*, 829 (1962)

Chapter 16

Cystinuria and Cystine Lithiasis

Calculi composed mostly of cystine $(SCH_2CH(COOH)NH_2)_2$, an amino acid which is a part of the protein molecule, are among the rarer stones found in the kidney. The disease which we call cystinuria is an ailment believed to have been present from birth and often present in the siblings [47]. It is characterized by excretion in the urine of large quantities of the amino acids cystine, lysine, arginine, ornithine and also of the mixed disulphide of cysteine and homocysteine, and by the tendency to form calculi in the urinary tract composed usually almost entirely of cystine, but occasionally admixed with apatite or calcium oxalate monohydrate. Cysteine, a component of the protein molecule, can be readily oxidized to form cystine, which, since the reaction is readily reversible, can be readily reconverted into cysteine. Methionine, a third sulphur-containing amino acid which is indispensable to the body and a cystic precursor, can be irreversibly converted into cysteine.

Cystine, being relatively insoluble, readily crystallizes out as thin hexagonal plate-like crystals which are insoluble in water, acetic acid, alcohol or ether, but are soluble in hydrochloric acid and in alkalis. Garrod [32, 33] in his monograph *The Inborn Errors of Metabolism*, referred to cystinuria and postulated that it resulted from a block in the oxidation of cystine to sulphate, an explanation subsequently shown to be erroneous. It has been shown that the patients have an abnormality of the transport of certain amino acids across the renal tubular epithelium and across the mucosa of the jejunum.

A considerable literature has accumulated dealing with the varied aspects of the disease and reviews have been published by Bartter et al. [3], Knox [41], Milne [49] and Watts [71].

I. Incidence of Cystinuria

In an examination of the urine of 10,534 students in the University of Michigan, Lewis [43] found the normal urinary excretion of cystine to be within the range 40–80 mg/day. His tests disclosed 18 students (1 in 600) who excreted an excess of urinary cystine consistently, and a further 22 who gave weakly positive results occasionally or consistently, giving a total incidence of 'cystinuria' as 1 in 250; 4 had repeated cystine crystalluria. None of the students who were examined had ever had renal symptoms suggestive of calculus, but a sister of one had had a cystine stone. Mallinson (quoted by Harris and Warren [45]) found four examples of cystinuria among 1000 London students (1 in 250); their urines contained 106–161 mg cystine/g creatinine and an increase of urinary lysine. Surveys of the incidence of urinary calculus in general agree that cystine stones form about 1% of all urinary calculi.

Crawhall and Watts [15] estimated the incidence of potential cystine stone-formers in Great Britain to be 1 in 20,000 of the population. Boström and Tottie [6] found among 7793 school children in Stockholm 19 incomplete (cystine–lysine) cystinuric heterozygotes (1 in 410), and three complete (cystine–lysine–arginine) cystinuric individuals (1 in 2600) in whom calculus formation would seem sooner or later to be inevitable, an incidence which is higher than the known frequency of cystine stone-formers in Sweden. In a series of 457 urinary stones seen in the author's department in Leeds during a given review period, there were 12 cystine stones (2.6%).

II. Cystinuria and Cystine Urolithiasis in Childhood

Pruzanski [57, 58], in a review of 56 cases of cystinuria, found 15 in pre-adolescent patients. Several had cystine calculi, and in these patients the disease tended to be severe. In all but one of these there was bilateral nephrolithiasis, impairment of renal function and ultimately uraemia. Seven patients between 8 and 15 years of age (five boys and two girls) had calculi; in six there were cystine crystals in the urine. In one child, large hard masses could be palpated in the left and right lumbar regions during life, while at autopsy there was bilateral hydronephrosis, the kidney containing up to 20 cystine stones, stones in both ureters and cystine crystals in the lumina of the renal tubules. Another patient who had bilateral renal stones and recurrent urinary infection at the age of 4, was shown at autopsy (at age 40) to have contracted pyelonephritic kidneys with cystine crystals in the renal tubules.

III. Pathology

1. Cystine Stone

Cystine as a component of urinary calculi was first described by Wollaston [74] who, in examining two stones removed from the bladder (one being from a child), noted the presence of a previously unknown substance which reacted with both acids and bases and which he believed to be an oxide which he called 'cystic oxide' because it had been found in a vesical calculus.

Typical cystine stones are honey-coloured and have a waxy semi-trans-lucence; they are usually firm but occasionally soft in consistency and may be small and multiple, or agglomerate to form a staghorn calculus. They are usually found in sterile urine. In thin sections the crystals usually consist of a compact mass of crystals which show marked cleavage one from another, though the hexagonal outlines of the crystals in thin sections may not always be obvious (Fig. 16.1). In one of our cases there was a suggestion of secondary crystallization within a hexagonal outline. Most commonly the stone is composed of pure cystine but occasionally other stone-forming substances such as apatite or calcium oxalate monohydrate become incorporated.

In Prien's [56] series of 1000 cases of urinary calculus there were 29 examples of cystine calculi, in 7 of which the cystine was associated with other substances. In the 73 calculi reported by Boström and Hambraeus [5], removed from 34 cystinuric patients, the stones were composed of pure cystine in 36 and of cystine together with small amounts of hydroxyapatite and ammonium magnesium phosphate in 31, possibly suggesting that in those cases the urine was infected; in 4 others the stone was composed predominantly of ammonium magnesium phosphate with traces of cystine. Several cases have been reported in which a cystinuric patient has formed cystine-free stones.

Cystinuric patients with cystine calculi occasionally pass pure uric acid stones, even when the uric acid urinary excretion and clearances are normal. Meloni and Canary [48] reported hyperuricaemia, normal uric acid clearance and urinary excretion, normal renal function, and family backgrounds of hyperuricaemia in four of six cystinuric patients, two of these being brothers. Family studies suggested inheritance of two distinct abnormalities in these patients: the serum uric acid in the four patients varied between 7.7 and 9.4 mg/100 ml (normal 6.5 mg/100 ml); recurrent renal

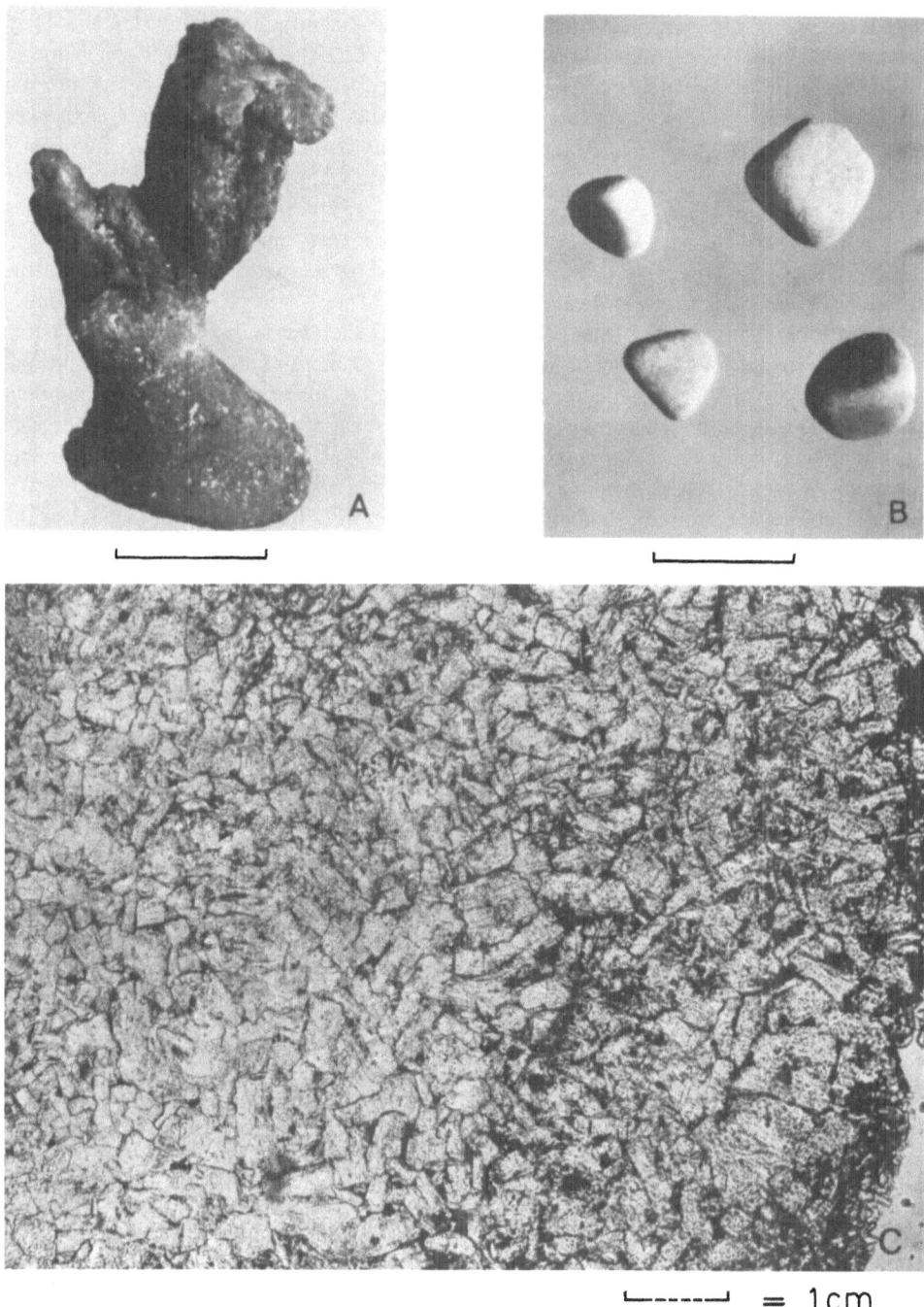

Fig. 16.1. **A.** A large cystine staghorn calculus with a yellowish surface showing the outlines of large cystine crystals. **B.** A few faceted tetrahedral vesical calculi composed of cystine. **C.** Photomicrograph of a cystine calculus showing a mass of small interlocking cystine crystals; there is little suggestion that the crystals have hexagonal outlines

calculi (recovered after nephrectomy in one patient in the series) were found on analysis to contain cystine, uric acid and calcium. Possibly cystinuria and hyperuricaemia coexist more often than has been thought.

2. The Kidney

In kidneys containing cystine calculi removed at operation, some at least of which will have been infected, pyelonephritis and hydronephrosis of varying degrees have been found, and the peripheral parts of the cortex often show scars; glomerular hyalinization, interstitial fibrosis, necrosis of the tubular epithelium, round-cell infiltration and often marked thickening of the arterioles can be seen. Renal papillary necrosis was found in three of the cases of Boström and Hambraeus [5], and in nine there was nephrocalcinosis associated with small calcium phosphate calculi in the distal portion of the renal collecting tubules. Cystine crystals in the renal tubules were found in the kidneys of two children reported by Pruzanski [57, 58].

IV. Pathogenesis and Genetics of Cystinuria

Researches carried out mainly since 1951 have shown that two distinct and apparently separate mechanisms are responsible for the condition known as cystinuria: firstly an abnormality in the transport of certain amino acids across the renal tubules, and secondly a failure of transport of amino acids across the mucosa of the jejunal epithelium.

1. Renal Transport Defect

Dent and co-workers [22, 24, 59] showed that there was a defective absorption of the basic amino acids in cystinuric patients by way of the proximal renal tubules. They showed that the plasma level of cystine in the cystinuric patient was below normal while that of the other amino acids was either normal or subnormal, in spite of their increased output in the urine. It was later shown [9] that the plasma levels of cysteine were reduced in the cystinuric patient, though no cysteine was excreted in the urine. They showed that in cystinuric patients the clearance of cystine was equal to the glomerular filtration rate (approximately 100 ml/min), while in normal individuals it was only about 4 ml/min. They also found elevated renal clearances of arginine, lysine and ornithine.

Infusions of lysine did not increase the urinary output of cystine, ornithine and arginine in cystinurics, since they were already near the glomerular filtration rate, but in normal individuals and in heterozygotes infusion of lysine caused transient increases in the clearances of cystine, arginine and ornithine. The investigations suggested the presence of a common reabsorptive system through the proximal renal tubules for the four dibasic amino acids, cystine, arginine, lysine and ornithine (with competition between the different amino acids).

Frimpter et al. [30, 31] also reported clearances of cystine in some cystinurics (homozygotes) to levels exceeding the glomerular filtration rate, indeed the amount of cystine excreted appeared to be almost twice the filtered load. They calculated the concentration of cystine and other amino acids in renal venous blood and compared it with that of the arterial blood, and found that the amino acid whose blood level fell most on its passage through the kidney was cysteine while that of cystine was hardly altered; they concluded that urinary cystine arises largely from plasma cysteine.

Subsequent evidence has suggested that simple competition for a common renal tubular transport system for the four amino acids does not account for all the observed abnormalities found in the cystinuric patient.

Rosenberg et al. [62] showed that lysine, ornithine and arginine, but not cystine, were concentrated in slices of rat kidney examined in vitro, but that cystine was not. Similar results were found in slices of renal tissue from normal and cystinuric human subjects [29]. Thier et al. [67, 68] described experiments using thin slices of renal tissue (obtained from cystinuric patients during operations for the removal of calculi), which were incubated for 30–90 min at 37°C in Krebs–Ringer bicarbonate buffer containing C^{14}-labelled l-lysine or l-arginine or S^{35}-labelled cystine; impaired transport of lysine and of arginine was found, the accumulation of these amino acids being reduced approximately 50% below control levels. There was mutual inhibition of uptake between lysine and arginine when the concentration of one of them was raised, but not when the concentration of cystine was raised.

Studies on the accumulation of S^{35} cystine indicated that its transport was unimpaired in cystinuric subjects. The studies indicated that in renal slices taken from control as well as from cystinuric subjects, lysine, arginine and probably ornithine compete for a common renal transport mechanism that is not shared by cystine. It was concluded that there is a defective renal tubular reabsorption of lysine, arginine and probably ornithine, which probably share a common transport mechanism, but there is increasing evidence that cystine reabsorption is unimpaired and does not share the same transport mechanism.

It was shown by Crawhall and Segal [14] that cystine absorbed by the renal cells is mostly reduced to cysteine; any apparent uptake of cystine into tissue slices in vitro represents the difference between cystine influx and cysteine efflux. The absorption of the isotopically labelled amino acids by the kidney of the rat was examined by Silber-

nagl and Deetjen [65], who suggested that lysine, ornithine and arginine are possibly reabsorbed from the renal tubular lumina by two separate mechanisms, one of which is shared by cystine.

2. Intestinal Transport Defect

The abnormal intestinal transport of amino acid in cystinuric patients was reviewed by Milne [49]. Stimulated by certain analogies between cystinuria and Hartnup disease (hereditary pellagra), Milne et al. [50, 51] showed that when tryptophane was fed to patients with Hartnup disease, a large proportion of the amino acid was not absorbed in the jejunum, but was degraded in the colon to indole and indolyl acetic acid, much of which was absorbed and excreted in the urine.

In the cystinuric (but not in normal subjects) they showed that after feeding lysine, a large amount of piperidine and occasionally small amounts of cadaverine were excreted in the urine. After feeding ornithine the urinary pyrollidine was increased but no putrescine was detected [49]. After the ingestion of arginine there was a considerable increase of urinary pyrollidine [1] and also an increase of faecal citrulline and putrescine from the metabolism of the unabsorbed amino acid by bacteria. When a given amount of arginine was fed, its level in the plasma was increased to a smaller extent in the cystinuric than in the normal patient. When the intestinal contents were sterilized by the administration of neomycin by mouth, the formation of piperidine and pyrollidine was completely prevented and could not then be found in the urine. The increase of the heterocyclic hydrocarbons piperidine and pyrollidine was a more constant finding in cystinurics than the urinary diamines, the presence of which had been observed by earlier workers and which were merely labile intermediates in the formation by bacteria of the more stable heterocyclic hydrocarbons [49].

These studies established that there is a defect in the cystinuric patient in the intestinal absorption of the dibasic amino acids. A further observation supported the view that there is competition between the amino acids for intestinal transport: the ingestion of lysine in cystinurics caused an increase in faecal arginine together with a slight increase of the urinary pyrollidine; whereas the ingestion of arginine caused a rise of faecal lysine with some increase of urinary piperidine [49]. The intestinal absorption of the dibasic amino acids in cystinurics, although less efficient than in normal subjects, is not simply a passive process mediated by simple diffusion.

The existence of the intestinal transport defect was confirmed by Thier et al. [68] and by London and Foley [44]. The latter workers showed that the level of plasma cystine was increased to a smaller extent in cystinurics than in normal individuals after identical oral cystine loads, suggesting that the cystinuric patient could not absorb cystine from the gut. The output of sulphate in the urine after the ingestion of cystine was delayed in cystinurics as compared with that in normal individuals, suggesting that the oxidation of the oral cystine was determined chiefly by bacterial decomposition in the intestine rather than by oxidation in the tissue cells in the body after it had been absorbed; the intestinal absorption of cysteine, however, appeared to be the same in cystinurics as in normal controls [28, 63].

The uptake from the jejunum of labelled samples of all four of the dibasic amino acids was examined in normal individuals and in cystinuric patients using small pieces of jejunal mucosa obtained by per-oral biopsy. In contrast to the results obtained with renal tissue, the uptake of lysine, arginine and also of cystine was markedly impaired in the intestine from eight cystinuric patients but was normal in normal

individuals [63]. Further experiments to determine relative competition between the different amino acids showed that arginine inhibited the uptake of lysine, and lysine and cystine were shown to be mutually inhibitory [63, 68].

3. Genetic Considerations

Because of the familial incidence among siblings Garrod [33] suggested that cystinuria was inherited, possibly as a dominant or alternatively as a rare recessive trait. In order to try to resolve the problem of the genetics of cystinuria, quantitative studies of the various amino acids excreted in the urine by cystinurics of 21 cystinuric families were carried out by Harris and his coworkers [21, 36, 37].

In some of the families the expected clear separation into cystinurics and normal individuals was found, but in other families there was a gradation in different individuals from normal to very abnormal cystine excretion. It seemed, therefore, that the disease existed in two distinctly separate inherited forms. The first, designated 'completely recessive cystinuria', was found in families in which all the individuals excreted either normal, or grossly abnormal amounts of cystine in the urine and no individuals excreted intermediary amounts. The familial distribution here was that which would be expected if the cystinuria occurred in individuals homozygous for a rare gene; the parents were normal and were heterozygotes but some of the offspring were homozygotes.

In families of the second type designated 'incompletely recessive cystinuric' [41] cystine excretion varied from normal to moderate and then to high levels. The distribution of the individuals in the family suggested that those with moderately raised values were heterozygous, and those with high values were homozygous for a rare gene. It was concluded from their studies of the lysine, arginine and cystine excretion of 28 stone-forming cystinurics and 121 of their relatives, that the variations in renal transport of the amino acids originated from the inheritance of different degrees of the renal tubular defect. Stone formation was found only in individuals who excreted more than 250 mg cystine/g creatinine, at which level saturation of the urine with cystine would occur. All degrees of cystinuria from 20 to 800 mg cystine/g creatinine were found.

The excretion of lysine was parallel quantitatively to the amount of urinary cystine, and was twice the amount. Not until cystine and lysine reabsorptions were seriously impaired (with a cystine excretion of 250 mg/g creatinine/day), were arginine and ornithine excreted in abnormal amounts, when the amounts of these amino acids increased in proportion to the rise in the amounts of cystine and lysine excreted. These relationships were observed in families with both the genetic types of the disorder [38, 39].

The explanation of the two variant forms may be that there are at least two mutant conditions of one gene, one having a mild and one having a severe effect on the renal tubular reabsorption of the four amino acids in the heterozygous state [41].

Subsequent investigations by Rosenberg and his co-workers have indicated that the genetic factor is even more complicated than that outlined above, and that what is known as cystinuria comprises at least three biochemically distinct inheritable diseases. In one form, active or mediated transport of cystine, lysine and arginine by the intestinal mucosa is totally abolished, a finding which is compatible with functional or structural absence of a specific enzymatic carrier protein. In the second type there is no intestinal transport of lysine and reduced transport of cystine; the excretion of cystine and lysine in heterozygotes is increased and there is a slight rise in the response of the plasma cystine to an oral load. In the third type there is a less than normal quantitative transport of cystine and lysine, but an increased urinary excretion of cystine and lysine. The second and third types are included in the 'incompletely recessive cystinuria' referred to above. Investigation of the final genetic picture of the cystinuric is still incomplete [61, 63].

With the availability of quantitative amino acid analyses and of new methods of genetic analysis Crawhall et al. [15, 17, 19] tried to define more clearly the homozygous and heterozygous states. They showed that there was an excess in the arginine excretion in the homozygote over that in the heterozygote; hyperlysinaemia was also sometimes found in the heterozygote. There was an overlap in the ranges of the amino acid excretion except in that of cystine (which was expected because of cystine stone formation, which results from a high cystine excretion).

V. Clinical Picture

Cystinuria is usually first seen in early or middle adult life though occasionally in children, and is commoner in the male sex; thus in the series of Boström and Hambraeus [5], of 98 patients 57 were male and 41 female. Patients with cystinuria present no clinical symptoms unless and until urinary calculi have been formed when the complaints are those common to all urinary calculi. Cystinuria does not usually appear to influence the general health and but for the accident of calculus formation with its complications, most patients would apparently lead a normal life to the allotted span.

Occasionally in young patients and in older patients who have had a severe loss of amino acids since childhood, there is a loss of stature, presumably consequent upon interference with general nutrition and impaired renal function. There is a similar loss of stature in some patients with Hartnup disease (in which there is an aminoaciduria, including lysine) and/or failure to absorb tryptophane [11].

The first symptoms usually appear before the age of 40. In the 98 cases reported by Boström and Hambraeus [5], in 22 patients the first symptom appeared before the age of 20, and in six males, before the age of 10. The incidence of urinary infection in 21 of the 98 patients was higher than in the experience of most surgeons including our own and that of Dent and Senior [23]. In most patients the urine is sterile, though attacks of infection associated with pain and frequency of micturition may lead to chronic pyelonephritis, impairment of renal function and hypertension.

Calculi from the kidney may be voided spontaneously if small or may be arrested in the ureter, the bladder or the urethra, such conditions sometimes calling for surgical intervention. In the absence of effective postoperative medical treatment, stones continue to recur through life. The long-term survival of cystinuric patients depends upon the extent of the calculous disease, the severity of any associated renal infection and the incidence of impairment of renal function. The improved treatment of recent years should enable co-operative patients to survive almost to the normal span. In Boström and Hambraeus's [5] 98 cases 26 died, renal failure being the immediate cause of death in 12 with an average age at death of 68.6 years.

The normal concentration of cystine in the plasma is about 0.8 mg (3.3 μmol) per 100 ml while in cystinurics it is below normal, with values ranging from 0.15 to 0.75 mg (0.5–2.5 μmol) per 100 ml [18, 22]. Adults normally excrete 40–80 mg of urinary cystine daily [37]. When in the cystinuric the daily output of urinary cystine exceeds 250–300 mg it precipitates out and stone formation is likely. Following a protein meal there is an increase of urinary cystine.

In the normal subject 96%–98% of the cystine filtered through the glomerulus and was reabsorbed by the renal tubules. In the cystinuric the clearance of cystine approaches that of inulin and may exceed it. It had long been known that excessive amounts of putrescine and cadaverine (in daily amounts between 0.2 and 0.4 g of the dibenzoyl derivatives of the diamines), arising presumably from the decomposition of lysine and arginine, were sometimes found in the urine of patients with cystinuria but not in normal subjects; but it was not understood that the enzymes responsible for the production of these substances were present not in the tissue cells, but in intestinal bacteria [49].

Radiography nowadays usually enables the presence of the stones to be detected though they may be less radio-opaque than calcium-containing stones. They cannot be distinguished radiographically from stones composed of any other substance.

The discovery of the hexagonal crystals of cystine in the urine is a useful diagnostic test for cystinuria (and helps to identify the homozygotes) and should be looked for in the concentrated urine passed first thing in a morning, the sample being allowed to stand and cool for some hours before centrifugalization. Crystals will be deposited when the volume of the 24-h output of urine of a potential stone-former falls below 1 litre.

Cystinuria may be present without the appearance of crystals in the urinary sediment. Stone formation occurs (in adults) only in individuals who excrete at least 400 mg cystine daily [38]. Since not more than 1% of all urinary calculi are cystine stones, their presence and composition may be overlooked unless the appropriate tests for urinary cystine are done for all calculous patients, as well as an examination of their stones.

A large staghorn calculus in a child or young adult in whom the urine is uninfected, could well be a cystine stone. In patients found to have cystinuria, the urinary content of the four amino acids, cystine, lysine, arginine and ornithine, should ideally be assessed quantitatively. Siblings and members of the patient's family should be examined so that they can have medical treatment (if appropriate) to prevent stone formation. If the inherited recessive trait is present on two sides of the family, several members will probably form stones [37, 39]. Very occasionally patients who are heterozygous for the incompletely recessive form of cystinuria may form stones [25].

Brand's test is positive in cases in which the urinary excretion of cystine is at an abnormally high level: 2 ml of a 5% solution of sodium cyanide is added to 3–5 ml urine and allowed to stand for a few minutes; a few drops of a freshly prepared 5% solution of sodium nitroprusside is added; if the urine gives a magenta colour the reaction is positive [8].

1. Spontaneous Dissolution of Cystine Calculi

The long-continued passage of very dilute urine can bring about the gradual dissolution of cystine calculi. Dent and Senior [23] described a cystinuric patient who had only one kidney, which contained many cystic calculi and which was showing gradual functional deterioration; the output of ordinary cystine fell from 645 to 161 mg/day during a period of 18 months in which the blood urea rose from 90 to 267 mg/100 ml. Owing to the decrease in the amount of urinary cystine, combined with the inability of the patient to pass a concentrated urine, as a consequence of grossly impaired renal function, the calculi were exposed to the solvent action of a urine which was now undersaturated with cystine, and were shown by successive periodic radiographs to be slowly undergoing dissolution. This finding, which was confirmed at subsequent autopsy when only a small number of residual calculi were found, compared with the large number demonstrated on radiography 18 months before. A similar case under the care of the author is illustrated in Figure 16.2 (see p. 348).

2. Associated Diseases

No other disease has been recognized to be commonly associated with cystinuria, but the following have been found in chance association with it:

1. Hereditary relapsing pancreatitis [34].
2. Mental deficiency and atypical osteogenesis imperfecta [4].
3. Severe mental deficiency and epilepsy [70].
4. Haemophilia [21].
5. Retinitis pigmentosa has been reported in two members of one family, one of whom had cystinuria and one not [10].

Cystinuria has been associated with severe steatorrhoea [27] and with coeliac disease [35] in children. In the series of 98 cystinurics reported by Boström and Hambraeus [5], peptic ulcer or gastritis was diagnosed in 15 (on clinical or radiological grounds), cardiac or vascular disease in 12, pulmonary tuberculosis in 3 and renal tuberculosis in 3. Various congenital defects have been found occasionally in cystinuric patients.

Cystinuria and gout, both genetically determined, are occasionally found in the same patient or in members of the same family. Atsmon et al. [2] observed one patient who had cystinuria as well as uric acid stones; in another cystinuric family, a brother and a sister had cystine stones, a second brother had uric acid stones, the father had gout and the mother cystinuria.

VI. Treatment

Efforts at treatment have been concerned to reduce the greatly increased amount of cystine excreted in the urine, and to create

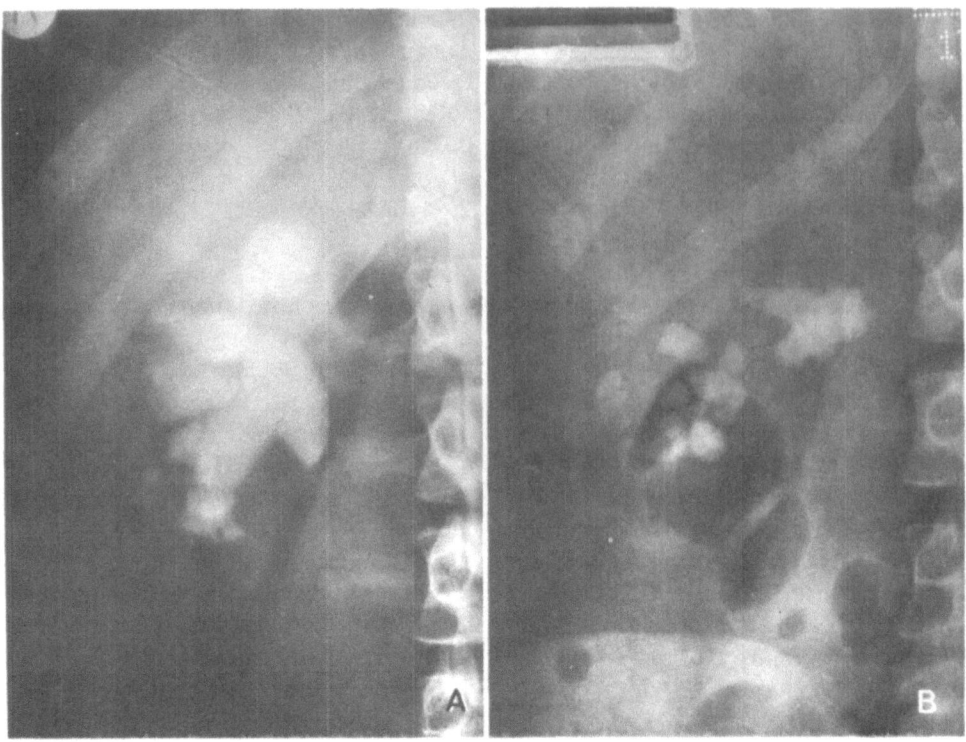

Fig. 16.2. **A.** Plain radiograph in a man aged 45 who had had the left kidney removed, showing massive staghorn cystine calculi in the right kidney; he was treated by a regulated intake of fluids and alkalis. **B.** He was admitted to hospital 4 years later with renal colic followed by calculous anuria; the blood urea was 450 mg/100 ml. The plain radiograph now showed a considerable reduction in size of the calculi seen in the earlier radiograph; the calculi were removed by operation. The reduction in size of the stones during the 4-year period between the two pictures was the result of gross impairment of his renal function leading to the voiding of a dilute urine with a low content of cystine, a situation which allowed much of the cystine to pass into solution. Following the operation he was followed up for a further 4 years but there was no recurrence of his cystine calculi, the concentration of cystine in the urine not now being sufficient to promote such a recurrence

conditions in the urine favourable to its solution (and the dissolution of cystine calculi), by artificially reducing its concentration and by raising the urinary pH. The stone-formers are to be found among those patients with the highest urinary output of cystine [37]. Dent and Senior [23] found that the incidence of stone formation among their cystinuric patients was more than 50%, figures which are at variance with those of some earlier observers.

1. Dietary Measures

Since cystine is included in the protein molecule, restriction in the amount of protein ingested has been recommended to bring about a moderate reduction in the urinary cystine. The diet is unappetizing, difficult to prepare and not easy for the patient to accept. Since the patient is already losing other amino acids in the urine (as much as 2.5 g lysine/24 h is lost) severe protein restriction by way of the diet may even be harmful [23].

Since methionine is the principal precursor of cystine, a low-methionine diet has been advocated [42, 54]. With such a diet the urinary cystine level of the urine was reduced though ornithine, lysine and arginine continued to be excreted; renal function remained normal and there were no side-effects.

Oral loading with methionine to a patient fed with the diet has resulted in the reappearance of large amounts of urinary cystine. In one patient who had had cystine calculi, reported by Kolb et al. [42] initially the average daily cystine excretion had varied from 3000 to 3600 mg/24 h, but following treatment with the diet for 10 years it had been progressively reduced to levels of 600 mg/day and later to 100–150 mg/day. Residual calculi decreased in size; the diet prevented the usual wide fluctuations in urinary cystine.

The forbidden articles of diet are rich meat, soups, fish, milk, eggs, cheese and nuts (except peanuts). Patients are allowed vegetable soup, peanut butter, spaghetti (but not with cheese or milk), all vegetables and fruits, whole wheat or rye bread, sugar and jam, butter and margarine and one serving daily of most meats.

Alkalis. Since cystine is soluble in urine of a high pH, treatment of cystinuric patients with alkali has been used as a method of preventing the recurrence of stones after operative removal, and possibly in assisting the dissolution of existing stones. A constant urinary pH of over 7.6 (a level which would require big doses of alkali) is needed before obvious increase in the solubility of cystine can occur. A total of 30 g sodium bicarbonate/day in divided doses throughout the 24 h (not easy for the patient to accept) is needed to ensure a constantly alkaline urine of pH 7.6 or higher, and will increase the solubility of cystine in the urine. A highly alkaline urine could predis-

pose to the formation of calculi composed of calcium phosphate and magnesium ammonium phosphate if the urine is infected; moderate doses may be given in combination with a high fluid regime, but it is not recommended as a routine measure.

2. Medicinal Measures

The administration of choline has been recommended in order to provide methyl groups for biological methylation, thereby exerting a methionine-sparing action and reducing the amount of cysteine derived from methionine, which would later be excreted as cystine [55, 75]. Dent and Senior [23], however, found that the administration of choline dihydrogen citrate, as recommended by some workers, failed to reduce the urinary cystine level in a cystinuric patient. Similar negative results were found with the administration of naphthalene, or of ascorbic acid or vitamin A.

High-Fluid Regime. Since cystine is an amino acid of low solubility there is a possibility that existing cystine stones could pass into solution in dilute urine undersaturated with cystine and that the formation of cystine stones could be prevented in some cystinuric patients.

In a cystinuric patient with renal calculi Dent and Senior [23] found that the cystine clearance was constant in minute volumes of urine, but that there was a fourfold rise in cystine clearance during high diuresis. This finding was interpreted as showing that the increased cystine must have come from the cystine stones which, therefore, should gradually pass into solution if a high output of dilute urine could be maintained for a long period. It was shown that the concentration of cystine in the urine of a cystinuric patient by day (when fluid was being freely taken by mouth) was much less than that passed by night (when the urine was supersaturated), and it was concluded that in many patients stone formation takes place during the night period.

In another patient on a constant diet and an intake of fluids of 3.5 litres evenly administered during the day and the night, it was found possible to maintain the urinary cystine concentration at about 300 μg/ml throughout, at which level, given a urinary pH higher than 6, the urine was just undersaturated with respect to cystine. They therefore advised a total intake of fluids of approximately 600 ml (1 pt) every 4 h throughout the day and night, an amount which should ensure a total daily output of urine of 3 litres. Two glasses of water were to be taken on retiring in bed and a further two glasses at about 2.00 a.m.

The results of treatment in 18 patients with cystinuria who had had the high-fluid regime for periods of between 4 and 14 years were reported [25]. Six were cysti-nurics who were stone-free at the beginning of treatment but all the others had stones. Alkali was given in varied dosage and the co-operation of the patients in a rather tedious regime was sought. The process was slower than had been theoretically expec-ted; in 9 patients the stones at first increased in size but later began to go into dissolution, circumstances which suggested an early failure to co-operate. The regime appeared to assist in the spontaneous voiding of multiple small calculi (possibly by reducing their size and so allowing them to migrate down the ureter), a sequence which was suggested by the radiographs of some stones, which showed pits and zones of diminished density.

D-Penicillamine. Urinary cystine is a rela-tively insoluble symmetrical disulphide. Mixed disulphides have different properties from those of the corresponding sym-metrical disulphide, and an examination of disulphide exchange-reactions with thiols and other disulphides suggested to Craw-hall and his co-workers [16, 18] that the excessive excretion and deposition in the

urine of the relatively insoluble cystine might be modified by the administration of a suitable thiol. Following experiments in vitro they showed that the urinary cystine in cystinuric patients could be abolished or reduced in amount (according to the dose given by the administration of D-peni-cillamine) and that two new highly soluble substances, namely penicillamine-cysteine disulphide and penicillamine disulphide appeared in the urine. A suitable dosage of penicillamine is required to keep the uri-nary cystine excretion below about 200 mg/g creatinine; with most patients a suit-able dose is between 1 and 2 g/24 h in three divided doses [71]. A reduction of the urinary cystine is usually achieved within 1 or 2 days. The mixed penicillamine–cysteine disulphide is at least 20 times as soluble in urine as cystine.

They advocated the use of D-peni-cillamine to prevent or modify cystinuria and satisfactory results in patients given treatment with D-penicillamine have been achieved. Crawhall et al. [18] reported a case of cystinuria in which renal calculi disappeared after 12 months' treatment. McDonald and Henneman [47] treated three patients who had urinary cystine levels of between 481 and 1334 mg/24 h with D-penicillamine and found a dramatic reduction in the urinary cystine maintained during 8, 10 and 12 months respectively; a cystine stone present in one patient was reduced in size after 6 months, and was completely dissolved after the year's treat-ment. Cystine stones gradually become smaller after 6–12 months of treatment, and ultimately disappear; this results be-cause the urine is no longer saturated with cystine, which has been converted into cysteine–penicillin before it reaches the kidney. The stone matrix remains behind and may cause trouble [13, 71].

Toxic skin reactions, presenting as a morbilliform rash coming on a week or 10 days after the commencement of treat-ment, are found in a considerable proportion of patients treated. They can be controlled by the administration of prednisolone, when treatment with penicillamine can be resumed. Albuminuria may develop after some months of treatment, a complication which calls for withdrawal of the penicillamine; corticosteroids may assist recovery. The subject of toxic changes and possible sensitivity to penicillamine is discussed by Rosenberg [60] and by Watts [71].

Penicillamine has been used with some success in the treatment of Wilson's disease, in which there is a disturbance of copper metabolism. An increased urinary excretion of copper and of zinc in two cystinurics receiving 2 g D-penicillamine daily was reported by Boström and Wester [7]. Studies of the excretion of copper, zinc and other elements in eight cystinuric patients in our clinic receiving 0.8–1.8 g D-penicillamine daily yielded less consistent results though the dosage used was only moderate [40, 64].

3. Surgery

In the past most patients with cystine stone came to operation for the relief of pain and obstruction, and many continue to do so. In the absence of effective non-surgical treatment in the past, many operations used to be needed for the almost certain recurrence of stone after removal. In the Swedish series of Boström and Hambraeus [5] of 98 cases operation was unnecessary in 39 patients, 22 had one operation and 36 underwent between two and eight operations each for the removal of stones (kidney, bladder and urethra). In 14 patients (10 male and 4 female) one kidney was removed, 7 having had no previous operation for urinary calculus; the interval between the onset of urinary symptoms and nephrectomy varied between 7 months and 36 years, 16 years being the average.

If conservative measures of treatment, especially the high-fluid regime and treatment by D-penicillamine, prove to be successful, the number of operations for recurrent cystine stones (performed in earlier years) should be reduced. If a stone of moderate size is causing troublesome symptoms there is much to be said for removing it surgically and then giving supervised medical treatment thereafter, as a permanent discipline [26, 72]. Attempts at dissolution of large staghorn calculi can only be successful if the kidney retains at least a moderate degree of function to enable the dilute urine to act as a solvent for the stone. A completely non-functioning kidney with a staghorn calculus may be an indication for nephrectomy, provided that the other kidney is healthy.

VII. Cystinuria in Animals

Cystine stones or cystinuria have been found at autopsy in several species of animals, including the dog and the mink. In earlier years the stones were recognized only at autopsy but in recent years they have been recognized as a cause of acute urinary retention, the stone being found either in the bladder [52] or in the urethra where a stone had become impacted [53] An incidence of 6.8% of cystine calculi in a series of 163 stones obtained from dogs has been recorded [69]. White et al. [73] found an incidence of 18% of cystine stones in dogs in England, most having caused urethral impaction. Crane and Turner [12] found the urinary pattern of amino acids in the urine of a Labrador retriever, which had had urethral impaction from cystine calculi, was the same as that expected in the heterozygous form of the incompletely recessive type of cystinuria in man (cystine and lysine predominating).

Cystinuria (but not cystine calculi) has been found very commonly in the blotched Kenya genet (Genetta tigrina), which is a

wild cat; using paper chromatography
Datta and Harris [20] found cystinuria in
every genet that they examined and also in
a number of other unrelated members of the
species. The abnormality appears to be a
species characteristic and not restricted to
certain families within the species.

References

1. Asatoor,A.M., Lacey,B.W., London,D.R., Milne,M.D.: Amino acid metabolism in cystinuria. Clin. Sci. *23*, 285 (1962)
2. Atsmon,A., De Vries,A., Frank,M.: Uric acid lithiasis. Amsterdam, London, New York: Elsevier 1963
3. Bartter,F.C., Lotz,M., Thier,S., Rosenberg,L.E., Potts,J.: Studies in cystinuria; a symposium. Ann. Int. Med. *62*, 796 (1965)
4. Berry,H.K.: Cystinuria in mentally retarded siblings with atypical osteogenesis imperfecta. Am. J. Dis. Child. *97*, 196 (1959)
5. Boström,H., Hambraeus,L.: Cystinuria in Sweden. VII. Clinical, histopathological and medico-social aspects of the disease. Acta Med. Scand. (Suppl. No. 411) (1964)
6. Boström,H., Tottie,K.: Cystinuria in Sweden. II. The incidence of homozygous cystinuria in Swedish school children. Acta Paediatr. *48*, 345 (1959)
7. Boström,H., Wester,P.O.: Excretion of trace elements in two penicillamine treated cases of cystinuria. Acta Med. Scand. *181*, 475 (1967)
8. Brand,E., Harris,M.M., Bildon,S.: Cystinuria: excretion of a cystine complex which decomposes in the urine with the liberation of free cystine. J. Biol. Chem. *86*, 315 (1930)
9. Brigham,M.P., Stein,W.H., Moore,S.: The concentrations of cysteine and cystine in human blood plasma. J. Clin. Invest. *39*, 1533 (1960)
10. Brooke,W.D.W., Heasman,M.A., Lovell, R.R.H.: Retinitis pigmentosa associated with cystinuria. Lancet *I*, 1096 (1949)
11. Colliss,J.E., Levi,A.J., Milne,M.C.: Stature and nutrition in cystinuria and Hartnup disease. Br. Med. J. *I*, 590 (1963)
12. Crane,C.W., Turner,A.W.: Amino acid patterns of urine and blood plasma in a cystinuric Labrador dog. Nature (London) *177*, 237 (1956)
13. Crawhall,J.C.: Canadian experience with penicillamine therapy for cystinuria. In: Penicillamine and its place in therapeutics now. Proc. R. Soc. Med. *70* (Suppl. No. 3) p. 34 (1977)
14. Crawhall,J.C., Segal,S.: The intracellular ratio of cysteine and cystine in various tissues. Biochem. J. *105*, 89 (1967)
15. Crawhall,J.C., Watts,R.W.E.: Cystinuria. Am. J. Med. *45*, 736 (1968)
16. Crawhall,J.C., Scowen,E.F., Watts,R.W.E.: Effect of penicillamine on cystinuria. Br. Med. J. *I*, 588 (1963)
17. Crawhall,J.C., Saunders,E.P., Thompson, C.J.: Heterozygotes for cystinuria. Ann. Hum. Genet. *29*, 257 (1966)
18. Crawhall,J.C., Scowen,E.F., Thompson, C.J., Watts,R.W.E.: Dissolution of cystine stones during D-penicillamine treatment of a pregnant patient with cystinuria. Br. Med. J. *I*, 216 (1967)
19. Crawhall,J.C., Purkiss,P., Watts,R.W.E., Young,E.P.: The excretion of amino acids by cystinuric patients and their relatives. Ann. Hum. Genet. *33*, 149 (1969)
20. Datta,S.P., Harris,H.: Urinary amino acid patterns of some mammals. Ann. Eugen. *18*, 107 (1953)
21. Dent,C.E., Harris,H.: The genetics of 'cystinuria'. Ann. Eugen. *16*, 60 (1951)
22. Dent,C.E., Rose,G.A.: Amino acid metabolism in cystinuria. Q. J. Med. *20*, 205 (1951)
23. Dent,C.E., Senior,B.: Studies on the treatment of cystinuria. Br. J. Urol. *27*, 317 (1955)
24. Dent,C.E., Heathcote,J.G., Joron,G.E.: The pathogenesis of cystinuria. I. Chromatographic and microbiological studies of the metabolism of sulfur-containing amino acids. J. clin. Invest. *33*, 1210 (1954)
25. Dent,C.E., Friedman,M., Green,H., Watson,L.C.A.: Treatment of cystinuria. Br. Med. J. *I*, 403 (1965)
26. Farr,J.J., Newling,D.W., Eldrissey,A.A., Marghani,G.A.: Anuria due to cystine stones in a body. Br. Med. J. *I*, 562 (1976)
27. Fleming,W.J., Avery,G.B., Morgan,R.T., Gone,jr.,T.E.: Gastrointestinal malabsorption associated with cystinuria. Report of a case in a negro. Pediatrics *32*, 358 (1963)

28. Foley,T.H., London,D.R.: Cysteine metabolism in cystinuria. Clin. Sci. 29, 549 (1965)

29. Fox,M., Thier,S., Rosenberg,L., Kiser,W., Segal,S.: Evidence against a single renal transport defect in cystinuria. N. Engl. J. Med. 270, 556 (1964)

30. Frimpter,G.W., Horwith,M., Furth,E., Fellows,R.E., Thompson,D.D.: Inulin and endogenous amino acid renal clearances in cystinuria: evidence for tubular secretion. J. Clin. Invest. 41, 281 (1962)

31. Frimpter,G.W., Haymovitz,A., Horwith, M.: Cystathioninura. N. Engl. Med. 268, 333 (1963)

32. Garrod,A.E.: Inborn errors of metabolism. Lancet II (1908) (Lecture I, p. 1; Lecture II, p. 73; Lecture III, p. 142; Lecture IV, p. 214)

33. Garrod,A.E.: Inborn errors of metabolism. 2nd ed. London 1923

34. Gross,J.B., Comfort,M.W., Ulrich,J.A.: The current status of hereditary pancreatitis. Minn. Med. 41, 78 (1978)

35. Hambraeus,L., De Hevesy,G.: Cystinuria in Sweden. VIII. A case of coeliac disease associated with cystine lysinuria. Acta Paediatr. Scand. 53, 213 (1964)

36. Harris,H., Robson,E.B.: Variation in homozygous cystinuria. Acta Genet. 5, 381 (1955)

37. Harris,H., Warren,F.L.: Quantitative studies on the urinary cystine in patients with cystine stone formation and in their relatives. Ann. Eugen. 18, 125 (1953)

38. Harris,H., Mittwoch,V., Robson,E.B., Warren,F.L.: The pattern of amino acid excretion in cystinuria. Ann. Hum. Genet. 19, 196 (1955a)

39. Harris,H., Mittwoch,V., Robson,E.B., Warren,F.L.: Phenotypes and genotypes in cystinuria. Ann. Hum. Genet. 20, 57 (1955b)

40. Hodgkinson,A., Pyrah,L.N.: Certain cations in the urine following the administration of D-penicillamine. Unpublished observations (1967)

41. Knox,W.E.: Cystinuria. In: The metabolic basis of inherited disease. Stanbury.J.B., Wyngaarden,J.W., Fredrickson,D.S. (eds.), 2nd ed., Ch. 56, p. 1262. New York: McGraw-Hill 1966

42. Kolb,F.O., Earll,J.M., Harper,H.A.: Disappearance of cystinuria in a patient treated with prolonged low methionine diet. Metabolism 16, 378 (1967)

43. Lewis,H.B.: The occurrence of cystinuria in healthy young men and women. Ann. Int. Med. 6, 183 (1932)

44. London,D.R., Foley,T.H.: Cystine metabolism in cystinuria. Clin. Sci. 29, 129 (1965)

45. Mallinson. Quoted by Harris,H., Warren, F.G.: Quantitative studies on the urinary cystine in patients with cystine stone formation and in their relatives. Ann. Eugen. 18, 125 (1953)

46. Marcet,A.: An essay on the chemical history and medical treatment of calculous disorders. London 1817

47. McDonald,J.E., Henneman,P.H.: Stone dissolution in vivo and control of cystinuria with D-penicillamine. N. Engl. J. Med. 273, 578 (1965)

48. Meloni,C.R., Canary,J.J.: Cystinuria with hyperuricemia. J. Am. Med. Assoc. 200, 169 (1967)

49. Milne,M.D.: In: The scientific basis of medicine. Annual reviews. London: Athlone Press 1967

50. Milne,M.D., Crawford,M.A., Girae,C.B., Loughridge,L.W.: The metabolism disorder in Hartnup disease. Q. J. Med. 29, 407 (1960)

51. Milne,M.D., Asatoor,A.M., Edwards, K.D.G., Loughridge,L.W.: The intestinal absorption defect in cystinuria. Gut 2, 323 (1961)

52. Morris,M.L., Green,D.F., Dinkel,J.H., Brand,E.: Canine cystinuria. North Am. Vet. 16, 16 (1935)

53. Oldfield,J.E., Allen,P.H., Adair,J.: Identification of cystine calculi in mink. Proc. Soc. Exp. Biol. Med. 91, 560 (1956)

54. Patch,F.S.: Cystinuria and cystine lithiasis. Can. Med. Assoc. J. 31, 250 (1956)

55. Prackken,H.: Case of congenital cystinuria. J. Pediatr. 40, 186 (1952)

56. Prien,E.L.: Studies in urolithiasis; relationships between pathogenesis, structure and composition. J. Urol. 61, 821 (1949)

57. Pruzanski,W.: Cystinuria—report on 56 cases. Urol. Int. 20, 154 (1966a)

58. Pruzanski,W.: Cystinuria and cystine lithiasis in childhood. Acta Pediatr. Scand. 55, 97 (1966b)

59. Robson,E.B., Rose,G.A.: The effect of intravenous lysine on the renal clearance of cystine, arginine and ornithine in normal subjects, in patients with cystinuria and Fanconi syndrome and in their relatives. Clin. Sci. 16, 75 (1957)

60. Rosenberg,L.E.: Extrarenal defect in

aminoacid transport in cystinuria. In: Clinical Staff Conference on Cystinuria at National Institutes of Health, Bartter,F.C., Lotz,M., Thier,S., Rosenberg,L.E., Potts, J.T. (eds.). Ann. Int. Med. *62*, 806 (1963)

61. Rosenberg,L.E.: Genetic homogeneity in cystinuria. In: Aminoacid metabolism and genetic variation. Nyhan,W.L. (ed.), p. 341. New York: McGraw-Hill 1967

62. Rosenberg,L.E., Downing,S.J., Segal,S.: Competitive inhibition of dibasic amino acid transport in rat kidney. J. Biol. Chem. *237*, 2265 (1962)

63. Rosenberg,L.E., Downing,S., Durant,J.L., Segal,S: Cystinuria: biochemical evidence of three genetically distinct diseases. J. Clin. Invest. *45*, 365 (1966)

64. Shaw,D.G., Sutor,D.J.: Cystine stone dissolution. Br. J. Radiol. *45*, 664 (1972)

65. Silbernagl,S., Deetjen,P.: The tubular reabsorption of L-cystine and L-cysteine. A common transport system with L-arginine or not? Pflugers Arch. *337*, 277 (1927)

66. Thier,S.: The renal transport defect in cystinuria. In: Clinical Staff Conference on Cystinuria at the National Institutes of Health, Bethesda. Ann. Int. Med. *62*, 806 (1965)

67. Thier,S., Fox,M., Segal,S., Rosenberg,L.E.: Cystinuria: in vitro demonstration of an intestinal transport defect. Science *143*, 483 (1964)

68. Thier,S., Segal,S., Fox,M., Blair,A., Rosenberg,L.E.: Cystinuria: defective intestinal transport of dibasic amino acids and cystine. J. Clin. Invest. *44*, 442 (1965)

69. Uller,E.: Ein Beitrag zur chirurgischen Behandlung des Harnsteinleidens der kleinen Haustiere. Wein. Tierarztl. Monatsschr. *46*, 130 (1959)

70. Visakorpi,J.K., Hyrske,I.: Urinary amino acids in mentally retarded patients. Ann. Paediatr. Fenn. *6*, 112 (1960)

71. Watts,R.W.E.: Cystinuria and cystine stone disease. In: Scientific foundations of urology. Williams,D.I., Chisholm,G.D. (eds.). London: Heinemann 1976

72. Weinburger,A., Oliver,I., Pinkhas,J., de Vries,A.: Treatment of renal obstruction caused by cystine crystals or stones. J. Am. Med. Assoc. *229*, 1045 (1974)

73. White,E.G.T., Treacher,R.J., Porter,P.: Urinary calculi in the dog. Incidence and chemical composition. J. Comp. Pathol. *71*, 201 (1961)

74. Wollaston,W.H.: On cystic oxide: a new species of urinary calculus. Trans. R. Soc. Lond. *100*, 223 (1810)

75. Zinsser,H.H.: Effect of urinary choline on cystine excretion in cystinuria. J. Urol. *63*, 929 (1950)

Chapter 17

Xanthine Calculi and Xanthinuria

Xanthine is a purine base and is closely related to hypoxanthine and uric acid. The main precursor of xanthine is inosinic acid, a substance which, if it is synthesized by the body to an amount in excess of that needed for nucleoprotein synthesis, can be metabolized ultimately to uric acid by one of three pathways: (1) by way of xanthylic acid and xanthosine (2) by way of guanylic acid, guanosine and guanine by irreversible deamination; or (3) by way of hypoxanthine by irreversible oxidation, a route which requires the presence of xanthine oxidase. These bases are derived by the action of ·purine nucleoside phosphorylase, from their respective nucleosides; the same enzyme breaks down inosine.

I. Xanthinuria and Xanthine Oxidase

In xanthinuria, xanthine is excreted as the major end-product of purine metabolism in the urine. The metabolic defect in xanthinuria is a gross deficiency of the activity of xanthine oxidase, an enzyme normally found in the liver and in the mucosa of the small intestine where its activity is now reduced. The uric acid in the urine is almost completely replaced by xanthine. When the patient is given a low-purine diet, the serum uric acid is less than 1.0 mg/100 ml, and the urinary uric acid is less than 50 mg/24 h. There is a slight elevation of oxypurines in the serum and an increased renal clearance. Xanthinuria is sometimes accompanied by xanthine stones in the urine.

Xanthine Oxidase is a flavoprotein of molecular weight approximately 320,000 which contains molybdenum and iron. This en-

zyme catalyzes the oxidation of hypoxanthine to xanthine, and of xanthine to uric acid and it therefore regulates the production of uric acid from its immediate precursors.

The enzyme is normally present in the liver and the mucosa of the small intestine [19] and possibly in the bone marrow [17]. The enzyme is usually measured colorimetrically, but for the very low levels of the enzyme present in small amounts of human tissue a highly sensitive enzymatic radiochemical method has been developed for the purpose by Watts et al. [23, 24]. It was shown that there is a gross deficiency of xanthine oxidase in xanthinuria, with less than 0.1% of the normal activity towards hypoxanthine, xanthine or xanthopterin in the liver or the mucosa of the jejunum. They showed that in xanthinuria the oxidation of the three physiological substrates xanthine, hypoxanthine and xanthopterin were virtually absent. The rapid renal clearance of the oxypurines in the xanthinuric patient was due to the high level of oxypurines in the plasma and not to a serious biochemical lesion in the kidney [9, 11].

In some patients uric acid and xanthine stones have co-existed. Some patients with xanthine stones, therefore, have only a partial lack, or no lack of xanthine oxidase activity. Hypouricaemia in addition to being found in xanthinuria is also observed in Wilson's disease and in the de Toni–Fanconi syndrome. Xanthinuria has been found in association with haemochromatosis by Ayvazian [1] though the association was probably one of chance. Further details of the chemistry of xanthine oxidase have been given by Watts [22]. Cifuentes Delatte and Castro-Mendoza [5] found xanthinuria in two brothers, only one of whom had xanthine calculi.

Renal Handling of Xanthine. The normal human kidney handles xanthine and hypoxanthine in a manner similar to that in which it handles uric acid, four-fifths or more of these substances present in glomerular filtrate being reabsorbed by tubules presumably by active transport; these processes can be prevented in man by blockage with organic mercurials [8].

In the xanthinuric patient the serum uric acid level is less than 1.0 mg/100 ml and the urinary uric acid is less than 50 mg/24 h, being almost completely replaced by xanthine. The levels of oxypurines (hypoxanthine with xanthine) in the plasma in xanthinuric patients is 0.5–0.9 mg/100 ml (normal values being 0–0.25 mg/100 ml); the level of oxypurines in the urine is 100 to 600 mg/24 h (normal values being 11 to 22 mg/24 h), the level of the xanthine especially being increased. The values are still lower when the patient is taking a purine-free diet [22].

The clearance of hypoxanthine ranges from 15 to 40 ml/min in man, being therefore three to five times the clearance of urate [9, 26]. Dickinson and Smellie [8] in their patient with xanthinuria found a renal clearance of oxypurines almost equal to that of the glomerular filtration rate. When the level of the serum oxypurine is raised in normal subjects to that found in patients with xanthinuria, by the administration of a xanthine oxidase inhibitor or by the infusion of xanthine, the clearance of oxypurine rises to a level higher than the creatinine clearance so that it can be regarded as a response to the raised serum level of oxypurine and not a primary renal abnormality in xanthinuria.

II. Xanthine Stones

Xanthine is the least soluble and the least common of the purines which occur naturally in the urine. Xanthine stone formation is the principal clinical symptom of the rare inherited metabolic disorder xanthinuria [7]. Xanthine calculi, though extremely rare, have been reported occasionally since Marcet [18] referred to them in his essay in 1817, in patients between the ages of 2 and 72 years, males being affected in three-quarters of the cases. Taylor and Taylor [21] found that 23 examples of xanthine stone had been reported in the literature up to 1952; they added a further case, a man of 60 who had had symptoms of renal stone and who illustrated many of the clinical features of these cases.

Ichikawa [14] referred to four cases reported by Japanese surgeons, his own patient being a male aged 44, who had had haematuria from the left kidney, which was removed at operation. The kidney after removal was found to be studded with numerous small nodules, which were shown on section to be cavities containing small granular brownish round or ovoid pure xanthine stones; some renal tubules contained hyaline or xanthine casts. The great rarity of the calculi is shown by the fact that only four stones which contained xanthine (one pure xanthine and three with varying percentages of xanthine) were found in the 10,000 cases of urinary calculi examined by X-ray diffraction by Herring [12].

Seven cases of xanthine stone have been observed in children under the age of 15 years including a girl aged 2 from Taiwan from whom a pure xanthine stone weighing 0.2 g was removed [13]. Seegmiller [20] stated that over 40 cases of xanthine stone had been reported in the literature, two-thirds of them being composed of pure xanthine and Watts [22] stated that there are now reports of 20 well-documented cases in the literature. In the author's department only one case of xanthine stone (a small one voided spontaneously per urethram) has been seen.

Xanthine stones are brownish or yellowish-brown in colour, round or ovoid, smooth on the surface, friable and when cut with a knife show a laminar whitish structure; they have varied in size from a few millimetres in diameter to that of a hen's egg [16]. The stones are composed of pure xanthine in two-thirds of the cases and are of a mixed composition (with uric acid, calcium oxalate or calcium phosphate) in one-third. They are not radio-opaque but their presence may be suspected from the presence of filling defects on the plain urogram, being similar in that respect to uric acid calculi. Mixed stones which contain calcium as well as xanthine may cast a shadow; a negative shadow in the urogram may therefore be a xanthine calculus or a uric acid stone or it may result from the presence of a solid tumour of the renal pelvis or the ureter.

The presence of xanthine in a urinary calculus may be proved by submitting the powdered stone to X-ray diffraction studies, when the characteristic powder pattern is obtained; by the use of paper chromatography [7]; by the use of ion exchange columns [25]; and by spectrophotometry [20].

The incidence of xanthine calculi may not be restricted to patients who have xanthinuria [20]; normal or high levels of serum uric acid have been reported in a few patients with xanthine stones. A slightly elevated urinary oxypurine level (classed therefore as a xanthinuria) was found in one of the siblings (a female) in the xanthinuric family reported by Cifuentes Delatte and Castro-Mendoza [6], the brothers who were affected having primary oxypurine levels between 504 and 517 mg/24 h; normal subjects excrete 11–22 mg daily. Her average daily uric acid excretion was 402 mg; she may have been a heterozygote carrier of the enzymatic defects.

III. Clinical Picture

Dent and Philpots [7] reported a patient who had xanthinuria and xanthine stones and who was shown to have a congenital deficiency of the enzyme xanthine oxidase. The case was followed up and a further report by Dickinson and Smellie [8], using more sophisticated techniques for analyses, was published. The patient was a female child aged 4.5 years, who had had haematuria and incidents of frequency of micturition which had usually resolved. The urine was sterile, the plain abdominal radiograph showed no evidence of stone and the intravenous pyelograms showed clubbing of some calyces of the left kidney (with some reduction of the thickness of the renal cortex), the changes being suggestive of chronic pyelonephritis; the right kidney was normal. Shortly afterwards she voided a small, pale brown, soft, smooth, ovoid stone which had concentric lamination, and which on analysis was found to consist of xanthine with traces of calcium and magnesium. The urine was found to contain 176 mg xanthine/24 h or 607 mg for every gram creatinine. In a female adult control subject, using the same method of estimation, the urine contained 25 mg xanthine/24 h; the blood plasma was shown to contain neither uric acid nor xanthine, a finding which was taken to mean that there was less than 1 mg/100 ml of these substances. No xanthinuria was detected in other members of the family.

The patient was clinically well in 1959 when she was reinvestigated by Dickinson and Smellie [8], who found that the plasma concentration of xanthine and of hypoxanthine was moderately increased (0.74 mg/100 ml, expressed as xanthine), and also that in the urine (13.3 mg/100 ml expressed as xanthine). The corresponding figures for creatinine were 0.75 and 16.6; the renal clearance of xanthine and hypoxanthine (that is of oxypurines estimated together), was 82% of the creatinine clearance instead of the normal 10%–20%, a level which helps to keep the plasma xanthine level low; it was believed that there had been a complete failure of the renal tubular reabsorption of xanthine and probably of hypoxanthine. It was thought that the findings could be explained by a congenital absence of the enzyme xanthine oxidase, which is normally present in the liver.

A form of myopathy in xanthinuric patients, giving rise to slight feelings of distension in the muscles of the thighs, calves and deltoid region, has been reported; in one patient the affected muscles contained increased amounts of oxypurines and xanthine crystals [2–4].

IV. Genetic Considerations

In the patient with xanthine stones, reported by Dent and Philpot [7], 13 relatives had normal outputs of uric acid in the urine and showed no abnormal excretion of xanthine; the relatives examined included a sister, both parents and three surviving grandparents, none of whom gave a history of renal stone. A patient with a familial incidence of xanthinuria, a boy of 17, was reported by Cifuentes Delatte and Castro-Mendoza [6]; he had a hydronephrosis and radiotranslucent stones in the ureter which were thought to be uric acid calculi. The presence of only a trace of uric acid in the urine and a low concentration in the blood led to a preoperative diagnosis of xanthinuria for which nephroureterectomy was done; 1 year later a large red-orange vesical calculus shown to be composed of xanthine was removed suprapubically. One brother, aged 21, who had no symptoms, was found to have 80 times the normal amount of xanthine and almost no uric acid in the urine; one sister, who was apparently normal, passed simultaneously uric acid and 16 times the normal amount of xanthine in the urine. The data are consistent with the autosomal recessive pattern of inheritance.

Watts [22] suggests that there are two pedigree charts for xanthinuric families: in some families the pattern of inheritance is that of the autosomal recessive, and the

presumably heterozygous individuals are clinically normal, with normal levels of uric acid and oxypurines in the blood and the urine; xanthine oxidase activities have been shown to be normal [10]. In other families the pattern is that of an incompletely recessive disorder and the levels of uric acid in the blood and the urine are normal (or low normal) while the oxypurines are intermediate between that in normal subjects and that in presumed homozygotes.

V. Treatment

It is not known how frequently the formation of xanthine stones takes place in patients with xanthinuria. If xanthinuria is recognized in a patient, one should assume that urolithiasis may ultimately occur, so that such preventive treatment as is possible should be administered as well as to patients known to have had xanthine calculi. It may be necessary to remove the stones surgically, especially if they are causing pain or obstruction [15]. A high intake of fluids together with alkalis should be advised as a permanent regime, since xanthine has a low solubility in acid solutions and some of the affected subjects may excrete a highly acid urine. Patients with xanthinuria associated with calculi should have a low intake of dietary purines.

Engelman et al. [9] found that in a patient with xanthinuria a considerable decrease in the urinary excretion of xanthine and compensating increase of hypoxanthine, followed treatment with 800 mg allopurinol daily; their patient had no calculi, so that the effectiveness of this form of treatment in the prevention of further stone formation could not be assessed. Seegmiller [20] pointed out that there are theoretical reasons why the introduction of the use of allopurinol for the treatment of hyperuricaemic states might eventually result in an increase of xanthine-containing stones, though so far such stones do not appear to have been reported as a consequence of the routine treatment of gouty patients [27].

References

1. Ayvazian,J.H.: Xanthinuria and hemochromatosis. N. Engl. J. Med. *270*, 18 (1964)
2. Chalmers,R.A.: Crystals in skeletal muscle in xanthinuria and in allopurinol-treated gout patients. S. Afr. Med. J. *49*, 2072 (1975)
3. Chalmers,R.A., Johnson,M., Pallis,C., Watts,R.W.E.: Xanthinuria with myopathy. Q.J. Med. *38*, 493 (1969a)
4. Chalmers,R.A., Watts,R.W.E., Bitensky,L., Clayson,J.: Microscopic studies on crystals in skeletal muscle from two cases of xanthinuria. J. Pathol. *99*, 45 (1969b)
5. Cifuentes Delatte,L., Castro Mendoza,H.: Lithiase xanthinique et xanthinurie familiale. J. Urol. *72*, 402 (1966)
6. Cifuentes Delatte,L., Castro Mendoza,H.: Xanthinuria familiale. Rev. Clin. Esp. *107*, 244 (1967)
7. Dent,C.E., Philpot,G.R.: Xanthinuria: an inborn error (or deviation) of metabolism. Lancet *I*, 182 (1954)
8. Dickinson,C.J., Smellie,J.M.: Xanthinuria. Br. Med. J. *II*, 1217 (1959)
9. Engelman,K., Watts,R.W.E., Klinenberg, J.R., Sjoerdsma,A., Seegmiller,J.E.: Clinical, physiological and biochemical studies of a patient with xanthinuria and pheochromocytoma. Am. J. Med. *37*, 839 (1964)
10. Frayha,R.A., Salti,I.S., Haidar,G.I.A., Al-Khalidi,V., Hemedy,K.: Hereditary xanthinuria and xanthine urolithiasis: an additional three cases. J. Urol. *109*, 87 (1973)
11. Goldfinger,S.E., Klinenberg,J.R., Seegmiller,J.E.: The renal excretion of oxypurines. J. Clin. Invest. *44*, 623 (1965)
12. Herring,L.C.: Observations on the analysis of 10,000 urinary calculi. J. Urol. *88*, 545 (1962)
13. Hsieh,Y.F., Hsu,T.C.: Xanthine calculus: a case report. J. Formosan Med. Assoc. *62*, 83 (1963)
14. Ichikawa,T.: Xanthine renal calculi. J. Urol. *72*, 770 (1954)
15. Kenawi,M.M.: Xanthinuria and xanthine calculous pyonephrosis. J. R. Coll. Surg. *21*(2), 95 (1976)
16. Kretschmer,H.L.: Xanthine calculi: report of case and review of literature. J. Urol. *38*, 183 (1937)
17. Mackler,B., Mahler,H.R., Green,D.E.: Studies on metalloflavoprotein. J. Biol. Chem. *210*, 149 (1954)
18. Marcet,A.: An essay on the chemical history and medical treatment of calculous disorders. London 1817
19. Morgan,E.J.: The distribution of xanthine oxidase I. Biochem. J. *20*, 1282 (1926)
20. Seegmiller,J.E.: Xanthine stone formation. Am. J. Med. *45*, 780 (1968)
21. Taylor,W.N., Taylor,J.N.: Xanthine calculus: case report. J. Urol. *68*, 659 (1952)
22. Watts,R.W.E.: Xanthinuria and xanthine stone formation. In: Scientific foundations of urology. Williams,D.I., Chisholm,G.D. (eds.), Vol. I, p. 310. Heinemann: London 1976
23. Watts,R.W.E., Engelman,K., Klinenberg, J.R., Seegmiller,J.E., Sjoerdsma,A.: The enzyme defect in a case of xanthinuria. Biochem. J. *90*, 40 (1964)
24. Watts,R.W.E., Watts,J.E.M., Seegmiller, L.E.: Xanthine oxidase activity in human tissue and its inhibition by allopurinol. J. Lab. Clin. Med. *66*, 688 (1965)
25. Weissmann,B., Bromberg,P.A., Gutman, A.B.: The purine bases of human urine. II. Semi-quantitative estimation and isotope incorporation. J. Biol. Chem. *224*, 423 (1937)
26. Wyngaarden,J.B.: Xanthinuria. In: The metabolic basis of inherited disease. 2nd ed. Stanbury,J.B., Wyngaarden,J.B., Fredrickson,D.S. (eds.), p. 729. New York: McGraw-Hill 1966
27. Wyngaarden,J.B.: Allopurinol and xanthine nephropathy. N. Eng. J. Med. *283*, 371 (1970)

Subject Index

A Journal of Clinical and Laboratory Investigation

Urological Research

Executive Editors:
G. D. Chisholm (Managing Editor), Edinburgh;
L. Andersson, Stockholm; D. F. Paulson, Durham;
G. Rutishauser, Basle; F. Truss, Göttingen; W. Vahlen-
sieck, Bonn

Editorial Board:
J. Auvert, Paris; N. J. Blacklock, Manchester;
A. T. K. Cockett, Rochester; K. B. Cummings, Seattle;
J. Frick, Salzburg; D. Grasset, Montpellier; R. Hohen-
fellner, Mainz; W. Lutzeyer, Aachen; P. O. Madsen,
Madison; M. Pavone-Macaluso, Palermo; P. G. Ransley,
London; S. Rummelhardt, Wien; F. H. Schröder, Rotter-
dam; P. O. Schwille, Erlangen; R. Scott, Glasgow;
J. Shimazaki, Chiba; R. L. Vereecken, Leuven; H. J.
de Voogt, Leiden; P. C. Walsh, Baltimore; E. Zingg, Bern

UROLOGICAL RESEARCH contains original articles
on research in the fields of clinical medicine, animal
experimentation, and laboratory techniques. The journal
will increase the reader's understanding of the functions
of the genitourinary system in normal and diseased
states. Preference is given to critical articles dealing with
the diagnosis and treatment of urological disorders.

North America
Please send your order or request to your bookseller or
directly to:
Springer-Verlag New York Inc.,
175 Fifth Avenue, New York, NY 10010, USA

All countries (except North America)
Please send your order or request to your bookseller or
directly to:
Springer-Verlag, Promotion Department
P.P. Box 105280, D-6900 Heidelberg 1

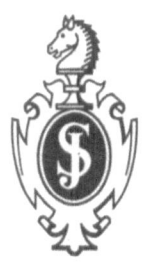

Springer-Verlag
Berlin
Heidelberg
New York

P. Deetjen, J. W. Boylan, K. Kramer

Physiology of the Kidney and of Water Balance

Translator: R. V. Coxon

1975. 63 figures. IX, 141 pages
(Springer Study Edition)
DM 26,–; US $ 13.00
ISBN 3-540-90048-9

W. M. Manger, R. W. Gifford Jr.

Pheochromocytoma

1977. 132 figures, 28 color plates, 40 tables
XXIV, 398 pages
Cloth DM 118,80; US $ 59.40
ISBN 3-540-90217-1

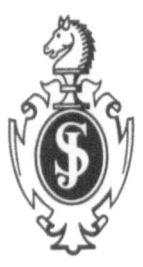

Springer-Verlag
Berlin
Heidelberg
New York

H. J. De Voogt, P. Rathert,
M. E. Beyer-Boon

Urinary Cytology

Phasecontrast, Microscopy and Analysis
of Stained Smears
Foreword by L. G. Koss

1977. 79 mostly colored figures in 327
separate illustrations, 12 tables.
X, 194 pages.
Cloth DM 98,–; US $ 49.00
ISBN 3-540-08042-2

Urinary Tract Infection

Proceedings of a Symposium on
"Urinary Tract Infection", London,
England, September 23–24, 1974
Guest Editors: A. W. Asscher, W. Brumfit

1975. III, 149 pages
(Kidney International Supplementa 4)
DM 52,–; US $ 26.00
Reduced price for subscribers to "Kidney
International"
DM 44,20; US $ 22.10
ISBN 3-540-90147-7

H. U. Zollinger, M. J. Mihatsch

Renal Pathology in Biopsy

Light, Electron and Immunofluorescent
Microscopy and Clinical Aspects
With the collaboration of F. Gudat,
U. Riede, G. Thiel, J. Torhorst
Translated from the German by
E. Castagnoli

1978. 949 figures, 82 tables.
XIII, 684 pages
Cloth DM 184,80; US $ 92.40
ISBN 3-540-08382-0
Distribution rights for Japan:
Igaku Shoin Ltd. Tokyo